Vinod H. Nargund, Derek Raghavan, and
Howard M. Sandler (Eds)

Urological Oncology

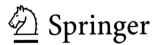 Springer

Vinod H. Nargund, PhD, FRCS (Urol), FEBU
Chair, Uro-Oncology MDT and
  Consultant Urological Surgeon
St. Bartholomew's and Homerton
  Hospitals
Queen Mary Barts and the London
  School of Medicine and
  Dentistry
University of London
London, UK

Derek Raghavan, MD, PhD, FACP, FRACP
Chairman and Director
Cleveland Clinic Taussig Cancer Center
Cleveland, OH
USA

Howard M. Sandler, MD
Professor and Senior Associate Chair
Department of Radiation Oncology
University of Michigan
Ann Arbor, MI
USA

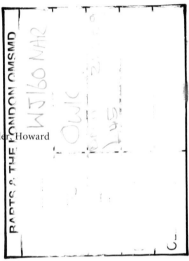

British Library Cataloguing in Publication Data

Urological oncology
  1. Urinary organs—Cancer   2. Prostate—Cancer
  I. Nargund, Vinod   II. Raghavan, Derek   III. Sandler, Howard
  M. (Howard Mark), 1956–
  616.9′9461

ISBN-13: 9781846283871

Library of Congress Control Number: 2007921871

ISBN: 978-1-84628-387-1   e-ISBN: 978-1-84628-738-1

Printed on acid-free paper

9 8 7 6 5 4 3 2 1

Springer Science+Business Media
springer.com

Urological Oncology

To Patients and Teachers

Foreword

Urological oncology is a subject of enormous interest to large numbers of urologists throughout the world, particularly with our increasing understanding of the possible causes and pathogenesis of the condition. As Editor-in-Chief of one of the urological journals, I can attest to this interest; the largest percentage of the papers I receive for review each year relate to either clinical or experimental urological oncology. It used to be that the manuscripts concerned mainly surgical techniques, but now this has extended to new technologies, diagnostic methods, randomized pharmaceutical clinical trials, and thoughtful and complex experimental studies into the genesis of urological cancer. This is all evidence of our increasing interest in the topic.

In addition to this, we have come to understand the management of urological cancer is not in the hands of a single discipline. The advent of multidisciplinary team meetings has made us realize that there is a hugely significant role to be played by urologists, medical oncologists, radiation oncologists, pathologists, and radiologists. This new dimension has been driven by the advent of new therapies and by closer interaction among all of these groups at academic meetings. This is to be applauded and has inevitably lead to improvements in the management of our patients.

One thing is of note which perhaps detracts from our overall feeling of satisfaction at these improvements. Although our understanding of the mechanisms of disease and of the pathogenesis and molecular pathways in urological cancer has increased exponentially, there is a slower rise in the advent of pharmaceutical agents which will, for example, reduce the need for surgical therapies which may be considered to have an associated morbidity. Much of this is due to delays in the development of such drugs and can perhaps best be advanced by involving pharmaceutical companies earlier on in the investigational loop.

This book, edited by Vinod Nargund, Derek Raghavan, and Howard Sandler is a very timely and significant volume. It contains the whole panoply of urological oncology from basic science through clinical investigations to clinical management of the various cancers. Each chapter is written by an acknowledged expert in the field. There is a widespread authorship from all parts of the world.

It is a pleasure to have been asked to introduce it and I congratulate the editors on having put together such an excellent book.

John Fitzpatrick
MCh FRCSI FC Urol (SA) FRCSGlas FRCS
University College Dublin
School of Medicine and Medical Science

Preface

I keep six honest serving men
(They taught me all I knew);
Their names are What and Why and When
And How and Where and Who.
　　　　　　—Rudyard Kipling ("The Elephant's Child," in *The Just-So Stories*, 1902)

Clinical knowledge is based on three components: meticulous observation, detailed recording, and an understanding of basic science relevant to the clinical situation. The first two come with apprenticeship and the last one with personal research or inquisitive reading. It is the last component that is the basis for this book. Although most general urology books contain a fair amount of urological oncology, most of them are written by urologists for urologists. There is increasing realization, however, that a multidisciplinary approach is required for the management of all cancers including urological cancers. In particular, there is a need for surgeons and oncologists to have an integrated strategy for the management of complex cancer cases. A multidisciplinary team will include anesthetists, radiologists, minimally invasive surgeons, intensivists, nutritionists, support and social work staff, in addition to the cancer clinicians. We aim, in this book, to provide this integrated approach as it has contributions from specialists from these different disciplines. All these specialists should have a role in the management of patients to provide them with the optimal chances of recovery. They have also a key role in counseling patients in a coordinated way, for otherwise patients would gain piecemeal information of variable quality from a number of sources including the Internet. The media and the Internet have increased cancer awareness among patients who demand more and more answers to questions such as: What caused my cancer? How can I prevent a recurrence? Will my children get it? How do I get the best up-to-date treatment for my cancer?

Patients have a greater understanding that there may be choices in the management of their condition, and oncologists, both surgical and medical, have to listen to and include the patient's views in the decision-making process. We hope this book will assist in both the management and the counseling of patients with urological cancer. The book also includes chapters on basic science, research, and trials related to urological cancers, which will help those students with an interest in research. Relevant surgical anatomy and other details of basic science are included wherever necessary.

Initially, this book was intended to be a pocket guide on adult urological cancer, but the book quickly metamorphosed into a mini-textbook. The authorship is truly international and therefore reflects a consensus approach to investigation and treatment across the world. The text is didactic and should provide the basis for further reading from journals or more detailed review papers. The book is aimed at residents and urological specialists at all levels of training in urology and oncology.

Vinod H. Nargund, London
Derek Raghavan, Cleveland, Ohio
Howard M. Sandler, Ann Arbor, Michigan

Acknowledgments

The authors acknowledge Sohail Baithun, FRCPath, consultant and reader in histopathology, Royal London Hospital, Whitechapel, London, UK, for his assistance with histopathology, and Anju Sahadev, FRCR, consultant radiologist, St. Bartholomew's Hospital, London, UK, for her assistance with ultrasound and computed tomography.

Vinod H. Nargund
Derek Raghavan
Howard M. Sandler

Contents

Contributors

Denise C. Babineau, PhD
Department of Quantitative Health
  Sciences
Glickman Urological Institute
Cleveland Clinic Foundation
Cleveland, OH, USA

Dean F. Bajorin, MD
Division of Solid Tumor Oncology
Department of Medicine
Memorial Sloan-Kettering Cancer
  Center
and
Joan and Sanford I. Weill Medical
  College of Cornell University
New York, NY, USA

Jeetesh Bhardwa, MRCS
Department of Urology
University Hospital
Birmingham, UK

Ronald M. Bukowski, MD
Cleveland Clinic Taussig Cancer
  Center
Cleveland Clinic Foundation
Cleveland, OH, USA

John Buscombe, MD, MSc, FRCP,
  FRCPEd
Department of Nuclear Medicine
Royal Free Hospital
London, UK

Cag Cal, MD
Department of Urology
Ege University
Izmir, Turkey

Lewis W. Chan, MBBS, FRACS, DDU
Department of Urology
Concord Repatriation General
  Hospital
Sydney, NSW, Australia

Shern L. Chew, BSc, MB BChir,
  MD FRCP
Department of Endocrinology
St. Bartholomew's Hospital
London, UK

Frank Chinegwundoh, MBBS, MS,
  FRCS(Urol), FEBU
Department of Urology
St. Bartholomew's Hospital
London, UK

Jose R. Colombo, Jr., MD
Section of Laparoscopic and Robotic
  Surgery
Glickman Urological Institute
Cleveland Clinic Foundation
Cleveland, OH, USA

E. David Crawford, MD
Division of Urologic Oncology
Department of Surgery
University of Colorado
Denver, CO, USA

Sophie D. Fosså, MD, PhD
Unit for Long Term Studies of
  Cancer Patients
Clinical Cancer Research
Rikshospitalet-Radiumhospitalet
  Medical Centre
Oslo, Norway

Matthew D. Galsky, MD
Division of Solid Tumor Oncology
Department of Medicine
Memorial Sloan-Kettering
  Cancer Center
New York, NY, USA

*Khurshid R. Ghani, BSc (Hons),
  MBChB, MRCS (Ed)*
Department of Urology
St. Bartholomew's Hospital
London, UK

Inderbir S. Gill, MD, MCh
Section of Laparoscopic and
  Robotic Surgery
Glickman Urological Institute
Cleveland Clinic Foundation
Cleveland, OH, USA

*T.R. Leyshon Griffiths, BSc, MD,
  FRCSEd (Urol)*
Urology Group
Department of Cancer Studies
  and Molecular Medicine
University of Leicester
Clinical Sciences Unit
Leicester General Hospital
Leicester, UK

Georges-Pascal Haber, MD
Section of Laparoscopic and
  Robotic Surgery
Glickman Urological Institute
Cleveland Clinic Foundation
Cleveland, OH, USA

Heather Hackett, FRCA
Department of Anaesthesia
St. Bartholomew's Hospital
London, UK

Freddie C. Hamdy, MS, FRCS (Urol)
Department of Urology
Royal Hallamshire Hospital
Sheffield, UK

Simon Horenblas, MD, PhD, FEBU
Netherlands Cancer Institute
Antoni van Leeuwenhoek Hospital
Amsterdam, The Netherlands

*Ray K. Iles, BSc, MSc, PhD, CBiol,
  MIBiol*
School of Health and Social Sciences
Middlesex University
London, UK

*Audrey E.T. Jacques, MBBS, BSc,
  MRCP, FRCR*
Department of Radiology
Guy's and St. Thomas's Hospital
London, UK

Dag Josefsen, MD, PhD
Department of Cell Therapy
  and Oncology
Rikshospitalet-Radiumhospitalet
  Medical Centre
Oslo, Norway

Sujith Kalmadi, MD
Department of Hematologic
  Oncology and Solid Tumor
  Oncology
Taussig Cancer Center
Cleveland Clinic
Cleveland, OH, USA

Sona Kapoor, MSc(Urol), MRCS
Department of Urology
Addenbrokes Hospital
Cambridge UK

Michael W. Kattan, PhD
Department of Quantitative
  Health Sciences
Glickman Urological Institute
Cleveland Clinic Foundation
Cleveland, OH, USA

Ziya Kirkali, MD, PhD
Department of Urology
Dokuz Eylül University
School of Medicine
Izmir, Turkey

Bin K. Kroon, MD, PhD
Netherlands Cancer Institute
Antoni van Leeuwenhoek Hospital
Amsterdam, The Netherlands

Priyadarshi Kumar, MRCS
St. Bartolomew's and Homerton
  Hospitals
London, UK

Irwin H. Lee, MD, PhD
University of Michigan
Ann Arbor, MI, USA

W. Robert Lee, MD, MS
Department of Radiation Oncology
Wake Forest University School
  of Medicine
Winston-Salem, NC, USA

Hing Y. Leung, PhD, FRCS(Urol)
Department of Surgical Oncology
Beatson Institute for Cancer Research
Glasgow, UK

*Murugesan Manoharan, MD, FRCS
  (Eng), FRACS (Urol)*
Department of Urology
Neobladder and Urostomy Center
Miller School of Medicine
University of Miami
Miami, FL, USA

Alistair F. McNarry, FRCA
Department of Anaesthesia, Critical
  Care, and Pain Medicine
Western General Hospital
Lothian University Hospitals Division
Edinburgh, UK

J. Kilian Mellon, MD, FRCS (Urol)
Urology Group
Department of Cancer Studies and
  Molecular Medicine
University of Leicester
Clinical Sciences Unit
Leicester General Hospital
Leicester, UK

Veronica Moyes, BSc, MBBS, MRCP
Department of Endocrinology
St. Bartholomew's Hospital
London, UK

*Vinod H. Nargund, PhD, FRCS (Urol),
  FEBU*
Chair, Uro-Oncology MDT and
  Consultant Urological Surgeon
St. Bartholomew's and Homerton
  Hospitals
Queen Mary Barts and the London
  School of Medicine and Dentistry
University of London
London, UK

Alan M. Nieder, MD
Department of Urology
Miller School of Medicine
University of Miami
Miami, FL, USA

R.T.D. Oliver, MD FRCP
Department of Oncology
St. Bartholomew's Hospital
Queen Mary Barts and the London
  School of Medicine and Dentistry
University of London
London, UK

Michael A. Papagikos, MD
Department of Radiation Oncology
Wake Forest University School
   of Medicine
Winston-Salem, NC, USA

*Christopher C. Parker, BA, MRCP,
   MD, FRCR*
Academic Unit of Radiotherapy &
   Oncology
The Institute of Cancer Research and
   the Royal Marsden Hospital Sutton
Surrey, UK

Melanie E.B. Powell, MD, FRCP, FRCR
Department of Radiotherapy
St. Bartholomew's Hospital
London, UK

*Suresh Radhakrishnan, MBBS, MS,
   MRCS*
Department of Urology
St. Bartholomew's Hospital
West Smithfield
London, UK

*Derek Raghavan, MD, PhD, FACP,
   FRACP*
Taussig Cancer Center
Cleveland Clinic
Cleveland, OH, USA

*Prabhakar Rajan, MA, MBBChir,
   MRCS*
Institute of Human Genetics
University of Newcastle-Upon-Tyne
Central Parkway
Newcastle-Upon-Tyne, UK

Sheilagh V. Reid, MD, FRCS(Urol)
Department of Urology
Royal Hallamshire Hospital
Sheffield, UK

Rodney H. Reznek, FRCP, FRCR
Department of Diagnostic Imaging
St. Bartholomew's Hospital
London, UK

*Andrew J. Richards, MBBS, MS,
   FRACS*
Department of Urology
Concord Repatriation General
   Hospital
Sydney, NSW, Australia

Brian I. Rini, MD
Department of Hematology
   and Oncology
Cleveland Clinic Foundation
Cleveland, OH, USA

Howard M. Sandler, MD
Department of Radiation Oncology
University of Michigan
Ann Arbor, MI, USA

Jonathan Shamash, MD, MRCP
Department of Oncology
St. Bartholomew's Hospital
London, UK

Raj C. Thuraisingham, MRCP
Department of Renal Medicine
   and Transplantation
Bart's and the London National
   Health Service Trust
London, UK

*Nicholas J. Van As, MBBCH, MRCP,
   FCCR*
Academic Unit of Radiotherapy &
   Oncology
The Institute of Cancer Research and
   the Royal Marsden Hospital Sutton
Surrey, UK

D. Michael A. Wallace, MBBS, FRCS
Department of Urology
Queen Elizabeth Hospital
Birmingham, UK

Julie C. Walther, MRCP, FRCR
Department of Oncology and
  Radiotherapy
St. Bartholomew's Hospital
London, UK

Shandra S. Wilson, MD
Department of Surgery
Division of Urology
University of Colorado
Denver, CO, USA

Part I
Basic Science

1
The Cell

Ray K. Iles

Cell and Molecular Biology

Knowledge of normal cell biology is crucial to understanding how functions of the normal cell are deregulated in cancer. This chapter describes the salient cellular and molecular features of a normal and malignant human cells, with particular reference to genitourinary cancers.

Cell Biology: Cell Structure and Function

The *cell (plasma) membrane* is a bilayer consisting of amphipathic phospholipids—a polar hydrophilic head (e.g., phosphatidyl choline) and a lipid hydrophobic tail (commonly two long chain fatty acids). The phospholipids spontaneously form an effective bilayer barrier impermeable to most water-soluble molecules; the barrier also defines cellular internal environment. The membrane exchanges are regulated by proteins embedded within the lipid bilayer. The *cytoskeleton* is a complex network of structural proteins that regulates not only the shape of the cell but its ability to traffic internal organelles. The major components are microtubules, intermediate filaments, and microfilaments. The *cytoplasm* contains organelles and defines the interior of the cell. Although a fluid compartment, the organelles are held within a scaffolding or cytoskeleton that regulates the passage and direction in which the interior solutes and storage granules flow.

The *basement membrane* (BM) is a specialized form of extracellular matrix (ECM) that has been recognized as a key regulator of cell behavior. In addition to structural support and cell compartmentalization, BM sends a signal to cells about the extracellular microenvironment, thereby regulating cell behavior (1). The role of BM in angiogenesis is described later.

The *nucleus* is an organelle containing the human genome and it is bound by two bilayer lipid membranes. The outer of the two is continuous with the endoplasmic reticulum (ER). Nuclear pores are present in the membranes, allowing the passage of nucleotides and deoxyribonucleic acid (DNA) interacting proteins in and messenger ribonucleic acid (RNA) (mRNA) out. *Nucleoli* are dense areas within the nucleus rich in proteins and RNA chiefly concerned with the synthesis of ribosomal RNA (rRNA) and ribosomes.

The *endoplasmic reticulum* (ER) is interconnecting tubules or flattened sacs (cisternae) of lipid membrane bilayer. It may contain ribosomes on the surface [rough endoplasmic reticulum (RER) when present, or smooth endoplasmic reticulum (SER) when absent]. *Ribosomes* are complexes of protein and RNA that translate mRNA into a primary sequence of amino acids of a protein peptide chain. This chain is synthesized into the ER where it is first folded and modified into mature peptides.

The *Golgi apparatus* is characterized as a stack of flattened cisternae from which vesicles bud off from the thickened ends. The primary processed peptides of the ER are exported to the Golgi for maturation into functional proteins (e.g., glycosylation of proteins, which are to be excreted, occurs here) before packaging into secretory granules and cellular vesicles, which bud off the ends.

Lysosomes are dense cellular vesicles containing acidic digestive enzymes.

Mitochondria are semiautonomous organelles responsible for cellular energy metabolism, free radical generation, and apoptosis (2). They have two lipid bilayer membranes and a central matrix. The *outer membrane* contains gated receptors for the import of raw materials [pyruvate and adenosine diphosphate (ADP)] and the export of precursor of amino acids and sugars (oxaloacetate) and adenosine triphosphate (ATP). Proteins of the Bcl-2-Bax family are incorporated in this membrane and can release cytochrome C that triggers apoptosis (3). The *inner membrane* is infolded (cristae) to increase its effective surface area, and it contains transmembrane enzyme complexes of the electron transport chain, generating an H^+ ion gradient. *The inner matrix* contains the enzymes of the Krebs' cycle. Mitochondria also possess their own DNA in a circular genome and thereby maintain genomic independence from the nucleus (4).

Mitochondrial Deoxyribonucleic Acid Alterations in Genitourinary Cancer

Mutations in mitochondrial DNA (mtDNA) have been identified in renal cell carcinoma (RCC) and prostate cancer. In RCC there is evidence to suggest alterations of mtDNA (mutation of the *ND1* gene) and mRNA coding for the subunit *ND3* gene (5,6). In prostate cancer there is evidence of mtDNA deletions that increase with advanced age (7).

Cell Dynamics

The cell component proteins and organelles are continually being formed and degraded. Old cellular proteins are mopped up by a small cofactor molecule called ubiquitin. Ubiquitination acts as a signal for destruction, and a complex containing more than three ubiquitin molecules is rapidly degraded by a macromolecule called 26S proteasome. Failure to remove worn protein can result in the development of chronic debilitating disorders. This is well demonstrated in von Hippel–Lindau (VHL) disease, which is caused by mutation of the *VHL* gene (3p26-p25). There is increased activity in hypoxia inducible factors 1 and 2 (HIF-1 and HIF-2) with *VHL* gene mutation (8). The HIFs are transcription factors in angiogenesis and tumor growth. The VHL protein is thought to form an E3 ligase (ubiquitin-activating enzyme) (8).

Cytoskeleton

The major cytoskeleton components are microtubules, intermediate filaments, and microfilaments. *Microtubules* are made up of polymerized α- and β-tubulin and continuously changing length. They form a "highway" transporting organelles through the cytoplasm. Two motor microtubule-associated proteins, dynein and kinesin, allow antegrade and retrograde movements. During the *interphase*, the microtubules are rearranged by the microtubule-organizing center (MTOC), which provides a structure on which the daughter chromosomes can separate.

Intermediate filaments form a network around the nucleus and extend to the periphery of the cell. They make cell-to-cell contacts with the adjacent cells via desmosomes and basement matrix via hemidesmosomes. Their function appears to be in structural integrity, being prominent in cellular tissues under stress. The intermediate filament fiber proteins are specific; for example, keratin is intermediate fibers only found in epithelial cells, whereas vimentin is only found in mesothelial (fibroblastic) cells.

Microfilaments

The muscle contractile actin and myosin filaments are also present throughout the nonmuscle cells, as truncated myosins (e.g., myosin 1), in the cytosol (forming a contractile actomyosin gel) beneath the plasma membrane. The calcium-dependent actin-binding proteins modulate the behavior of microfilaments. Alterations in the cell's actin architecture are also controlled by the activation of small Ras-like guanosine triphosphate (GTP)-binding proteins Rho and Rac. These are important in the rearrangement of the cell during division, and dysfunctions of these proteins are associated with malignancy.

Intercellular Connections

The cytoskeleton and plasma membrane interconnect, and extracellular domains form junctions between cells to form tissues—tight, adherent, and gap junctions.

Tight junctions (TJs) (zonula occludens) hold cells together with the proteins called *claudins*. They show selective tissue expression and regulate what small ions may pass through the gaps between cells. These are particularly important in the lining urothelium as they create a physiological barrier between urine and blood (9). Increased urinary concentration of hepatocyte growth factor/

scatter factor (HGF/SF) is associated with high grade and muscle invasive bladder cancer (10,11); HGF/SF and interleukin-8 disrupt tight junctions and have been thought to cause progression of transitional cell carcinoma (TCC) (12). *Adherent junctions* (zonula adherens) are continuous on the basal side of cells and contain cadherins. Cadherins comprise a family of calcium-dependent transmembrane cell-to-cell adhesion molecules, and reduced expression of subclass E-cadherin is associated with increased urothelial tumor recurrence and invasiveness (13). Similarly aberrations in E-cadherin are associated with prostate cancer progression (14). *Desmosomes* are apposed areas of thickened membranes of two adjacent cells attached to intermediate filaments of cytokeratin. Desmosomal adhesion inhibits invasive behavior of cancer cells. Invasive TCCs show decreased desmosomal density compared to noninvasive TCCs (15). *Gap junctions* allow substances to pass directly between cells without entering the extracellular fluids.

Cell Adhesion Molecules

Adhesion molecules and adhesion receptors are essential for tissue structure organization. Differential expression of such molecules is implicit in the processes of cell growth and differentiation, such as wound repair and embryogenesis. There is increasing evidence to suggest that the adhesion properties of neoplastic cells play a key role in the development and progression of cancer (16). Some of these molecules are involved in cell signaling and tumor suppression. There are four major families of adhesion molecules: cadherins, integrins, the immunoglobulin superfamily, and the selectins.

The role of *cadherins* has already been described (zonula adherens). At desmosomal junctions cadherins mediate cell-to-cell connection.

Integrins are transmembrane glycoproteins with α- and β-subunits that dimerize to yield different heterodimers, each with distinct ligand binding and signaling properties. They principally bind to extracellular matrix components such as fibrinogen, elastase, and laminin. Their intracellular domains connect to the actin cytoskeleton. They also affect migration, proliferation, and survival of both normal and neoplastic cells. The $\alpha_6\beta_4$ integrin is associated with collagen VII on the basement membrane of urothelium forming a hemidesmosomal anchoring complex, which acts as an effective barrier to cell migration (17). Loss of the $\alpha_6\beta_4$ integrin is associated with collagen VII, which explains the defects in the loss of the urothelial barrier in bladder cancer (18).

The *immunoglobulin* superfamily cell adhesion molecules (CAMs) contain domain sequences, which are immunoglobulin-like in structures. The neural CAM (N-CAM) is found predominantly in the nervous system mediating a homophilic (like with like) adhesion. Their function in the urinary tract is not completely understood. The *selectins*, unlike most adhesion molecules that bind to other proteins, interact with carbohydrate-ligands and mucin complexes on leukocytes and endothelial cells (vascular and hematological systems).

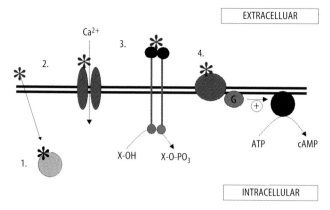

FIGURE 1.1. Diagrammatic illustration of the four types of receptor found in a cell: 1, cytoplasmic; 2, ion channel; 3, enzyme linked; 4, G-protein linked. ATP, adenosine triphosphate; cAMP, cyclic adenosine monophosphate; *, receptor ligand.

Receptors (Fig. 1.1)

Cellular interpretation and translation of extracellular signals into an appropriate response is achieved through a diversity of receptors. These signals could be soluble factors (e.g., chemicals, polypeptides, proteins, sugars), a ligand bound to another cell, or the extracellular matrix itself (19). The receptors then transduce these extracellular signals across the cell wall to activate intracellular pathways, thereby bringing desired change (19). There are three types of intercellular signaling: autocrine (cells respond to the substances secreted by themselves), paracrine (cells respond to signaling substance from adjacent cells); and endocrine (cells respond to signaling substances produced from distant sites). The malignant cells use signaling systems in all possible combinations. Major signaling systems are summarized in Table 1.1.

TABLE 1.1. Major signaling pathways

G-protein linked	Activated by a ligand, binds a trimeric complex and anchored to the inner surface of the plasma membrane. This complex is a guanosine triphosphate (GTP)-binding protein, or G-protein. These complexes in turn activate one or all three of the secondary messengers [cyclic AMP (cAMP), Ca^{2+} ions, and inositol 1,4,5-triphosphate/ diacylglycerol (IP_3/DAG)	Inflammatory chemokines
Intrinsic kinase activity	Extracellular domain for ligand binding; intrinsic tyrosine kinase activity in the cytoplasm	Cell proliferation, maturation EGF, PDGF, FGF
Ion channel linked	Mostly synaptic transmission in CNS	GABA, 5-HT, glycine

CNS, central nervous system; EGF, epithelial growth factor; FGF, fibroblast growth factor; GABA, γ-aminobutyric acid; 5-HT, 5-hydroxytryptamine; PDGF, platelet-derived growth factor.

Secondary Messengers

Cyclic AMP, IP₃/DAG, and Ca²⁺ ions

Cyclic adenosine monophosphate (cAMP) is derived from ATP. It functions in intracellular signal transduction (e.g., effects of hormones like glucagon and adrenaline). Its activates protein kinases and regulates the passage of Ca^{2+} through ion channels. The G-protein–coupled transmembrane receptors (GPCs) form one of the largest families of cell receptors. G-protein complexes activate inner membrane-bound phospholipase complexes. These in turn cleave membrane phospholipid—polyphosphoinositide (PIP₂)—into inositol triphosphate (IP₃) (water soluble) diacylglycerol (DAG) (lipid soluble). The former interacts with gated ion channels in the ER, causing a rapid release of Ca^{2+}, and the latter remains at the membrane, activating a serine/threonine kinase, protein kinase C.

Protein Phosphorylation

Although phosphorylation of the cytoplasmic secondary messengers is often a consequence of secondary activation of cAMP, Ca^{2+}, and DAG, the principal route for the protein phosphorylation cascades is from the dimerization of surface protein kinase receptors. The tyrosine kinase receptors phosphorylate each other when ligand binding brings the intracellular receptor components into close proximity. The inner membrane and cytoplasmic targets of these activated receptor complexes are Ras, protein kinase C, and ultimately the mitogen-activated protein (MAP) kinase, Janus Stat pathways (family of intracellular tyrosine kinase), or phosphorylation of inhibitor kappa B (IKB), causing it to release its DNA-binding protein nuclear factor κB (NF-κB). These intracellular signaling proteins usually contain conserved noncatalytic regions called the Serc homology regions 2 and 3 (SH2 and SH3). The SH2 region binds to phosphorylated tyrosine. The SH3 domain has been implicated in the recruitment of intermediates, which activate Ras proteins. Like G proteins, Ras (and its homologous family members Rho and Rac) switches between an inactive GDP-binding state and an active GTP-binding state. This starts a phosphorylation cascade of the MAP kinase, Janus-Stat protein pathways, which ultimately activate a DNA binding protein. This protein undergoes a conformational change, enters the nucleus, and initiates transcription of specific genes.

Free Radicals

A free radical is any atom or molecule containing one or more unpaired electrons, making it more reactive than the native species. They have been implicated in a large number of human diseases. The hydroxyl (OHO) radical is by far the most reactive species, but the others can generate more reactive species as breakdown products. When a free radical reacts with a nonradical, a chain reaction ensues resulting in direct tissue damage by lipid peroxidation of membranes. Hydroxyl radicals can cause mutations by attacking DNA.

Superoxide dismutases (SOD) convert superoxide (O_2^-) to hydrogen peroxide. Glutathione peroxidases are major enzymes that remove hydrogen peroxide generated by SOD in cytosol and mitochondria. Free radical scavengers bind reactive oxygen species. α-Tocopherol, urate, ascorbate, and glutathione remove free radicals by reacting directly and noncatalytically. There is growing evidence that cardiovascular diseases and cancer can be prevented by a diet rich in substances that diminish oxidative damage. Principal dietary antioxidants are vitamin E, vitamin C, β-carotene, and flavonoids.

Heat Shock Proteins

Heat shock proteins (HSPs) are induced by heat shock and other chemical and physical stresses (20), and their functions include the export of proteins in and out of specific cell organelles, acting as molecular chaperones (the catalysis of protein folding and unfolding), and the degradation of proteins (often by ubiquitination pathways). The unifying feature, which leads to the activation of HSPs, is the accumulation of damaged intracellular protein. Tumors have an abnormal thermo-tolerance, which is the basis for the observation of the enhanced cytotoxic effect of chemotherapeutic agents in hyperthermic subjects. The HSPs are expressed in a wide range of human cancers and are implicated in cell proliferation, differentiation, invasion, metastasis, cell death, and immune response (20). Although HSP detection by immunocytochemistry has been an established practice, serum detection of HSP and its antibodies is still a new research area. Various types of HSP have been demonstrated in urogenital cancers including kidney, prostate, and bladder. For example, HSP27 expression in prostate cancer indicates poor clinical outcome (21,22).

Programmed Cell Death

In necrotic cell death external factors damage the cell with influx of water and ions leading to the swelling and rupture of cellular organelles. Cell lysis induces acute inflammatory responses in vivo (Table 1.2). In apoptosis, cell death occurs through the deliberate activation of constituent genes whose function is to cause their own demise. Apoptotic cell death has the following characteristic morphological features:

TABLE 1.2. Contrasting morphological features of necrotic and apoptotic cell death

Necrosis	Apoptosis
Swelling of cell	Shrinkage of cell
Rupture of plasma membrane	Intact plasma membrane
Nucleus relatively intact	Chromatin condensation, mDNA cleavage
Nonspecific proteolysis	Specific coordinated proteolysis
Swelling of cell organelles	Normal size cell organelles
Occurs because no energy available	Energy requirement

- Chromatin aggregation, with nuclear and cytoplasmic condensation into distinct membrane-bound vesicles, which are termed apoptotic bodies
- Organelles remain intact
- Cell blebs (which are intact membrane vesicles)
- No inflammatory response
- Cellular blebs and remains are phagocytosed by adjacent cells and macrophages

Molecular Biology of Apoptosis

Most cells rely on a constant supply of survival signals without which they will undergo apoptosis. Neighboring cells and the extracellular matrix provide these signals. Cancer, autoimmunity, and some viral illnesses are associated with inhibition of apoptosis and increased cell survival. Metastatic tumor cells circumvent the normal environmental cues for survival and can survive in foreign environments. The molecular basis of steps of apoptosis—death signals, genetic regulation, and activation of effectors—has been identified (23). Apoptosis requires energy (ATP), and several Ca^{2+}- and Mg^{2+}-dependent nuclease systems are activated, which specifically cleave nuclear DNA at the interhistone residues. This involves the enzyme cysteine-containing aspartase-specific protease (CASPASE), which activates the caspase-activated DNAase (CAD)/inhibitor of CAD (ICAD) system. Apoptotic signals affect mitochondrial permeability, resulting in reduction in the membrane potential and mitochondrial swelling. The apoptotic trigger cytochrome c is released from mitochondria into cytosol (24).

Bcl-2, *p53*, and the Proapoptotic Gene *bax*

Several proteins including members of the Bcl-2 family regulate mitochondrial permeability. Bcl-2 (24 kd) is associated with the internal membrane of the mitochondria and the nucleus. Bcl-2 suppresses apoptosis by directly preventing mitochondrial permeability and by interacting with other proteins (25). The other gene that has been studied extensively is the tumor suppressor gene *p53*. It has an important role in cell cycle regulation and acts as a transcription factor that controls other gene products. Normal wild-type *p53* limits cell proliferation after DNA damage by arresting the cell cycle or activating apoptosis (25). Also, *p53* has a complex role in chemosensitivity; it can increase apoptosis or arrest growth, thereby increasing drug resistance (26).

Drugs like taxanes and vinca alkaloids induce apoptosis independent of *p53*, as they do not damage DNA (26). The proapoptotic gene *bax* has also been extensively investigated. In contrast to Bcl-2, *bax* is a promoter of apoptosis. Different pathways are discussed later.

Molecular Genetics

Genetic information is stored in the form of double-stranded deoxyribonucleic acid (DNA). Each strand of DNA is made up of a deoxyribose-phosphate backbone and a series of *purine* [adenine (A) and guanine (G)] and *pyrimidine* [thymine (T) and cytosine (C)] bases of the nucleic acid. For practical purposes, the length of DNA is generally measured in numbers of base pairs (bp). The monomeric unit in DNA (and in RNA) is the nucleotide, which is a base joined to a sugar-phosphate unit. The two strands of DNA are held together by hydrogen bonds between the bases. There are only four possible pairs of nucleotides: TA, AT, GC, and CG. The two strands twist to form a double helix with major and minor grooves, and the large stretches of helical DNA are coiled around histone proteins to form nucleosomes and are further condensed into the chromosomes that are seen at metaphase.

Human Chromosomes (Fig. 1.2)

The nucleus of each diploid cell contains 6×10^9 bp of DNA. Chromosomes are massive structures containing one linear molecule of DNA that is wound around histone proteins, which are further wound to make up the structure of the chromosome itself. Diploid human cells have 46 chromosomes, 23 inherited from each parent; 22 pairs of autosomes, and two sex chromosomes (XX female and XY male).

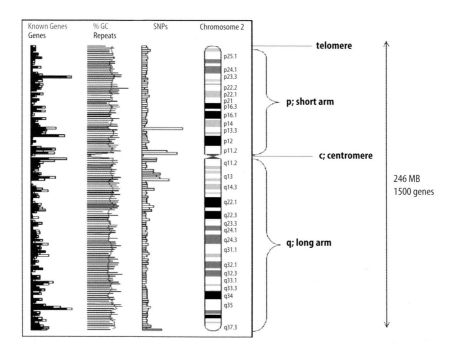

FIGURE 1.2. Chromosome structure (ch2) showing the position of the centromere telomeres, and short (p) and long arms (q). A G-banding pattern is shown and how this maps to known sites of genes and genetic markers such as single nucleotide polymorphisms (SNPs) and the CG rich island, which are characteristic of gene control elements.

Chromosomes can be classified according to their size and shape, the largest being chromosome 1. The constriction in the chromosome is the *centromere*, which may be in the middle of the chromosome (metacentric) or at one extreme end (acrocentric). The centromere divides the chromosome into a short arm (*p* arm) and a long arm (*q* arm). In addition, chromosomes can be stained when they are in the metaphase stage of the cell cycle and are very condensed. The stain gives a different pattern of light and dark bands that is diagnostic for each chromosome. Each band is given a number, and gene mapping techniques allow genes to be positioned within a band within an arm of a chromosome. During cell division, *mitosis*, each chromosome replicates so that each daughter nucleus has the same number of chromosomes as its parent cell. During gametogenesis, however, the number of chromosomes is halved by *meiosis*.

Telomeres and Immortality

The ends of eukaryotic chromosomes, *telomeres*, do not contain genes but rather many repeats of a guanine-rich hexameric sequence TTAGGG. Telomeres are specialized DNA structures that protect the ends of chromosome from fusion and recombination events (27). *Telomerase* is a ribonucleoprotein that is necessary to repair the telomeric losses. Replication of linear chromosomes starts at coding sites (origins of replication) within the main body of chromosomes and not at the two extreme ends. The extreme ends are therefore susceptible to single-stranded DNA degradation back to double-stranded DNA. As a consequence of multiple rounds of replication, the telomeres shorten, leading to chromosomal instability and ultimately cell death.

Stem cells have longer telomeres than their terminally differentiated daughters. However, germ cells replicate without shortening of their telomeres because of telomerase. Most somatic cells (unlike germ and embryonic cells) switch off the activity of telomerase after birth and die as a result of apoptosis. Many cancer cells, however, reactivate telomerase, contributing to their immortality. Conversely, cells from patients with progeria (premature ageing syndrome) have extremely short telomeres (28). Telomerase activity is detected in nearly all cancer cells (29). Likewise, prostate cancer but not normal prostate or benign prostatic hyperplasia (BPH) tissue, expresses telomerase activity (30).

Inhibition of telomerase with DNA-damaging chemotherapy drugs seems a possibility in prostate cancer (31). Telomerase from exfoliated transitional cell carcinoma cells has been used as a urinary marker in bladder cancer (32).

The Mitochondrial Chromosome

The mitochondrial chromosome is a circular DNA (mtDNA) molecule (16.5 kb), and every base pair makes up part of the coding sequence. These genes principally encode proteins or RNA molecules involved in mitochondrial function. These proteins are components of the mitochondrial respiratory chain involved in oxidative phosphorylation (OXPHOS) producing ATP. The mtDNA mutations are generated during OXPHOS through pathways involving *reactive oxygen species* (ROS), and unlike the nucleus these mutations may accumulate in mitochondria because they lack protective histones (33). There are many reasons to believe that the biology of mitochondria could drive tumorigenesis: 1. mitochondria generate ROSs, which in high concentrations are highly mitogenic to the nuclear and mitochondrial genomes; 2. mitochondria have a key role in effecting apoptosis; and 3. mitochondria accumulate in high density in some malignant tumors (renal cell carcinoma) as tumor cells have lesser dependence on mitochondria for their oxidative phosphorylation (34). The mutations of mtDNA have been demonstrated in renal cell, prostate, and bladder cancers.

Genes

A gene is a portion of DNA that contains the codes for a polypeptide sequence. Three adjacent nucleotides (a codon) code for a particular amino acid, such as AGA for arginine, and TTC for phenylalanine. There are only 20 common amino acids, but 64 possible codon combinations that make up the genetic code. This means that more than one triplet encodes for some amino acids; other codons are used as signals for initiating or terminating polypeptide-chain synthesis. Genes consist of lengths of DNA that contain sufficient nucleotide triplets to code for the appropriate number of amino acids in the polypeptide chains of a particular protein. In bacteria the coding sequences are continuous, but in higher organisms these coding sequences (exons) are interrupted by intervening sequences that are noncoding (introns) at various positions.

Some genes code for RNA molecules, which will not be further translated into proteins. These code for functional ribosomal RNA (rRNA) and transfer RNA (tRNA), which play vital roles in polypeptide synthesis.

Transcription and Translation (Fig. 1.3)

The conversion of genetic information to polypeptides and proteins relies on the transcription of sequences of bases in DNA to mRNA molecules; mRNAs are found mainly in the nucleolus and the cytoplasm, and are polymers of nucleotides containing a ribosephosphate unit attached to a base. RNA is a single-stranded molecule but it can hybridize with a complementary sequence of single-stranded DNA (ssDNA). Genetic information is carried from the nucleus to the cytoplasm by mRNA, which in turn acts as a template for protein synthesis.

Each base in the mRNA molecule is lined up opposite to the corresponding base in the DNA: C to G, G to C, U to A, and A to T. A gene is always read in the 5′-3′ orientation and at 5′ promoter sites, which specifically bind the enzyme RNA polymerase and so indicate where transcription is to commence.

Eukaryotic genes have two AT-rich promoter sites. The first, the TATA box, is located about 25 bp upstream of (or before) the transcription start site, while the second, the CAAT box, is 75 bp upstream of the start site.

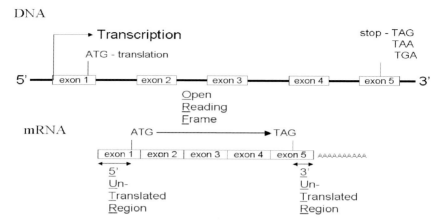

FIGURE 1.3. The intronic and exonic structure of a gene coded on chromosomal DNA and the structural correspondence as a processed mRNA.

The initial or primary mRNA is a complete copy of one strand of DNA and therefore contains both introns and exons. While still in the nucleus, the mRNA undergoes posttranscriptional modification whereby the 5′ and 3′ ends are protected by the addition of an inverted guanidine nucleotide (CAP) and a chain of adenine nucleotides (Poly A), respectively. In higher organisms, the primary transcript mRNA is further processed inside the nucleus, whereby the introns are spliced out. Splicing is achieved by small nuclear RNA in association with specific proteins. Furthermore, alternative splicing is possible whereby an entire exon can be omitted. Thus more than one protein can be coded from the same gene. The processed mRNA then migrates out of the nucleus into the cytoplasm. Polysomes (groups of ribosomes) become attached to the mRNA. Translation begins when the triplet AUG (methionine) is encountered. All proteins start with methionine, but this is often lost as the leading sequence of amino acids of the native peptides is removed during protein folding and post-translational modification into a mature protein. Similarly the Poly A tail is not translated and is preceded by a stop codon, UAA, UAG, or UGA.

The Control of Gene Expression (Fig. 1.4)

Gene expression can be controlled at many points in the steps between the translation of DNA to proteins. Proteins and RNA molecules are in a constant state of turnover; as soon as they are produced, processes for their destruction are at work. For many genes transcriptional control is the most important point of regulation. Deleterious, even oncogenic, changes to a cell's biology may arise through no fault in the expression of a particular gene. Apparent overexpression may be due to non-breakdown of mRNA or protein product.

Transcriptional Control

Gene transcription (DNA to mRNA) is not a spontaneous event and is possible only as a result of the interaction of a number of DNA-binding proteins with genomic DNA. Regulation of a gene's expression must first start with the opening up of the double helix of DNA in the correct region of the chromosome. To do this, a class of protein molecules that recognize the outside of the DNA helix have evolved.

These DNA-binding proteins preferentially interact with the major groove of the DNA double helix. The base-pair composition of the DNA sequence can change the geometry of a DNA helix to facilitate the fit of a DNA-binding protein with its target region: CG-rich areas form the Z-structure DNA helix; sequences such as AAAANNN cause a slight bend, and if this is repeated every 10 nucleotides it produces pronounced curves. DNA-binding proteins that recognize these distorted helices result either in the opening up of the helix so that the gene may be transcribed, or in the prevention of the helix being opened.

Structural Classes of Deoxyribonucleic Acid-Binding Proteins

The regulation of gene expression is controlled by DNA binding proteins. There are four basic classes of DNA-binding protein, classified according to their structural motifs: helix-turn-helix, zinc finger, helix-loop-helix, and leucine zipper.

Transcription Factors

The *promoter* is a modular arrangement of different elements that act as a binding site for RNA polymerase II and the initiation of transcription. The initiation of transcription involves a large complex of multimeric proteins [RNA polymerase (I or II)] plus the general transcription factors (GTFs). The GTFs can activate transcription of any gene that has a GTF recognition sequence such

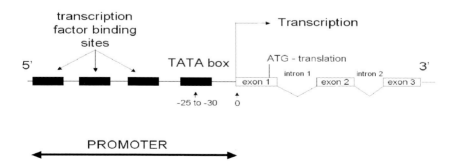

FIGURE 1.4. Diagrammatic representation of the location of DNA binding sequence, which constitute the promoter recognition and assembly site in relationship to the site of gene transcription.

as the TATA box. The TATA box is a promoter element that is always located 25 to 30 base pairs from the start of transcription and serves to anchor RNA polymerase II.

Operators are proteins that bind to DNA sequences in the spatial areas where the large complex of proteins of the GTFs (such as the RNA polymerase II complex) assemble. Their mere presence stoichiometrically inhibit or enhance promoter protein assembly.

Enhancers are elements that can be at the 5′ or the 3′ end of genes and can vary in distance from the coding sequence itself. Enhancers are not obligatory for the initiation of transcription but alter its efficiency in such a way as to lead to the upregulation of genes. Looping of the DNA helix allows distantly located enhancers to interact with the promoter site.

Transcription factors are proteins that bind to sequence specific regions of DNA at the 5′ end of genes called response elements to regulate gene expression. These elements can form a part of the promoters or enhancers. They can be divided into basal transcription factors, which are involved in the constitutive activation of so-called housekeeping genes, and inducible transcription factors, which are involved in the temporal and spatial expression of genes that underlie tissue phenotype and developmental regulation.

Genetic Disorders in Genitourinary Cancer

Normal cell growth and survival require genomic stability. One of the hallmarks of all neoplasms is genetic instability (35). Gross chromosomal rearrangements (GCRs) such as translocations, deletions of a chromosome arm, interstitial deletions, inversions, and gene amplification have been consistently reported in different cancers (36). Genomic instability in cells leads to the activation of proto-oncogenes or inactivation of tumor suppressor genes leading to transformation and development of cancer phenotypes (see below). Knowledge of the mechanism by which genome stability is maintained is crucial for the development of therapeutic applications in cancer management

Definitions of Chromosomal Disorders

Aneuploidy refers to the state of an abnormal number of chromosomes (differing from the normal diploid number). Abnormalities may occur in either the number or the structure of the chromosomes.

Abnormal Chromosome Numbers

Nondisjunction

If chromatids fail to separate either in meiosis or mitosis, one daughter cell would receive two copies of that chromosome and other cells receive no copies of the chromosome. Nondisjunction during meiosis can lead to an ovum or sperm having either 1. an extra chromosome (trisomic), resulting in three instead of two copies of the chromosome [e.g., trisomy 7 bladder and ureteral tumors (37)]; or 2. no chromosome (monosomic), resulting in one instead of two copies of the chromosome.

Full autosomal monosomies are extremely rare and deleterious. Sex-chromosome trisomies (e.g., Klinefelter's syndrome, XXY) are relatively common. The sex-chromosome monosomy in which the individual has an X chromosome only and no second X or Y chromosome is known as Turner's syndrome. Occasionally, nondysjunction can occur during mitosis shortly after two gametes have fused. It will then result in the formation of two cell lines, each with a different chromosome complement. This occurs more often with the sex chromosome, and results in a *mosaic* individual. Rarely the entire chromosome set may be present in more than two copies, so the individual may be triploid rather than diploid and have a chromosome number of 69. Triploidy and tetraploidy (four sets) are nonviable.

Abnormal Chromosome Structures

Abnormal constitution of chromosomes can lead to the disruption to the DNA and gene sequences, giving rise to genetic diseases. *Deletions* of a portion of a chromosome may give rise to a disease syndrome if two copies of the genes in the deleted region are necessary, and the individual will not be normal with the one copy remaining on the nondeleted homologous chromosome. For example, Wilms' tumor is characterized by deletion of part of the short arm of chromosome 11.

Duplications occur when a portion of the chromosome is present on the chromosome in two copies, in that there is an extra set of chromosomes present. *Inversions* involve an end-to-end reversal of a segment within a chromosome; e.g. abcdefgh becomes abcfedgh. *Translocations* occur when two chromosome regions join together, when they would not normally. Chromosome translocations in somatic cells may be associated with tumorigenesis.

Mitochondrial Chromosome Disorders

Most mitochondrial diseases are myopathies and neuropathies with a maternal pattern of inheritance. Other abnormalities include retinal degeneration, diabetes mellitus, and hearing loss.

Analysis of Chromosome Disorders

The analysis of gross chromosomal disorders has traditionally involved the culture of isolated cells in the presence of toxins such as colchicine. It arrests the cell cycle in mitosis, and with appropriate staining, the chromosomes with their characteristic banding can be identified and any abnormalities detected. New molecular biology techniques, such as yeast artificial chromosome

(YAC)-cloned probes, have made it simpler and cover large genetic regions of individual chromosomes. These probes can be labeled with fluorescently tagged nucleotides and used in in situ hybridization of the nucleus of isolated tissue from patients, as in fluorescent in-situ hybridization (FISH). These tagged probes allow rapid and relatively unskilled identification of metaphase chromosomes, and allow the identification of chromosomes dispersed within the nucleus. Furthermore, tagging two chromosome regions with different fluorescent tags allows easy identification of chromosomal translocations.

Gene Defects

Mutations

Although DNA replication is a very accurate process, occasionally mistakes occur to produce changes or mutations. These changes can also occur due to other factors such as radiation, ultraviolet light, or chemicals. Mutations in gene sequences or in the sequences that regulate gene expression (transcription and translation) may alter the amino acid sequence in the protein encoded by that gene. In some cases protein function will be maintained; in other cases it will change or cease, perhaps producing a clinical disorder.

Point mutation involves the substitution of one nucleotide for another, thereby changing the codon in a coding sequence. For example, the triplet AAA, which codes for lysine, may be mutated to AGA, which codes for arginine. Whether a substitution produces a clinical disorder depends on whether it changes a critical part of the protein molecule produced. Fortunately, many substitutions have no effect on the function or stability of the proteins produced, as several codons code for the same amino acid.

Insertion or *deletion* of one or more bases is a more serious change, as it results in the alteration of the rest of the following sequence to give a frame-shift mutation. For example, if the original code was TAA GGA GAG TTT and an extra nucleotide (A) is inserted, the sequence becomes TAA AGG AGA GTT T. Alternatively, if the third nucleotide (A) is deleted, the sequence becomes TAG GAG AGT TT. In both cases, different amino acids are incorporated into the polypeptide chain. This type of change is seen in some forms of thalassemia. Insertions and deletions can involve many hundreds of base pairs of DNA. For example, some large deletions in the dystrophin gene remove coding sequences, and this results in Duchenne muscular dystrophy.

Splicing Mutations

If the DNA sequences that direct the splicing of introns from mRNA are mutated, then abnormal splicing may occur. In this case the processed mRNA, which is translated into protein by ribosomes, may carry intron sequences, thus altering which amino acids are incorporated into the polypeptide chain.

Termination Mutations

Normal polypeptide chain termination occurs when the ribosomes processing the mRNA reach one of the chain termination or stop codons (see above). Mutations involving these codons result in either late or premature termination. For example, hemoglobin constant spring is a hemoglobin variant where, instead of the stop sequence, a single base change allows the insertion of an extra amino acid.

Single-Gene Disease

Monogenetic disorders involving single genes can be inherited with dominant, recessive, or sex-linked characteristics. Inheritance occurs according to simple mendelian laws, making predictions of disease in offspring and therefore genetic counseling more straightforward.

Autosomal Dominant Disorders

Autosomal dominant disorders (incidence, 7 per 1000 live births) occur when one of the two copies has a mutation and the protein produced by the normal form of the gene is unable to compensate. In this case a heterozygous individual will manifest the disease. The offspring of heterozygotes have a 50% chance of inheriting the chromosome carrying the disease allele, and therefore also of having the disease (as in polycystic kidney disease).

These disorders have great variability in their manifestation and severity. Incomplete penetrance may occur if patients have a dominant disorder that does not manifest itself clinically. This gives the appearance of the gene having skipped a generation. New cases in a previously unaffected family may be a result of a new mutation. If it is a mutation, the risk of a further affected child is negligible. *Li-Fraumeni syndrome* (LFS) is an autosomal dominant disorder associated with cancer predisposition syndrome. Affected individuals have a *p53* mutation and have a predisposition to a number of malignancies including soft tissue sarcoma, breast cancer, leukemia, adrenocortical tumors, melanoma, and colon cancer (38). Similarly, *hereditary nonpolyposis colorectal carcinoma* (HNPCC) is an autosomal dominant predisposition to develop colorectal, endometrial, ovarian, urinary tract, stomach, small bowel, and biliary tract carcinomas, as well as brain tumors (Lynch syndrome I and II) (39).

Autosomal Recessive Disorders

These disorders manifest themselves only when an individual is homozygous for the disease allele. In this case the parents are generally unaffected, healthy carriers (heterozygous for the disease allele). There is usually no family history, although the defective gene is passed from generation to generation. The offspring of an affected person will have healthy heterozygotes unless the other parent is also a carrier. If both parents are carriers, the offspring have a one in four chance of being homozygous and affected, a one in two chance of being a carrier, and a one in four chance of being genetically normal. Consanguinity increases the risk. The clinical features of autosomal recessive disorders are usually severe; patients often present in the first few years of life and have a high mortality. Many inborn errors of metabolism are recessive diseases.

Sex-Linked Disorders

Genes carried on the X chromosome are said to be X-linked, and can be dominant or recessive in the same way as autosomal genes. As females have two X chromosomes, they will be unaffected carriers of X-linked recessive diseases. However, since males have just one X chromosome, any deleterious mutation in an X-linked gene will manifest itself because no second copy of the gene is present.

Imprinting

It is known that for normal function a diploid number of chromosomes, 46, are required. In some way the chromosomes are imprinted so that the maternal and paternal contributions are different. The expression of a gene depends on the parent who passed on the gene. Imprinting is relevant to human genetic disease because different phenotypes may result, depending on whether the mutant chromosome is maternally or paternally inherited. It has been suggested that *DNA methylation* may be the epigenetic marking for imprinting phenomenon in mammals (40). DNA methylation is involved in the activation of tumor suppressor and other genes in prostate, renal, and bladder cancer. Loss of imprinting may be a primary event in Wilms' and testicular tumors (41).

Complex Traits: Multifactorial and Polygenic Inheritance

Characteristics resulting from a combination of genetic and environmental factors are said to be multifactorial; those involving multiple genes can also be said to be polygenic. Measurements of most biological traits (e.g., height) show a variation between individuals in a population. This variability is due to variation in genetic factors and environmental factors. Environmental factors may play a part in determining some characteristics, such as weight, while other characteristics such as height may be largely genetically determined. This genetic component is thought to be due to the additive effects of a number of alleles at a number of loci, many of which can be individually identified using molecular biological techniques (42).

Cancer Cell Biology and Genetics

Cancer cells are a clonal population of cells in which the accumulation of mutations in multiple genes has resulted in escape from the normally strictly regulated mechanisms that control growth and differentiation of somatic cells. The malignant phenotype acquired by cancer cells have the following properties (43):

1. Loss of growth control
2. Resistance to apoptosis
3. Ability to create new blood supply (angiogenesis)
4. Infiltration into the surrounding tissues
5. Metastasis: ability to colonize and survive in an ectopic environment

The process of oncogenesis can be thought of as a stepwise process, with mutations in particular genes being required for progression from one phase to another, that is, from transformed cell to metastatic cell; these gene mutations are rate-limiting. Rarely, if ever, is a single event responsible for conversion of a normal cell to a malignant cell. Mutations may be a combination of inherited, spontaneous, and environmentally induced factors. *Oncogenes* are mutated genes that cause normal cell to grow out of control and become cancer cells. *Tumor suppressor genes* slow down cell division, repair DNA, and induce apoptosis. Often several oncogenes may be found within the same receptor-signaling pathway (Fig. 1.5).

The study of mechanisms and genes that are responsible for the loss of regulation of the cell cycle control does not in itself explain invasion and metastasis. There are events arising from expression of proteases to digest tissue stroma,

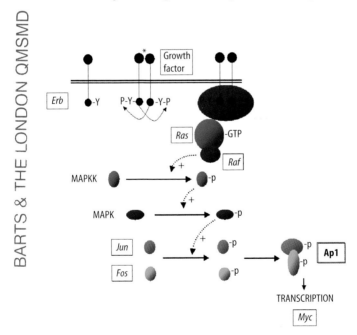

FIGURE 1.5. Diagrammatic illustrations of proto-oncogene positions within the growth factor receptor signal transduction pathway. GTP, guanosine triphosphate; MAPK, mitogen-activated protein kinase; MAPKK, mitogen-activated protein kinase kinase.

downregulation of certain cell adhesion molecules such as cadherins that anchor cells, and the expression of those adhesion molecules that regulate cytoskeletal changes and cell migration, such as the integrins. Most important is the deregulation of apoptotic pathways, both intrinsic and extrinsic, which would signal a cell that has lodged in an inappropriate tissue to undergo altruistic apoptosis.

Apoptosis (Fig. 1.6)

Apoptosis was mentioned earlier in this chapter (programmed cell death). It is triggered by a number of factors, such as ultraviolet rays, γ-radiation, chemotherapeutic drugs, and death receptors (DRs) (44). In oncology it has become clear that chemotherapy and radiotherapy regimes work effectively if they can trigger the tumor cells' own apoptotic pathways. Failure to do so may result in resistant tumors.

Several factors initiate apoptosis, but in general there are two signaling pathways: the extrinsic apoptotic pathway triggered by death receptors on the cell surface, and the intrinsic pathway initiated at the mitochondrial level. Death receptors are all members of the tumor necrosis factor (TNF) receptor superfamily [TNF-related apoptotic inducing ligand receptor-1 family: TRAIL-R1 or D4, APO-2, and TRAIL-2; DR5, TRICK2 (TRAIL inducer of cell killing), and Fas ligands (CD95) (APO-1/Fas)] (44).

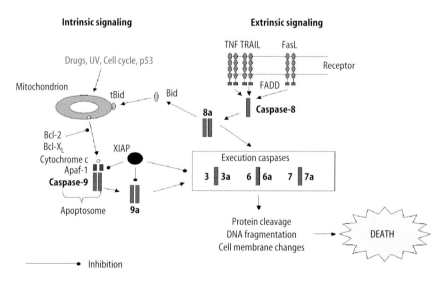

FIGURE 1.6. Intrinsic and extrinsic apoptosis pathways and their linkage. FADD, fas associated protein with death domains; TNF, tumor necrosis factor; TRAIL, TNF-related apoptotic inducing ligand; XIAP, inactivator of inhibitors of apoptosis.

Apoptotic Pathways

Cysteine Proteases

The capsases are secondary messenger regulators and effectors of cell destruction, characteristic of apoptosis. They couple proapoptotic signals, receptor activation, or gene expression as a result of cellular damage with effector capsases.

The extrinsic pathway is important in processes such as tissue remodeling and induction of immune self-tolerance. Activated receptors with internal death domains complex multiple pro-caspase 8 molecules whose autocatalytic activity results in release of the initiator caspase 8. In turn, caspase 8 cleaves pro-caspases 3 and caspase 3, in combination with the other effector caspases, activates DNA cleavage, cell condensation, and fragmentation.

The intrinsic pathway centers on the release of mitochondrial cytochrome c. Cellular stress, such as growth factor withdrawal and p53 gene expression, induces the expression of the proapoptotic Bcl-2 family of proteins, Bax and Bak. Bax is normally localized in the cytosol or loosely associated with the outer mitochondrial membrane, whereas Bak is mostly localized in the outer mitochondrial membrane and remains inactive. Bak and Bax polymerize and form holes in the mitochondrial membrane that allows cytochrome C to be released into the cell cytosol. Cytochrome C binds Apaf1, and forms a complex known as the apoptosome, which then activates an initiator caspase, in this case, caspase 9, which activates the effector caspase, caspase 3. Other proteins released from damaged mitochondria, Smac/DIABLO and Omi/HtrA2, counteract the effect of inhibitor of apoptosis proteins (IAPs), which normally bind and prevent activation of pro-caspase 3. Antiapoptotic Bcl-2 protein, when incorporated as a member of the Bak/Bax pore complex, render the mitochondrial pore non-permissive to release of cytochrome c and the anti-IAPs.

There is an amplification link between the extrinsic and intrinsic apoptotic pathways in that caspase 8 cleaves a Bcl-2 family member, tBid, which then aids formation of the Bcl-2/Bax/Bak pore complexes. If this complex is predominately formed from proapoptotic members of the Bcl-2 family of proteins, then apoptosome/caspase 9, along with mitochondrial anti-IAPs, amplifies the apoptotic activation of effector caspases 3. Conversely, overexpression of antiapoptotic Bcl-2 will not only inhibit intrinsic but also dampen down extrinsic apoptotic signaling.

Cell Cycle Control Oncogenes and Tumor Suppressors

Regulation of the cell cycle is complex. Cells in the quiescent G0 phase (G, gap) of the cycle are stimulated by the receptor-mediated actions of growth factors [e.g., epithelial growth factor (EGF); platelet-derived growth factor (PDGF); insulin-like growth factor (IGF)] via intracellular second messengers. Stimuli are transmitted to the nucleus, where they activate transcription factors and lead to the initiation of DNA synthesis, followed by mitosis and cell division. Cell cycling is modified by the cyclin family of proteins that activate or deactivate proteins involved in DNA replication by phosphorylation

TABLE 1.3. Examples of oncogenes

Gene	Function of product
Sis	PDGF growth factor
ErbB/Neu	EGF receptor
	Truncated
Erb A	Thyroid hormone cytoplasmic receptor
Ras	G protein
Src	Membrane/cytoskeleton-associated tyrosine kinase
Fes	Cytoplasmic tyrosine kinase
Raf	Serine/threonine protein kinase
Myc	Transcription factor nuclear proteins
Fos, Jun	

(via kinases and phosphatase domains). Thus from G0 the cell moves on to G1 (gap1) when the chromosomes are prepared for replication. This is followed by the synthetic (S) phase, when the 46 chromosomes are duplicated into chromatids, followed by another gap phase (G2), which eventually leads to mitosis (M).

As shown in Figure 1.6, mutations leading to deregulation of expression or function of any protein in the pathway from growth factor to target replication gene expression can be an oncogene (Table 1.3).

However, although multiple mutations may arise to give enhanced replication signaling, the cell cycle itself is regulated by two gatekeepers, which would normally halt the aberrant signal. Tumor suppressor gene products are intimately involved in control of the cell cycle (Table 1.4). Progression through the cell cycle is controlled by many molecular gateways, which are opened or blocked by the cyclin group of proteins that are specifically expressed at various stages of the cycle. The RB and p53 proteins control the cell cycle and interact specifically within many cyclin proteins. The latter are affected by inhibitor of cyclin-

TABLE 1.4. Examples of tumor suppressor genes in urological cancers

Gene	Function of product	Hereditary tumors	Sporadic tumors
RB1	Transcription factor	Retinal and sarcoma	SCLC, breast, prostate, bladder, retinal and sarcoma
p53	Transcription factor	Li-Fraumeni syndrome—breast, osteosarcoma, leukaemia, soft tissue sarcoma	50% of all cancers
WT1*	Transcription factor	Nephroblastoma (Wilms' tumor)	Nephroblastoma
BRCA1 + 2	DNA repair	Prostate	Prostate
VHL	Stabilization of hypoxia inducible factor (HIF), vascular endothelial growth factor (VEGF), transforming growth factor (TGFα and β)	Hemangioblastoma of the brain, spinal cord, retina; renal cysts and renal cell carcinoma; cystadenomas of epididymis, broad ligament, pancreas, liver and pheochromocytoma	Renal

SCLC, small-cell lung cancer.

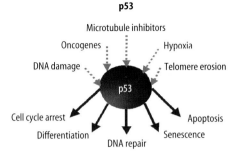

FIGURE 1.7. Cellular events that induce tumor suppressor gene *p53* expression (blue arrows) and the cellular consequences of p53 activation (red arrows).

dependent kinase (INK) 4A acting on cdc 4 and 6. The general principle is that being held at one of these gateways will ultimately lead to programmed cell death. p53 is a DNA-binding protein that induces the expression of other genes and is a major player in the induction of cell death. Its own expression is induced by broken DNA.

The induction of *p53* gene transcription by damage initially causes the expression of DNA repair enzymes. If DNA repair is too slow or cannot be effected, then other proteins that are induced by p53 will effect programmed cell death (Fig. 1.7).

One gateway event that has been largely elucidated is that between the G1 and the S phase of the cell cycle. The transcription factor dimer complex E2F-DP1 causes progression from the G1 to the S phase. However, the RB protein binds to the E2F transcription factor, preventing its induction of DNA synthesis. Other, cyclin D-related, molecules inactivate the RB protein, thus allowing DNA synthesis to proceed. This period of rapid DNA synthesis is susceptible to mutation events and will propagate a preexisting DNA mistake. Damaged DNA-induced *p53* expression rapidly results in the expression of a variety of closely related (and possibly tissue-specific) proteins, WAF-1/p21, p16, and p27. These inhibit the inactivation of RB by cyclin D-related molecules. As a result, *RB*, the normal gate that stops the cell cycle, binds to the E2F-DP1 transcription factor complex, halting S phase DNA synthesis. If the DNA damage is not repaired, apoptosis ensues (Fig. 1.8).

Viral Inactivation of Tumor Suppressors

The suppression of normal tumor suppressor gene function can be achieved by disabling the normal protein once it has been transcribed, rather than by mutating the gene. Viruses have developed their own genes, which produce proteins to do precisely this. The main targets of these proteins are RB and p53, to which they bind and thus disable. The best understood are the adenovirus E1A and human papillomavirus (HPV) E7 gene products, which bind RB, while the

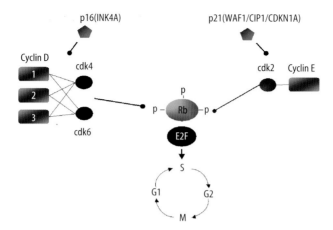

FIGURE 1.8. Tumor suppressor RB protein gatekeeper role in preventing cell cycle progression from G1–S phase until progressive phosphorylation by cyclin molecules renders RB unable to bind the cycle-specific E2F transcription factor.

adenovirus E1B and HPV E6 gene products bind p53. The simian virus 40 (SV40) large T antigen binds both RB and p53.

Hereditary Predisposition to Cancer

Some cancers have a hereditary nature, although this is manifest via a more subtle genetic predisposition. Only one hit is required to lose the function of the tumor suppressor gene if there is already a hereditary mutation on the other allele. Compared to patients with sporadic tumors, those with inherited predisposition to cancer tend to develop tumors at an earlier age and more commonly bilaterally or multifocal, and often with a more restricted tissue origin (Table 1.4).

Approximately 5% to 10% of all prostate cancer seems to be due to autosomal dominant cancer susceptibility genes (45). Inherited oncogenes would be expected to be lethal, although two are recognized: multiple endocrine neoplasia type II (MEN-II) and hereditary papillary renal cancer.

Genomic Imprinting and Cancer

Genomic imprinting is the epigenetic marking of a gene, based on parental origin that results in monoallelic expression. This phenomenon differs from the classical sequence-based qualitative changes in that gene expression and effective gene dosage are controlled by epigenetic dysregulation of parental alleles of an imprinted gene. Imprinting dysregulation may contribute to tumorigenesis either by activating a transcriptionally repressed allele, resulting in gene activation, or by inactivating an expressed allele of an imprinted tumor suppressor gene, leading to loss of function. Evidence implicating this process in tumorigenesis is based on the finding of selective loss of parental heterozygosity (LOH) at certain imprinted domains in several pediatric tumors. The p57 KIP2 protein is a cell cycle inhibitor of several G1 cyclin complexes and is a negative regulator of cell proliferation. The p57KIP2 is located on 11p15.5, a region implicated in Beckwith-Wiedemann syndrome, which is characterized by childhood tumors including Wilms' tumor, rhabdosarcoma, and adrenal carcinoma, which display a specific loss of maternal 11p15 alleles, suggesting that genomic imprinting plays an important role (46).

Microsatellite Instability

Microsatellites are short (50 to 300 bp) sequences composed of tandemly repeated segments of DNA two to five nucleotides in length (dinucleotide/trinucleotide/tetranucleotide repeats). Often used as markers for linkage analysis because of high variability in repeat number between individuals, these regions are inherently unstable and susceptible to mutations during DNA synthesis. Somatic microsatellite instability (MSI) has been detected in a number of cancers including bladder and upper urinary tract tumors. It has been assessed as a predictor of survival in patients with invasive upper urinary tract transitional cell carcinoma (47). Detecting MSI involves comparing the length of microsatellite alleles amplified from tumor DNA with the corresponding allele in normal tissue from the same individual.

Tumor Angiogenesis

Once a nest of cancer cells reaches 1 to 2 mm in diameter, it must develop a blood supply in order to survive and grow larger, as diffusion is no longer adequate to supply the cells with oxygen and nutrients. As with all tissues, solid tumor cancer cells secrete substances that promote the formation of new blood vessels, a process called angiogenesis. The factors that favor and inhibit angiogenesis are summarized in Table 1.5 (48,49).

Angiogenic Switch

Due to rapid growth and increased cell mass, oxygen and nutrient deprivation leads to promotion of neovascularization. Tumor cells induce angiogenesis via expression of angiogenic cytokines such as the vascular endothelial growth factor (VEGF); a potent and unique angiogenic protein that induces endothelial cell (EC) proliferation, EC migration, and vascular permeability, and acts as a crucial survival factor for endothelial cells (50).

TABLE 1.5. Proangiogenic and antiangiogenic factors

Proangiogenic	Antiangiogenic
Activators of endothelial cell proliferation and migration: vascular endothelial growth factor, fibroblast growth factor (FGF); platelet-derived growth factor (PDGF); epidermal growth factor (EGF)	Endogenous regulators
	Laminin: binds with endostatin
	Endostatin: inhibitor of endothelial cell proliferation and migration
	Tumostatin: induction of apoptosis of endothelial cells
Chemokines	BM components: perlecan, laminin, and collagen
Matrix metalloproteinase (MMP)-mediated degradation	Genes upregulated by p53: thrombospondin-1 (TSP1) and matrix metalloproteinase 2 (MMP2)
Cyclooxygenase 2	

Oncogenes and Angiogenesis

The recruitment process of host blood vessels to the tumor site is triggered by the very same set of genetic alterations (activated oncogenes and inactivated tumor suppressor genes, inhibition of apoptosis, and aberrant mitogenesis) (51). For example, mutant *Ras* expression is associated with increased production of VEGF and increases the bioavailability of metalloproteinases (52).

Angiogenesis and Urological Cancers

Several therapeutic vaccine preparations are under development to produce a range of host immune (humoral, cellular) against proangiogenic factors and their receptors in tumors.

Renal Cell Carcinoma

Many angiogenic factors have been found to have increased expression in renal cell carcinoma. Increased expression of VEGF and VEGF mRNA is seen (53). *VHL* mutation in relation to angiogenesis has already been discussed. The anti-angiogenesis therapy of RCC is discussed in Chapter 15.

Bladder Cancer

Microvessel density is an independent prognostic indicator for muscle invasive TCC (54). High serum levels of VEGF indicate metastatic disease (55), and high urinary levels correlate with tumor recurrence (56). The therapeutic applications are discussed in Chapter 16.

Prostate Cancer

Vascular endothelial growth factor expression is low in the normal prostate but increased in cancer, and shows a positive association with microvascular density (MVD), tumor stage, Gleason grade, and disease-specific survival (57).

Testicular Cancer

Increased VEGF expression is seen in germ cell tumors. There is evidence to suggest that VEGF expression is involved in tumor development, angiogenesis, and metastasis (58).

Important Techniques in Molecular Cell Biology

Monoclonal Antibodies

Myeloma is a malignancy of transformed B-cell lineage that secretes a specific antibody. This fact is used to produce specific antibodies directed toward an antigen of choice. A laboratory animal is injected with the antigen of choice against which it mounts an immune response. B cells are then harvested from the spleen. The cells are fused en masse to a specialized myeloma cell line that no longer produces its own antibody. The resulting fused cells, or *hybridomas*, are immortal and produce antibodies specified by the lymphocytes of the immunized animal. These cells can be screened to select for the antibody of interest, which can then be produced in limitless amounts. Modification of the mouse antibody is then required for the recognition of the Fc (effector) region of the antibody to initiate human defense mechanisms and to avoid an immune response against the antibody shortening its half-life. Attachment of a human Fc fragment to the mouse Fab fragment to create a chimeric antibody is called humanization.

Southern Hybridization

DNA, which has first been digested with restriction endonucleases (e.g., Eco-R1), can be separated by virtue of the differential mobility of fragments of varying size in an electrical field. This is done in an agarose gel. The gel is then placed on a nylon transfer membrane, and the DNA is absorbed onto it by capillary action; this is the process of Southern blotting. (Northern and Western blotting refer to essentially the same process but using mRNA and protein, respectively, rather than DNA.)

The nylon membrane can then be incubated with a short strand of DNA (the probe) that has been radiolabeled with 32p. If the DNA on the membrane contains sequences homologous to the probe, then Watson-Crick base pairing will occur and the probe will stick to the membrane. This can be visualized by exposing the membrane to a standard radiographic film. Thus a probe for a given region of the genome can be used to investigate the DNA of patients to determine the presence or absence of a given mutation if that mutation creates or destroys a restriction enzyme recognition site, thereby altering the size of a band on the exposed film.

Polymerase Chain Reaction

Polymerase chain reaction (PCR) has led to a revolution in molecular biology. Two unique oligonucleotide sequences on either side of the target sequence, known as *primers*, are mixed together with a DNA template, a thermostable DNA polymerase *(taq polymerase)*, and purine and pyrimidine bases attached to sugars.

In the initial stage of the reaction, the DNA template is heated to 90°C to make it single stranded (denature), and then as the reaction cools the primers will *anneal* to the template if the appropriate, complementary, sequence is present. Then the reaction is heated to 72°C for the DNA polymerase to synthesize new DNA between the two primer sequences. This process is then repeated on multiple occasions, up to about 30 or so cycles, amplifying the target sequence exponentially. Each cycle takes only a few minutes. The crucial feature of PCR is that to detect a given sequence of DNA it needs to be present only in one copy (i.e., one molecule of DNA); this makes it extremely powerful.

The sensitivity of the technique is dictated by the amount of amplification and thus the number of cycles performed. The specificity relies on the uniqueness of the oligonucleotide sequence of the primers (if the primers bind at multiple sites, then multiple DNA sequences will be amplified).

Refinements of PCR include the following:

Multiplex PCR, in which where multiple pairs of primers are used to amplify several target areas of DNA in parallel

Nested PCR, which improves the specificity of the reaction by including a second pair of primers just within the target sequence defined by the first set of primers.

Reverse transcription (RT)-PCR which uses reverse transcriptase to form cDNA from mRNA, which can then be used for the standard PCR reaction.

Real-time RT-PCR, which is a quantitative RT-PCR whereby relative levels of mRNA are determined by monitoring the simultaneous amplification of the cDNA of a target gene against that of a housekeeping gene mRNA.

Expression Microarrays/Gene Chips

This is a methodology developed to examine the relative abundance of mRNA for thousands of gene present in cells/tissue of different types or conditions, for example, to examine the changes in gene expression from normal colonic tissue to that of malignant colonic polyps. The basic technology is the ability to immobilize sequence of DNA complementary to specific genes or different regions of known genes, onto a solid surface in precise microdot arrays. Total mRNA is extracted from one tissue and labeled with fluorescent tag Cy3-green and the mRNA from the second tissue with fluorescent tag Cy5-red. The two fluorescent-tagged total mRNA samples are mixed in a 1:1 ratio and washed over the DNA gene chips. The mRNA for specific genes will bind to their complementary microdot and can be detected by laser-induced excitation of the fluorescent tag, and the position and light wavelength and intensity recorded by a scanning confocal microscope. The relative intensity of Cy5-red:Cy3-green is a reliable measure of the relative abundance of specific mRNAs in each sample. Yellow results from equal binding of both fluorescent-tagged mRNAs. If no hybridization occurs on a dot, then the area is black. The power of the system is that many thousands of genes can be screened not only for their expression but also for their relative expression in normal and diseased tissue. A considerable amount of computing power and analysis is required to interpret the thousands of dots on a microarray chip.

Proteomics and Genomics

A more direct route to understanding genetic and somatic disease is by studying the protein expression characteristics of normal and diseased cells—the proteome. This method relies on the separation of proteins expressed by a given tissue by molecular size and charge on a simple two-dimensional display and is achieved by using two-dimensional (2D) gel electrophoresis. The pattern of dots corresponds to the different proteins expressed. With the improvement in technology the patterns are reproducible and can be stored as electronic images. Non-, over-, and underexpression of a given protein can be detected by a corresponding change on the proteome 2D electrophoresis. Furthermore, posttranslational modifications of the protein show up as a change in either size or charge on the proteome picture. To positively identify the altered protein and the posttranslational modification it may contain, these protein spots are eluted and subjected to modern mass spectrometry techniques such as matrix-assisted laser desorption/ionization (MALDI) and electrospray ionization (ESI) time of flight (TOF), which not only give the precise mass of the protein, up to ~500,000 daltons, but also can sequence its amino-acid, phosphorylation and glycosylation structure, which cannot be detected by genome analysis. There is increasing interest in the proteomic and genomic study of urological cancers (prostate, bladder, and kidney) and their markers, which will help in early detection of the disease, to predict prognosis and response to therapy (59–61).

Metabolomics

In the postgenomic era, computing power, statistical software, separation science, and modern mass spectrometry have facilitated the analysis of complex mixtures as a complete entity and not merely the fluctuation in concentration of one analyte within it. To realize this potential, the metabolic pathways and networks can be traced by the flow of atoms through metabolites (isotopomer analysis) (62). Metabolomics is the study of the repertoire of nonproteinaceous, endogenously synthesized small molecules present in an organism. Such small molecules include well-known compounds like glucose, cholesterol, ATP, and lipid signaling molecules. These molecules are the ultimate product of cellular metabolism, and the metabolome refers to the catalogue of those molecules in a specific organism, for example, the human metabolome. In terms of clinical biochemistry, the analysis of the pattern of change of such molecules in urine samples of individuals with and without a particular disease and those treated with specific drugs represents a change in the metabolome. It is very likely that, in the future, medicine-regulating authorities will require metabolomic studies on all new drugs.

References

1. Paulson M. Basement membrane proteins: structure, assembly and cellular interaction. Crit Rev Biochem Mol Biol 1992;27:93–127.
2. Carew JS and Huang P. Review: mitochondrial defects in cancer. Mol Cancer 2002;1:9 (www.molecular.cancer.com).
3. Wong X. The expanding role of mitochondria in apoptosis. Genes Dev 2001;15: 2922–2933.
4. Frey TG, Mannella CA. The internal structure of mitochondria. Trends Biochem Sci 2000;25:319–324.
5. Horton TM, Petros JA, Heddi A. Novel mitochondrial genome in a renal cell carcinoma. Genes Chromosomes Cancer 1996;15:95–101.
6. Selvanayagam P, Rajaraman S. Detection of mitochondrial genome depletion by a novel cDNA in renal cell carcinoma. Lab Invest 1996;74:592–599.
7. Jessie BC, Sun CQ, Irons HR, et al. Accumulation of mitochondrial DNA deletions in the malignant prostate of patients of different ages. Exp Gerontol 2001;37: 169–174.
8. Ogura M, Shibata T, Junlin Yi, et al. A tumor-specific gene therapy strategy targeting dysregulation of the VHL/HIF pathway in renal cell carcinomas. Cancer Sci 2005; 96:288–294.
9. Haynes MD, Martin TA, Jenkins SA, et al. Tight junctions and bladder cancer (review). Int J Mol Med 2005;16:3–9.
10. Rosen EM, Joseph A, Jin L, et al. Urinary and tissue levels of scatter factor in transitional cell carcinoma of bladder. J Urol 1997;157:72–78.
11. Li B, Kanamaru H, Noriki S, et al. Differential expression of hepatocyte growth factor in papillary and nodular tumors of the bladder. Int J Urol 1998;5:436–440.
12. Inoue K, Slaton JW, Kim SJ, et al. Interleukin-8 expression regulates tumorigenicity and metastasis in human bladder cancer. Cancer Res 2000;60:2290–2299.
13. Lipponen PK, Eskelinen MJ. Reduced expression of E-cadherin is related to invasive disease and frequent recurrence in bladder cancer. J Cancer Res Clin Oncol 1995; 121:303–308.
14. Rashid MG, Sanda MG, Vallorosi CJ, et al. Posttranslational truncation and inactivation of human E-cadherin distinguishes prostate cancer from matched normal prostate. *Cancer Res* 2001;61:489–492.
15. Conn IG Vilela MJ, Garrod DR, et al. Immunohistochemical staining with monoclonal antibody 32–2B to desmosomal glycoprotein 1. Its role in the histological assessment of Urothelial carcinomas. Br J Urol 1990;65:176–180.
16. Okegawa T, Li Y, Pong RC, Hsieh JT. Cell adhesion proteins as tumor suppressors. J Urol 2002;167(4):1836–1843.
17. Jung I, Messing E. Molecular mechanisms and pathways in bladder cancer development and progression. Cancer Contr 2000;7:325–334.

18. Liebert M, Washington R, Wedemeyer G, et al. Loss of co-localization of alpha 6 beta 4 integrin and collagen VII in bladder cancer. Am J Pathol 1994;144:787–799.
19. Uings IJ, Farrow SN. Cell receptors and signalling. J Clin Path Mol Pathol 2000;53: 295–299.
20. Lindquist S, Craig EA. The heat shock proteins. Annu Rev Genet 1988;22:631–637.
21. Clocca DR, Calderwood SK. Mini-review: heat shock proteins in cancer: diagnostic, prognostic, predictive and treatment implications. Cell Stress Chaperones 2005;10: 86–103.
22. Cornford PA, Dodson AR, Parsons KF, et al. Heat shock protein expression independently predicts clinical outcome in prostate cancer. Cancer Res 2000;60:7099–7105.
23. Renehan AG, Booth C. What is apoptosis, and why is it important? BMJ 2001;322: 1536–1538.
24. Hengartner MO. Death cycle and Swiss army knives. Nature 1998;391:441–442.
25. Yang E, Korsmeyer SJ. Molecular thanaptosis: a discourse on the Bcl-2 family and cell death. Blood 1996;88:386–401.
26. Wallace-Brodeuer RR, Low SW. Clinical implications of p53 mutations. Cell Mol Life Sci 1999;55:64–75.
27. Sjostrom J, Bergh J. How apoptosis is regulated, and what goes wrong in cancer. BMJ 2001;322:1538–1539.
28. Flint J, Craddock CF, Villegas A, et al. Healing of broken human chromosomes by addition of telomeric repeats. Am J Hum Genet 1994;55:505–512.
29. Kim NW, Piatyszek MA, Prowse KR, et al. Specific association of human telomerase activity with immortal cell and cancer. Science 1994;266:2011–2015.
30. Sommerfield HJ, Meeker AK, Piatyszek MA, Bova GS, et al. Telomerase activity: a prevalent marker of malignant human prostate tissue. Cancer Res 1996;56: 218–222.
31. Biroccio A, Leonetti C. Review: telomerase as a new target for the treatment of hormone-refractory prostate cancer. Endo Rel Cancer 2004;11:407–421.
32. Yoshida K, Ugino T, Tahara H, et al. Telomerase activity in bladder carcinoma and its implication for non-invasive diagnosis by detection of exfoliated cancer cells in the urine. Cancer 1997;79:362–369.
33. Jones JB, Song JJ, Hempen PM, et al. Detection of mitochondrial DNA mutations in pancreatic cancer offers a "mass"-ive advantage over detection of nuclear DNA mutations. Cancer Res 2001;61:1299–1304.
34. Croteau DL, Bohr VA. Repair of oxidative damage to nuclear and mitochondrial DNA in mammalian cells. J Biol Chem 1997;272:25409–25412.
35. Vessey CJ, Norbury CJ, Hickson ID. Geneic disorders associated with cancer predisposition and genetic stability. Prog Nucleic Acid Res Mol Biol 1999;63: 189–221.
36. Matzke MA, Mette MF, Kanno T, Matzke AJ. Does the intrinsic instability of aneuploid genomes have a causal role in cancer? Trends Genet 2003;19:253–256.
37. Berrozpe G, Miro R, Caballin MR, et al. Trisomy 7 may be a primary changes in non-invasive transitional cell carcinoma of the bladder. Cancer Genet Cytogenet 1990;50: 9–14.
38. Birch JM, Hartley AL, Tricker KJ, et al. Prevalence and diversity of constitutional mutations in the p53 gene among 21 Li-Fraumeni families. Cancer Res 1994;54: 1298–1304.
39. Peltomäki P, Vasen H. Mutations associated with HNPCC predisposition—update of ICG-HNPCC/INSiGHT mutation database. Dis Markers 2004;20(4–5):269–276.

40. Sasaki H, Allen NA, Surani MA. DNA methylation and genomic imprinting in mammals. In: Jost JP, Saluz HP, eds. DNA Methylation: Molecular and Biological Significance. Basel, Switzerland: Birkhauser Verlag, 469–488.
41. Schilz WA. DNA methylation in urological malignancies (review). Int J Urol 1998; 13:151–167.
42. Drajani TA, Canzian F, Pierotti MA. A polygenic model of inherited predisposition to cancer. FASEB J 1996;10:865–870.
43. Campisi J. Cancer and aging: rival demons? Nature Rev Cancer 2003;3:339–349.
44. Lavrik I, Golks A, Krammer PH. Death receptor signalling. J Cell Sci 2005;118: 265–267.
45. Carter BS, Beatty TH, Steinberg GD, et al. Mendelian inheritance of familial prostate cancer. Proc Natl Acad Sci USA 1992;89:3367–3371.
46. Hatada I, Inazawa J, Abe T, et al. Genomic imprinting of human p57KIP2 and its reduced expression in Wilms' tumors. Hum Mol Genet 1996;5;783–788.
47. Roupret M, Fromont G, Azzouzi AR, et al. Microsatellite instability as predictor of survival in patients with invasive upper urinary tract transitional cell carcinoma. Urology 2005;65(6):1233–1237.
48. Bergers G, Benjamin LE. Tumorigenesis and angiogenic switch. Nature Rev Cancer 2003;3:401–410.
49. Kalluri R. Basement membranes: structure assembly and role in tumorigenesis. Nature Rev Cancer 2003;3:422–433.
50. Gerbert HP, McMurtrey A, Kowalski J, et al. Vascular endothelial growth factor regulates endothelial cell survival through the phosphatidylinositol 3'-kinase/Akt signal transduction pathway. Requirement for Flk-1/KDR activation. J Biol Chem 1998;273: 30336–30343.
51. Rak J, Yu JL, Kerbel RS. Oncogenes and angiogenesis: signalling three-dimensional tumor growth. J Invest Dermatol Symp Proc 2000;5:24–33.
52. Kerbel RS, Viloria-Petit A, Okada F, Rak J. Establishing a link between oncogenes and tumour angiogenesis. Mol Med 1998;4:286–295.
53. Nakagawa M, Emoto A, Hanada T, et al. Tubulogenesis by microvascular endothelial cells is mediated by vascular endothelial growth factor(VEGF) in renal cell carcinoma. Br J Urol 1997;79:681–687.
54. Jaeger T, Weidner N, Chew K, et al. tumor angiogenesis correlates with lymph node metastasis in invasive bladder cancer. J Urol 1995;154:69–71.
55. Inoue K, Slaton JW, Karashima T, et al. The prognostic value of angiogenesis factor expression for predicting recurrence and metastasis of bladder cancer after neoadjuvant chemotherapy and radical cystectomy. Clin Cancer Res 2000;6: 4866–4873.
56. Bernardini S, Fauconnet S, Chabannes E, et al. Serum levels of vascular endothelial growth factor as a prognostic factor in bladder cancer. J Urol 2001;166:1275–1279.
57. Borre M, Nerstrom B, Overgaard J. Association between immunohistochemical expression of vascular endothelial growth factor (VEGF), VEGF-expressing neuroendocrine-differentiated tumor cells, and outcome in prostate cancer patients subjected to watchful waiting. Clin Cancer Res 2000;6:1882–1890.
58. Fukuda S, Shiriham T, Imazono Y, et al. Expression of vascular endothelial growth factor in patients with testicular germ cell tumours as an indicator of metastatic disease. Cancer 1999;85:1323–1330.
59. Troyer DA, Mubiru J, Leach RJ, Naylor SL. Promise and challenge: markers of prostate cancer detection, diagnosis and prognosis. Dis Markers 2004;20:117–128.

60. Adam BL, Vlahou A, Semmes OJ, Wright GL Jr. Proteomic approaches to biomarker discovery in prostate and bladder cancers. Proteomics 2001;1:1264–1270.
61. Kashyap MK, Kumar A, Emelianenko N, et al. Biochemical and molecular markers in renal cell carcinoma: an update and future prospects. Biomarkers 2005;10: 258–294.
62. Fan TW, Lane AN, Higashi RM. The promise of metabolomics in cancer molecular therapeutics. Curr Opin Mol Ther 2004;6(6):584–592.

2
Animal Models in Genitourinary Malignancies

Prabhakar Rajan and Hing Y. Leung

Experimental Models in Cancer

In Vitro Models

In vitro cell culture techniques facilitate cultivation of human- and animal-origin cells for prolonged periods of time. Cell lines, harvested from primary or metastatic sites, maintain some of the phenotypical characteristics of the tumor of origin. However, establishing cell lines from early or premalignant disease, such as primary cultures, is more difficult. Cells can be immortalized inadvertently by exposure to environmental carcinogens or by repeated passage, transfection with viral or human oncogenes, and chemical or radiation exposure. Cell lines are vulnerable to significant interspecies and intercell-type contamination.

In Vivo Models

Interactions between adjacent cells and their biological microenvironment (e.g., endocrine and paracrine pathways) play an important role in cancer and hence manipulation of cell lines *in vitro* will not truly reflect the full spectrum of disease.

Xenografts

Human tissue can be transplanted into animals, usually an immune-deficient mouse, and studied *in vivo*. Xenografts can be orthotopic (in organ of origin) or ectopic (in another tissue or organ).

Transgenic Models

Transgenic animals, usually mice, express oncogenes under the control of promoters that drive gene expression in the tissue of interest and are created by two methods:

Pronuclear microinjection

This is a partially transgenic approach where the gene of interest is introduced directly into a mouse oocyte after fertilization and integrates at random into the genome. Germline transmission is necessary for the next generation to be fully transgenic.

Embryonic Stem Cells

The gene of interest is introduced into embryonic stem (ES) cells and undergoes homologous recombination. There is some germline transmission, and when transgenic sperm fertilize a normal oocyte, a transgenic mouse is produced with ubiquitous gene expression.

Syngeneic Model

Embryonic tissue is isolated, transfected with oncogenes, and then implanted into a genetically identical adult host.

Urological Cancer-Specific Models

Prostate Cancer

The use of animal models in prostate cancer is significantly limited by the fact that this disease is extremely rare in other species, even nonhuman primates. Therefore, studies have relied on human-derived models. Presently, a number of different models are in use (1), representative of prostatic intraepithelial neoplasia (PIN) or metastasis, and are derived from humans.

Cell Lines

The "classical" prostate cancer cell lines are the following: LNCaP, obtained from the supraclavicular lymph node metastasis of a 50-year-old Caucasians; DU-145, derived from a moderately differentiated brain metastasis of a 60-year-old Caucasian; and PC-3, derived from a bony metastasis of a 60-year-old Caucasian. A number of derivatives and sublines of these cell lines have been developed.

Human Xenografts

The major successes in serially transplantable xenografts were the Case Western Reserve (CWR) series. These were established from primary cell lines grown in mice with sustained-release testosterone pellets (CWR 21, 31, 91, 22). The CWR22 model has been used extensively. CWR22 regresses after androgen withdrawal, but can progress to hormone-refractory cancer (CWR22R). Further sublines have been derived from this model (e.g., 22Rv1).

Dunning Rat Model

The R-3327 tumor is a well-differentiated, slow-growing, nonmetastatic adeno-carcinoma that developed spontaneously in a rat and was subsequently transplanted into a syngeneic rat host. A number of sublines have been established with different distinct phenotypes, useful for studying androgen ablation and tumor metastasis.

Mouse Models

Mouse Prostate Reconstitution Model

The fetal urogenital sinus can differentiate into a mature prostate following grafting under the renal capsule of an adult isogeneic male host. Using retroviral transduction, *ras* and *myc* oncogenes are introduced into the mesenchymal and epithelial compartments of the syngraft.

Transgenic Models

A viral transgene, such as simian virus 40 (SV40), can be introduced under regulatory control of a prostate-specific promoter. Mice bearing this transgene develop prostatic hyperplasia that progresses to adenoma or adenocarcinoma.

Canine Model

Canines are the only species in which benign prostatic hyperplasia and prostate cancer are frequently seen. Prostate cancer spontaneously develops in the dog and can metastasize to bone. There is a high incidence of high-grade PIN in this species.

Bladder Cancer (2)

In Vitro Models

Experimental data and clinical studies have shown that *p53*, *Rb*, and *ras* genes play an important role in bladder carcinogenesis, and available experimental models reflect these genotypes (3). The *ras* genes were originally identified in the T24 human differentiated cell line derived from a recurrent bladder tumor. Examples of cell lines used to study superficial cancers include RT4 and RT112 (derived from a primary bladder tumor). Similarly, cell lines used to study invasive disease include EJ28 and 253J; the latter is derived from an orthotopic metastatic model.

In Vivo Models

Xenograft Models

Orthotopic xenografts are used to study superficial and invasive disease. Immunocompetent animals are used to study immunotherapy regimes.

Transgenic Models

A viral transgene, such as SV40, can be introduced under regulatory control of the uroplakin promoter. Mice bearing this transgene develop carcinoma-in-situ and highly invasive tumors through inactivation of *p53* and *Rb* pathways. The same promoter can be used to drive expression of mutant *ras* (resulting in superficial papillary lesions) or epidermal growth factor receptor (EGFR) (resulting in urothelial hyperplasia). Studies show that crossing *ras* transgenic mice with *p53*-null mice results in invasive tumors.

Renal Cancer

In Vitro Models

There are a number of cell line models of renal cancer. Examples include the *VHL*-positive RCC-1 and SN12C, and *VHL*-negative 786-0.

In Vivo Models (4)

RENCA

Murine RENCA (murine renal adenocarcinoma system) cells were originally obtained from a tumor that arose spontaneously in the kidney of Balb/c mice. Histologically, RENCA is a pleomorphic granular cell type adenocarcinoma. RENCA cells can be implanted into BALB/c athymic mice and exhibit a high degree of vascularization. Spontaneous metastases develop in abdominal lymph nodes, lungs, liver, and spleen.

Wistar-Lewis Model

This is a model of renal adenocarcinoma of spontaneous origin in the rat.

Hereditary Rat Models

Hereditary renal cell carcinoma develops in Eker rats heterozygous for an insertional germline mutation in the tuberous sclerosis *Tsc2* tumor suppressor gene (5). A germline mutation has been identified in the Birt-Hogg-Dube *(BHD)* gene of the Nihon rat, which is also predisposed to renal carcinoma, and may provide insight into human BHD syndrome (6).

Xenografts

Human cultured renal cell carcinoma cells can be implanted into athymic severe combined immunodeficiency disease (SCID) mice.

Clinical Application

Role of Molecular Biology in Tumor Diagnosis

Background

Morphological analyses of diseased tissue still remain the basis of tumor diagnoses. Developments in molecular biology have allowed scientists and clinicians to focus on genetic analysis of cancer and premalignant conditions, correlating gene expression with disease phenotypes. Molecular analyses can be useful for diagnostic and prognostic assessment, where tumor classification can guide the choice of and response to therapy. Novel serum proteomic patterns are being studied for potential biomarkers. Molecular analysis could target chemopreventive strategies, screening, risk assessment of premalignant disease, pathological classifications, clinical staging, treatment, and prognosis.

Molecular Techniques

Advances in molecular diagnostics in urological cancers range from DNA-based technologies to newer proteomic techniques (7–9). Urine cytology for lower grade bladder cancer lacks sensitivity and is subject to high variability in sample preparation and interpretation. Prostate-specific antigen (PSA) screening remains controversial as the test lacks sensitivity. For renal cancer, molecular analyses may help identify patients with sporadic renal cell carcinoma who are at high risk of relapse after initial treatment and those with inherited syndromes.

Polymerase Chain Reaction–Based Techniques

Reverse Transcription Polymerase Chain Reaction. Nucleic acid sequences can be rapidly amplified in vitro using a DNA polymerase. Reverse transcription polymerase chain reaction (RT-PCR) uses a DNA polymerase reverse transcriptase to create copy DNA (cDNA) sequences from RNA. It is highly sensitive, as minimal sample RNA is required. Aberrant cancer-specific transcripts can be identified and RT-PCR products can be sequenced to search for point mutations. Single nucleotide polymorphisms (SNPs) are single base-pair alterations that code for single amino-acid substitutions, generating differences in protein structure or function. They can also be detected by hybridization techniques.

Methylation-Specific Polymerase Chain Reaction. DNA methylation, catalyzed by DNA methyl-transferase, typically occurs at CpG islands where cytosine is directly followed by a guanine in the DNA sequence. CpG islands are found in promoter regions, and, if hypermethylated, have a major impact on gene expression, often silencing tumor suppressor genes. Methylation-specific PCR can distinguish methylated from unmethylated DNA. Hypermethylation of CpG island sequences at GSTP1, a glutathione S-transferase, has been reported in prostate cancer (10).

Fluorescence In Situ Hybridization

Fluorescence *in situ* hybridization (FISH) can identify chromosomal abnormalities in tissue sections, such as chromosomal numbers, translocations, deletions, rearrangements, and duplications. A fluorescent-labeled probe, complementary to the DNA or RNA of interest, is hybridized to metaphase chromosomes. Studies in prostate cancer have correlated increases in c-*myc* and loss of *p53* with Gleason grade and cancer progression, respectively. For the diagnosis of bladder cancer, a commercial FISH assay is available to detect aneuploidy of chromosomes 3, 7, and 17, and loss of the 9p21 band in exfoliated cells in urine (11).

Comparative Genomic Hybridization

Comparative genomic hybridization (CGH) provides an overview of DNA sequence copy number changes (amplifications, gains, deletions, and losses). Total genomic tumor DNA and normal reference DNA are differentially labeled and hybridized to normal human metaphase chromosomes. After fluorescent staining, copy number variations are detected by measuring the differential fluorescence intensity ratios for each locus. Numerous amplifications and losses have been identified in prostate cancer, with candidate genes such as *PTEN* and the androgen receptor.

Serial Analyses of Gene Expression

Serial analyses of gene expression (SAGE) can be used to produce a snapshot of the RNA in a tumor. Extracted RNA is digested into small "tags," linked and sequenced. Serial analyses of gene expression gives a list of short sequence tags and the number of times it is observed in the RNA transcript. Using SAGE, it is possible to identify differences in gene expression between normal tissue and tumors.

High-Throughput Array Technologies

A technological revolution in molecular biology has resulted in the emergence of a number of high-throughput automated array-based methods of gene and protein analyses and expression profiling.

Deoxyribonucleic Acid and Oligonucleotide Arrays. Microarrays facilitate simultaneous expression analysis of the whole or part of the human genome. RNA from a tumor sample is labeled with a fluorophore and hybridized to an array slide of synthetic oligonucleotides or cDNA, complementary to a specific gene. Comparison is made to normal controls to identify increases or decreases in gene expression. The CGH arrays can be used as genome-wide screens for DNA amplifications and losses. Expression profiling studies have identified a tumor suppressor role of *KiSS-1* in bladder cancer and increased expression of α-methylacyl–coenzyme A (CoA) racemase in prostate cancer, among other candidate genes. Clinically, array-based technologies could be used for molecular profiling of tumors to accurately classify tumor subtypes and determine the most effective therapeutic interventions.

Tissue Microarrays. Tissue microarrays (TMAs) are used to validate gene expression profiling and correlate expression with clinicopathological parameters. Small cores of tissue (0.6 to 2 mm) are taken from a number of parent tissue blocks and arrayed into a recipient block, which is sectioned. The TMAs can be used for *in situ* hybridization, FISH, and immunohistochemistry.

Protein Arrays. Microarrays constructed with purified or overexpressed proteins can be used for protein profiling and functional genomics. Protein arrays allow screening of thousands of interactions such as protein–antibody, protein–protein, protein–nucleic acid, and protein–drug. Since most protein arrays are made by recombinant methods, results can be correlated with DNA sequence information.

Proteomics

Proteomic analysis can be used to identify changes in expression, posttranslational modification, and structure of proteins irrespective of errors in encoded by DNA. These systems can be used to identify putative biomarkers in serum and urine for diagnostic purposes from spectral profiles (see Chapter 1).

Two-Dimensional Polyacrylamide Gel Electrophoresis and Mass Spectroscopy. In one-dimensional (1D) polyacrylamide gel electrophoresis (PAGE), proteins are separated in one dimension, usually by molecular weight (MW). Two-dimensional (2D) PAGE resolves proteins in two dimensions by isoelectric point at 90 degrees to MW. "Spots" of interest can be isolated and analyzed using mass spectroscopy (MS) to identify protein sequence, structure, and other molecular characteristics. Conventional proteome analysis using 2D PAGE and MS is highly effective but has limitations, and in particular may miss proteins of low molecular weight expressed at low abundance.

Matrix-Assisted Laser Desorption/Ionization Time-of-Flight. Matrix-assisted laser desorption/ionization (MALDI) captures proteins on a solid surface, and subsequent laser excitation or energy transfer results in fragmentation. An anode detects ionized peptides and the time of flight (TOF) to the anode is translated into molecular mass.

Surface-Enhanced Laser Desorption/Ionization Time-of-Flight. A protein pattern can be identified without knowledge of the protein identity, which can correlate with the presence or recurrence of cancer. Surface-enhanced laser desorption/ionization (SELDI) selectively captures protein subtypes interacting preferentially with hydrophobic, hydrophilic, ionic, metal binding, or mixed property surfaces. These techniques are particularly useful for proteins of lower MW.

Clinical Development of Gene Therapy and Its Limitations (12)

Background

Gene therapy is the intracellular delivery of genetic material for therapeutic purpose, such as to replace an absent or defective gene, to augment existing gene function, to create a specific sensitivity to a normally inert prodrug, or to affect the life cycle of an infectious agent. This can be performed in two ways:

Germline Manipulation

At present, germline manipulation, as homologous recombination in transgenic animals, is subject to ethical debate and considered by many to be unethical.

Somatic Cell Manipulation

Ex Vivo Delivery. Genetic material is explanted, manipulated *in vitro*, and subsequently reimplanted. The benefits include protein expression at therapeutic levels for extended period, reducing the need for readministration or adjuvant treatment. However, many reimplanted cells do not survive, and the approach is limited to certain diseases.

In Situ Delivery. The viral and nonviral vectors are delivered in situ, and this method is attracting the most clinical interest in cancer at present (Table 2.1).

Gene Therapy in Urological Malignancy (13–15)

Single gene therapy is relatively more feasible; however, cancer is caused by multiple genetic abnormalities. A specific genetic mutation or deletion can drive clonal expansion for a limited period before a further mutation takes over, creating a small therapeutic window for any particular gene. The most famous example of this is Vogelstein's adenoma to carcinoma sequence in colorectal tumorigenesis. In urological oncology, studies have revealed a number of potential targets for gene therapy:

Tumor Suppressor Genes

p53 mutations are the most commonly described genetic mutation in cancer. *p53* gene therapy *in vitro* and *in vivo*, and clinical trials have been established in a number of cancers. A modified E1B-deleted adenovirus has been engineered to specifically target tumor cells combating problems of vector efficiency; E1B functions to inactivate host *p53*-dependent apoptosis. Clinical trials using *p53* gene therapy in prostate and bladder cancer are currently underway. Other tumor suppressor genes under evaluation include *PTEN* and *nm23* (prostate), *p16* (prostate and bladder), and *Rb* (bladder).

Oncogenes

Oncogenes activated or mutated in urological malignancies include c-*myc*, bcl-2, and c-*met* (prostate), and *erbb2* and *ras* (prostate and bladder). Overexpressed

TABLE 2.1. Delivery systems

System	Example	Features	Advantages	Disadvantages
RNA virus	Retroviruses (RV) e.g., murine leukemia virus (MuLV)	Replicate using DNA -polymerase; integrate into host genome	Wide tissue trophism High target efficiency Stable integration into host genome with sustained transgene expression	Low titers MuLV immunogenic and causes complement inactivation Poor infection of postmitotic tissue or low mitotic rates (e.g., neurons) Limited transgene capacity (9–10 kb)
DNA virus	Adenoviruses (AV) e.g., AV serotypes 2, 5	Double-stranded DNA	High efficiency Wide tissue trophism Low pathogenicity and risk of insertional mutagenesis Infect quiescent and dividing cells High immunogenicity advantageous in cancer	Delivered genes are episomally maintained and lost due to genetic instability Repeated dosing necessary with limited efficacy due to immunization Limited capacity (7.8 kb)
	Adeno- associated virus (AAV)	Single-stranded DNA	High efficiency Not pathogenic Wide tissue trophism	Reduced propensity for site-direction integration Complicated production process and limited capacity (4.7 kb)
	Herpes simplex virus (HSV)	Single-stranded DNA	Wide trophism Able to infect dividing and nondividing cells Disabled infectious single copy (DISC) variants replicate in vivo and infects subsequent cells, but will not produce any further infectious particles	Gutless variant has large transgene capacity (150 kb) High copy numbers
Other viruses	Parvoviruses, baculoviruses	Chimeric variants with features of retroviral integration and adenoviral infectivity	Stable transduction and efficient delivery	
Lipid- mediated	Lipoplex or polyplex, e.g., N-[1-(2, 3-dioleyloxy)propyl] -N,N,N-trimethylammonium chloride (DOTMA)	DNA and lipid interact to facilitate formation of complexes	Safer than viral systems	Low efficiency transfer Ineffective in presence of certain serum proteins
Naked DNA	Biolistics, electroporation, microinjection	High-velocity injection of naked DNA on microcarriers (e.g., gold); *in vivo* electroporation	Simplicity of delivery Suitable for DNA vaccination	Low efficiency transfer improved by multiple dosing

oncogenes can be targeted using antisense technology, by generating nucleic acids complementary to the RNA or DNA sequence of interest, which hybridize and block transcription or translation.

Prodrugs

Prodrug or suicide gene therapy involves the transfer of a drug-metabolizing enzyme to tumor cells. An inactive prodrug is then systemically administered and converted to a cytotoxic agent, and catalyzed by the enzyme, in the tumor cells alone. Prodrug systems that have been trialed in urological oncology include HSV-thymidine kinase (HSV-TK), *Escherichia coli* cytosine deaminase, and nitroreductase. The respective prodrugs are ganciclovir, 5-fluorocytosine, and 5-(aziridin-1-yl)-2,4-dinitrobenzamide (CB1954).

Multidrug Resistance

Current chemotherapeutic regimes can confer drug resistance with multidrug resistant gene (MDR) expression. Identified MDRs can be transferred *ex vivo* to hematopoietic tissue prior to myelosuppressive chemotherapy.

Angiogenesis

Angiogenesis and tumor spread can be inhibited by suppression of positive regulators such as vascular endothelial growth factor (VEGF), induction of negative regulators, or suppression of receptor expression on endothelial cells (e.g., VEGF-receptor antagonists).

Effective Targeting (12)

Anatomical Targeting

In urological malignancies, anatomical targeting is usually intraprostatic or intravesical, although vectors can be introduced into bony or lymph node metastasis.

Ex Vivo Transfer

Target cells can be isolated from the patient, cultured in vitro, transduced, and reimplanted. Autologous tumor cells or fibroblasts can be transduced with immunostimulatory genes [e.g., interleukin-2 (IL-2), tumor necrosis factor-α (TNF-α)] to cause cell destruction *in vivo*. Natural vector trophism can be used to direct transduced tumor infiltrating lymphocytes (TILs), CD8$^+$ T cells that normally infiltrate tumors, to the site of cancer, thereby stimulating a larger T-cell response.

Transduction Targeting

Natural vector trophism can be used to direct gene therapy; however, in practice the efficacy of this technique is limited by a lower rate of cell division in human tumors. Targeted integration into known sites in the human genome (e.g., adeno-associated virus, AAV) improves vector safety and prevents direct gene disruption and potential activation of oncogenes. Hybrid virions can be generated to exploit specific trophisms exhibited by certain envelope proteins (e.g., gp120 of HIV for CD4$^+$ T cell). Existing envelope proteins can be engineered to exhibit increased specificity by physical coupling of molecules or viral envelope gene fusions.

Liposome Vectors

Liposomes are preferentially taken up by cells of the reticuloendothelial system due to matching of the lipid composition of the liposome and cell membrane. By altering liposome characteristics, transfection efficiency can be improved. Incorporating monoclonal antibodies and peptide ligands into the liposome complexes can improve cell targeting.

Endosomal Pathways

DNA can be compacted into toroids, small doughnut-like structures, coated with ligands with certain receptor specificities. This is dependent on endosomal pathways, and is limited by lysosomal degradation and in vivo immunogenic properties.

Transcriptional Targeting

Tissue-Specific Promoters. The therapeutic gene can be cloned upstream of a tumor-specific transcriptional regulatory element (TRE) such as the *PSA* gene; transcription only occurs in cells that express factors that bind to the TRE. Modifications of this technique include tissue-specific knockouts, Cre-recombinase system, and a *bcl-2*–dependent tamoxifen-dependent variant.

Vector Selection. Vectors can be selected to utilize a certain transductional characteristic of the target tissue. There is a significant "bystander" effect as not all cells are transduced, and therapeutic efficacy is dependent on a subsequent T-cell–mediated cytotoxic immune response.

The Future

The major limitations of gene therapy are efficiency of gene transfer, selectivity of tumor targeting, immunogenicity of the vectors, and other general safety considerations. In cancer any single remaining malignant cell following treatment would suffice to repopulate a whole tumor, and so vector efficiency is important. Outcomes from preclinical studies and phase I trials are promising, and provide hope for further studies and a future of gene-based therapeutics.

Tumor Immunotherapy and the Cancer Vaccine (16)

Background

Cancer immunotherapy is the modulation of the immune system to treat malignant disease. Tumors can be antigenic but not immunogenic, and modification of antigen presentation can result in tumor destruction. Cytokine infusions or adoptive T-cell transfer can result in antitumor responses, and monoclonal antibodies to growth factor receptors can hinder tumor growth (e.g., trastuzumab and cetuximab to block HER2/neu and EGFR, respectively). A nonvirulent strain of *Mycobacterium bovis* (bacille Calmette-Guérin, BCG) has been used for the treatment of superficial bladder cancer for many years. Antigen-containing cancer vaccines are able to utilize immunological "memory" to stimulate an effective and long-lasting immune response, although clinically this has been more difficult to elicit. In urological oncology, immunotherapy is an established treatment option for superficial bladder cancer and renal cell carcinoma.

Antigen Presentation (Fig. 2.1)

Normally, cells present intracellular and extracellular protein fragments as antigens via major histocompatibility complexes (MHCs) I and II to $CD8^+$ and $CD4^+$ T cells, respectively. All cells express MHC-I; however, MHC-II is expressed only on specialized antigen-presenting cells (APCs) (e.g.. dendritic cells, macrophages, and B cells). Co-stimulatory molecules on APCs interact with complementary ligands on the $CD4^+$ T cell (T-helper cells) to cause activation.

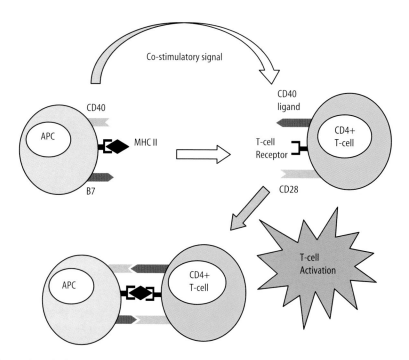

FIGURE 2.1. Antigen presentation. APC, antigen-presenting cell; MHC, major histocompatibility complex.

Immune Response to Cancer

Immunosurveillance

Tumors are regarded as non-self by the immune system, and are detected by the immunosurveillance mechanism, which identifies malignancy and eliminates tumor cells as they arise.

The Danger Model

Normally, APCs present antigens and stimulate a T-cell response in the presence of "danger signals" from distressed or injured cells. It is thought that a lack of "danger signals" in cancer results in immune tolerance of tumor cells (17).

Immune Escape Mechanisms in Cancer

A form of "natural selection" may take place as weakly immunogenic cells in a tumor may evade immune detection, differentiating into a more malignant phenotype (Table 2.2).

Types of Antigen

Unique antigens are exclusively produced by tumors and will not have been previously encountered by the immune system (e.g., mutations in *p53*). Immunotherapy against shared antigens, also expressed at low levels in normal tissue, involves risk of autoimmunity. Overexpressed self-antigens can be used diagnostically [e.g., hTERT (human telomerase reverse transcriptase) and PSA] or therapeutically via receptor blockade (e.g., HER2/neu). Stromal antigens

TABLE 2.2. Mechanism of immune escape in cancer (18)

Strategy	Mechanism
Ignorance	Lack of danger signals
	Lack of tumor antigens in lymphoid tissue
	Growth in immune privileged sites (e.g., brain, eye)
	Downregulation of adhesion molecules may result in physical barrier by stroma
Impaired antigen presentation	Mutation or downregulation of tumor antigens
	Mutation or downregulation of MHC
	Defective antigen processing
Expression of immunosuppressive factors	Cytokines
	Prostaglandins
Tolerance induction	Lack of co-stimulatory molecules rendering T cells anergic
	Immune deviation away from cytotoxic T-cell response
	Induction of regulatory T cells
	T-cell deletion by antigen-induced apoptosis
Apoptosis resistance	Expression of antiapoptotic molecules
	Downregulation and mutation of proapoptotic molecules
Counterattack	Expression of fas and other death receptor ligands that cause immune cell apoptosis

expressed on cells adjacent to the tumor are less likely to evade the immune response. Antigens may be derived from DNA, RNA, peptides and proteins, and cells and tissue lysates. Single epitope immunotherapy in cancer is predictable, but prone to immunological escape.

Types of Tumor Vaccine (16)

Deoxyribonucleic Acid or Ribonucleic Acid Vaccine

Nucleic acid sequences encoding cancer-specific peptides are taken up by endocytosis into tumor cells or APCs. Following transcription and translation, peptides are presented to the immune system. The use of shared peptide antigens risks autoimmunity.

Peptide or Protein Vaccine

Any foreign particle administered will be processed and presented to the immune system, which will mount a significant response if the individual has been immunized. However, sometimes newly encountered antigens may produce little or no effect, and secondary stimuli such as cytokines are necessary to assist APC activation.

Cell and Tissue Lysate Vaccines

Whole tumors and cells express multiple antigens that stimulate the innate and adaptive immune systems. To assist the immune response, cell lines can be transfected with genes encoding proinflammatory cytokines. There are limitations of using whole cells and tissue: first, this method is not applicable if tumor has already escaped immune surveillance; and second, using shared antigens with normal tissue may result in autoimmunity.

Tumor/Dendritic Cell Chimeras

Fusing dendritic cells with tumor cells may restore the MHC function and allow these chimeric cells to act as modified APCs.

Dendritic Cell Vaccines

Harvested dendritic cell (DC) precursors can be cultured *ex vivo* and forced to differentiate with cytokines. They can be pulsed with tumor antigens and used prior to vaccination. Treatment of DCs with unmethylated CpG oligodeoxynucleotides promotes the production of cytokines creating a T-helper (TH)-1 cytokine response [interferon-γ (IFN-γ); interleukins IL-2 and IL-12].

Immunotherapy and Urological Malignancies

Bladder Cancer

Background. Intravesical BCG therapy has been described as the successful immunotherapy to date and yet its precise mechanism of action remains

TABLE 2.3. Immune system components contributing to the antitumor action of bacille Calmette-Guérin (BCG) immunotherapy (19)

Immune system component	Stimulation of immune cells by BCG in vitro	Animal model of immunotherapy with BCG	Analysis of material from BCG-treated patients
T-helper (TH)1 cytokines	Required	Detected in urine and bladder of treated mice	Increased expression in urine of treated patients
T cells	Accessory function	Required for successful therapy	Induced in treated patients
Natural killer (NK) cells	Effector function	Required for successful therapy	Rare population (immunohistology is problematic)
Monocytic cells	Accessory function/ direct killing	Unclear	Unclear
Granulocytes	Unclear	Induced in treated mice	Induced in treated patients
Cellular cytotoxicity against tumor	Perforin is major killing mechanism	Unclear	Unclear (increased number of perforin positive cells in treated patients)
Nitric oxide (NO)	BCG induces nitric oxide synthase (NOS) activity in bladder cancer cells and NO production in splenocytes	NOS upregulated in a rat model of BCG immunotherapy	Nitrite locally induced in BCG treated patients (clinical relevance yet unclear)

unknown (Table 2.3). Current practice follows an induction schedule of weekly intravesical instillations for 6 weeks. Subsequent maintenance BCG has been shown to be superior to the standard induction course and may prevent disease progression.

Mechanism of Action (19)

Urothelial Cell Activation. A crucial step appears to be binding between fibronectin proteins on the mycobacterial and urothelial surfaces, resulting in urothelial cells activation and cytokine production. This appears to have tumor antiproliferative effects.

Localized Immune Response. There is activation of APCs, followed by migration of granulocytes and other mononuclear cells to the bladder wall. A TH-1 cytokine response predominates and there is formation of granuloma-like cellular foci. The TH-1 response appears to have an accessory role to natural killer (NK) cell-mediated cytotoxicity via perforins, which insert into the plasma membrane of target cells and allow lysosomal proteases to activate caspase-mediated apoptosis. The IL-2 response is thought to have clinical prognostic value.

The Future. The future should bring better understanding of the mechanism of action of BCG, as its efficacy appears to rely on persistent localized immunological activation. Alternative strategies being explored include the use of mycobacterial subfractions (to avoid risks associated with live organisms) and cytokine combination therapy, via engineered recombinant BCG strains.

Renal Cell Carcinoma (20)

Background. Cytoreductive nephrectomy followed by immunotherapy is considered standard practice for metastatic renal cell carcinoma, which is resistant to current chemotherapy and radiotherapy strategies.

Active Immunotherapy

Interferon-α. Systemic administration of IFN-α for metastatic renal cell carcinoma has been shown to improve survival. The mode of antitumor action is poorly understood but is thought to be mediated via a number of mechanisms: upregulation of MHC-I on tumor cells with enhanced antigen-presentation; activation of cell-mediated cytotoxicity promoting a TH-1 response; and direct cytostatic activity via reduction of cell proliferation, interference with cellular metabolism, modulation of 2′,5′-oligoadenylate synthase, and oncogenes. IL-2 may also confer a direct antiangiogenic benefit.

Interleukin-2. Intravenous administration of IL-2 has also been shown to improve survival. It is secreted by activated T-cells, causing self-help by producing further IL-2 but also increasing expression of high-affinity IL-2 receptors. The effects of IL-2 include proliferation of activated T cells; clonal expansion CD8$^+$ T cells; activation cell-mediated cytotoxicity via CD8$^+$ T-cells and NK cells; and release of cytokines such as IFN-α, TNF, granulocyte-macrophage colony-stimulating factor (GM-CSF), IL-1, and IL-6.

Other Cytokine/Chemotherapy Combinations. Combinations of IFN-α and IL-2 are thought to have synergistic antitumor effects as described above. Augmentation of immunogenicity caused by cellular killing has been suggested with cytokine therapy and chemotherapy such as 5-fluorouracil, vinblastine, and thalidomide. Thalidomide is thought to lower expression of angiogenic factors such as VEGF and TNF-α. Other combinations of cytokine and chemotherapy regimes are currently under evaluation.

Adoptive Immunotherapy

Lymphokine-Activated Natural Killer Cells. Autologous NK cells can be activated *ex vivo* with IL-2 and subsequently reinfused. Unfortunately, clinical trials using lymphokine-activated natural killer cells (LAKs) have been disappointing.

Tumor-Infiltrating Lymphocytes. Autologous tumor-infiltrating lymphocytes (TILs) can be activated *ex vivo* with IL-2. It is thought that activated TILs exhibit greater cytotoxicity in renal cell carcinoma than the general population of CD8$^+$ T cells. Again, clinical trials have been disappointing.

The Future

Tumor Vaccines. Vaccination with whole cell lysates has been used, with or without nonspecific immunotherapy (e.g., BCG), as adjuvant therapy or for metastatic disease. Other studies are examining the efficacy of dendritic cell vaccines and hybrid cell vaccines. Peptide vaccines (e.g., heat-shock protein–peptide complex vaccine-96) have also been evaluated in association with IL-2.

Allogenic Stem Cell Transplant. A recipient reduced-intensity conditioning regime, used for refractory hematological malignancies, allows transplantation of donor-derived CD8$^+$ T cells. Recognition of minor histocompatibility antigens on recipient tissues is thought to contribute a posttransplant "graft-versus-tumor" response. Early studies have been promising; however, the technique is labor-intensive, expensive, and associated with significant morbidity and mortality.

Prostate Cancer (14)

Cancer Vaccine. A recombinant PSA vaccine delivered by a modified vaccinia virus is currently under evaluation, administered with GM-CSF to augment the immune response.

Gene Therapy Strategies. Intraprostatic delivery of liposomal and adenoviral vectors expressing IL-2 are under clinical investigation. *Ex vivo* transduction of autologous prostate cancer cells with GM-CSF followed by intradermal injection has been shown to induce immunity to prostate cancer antigens.

Impact of Race, Ethnicity, and Aging: Molecular Pathways

Race and Ethnicity

Prostate Cancer

African-Americans have a higher incidence of prostate cancer and death rates compared to Caucasians. Asians have a lower incidence of clinically-diagnosed prostate cancer compared to African-Americans and Caucasians. This risk increases in Asian immigrants to the United States, although never reaching rates found in native-born Caucasians. Autopsy studies show that the rate of latent prostate cancer is similar in all ethnic groups worldwide, suggesting that this ethnic variability is due to differences in the diagnosis of, or progression to, clinically significant disease. African-Americans are diagnosed with later stage disease; however, they have lower survival rates even after correcting for stage, suggesting a more aggressive disease phenotype. Proposed mechanisms relating to race and ethnicity in prostate cancer include the following:

Ras *Oncogene Mutations*

A higher frequency of *ras* mutations is seen in Japanese men with prostate cancers as compared to Caucasians (21).

Vitamin D Theory (22)

The descriptive epidemiology of prostate cancer resembles that of vitamin D deficiency; namely age, black race, and residence at northern latitudes. A dark-skinned individual may require 10 to 50 times the exposure to ultraviolet B (UV-B) rays to produce the equivalent amount of vitamin D as a light-skinned person, and African-Americans have a higher rate of vitamin D deficiency. Prostate cancer cells express high-affinity vitamin D receptors (VDRs), and furthermore 1,25-dihydroxycholecalciferol has been shown to inhibit proliferation and metastasis of prostate cancer cells. There is also evidence to suggest that VDR polymorphisms are associated with advanced prostate cancer (23).

Androgen Receptor Mutations

The androgen receptor (AR) gene contains trinucleotide repeat sequences (CAG) and (GGC) coding for a polyglutamine and polyglycine tracts respectively, in exon 1 of the gene. The response of androgen receptor to androgen is inversely dependent on the length of CAG repeats. African-American males possess shorter CAG repeat lengths than other racial groups; it has been suggested that the racial differences seen in prostate cancer susceptibility may be due in part to variability in the AR CAG repeat length (24).

Dietary Fat and Steroid Hormones

Although higher serum testosterone levels are not always found in patients diagnosed with prostate cancer, African-American males have been found to have higher testosterone levels. The racial differences between Asian and Caucasian prostate cancers have been attributed to dietary fat intake, which may affect steroid hormone synthesis. Low-fat, high-fiber diets lower serum testosterone.

Bladder Cancer (25)

Bladder cancer is twice as common among American-Caucasian males as among African-American males, and roughly one and a half times as common among American-Caucasian females as among African-American females. The incidence among Hispanic-Americans and Native Americans is one-half and one-sixth, respectively, that of Caucasians of each gender. However, African-Americans (especially women) have a 60% to 100% higher mortality from bladder cancer than Caucasians. Some suggest that this reduced risk among Caucasians is limited to noninvasive cancers, and could be due to earlier diagnoses or less aggressive disease phenotypes than in African-Americans. Cultural reasons such as reluctance to accept therapy, or socioeconomic factors could be responsible for a delay in diagnosis among African-Americans. Furthermore, there appears to be preponderance of more aggressive cell types such as squamous cell and adenocarcinoma in these ethnic groups. A proposed explanation for Hispanic-Americans having lower incidence and mortality rates when compared to other minority ethnic groups is the lower rate of tobacco usage.

Aging

Background

Around 65% of cancers in the United Kingdom occur in people over 65 (Cancer Research U.K. Statistics), and therefore it is important to understand the relationship between aging and cancer. Age is the strongest risk factor for the two most common urological malignancies, prostate and bladder cancer. The underlying mechanisms of increased prevalence and incidence of cancer in old age are controversial and three hypotheses have been proposed (26,27).

Duration of Carcinogenesis

It takes several years for the cumulative sequential carcinogenic steps required for neoplastic transformation of normal tissue. Therefore, cancer is more likely to manifest in the elderly through a process of natural selection by accumulation of the dose of the environmental carcinogen.

Physiological Changes

Disease phenotypes can change with age, and can be more indolent or more aggressive depending on the type of cancer. Certain cancers are less aggressive in the old (e.g., breast), whereas others are less aggressive in the young (e.g., immunogenic tumors). Growth of less immunogenic tumors may be slowed in older patients due to a reduction in infiltrative TILs and cytokine expression. One might expect that endocrine senescence may cause slower growth of endocrine-dependent tumors; however, most prostate cancers, for example, occur in an environment characterized by diminished testosterone levels.

Carcinogenic Susceptibility

Aging tissues may be cancer-prone as a result of molecular changes that parallel carcinogenic changes and increase susceptibility to environmental carcinogens.

Molecular Changes

Procarcinogenic

A higher concentration of cells in advanced carcinogenesis makes them more likely to be random targets for environmental carcinogens. In animal models, a higher number of tumors are seen in older tissue following exposure of young and old tissues to the same dose of carcinogen. Predisposing changes include the following:

Accumulation of Deoxyribonucleic Acid Adducts. DNA is continuously exposed to a variety of chemical carcinogens that form covalent bonds with nucleic acids to then form adducts that cause local conformational changes in DNA architecture. Repair enzymes usually remove these adducts and restore the genome to its natural state. If, however, this does not occur in time, the damaged DNA sites will interfere with replication and may result in mutations.

Deoxyribonucleic Acid Hypermethylation. Aberrant methylation of gene promoter regions in cancer can disrupt tumor suppressor genes and inactivate DNA-repair genes.

Point Mutations. Mutations in noncoding regions of a gene are mostly without consequence. Promoter sequence point mutations may affect gene expression, and mutations in the intronic splicing seat can result in aberrant splicing

Anticarcinogenic

Replicative Senescence. Telomere dynamics are a critical component of both aging and cancer. Telomere shortening occurs with each cell generation resulting in a reproducible loss of proliferative potential as most human primary cells do not express high levels of telomerase. This eventually results in loss of chromosomal function, chromosomal loss, and replicative senescence (28). Telomere shortening may be a potent tumor suppressor mechanism, and telomerases can be reactivated or upregulated, resulting in immortalization.

Oncogenic Stress and Deoxyribonucleic Acid Damage. DNA damage and activated oncogenes can trigger senescence via D-type cyclin and *p53* pathways, mediated by mitogen-activated protein kinase (MAPK).

Cellular Changes

Stromal-Epithelial Interactions

Changes in paracrine effects exhibited by stromal cells may alter the microenvironment in which epithelial tumors form, thereby playing an important role in the age-related increase in cancer incidence. Furthermore, senescent stromal cells may lose apoptotic mechanisms, producing factors that disturb the stromal-epithelial milieu.

Premature Senescence

Premature senescence may be associated with a loss of apoptotic mechanisms and the development of immortal cells.

References

1. Navone NM, Logothetis CJ, von Eschenbach AC, Troncoso P. Model systems of prostate cancer: uses and limitations. Cancer Metastasis Rev 1998;17:361–371.

2. Dinney CP, McConkey DJ, Millikan RE, et al. Focus on bladder cancer. Cancer Cell 2004;6:111–116.
3. Brandau S, Böhle A. Review of bladder cancer: I. Molecular and genetic basis of carcinogenesis. Eur Urol 2001;39:491–497.
4. Hillman GG, Droz JP, Haas GP. Experimental animal models for the study of therapeutic approaches in renal cell carcinoma. In Vivo 1994;8:77–80.
5. Yeung RS, Xiao GH, Jin G, et al. Predisposition to renal carcinoma in the Eker rat is determined by germ-line mutation of the tuberous sclerosis 2 (TSC2) gene. Proc Natl Acad Sci USA 1994;91:11413–11416.
6. Okimoto K, Sakurai J, Kobayashi T, et al. A germ-line insertion in the Birt-Hogg-Dube (BHD) gene gives rise to the Nihon rat model of inherited renal cancer. Proc Natl Acad Sci USA 2004;101:2023–2027.
7. Montironi R, Mazzucchelli R, Scarpelli M. Molecular techniques and prostate cancer diagnostic. Eur Urol 2003;44:390–400.
8. Petricoin EF, Ornstein DK, Liotta LA. Clinical proteomics: applications for prostate cancer biomarker discovery and detection. Urol Oncol 2004;22:322–328.
9. Sanchez-Carbayo M. Recent advances in bladder cancer diagnostics. Clin Biochem 2004;37:562–571.
10. Lin X, Tascilar M, Lee W-H, et al. GSTP1 CpG island hypermethylation is responsible for the absence of GSTP1 expression in human prostate cancer cells. Am J Pathol 2001;159:1815–1826.
11. Sarosdy MF, Schellhammer P, Bokinsky G, et al. Clinical evaluation of a multi-target fluorescent in situ hybridization assay for detection of bladder cancer. J Urol 2002;168:1950–1954.
12. Lemoine NR, ed. Understanding Gene Therapy, 1st ed. Oxford: Bios, 1999.
13. Foley R, Lawler M, Hollywood D. Gene-based therapy in prostate cancer. Lancet Oncol 2004;5:469–479.
14. Mazhar D, Waxman J. Gene therapy for prostate cancer. BJU Int 2004;93:465–469.
15. Pagliaro LC. Gene therapy for bladder cancer. World J Urol 2000;18:148–151.
16. Gore M, Riches P, eds. Immunotherapy in Cancer, 1st ed. Chichester: Wiley, 1996.
17. Fuchs EJ, Matzinger P. Is cancer dangerous to the immune system? Semin Immunol 1996;8:271–280.
18. Igney FH, Krammer PH. Immune escape of tumors: apoptosis resistance and tumor counterattack. J Leukoc Biol 2002;71:907–920.
19. Bohle A, Brandau S. Immune mechanisms in bacillus Calmette-Guerin immunotherapy for superficial bladder cancer. J Urol 2003:170:964–969.
20. Mancuso A, Sternberg CN. What's new in the treatment of metastatic kidney cancer? BJU Int 2005;95:1171–1180.
21. Shiraishi T, Muneyuki T, Fukutome K, et al. Mutations of ras genes are relatively frequent in Japanese prostate cancers: pointing to genetic differences between populations. Anticancer Res 1998;18:2789–2792.
22. Giovannucci E. The epidemiology of vitamin D and cancer incidence and mortality: a review (United States). Cancer Causes Control 2005;16:83–95.
23. John EM, Schwartz GG, Koo J, Van Den Berg D, Ingles SA. Sun exposure, vitamin D receptor gene polymorphisms, and risk of advanced prostate cancer. Cancer Res 2005;65:5470–5409.
24. Coetzee GA, Ross RK. Re: prostate cancer and the androgen receptor. J Natl Cancer Inst 1994;86:872–873.

25. Madeb R, Messing EM. Gender, racial and age differences in bladder cancer incidence and mortality. Urol Oncol 2004;22:86–92.
26. Anisimov VN. The relationship between aging and carcinogenesis: a critical appraisal. Crit Rev Oncol Hematol 2003;45:277–304.
27. Balducci L, Ershler WB. Cancer and ageing: a nexus at several levels. Nat Rev Cancer 2005;5:655–662.
28. Serrano M, Blasco MA. Putting the stress on senescence. Curr Opin Cell Biol 2001; 13:748–753.

Part II
Clinical Aspects and Investigations

3
Radiological Investigations in Genitourinary Cancer

Audrey E.T. Jacques and Rodney H. Reznek

Noninterventional Radiology

Intravenous Urogram (Excretory Urography)

The intravenous urogram (IVU) forms part of the initial workup for patients with unexplained hematuria. With recent advances in computed tomography (CT) and magnetic resonance imaging (MRI) technology, the future of the IVU is a subject of ongoing debate (1), although at present it still remains integral to the diagnosis and surveillance of urothelial malignancy. It consists of a series of plain x-rays of the renal tract followed by intravenous administration of water-soluble, iodinated, contrast medium. The contrast medium is excreted by the kidneys, enabling visualization of high-density contrast-filled calyces, renal pelvis, ureters, and bladder. Tumors are demonstrated as filling defects (Fig. 3.1).

Patient Preparation

Ideally the patient fasts for at least 4 hours prior to the IVU and is ambulant for 2 hours, in order to reduce the amount of bowel gas overlying and obscuring the renal tract. The routine use of purgatives is no longer done, as it does not significantly improve the diagnostic quality of the examination. Fluid restriction is no longer advocated, as dehydration is associated with an increased risk of contrast medium nephrotoxicity. Patients are advised to empty their bladder prior to the examination.

Precautions and Contraindications

Patients with diabetes, multiple myeloma, or sickle cell disease, and infants are at increased risk of nephrotoxicity, and indeed, good hydration prior to the examination is advised in these patients. Renal impairment is a relative contraindication for the use of iodinated contrast medium due the risk of precipitating severe renal failure and poor contrast medium excretion limiting visualization of the collecting system. Those with mild renal impairment may be given iso-osmolar nonionic iodinated contrast medium (Iodixanol), which is less nephrotoxic than standard nonionic iodinated contrast agents in this group (2). Patients with a history of previous severe contrast medium reaction should be excluded (Table 3.1).

Technique

An initial full-length film, including the renal area and bladder, is taken to assess technical factors and identify renal calcification that may become obscured on

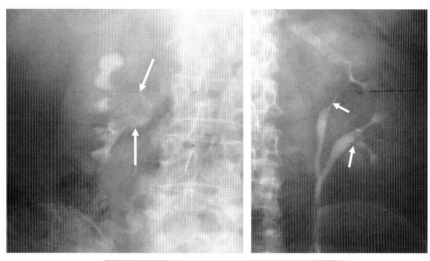

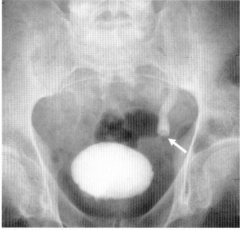

FIGURE 3.1. (A) Intravenous urography shows tumor as a large lucent filling defect within the renal pelvis (arrows) with calyceal dilation. (B) Intravenous urography in a different patient showing small filling defects (arrows) due to multifocal tumors in both pelvicaliceal systems of a left duplex kidney. (C) Intravenous urography in a third patient with a distal left ureteric transitional cell carcinoma seen as a rounded filling defect (arrow) with proximal ureteric obstruction.

TABLE 3.1.   Cautious use of iodinated intravenous contrast medium (ICM)

1. History of previous allergic reaction to ICM: absolute contraindication to use of ICM excluding those with previous mild flushing or nausea
2. Asthmatics: prophylactic oral steroid cover given prior to the procedure according to local policy
3. Those at risk of nephrotoxicity:

Renal impairment (can be given to patients with renal failure having regular dialysis when discussed with clinical team)
Known diabetic nephropathy and those on metformin (follow local guidelines regarding the use of ICM in patients on metformin)
Severely debilitated and dehydrated patients

later contrast-enhanced films. A standard adult dose of 50 mL of 350 to 370 g iodine/mL (I/mL) or 100 mL of 300 g I/mL contrast medium is administered intravenously. This can be altered for patients larger or smaller than the average-sized 70-kg adult. A standard sequence of films is obtained at timed intervals, with variations tailored to the individual. The series includes immediate, 5- and 10-minute postcontrast renal area films, and 15-minute full length and post-micturition films. The immediate postcontrast film demonstrates renal paren-chymal enhancement with contrast medium uptake in the proximal tubules and is termed the nephrographic phase. This enables renal size, position, contour, and parenchymal integrity to be evaluated. Excretion of contrast medium into the calyceal system is seen from the 5-minute film onward. Collecting system opacification can be augmented with the use of abdominal compression, and a variety of devices are available for this. Compression serves to impede ureteric emptying and enhance pelvicaliceal distention and is applied after the 5-minute film if the system is not obstructed. Compression is contraindicated in patients with acute abdominal pain, recent surgery, a known abdominal aortic aneu-rysm, or other large abdominal mass. Compression is released once adequate views of the upper tract have been achieved, and a full-length film obtained, to demonstrate contrast medium enhancement of the lower ureters. In practice, in an unobstructed system with normal ureteric peristalsis, the ureters are not usually visualized throughout their length. Additional views such as oblique projections and tomograms can be performed where needed.

Diagnostic Value

Deformity of the renal contour seen on the nephrographic phase of the IVU or calyceal compression or distortion may indicate the presence of a focal paren-chymal mass, such as a renal cell carcinoma. The nature of such a lesion cannot usually be determined further on the IVU, and the differential diagnosis includes a simple cyst or other benign lesion. In practice, ultrasound (US) or CT is indi-cated for the detection and characterization of focal renal masses. In the inves-tigation of hematuria, the IVU images must be carefully examined for the presence of any filling defect within the collecting system, ureter, or bladder, which may indicate urothelial tumor. These are frequently small and may be seen as a broad-based flat or polypoid filling defect arising from the wall.

In some cases, slight irregularity of the wall may be the only indication of the presence of a tumor (Fig. 3.1B). Large tumors may cause obstruction and dilatation of a single or group of calyces (Fig. 3.1A). As transitional cell carcinomas (TCCs) arise on a background of dysplastic urothelium, bilateral or multiple synchronous or metachronous lesions may occur in up to 38% (3,4). The IVU, therefore, still has a role in excluding multifocal disease in a patient with bladder TCC, and in the follow-up and surveillance of treated patients. The IVU can be used in the diagnosis of suspected fistulae, although MRI is more frequently performed.

Retrograde Pyelography

Retrograde pyelography can be used to visualize the lower ureters or vesicoureteric junction when not well demonstrated on IVU, or to demonstrate the lower limit of an obstructive lesion. Retrograde pyelography might be indicated to confirm the presence of uncertain filling defects seen on the standard IVU.

Technique

A 7-Ch ureteric catheter is passed cystoscopically into either the renal pelvis or to the lower level of an obstructing lesion. Under fluoroscopy, 5 to 20 mL of dilute contrast medium is gently injected, making sure that there are no air bubbles. A lower strength contrast medium than that used for a standard IVU is used to avoid obscuration of small filling defects by dense contrast. X-ray films of the opacified pelvicaliceal system and ureter are obtained. Only small (3 to 5 mL) volumes of contrast are injected at a time to avoid pelvicaliceal extravasation of contrast, particularly in an obstructed system. The catheter is gently withdrawn to the level of the ureteric orifice, and images are obtained in the oblique position to enable excellent visualization of the distal ureter and vesicoureteric junction.

The role of the retrograde pyelogram has diminished in recent years because it is invasive to the patient and carries the potential for ureteric and renal pelvis perforation. In practice, patients with fractionally visualized upper tracts on standard IVU are preferentially imaged with contrast-enhanced CT. Suspicious filling defects in the renal pelvis or ureter can be directly visualized ureteroscopically, particularly where the suspicion of urothelial tumor is high.

Alternatives to the Intravenous Urogram

Unenhanced CT through the renal tract has replaced IVU for the diagnosis of stone disease, but at present the standard IVU is still a useful tool in the workup of hematuria when renal tract malignancy is suspected. With recent advances in CT and MRI technology, newer techniques are being developed that may take over the role of the traditional IVU.

Computed Tomography Urography

Multidetector row CT (MDCT) has made a significant impact in all areas of radiology in recent years (see Computed Tomography, below). It enables the fast scanning of a large volume of the patient in a single breath-hold.

Thin slices as narrow as 1.25 mm can be reconstructed, resulting in much improved spatial resolution. These images can be further reconstructed into sagittal and coronal planes. Images of contrast-filled structures can be also reconstructed to produce CT angiographic images in three-dimensional planes. Excretory phase CT can now be used to evaluate the calyces, renal pelvis, and ureters, and to provide images akin to that of a standard IVU (5) (Fig. 3.2).

Computed tomography urography is performed with a combination of unenhanced nephrographic phase and excretory phase imaging. Renal tract calcification is detected on the unenhanced images and focal renal parenchymal lesions can be detected and characterized on corticomedullary (40-second) and nephrographic phase (90-second) imaging. Images obtained at 10 minutes post–intravenous contrast administration demonstrate enhancement of the calyces and ureter (excretory phase) and are ideal for evaluating the urothelium. The advantage of this technique is that comprehensive evaluation of the renal tract can now be achieved during a single examination (6,7). The disadvantages of the technique include cost and time implications as well as radiation dose considerations. The estimated dose equivalent for the CT urogram is approximately 13.2 mSv compared with about 3 mSv for a typical standard IVU (6). However,

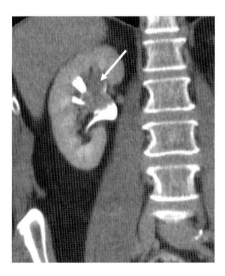

FIGURE 3.2. Computed tomography (CT) urogram. Coronal CT reformatted image from images acquired at 1.25-mm intervals at 10 minutes following intravenous contrast medium injection. The large right-sided transitional cell carcinoma is visible as a filling defect (arrow) within the right renal pelvis and upper pole calyces. (Courtesy of Dr. G. Rottenberg.)

in the investigation of hematuria the patient would undergo at least an US in addition to the IVU and in some cases proceed to CT also.

Magnetic Resonance Urography

Magnetic resonance (MR) urography combines the advantage of CT urography, in being able to investigate both the renal parenchyma and the urothelium in a single examination, with safety for patients with iodinated contrast allergies or radiation exposure considerations where standard IVU or CT urography are contraindicated. Both the dilated and nondilated renal collecting system can be visualized using MR urography, which is achieved by using either heavily T2-weighted (T2W) sequences or gadolinium-enhanced T1-weighted (T1W) sequences (8). Heavily T2W MRI sequences generate high signal intensity from simple fluids such as urine, while suppressing signal intensity from surrounding tissues.

Thin-section axial images of the urine-filled collecting system can be reconstructed into 3D coronal views to provide IVU like images. Gadolinium-enhanced MR urography relies on contrast excretion in the same way as standard or CT urography to visualize the collecting system.

Suboptimal collecting system opacification may limit this technique in the presence of markedly impaired renal function or high-grade urinary obstruction. While the presence and level of ureteric obstruction can be evaluated, the absence of signal from calculi makes them difficult to visualize with either MRI technique.

Interventional Radiology

Interventional radiology currently plays a significant role in the management of patients with genitourinary disease. Many minimally invasive diagnostic and therapeutic techniques such as percutaneous biopsy, percutaneous nephrostomy, ureteric stent placement, angiography, and tumor embolization are available. Although these procedures are much less invasive than open surgery, risks of hemorrhage and sepsis exist, and it is vital that blood count, coagulation profile, and serum electrolytes are available prior to the procedure.

Percutaneous Nephrostomy and Associated Procedures

Indications

Percutaneous nephrostomy (PCN) enables direct access to the renal collecting system via the skin surface and can be used as both a diagnostic and therapeutic procedure. Diagnostic indications involve accurate demonstration of collecting system anatomy and filling defects, delineation of the level of collecting system obstruction, and aspiration of urine for microscopy or cytology. The main therapeutic indications include the relief of ureteric obstruction or pyonephrosis. Percutaneous nephrostomy is also the first step for other procedures such as ureteric stent placement, ureteric stricture dilatation, percutaneous nephrolithotomy (PCNL) and chemo/immunotherapy for upper tract TCC. It may be performed as an emergency procedure in the case of an infected, obstructed system or in precipitant renal failure. In long-standing malignant or acute-on-chronic obstruction, there should be evidence that the kidney remains functioning before proceeding. This can be inferred on US or CT where good renal parenchyma is maintained, or assessed formally with an isotope renal function study.

Patient Preparation

Percutaneous nephrostomy is usually performed under local anesthesia alone, although some form of sedation may be given during the procedure. Intravenous antibiotics are administered prior to the procedure, particularly when there is suspicion of an infected system, as there is a risk of precipitating acute bacteremia.

Technique

The patient is positioned in an oblique-prone position. The procedure uses both US and fluoroscopic x-ray guidance. Initial US is performed to confirm hydronephrosis and plan a suitable entry point. Under US control an appropriate renal calyx is punctured with a fine needle.

Urine can then be aspirated for analysis and iodinated contrast medium injected to opacify the collecting system and delineate the nature and level of obstruction. The reminder of the procedure uses the well-known Seldinger technique to place an 8- or 10-French (F) catheter with the tip positioned within the renal pelvis. Locking catheters are often used, which are associated with less catheter displacement. It is essential that the ward staff be aware of the type of catheter used and familiar with techniques to remove such catheters; the radiology staff can provide advice.

Antegrade Stent Placement

A double-J ureteric stent may be placed antegradely via PCN when retrograde placement (via cystoscopy) is not possible. Stenting overcomes ureteric obstruction due to benign or malignant strictures or allows healing of ureteric injury or rupture. Benign strictures may develop following long-standing infection or stone disease or after pelvic radiotherapy. In malignant obstruction (prostate, bladder, rectal, and gynecological malignancies), the stent is usually left permanently indwelling, although it should be changed retrogradely every 3 to 4 months.

Technique

The procedure is performed via a PCN. An initial nephrostogram is performed to characterize the obstruction, and the nephrostomy catheter is then exchanged over a guidewire for a steerable catheter that can be manipulated into the ureter. The guidewire is then manipulated into the bladder, under fluoroscopic x-ray guidance, and the double-J stent is inserted over it. The distal tip of the stent is placed within the bladder with the proximal end in the renal pelvis.

Antegrade Ureteric Stricture Dilatation

It may be possible to dilate a focal benign stricture. This is often performed at the time of double-J stent insertion via PCN.

Technique

Using the Seldinger technique, a special balloon catheter is passed over a guide-wire and manipulated down the ureter to the level of the stricture. Radiopaque markers indicate the position of the balloon. The balloon is expanded to dilate the stricture prior to placement of a double-*J* stent.

Complications

Percutaneous nephrostomy carries a low rate of complications, 1% to 2%, although it is higher with stent placement or stricture dilatation.

Hemorrhage

A degree of hematuria is expected postprocedure, which normally tails off over 1 to 2 days. The catheter can be flushed with saline to keep it patent, especially when hematuria is present.

Clinically significant hemorrhage occurs in less than 2% of cases, leading to intrarenal hemorrhage with frank hematuria or expanding subcapsular or peri-renal hematoma with pain.

Urinary Leak

Injury to the collecting system may lead to urine leak and development of urinoma, which can become infected.

Catheter Displacement

Catheter displacement can be minimized with the use of a self-locking type, but close attention and care should be advised to both patient and ward staff.

Other

Other complications include *catheter occlusion* and *septicemia*.

Image Guided Biopsy Procedures

The need to obtain histological confirmation of malignancy is restricted to a number of specific situations in urologic oncology (Table 3.2). Certain lesions, namely solid renal or testicular masses have such a high suspicion of malignancy based on radiological appearances, that routine preoperative biopsy is rarely indicated and in addition, the risks of tumor seeding or hemorrhage may outweigh the need for histological confirmation. For cystic renal lesions with features suspicious of malignancy (Bosniak III lesions), we advocate surgical resection rather than biopsy, as the risk of retroperitoneal hemorrhage from

TABLE 3.2. Indications for image guided biopsy in genitourinary malignancy

Site	Indications	Special considerations
Renal	Indeterminate renal lesion where there is suspicion of lymphoma or metastases from another primary malignancy	Surgical resection rather than biopsy if high suspicion of renal cell carcinoma on imaging appearances
	Prior to radiofrequency ablation or chemotherapy for presumed renal cell carcinoma	
	Clinical or radiological suspicion of infective nature of lesion, particularly tuberculosis	
Adrenal	Indeterminate adrenal mass	Hormonal profile to exclude functioning adrenal pathology prior to biopsy
Bladder	Percutaneous biopsy not usually indicated	
Prostate	Patients with elevated prostate-specific antigen (PSA); transrectal ultrasound (TRUS) guided biopsy	Antibiotic prophylaxis
Testes	Biopsy not indicated	Urgent radical orchidectomy after US diagnostic of testicular cancer
Retroperitoneum	Retroperitoneal lymph node biopsy if doubt regarding nature in a patient with otherwise resectable urologic malignancy	

hypervascular tumors may complicate future surgery. Biopsy of indeterminate renal lesions is reserved when there is suspicion of lymphoma, metastases, or tuberculosis.

Technique

Image-guided biopsy is largely performed under CT or US visualization. Ultrasound has the advantages of being real-time imaging, being quicker, and enabling a more angled approach than does CT; CT guidance is reserved for areas not well visualized with US, particularly the retroperitoneum and deep in the pelvis. A CT-guided biopsy can be performed safely and with high accuracy as an outpatient procedure. Antibiotic prophylaxis is not routinely recommended, and any coagulation abnormalities should be corrected prior to biopsy. Biopsy is performed under local anesthesia. The patient is placed in the prone position and is advised to lie still for the duration of the procedure. An initial CT scan is performed to confirm the mass and select the most appropriate biopsy approach. Contrast medium enhancement is preferable to highlight the position of adjacent vessels. Repeated localized scanning is performed to confirm the position of the biopsy needle. Core biopsy can be performed with a single cutting needle or using a coaxial technique to obtain multiple cores. Fine-needle aspiration (FNA) can be performed if cytological confirmation only of malignancy is considered adequate. Overall accuracy for percutaneous biopsy is over 80%. False-negative results may be due to sampling error in an inhomogeneous tumor. A benign biopsy in a highly suspicious lesion should be interpreted with caution, and repeat biopsy considered. Complications rates are low, less than 2%. Hemorrhage may be occult and regular observations and bed rest is advised for at least 4 hours following biopsy of a deep lesion.

Interventional Angiography and Tumor Embolization

The role of renal angiography in routine diagnosis and staging of renal masses has largely been surpassed by US, CT, and MRI. However, angiography still has a specific role in tumor management, in particular for preoperative tumor embolization and in the management of acute hemorrhage (9,10).

Technique

Angiography involves acquiring percutaneous access into a central artery, usually the femoral artery, through which specific catheters can be inserted using the Seldinger technique, under x-ray guidance. Catheters are then manipulated into the relevant vascular tree. Arterial embolization of a tumor can be achieved with the injection of alcohol, small particles or coils to occlude capillaries or precapillary arterioles. This technique has been used for preoperative tumor embolization of large, hypervascular renal cell carcinomas (RCCs) or bladder transitional cell carcinomas. Surgical resection is then optimally performed 24 hours postembolization. Similar techniques are also used in the management of acute hemorrhage, occurring spontaneously from a tumor or partial nephrectomy-associated arteriovenous fistula or aneurysm.

Image-Guided Percutaneous Radiofrequency Ablation

Radical nephrectomy has long been the traditional treatment option for RCC, for which systemic chemotherapeutic options are often unsuccessful.

Over the past 20 years a steady increase in the frequency of small (≤4 cm), incidentally detected RCCs has been observed, paralleled by the increasing use of cross-sectional imaging (11). Therefore, treatment options aimed at avoiding nephrectomy for small tumors have been advocated. Percutaneous in situ tumor radiofrequency ablation (RFA) has emerged as one of the minimally invasive techniques (12,13).

Technique

Radiofrequency ablation involves placing a US/CT-guided electrode into the target tissue. A high-frequency alternating current is applied to induce heating or thermal injury of the target tissue. Coagulation necrosis of the tumor occurs when heated to between 50° and 100°C. The diameter of tissue ablated is influenced by the electrode diameter and duration of ablation, although increased target size can be achieved with overlapping RFA treatments. At least 0.5 to 1 cm of tissue beyond the tumor should be ablated to reduce the risk of recurrence

(14,15). The extent of coagulation necrosis is maximal after 7 days post-RFA. Contrast-enhanced CT is used to assess postablation response, and demonstration of nonenhancement of a previously enhancing lesion is an accurate indicator of success. Persistent enhancing tissue at the treatment site indicates viable tumor, and repeated ablation should be performed. Studies to date show promising results of RFA for small RCCs with low rates of complications, side effects, and recurrence (16–18). For success, careful patient selection is essential, and current recommended indications for percutaneous RFA include localized exophytic tumors less than 3 to 4 cm in diameter.

The patients most likely to benefit from this treatment include those unfit for surgery, those with a solitary kidney, and those with multiple and bilateral small RCCs (for example those with von Hippel–Lindau syndrome). Absolute contraindications include current sepsis, severe debilitation, and an uncorrectable coagulopathy.

The complication rate following RFA is low. Side effects specific to the treatment include the development of low-grade fever and flu-like symptoms 3 to 5 days posttreatment, termed postablation syndrome. This clinical picture has been well documented following tumor embolization and is thought to be the result of an inflammatory response to tumor necrosis. Postablation syndrome is self-limiting and reported in around 30% of patients, although up to 95% experience some degree of either fever or flu like illness (19).

Ultrasound

General Principles

Ultrasound imaging is based on the principle that when sound waves are directed into the body by a transducer placed on the skin surface, some waves will be reflected back to the body surface and detected by the same transducer. The transducer surface is made of material that has the unique property of expanding or contracting when a voltage is applied across it, known as the piezoelectric effect. When the transducer is in contact with the skin and voltage applied, the surface material expands and compresses an adjacent layer of the material. This pressure induces a corresponding voltage to the next layer of the material, which also expands.

The mechanical energy thus created by this wave of compression created in the probe is transmitted to the skin surface and propagates through the patient. The propagation and reflection of the sound wave through the patient is dependent on the density and elasticity of the tissues (acoustic impedance). Reflected echoes returning to the probe induce a voltage that can be detected by the transducer and converted into a gray-scale image. The reflection of sound waves is greatest where there is a large difference in acoustic impedance of two tissues. Thus soft tissue structures reflect more echoes than fluid and appear bright or echogenic. Fluid appears dark, or hypoechoic. The time delay between the initiated pulse and that returning to the probe is proportional to the distance the beam has passed, and spatial information as to the position and depth of tissues are incorporated into the image composition. Constant pulses of sound waves are produced to generate fast real-time images of moving body tissues, including flowing blood (Doppler US). Bone and air reflect sound and cannot be imaged, whereas fluid in simple cysts or bladder does not reflect sound waves, which pass through and are available for imaging deeper structures, a phenomenon termed acoustic enhancement. This is of use in the pelvis where the urine-filled bladder is used as an acoustic window for visualizing the deeper pelvic organs such as the prostate gland and uterus.

Advantages

Ultrasound is a noninvasive real-time imaging method; it does not use ionizing radiation and thus is well tolerated by patients. The examination does not require special preparation. It poses no real risk to the patient, making it ideal for repeated surveillance imaging without the radiation burden associated with CT.

The ability to image flowing blood in real time is a major advantage of US, which can detect tumor extension into the renal vein and inferior vena cava (IVC) in the case of renal and adrenal carcinomas. The demonstration of vascularity (testis; Fig. 3.3B) within a lesion can aid its characterization (kidney; Fig. 3.4E,F). The real-time aspect of US is well suited to guide procedures such

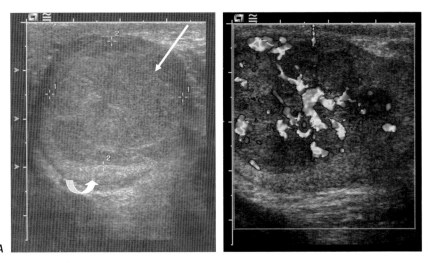

A   B

FIGURE 3.3. Testicular seminoma. (A) Ultrasound of the right testis revealing a focal heterogeneous mass (arrow) surrounded by normal testicular tissue (curved arrow). (B) Doppler ultrasound demonstrates marked vascularity of the mass. (Courtesy of Dr. A.P.K.Lim.)

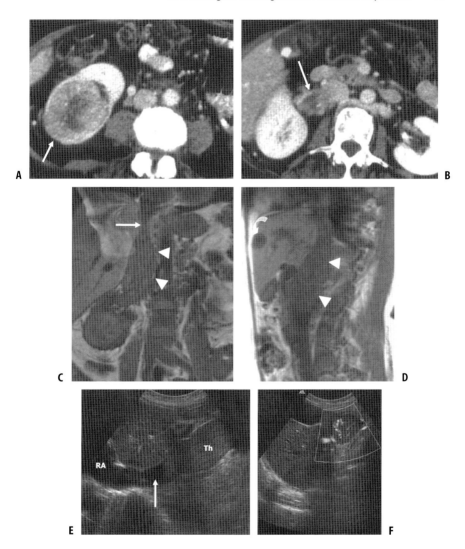

FIGURE 3.4. Right renal cell carcinoma with intracaval tumor extension. (A) Axial enhanced CT scans showing well-defined enhancing tumor in right kidney (arrow). (B) The right renal vein is expanded with thrombus and there is the suggestion of RCC extending into the IVC. (C) Coronal T1-weighted MRI. (D) Sagittal T1-weighted MRI confirming IVC extension of RCC (white arrowheads) markedly expanding the IVC. The superior border of the lesion (arrow) is identified well below the level of the diaphragm and insertion of the middle hepatic vein. Incidental cyst in liver (curved arrow). (E) Longitudinal ultrasound (US) images showing thrombus (Th) within the IVC. The superior level of the thrombus is clearly seen and the suprahepatic IVC above this level is patent (arrow). Thrombus does not extend into the right atrium (RA). (F) Doppler US shows vascularity within the thrombus, confirming tumor rather than bland thrombus.

as FNA, biopsy, and drain insertions. The echogenic tip of a biopsy needle, for example, can be easily demonstrated with US, providing a clearly visible route for safe insertion. Intraoperative US probes have also been designed that can be used to localize tumors during an RFA and partial nephrectomy.

Disadvantages

The success of a US scan is very operator dependent, and images may not always be reproducible between different operators. Although a representative sample of reference images is usually saved onto hardcopy or digital archiving, images are generally best appreciated dynamically during the scan. Comparing a current study with saved hardcopy images from a previous study is not as accurate as it is with CT or MRI.

Patient factors such as body habitus may influence the quality of the images produced, with greater attenuation of the US beam occurring in larger patients, resulting in poor visualization of deeper structures. As the US beam is absorbed by air, the presence of prominent bowel gas in the abdomen or pelvis may limit visualization of deeper organs.

Ultrasound in Genitourinary Cancers

Ultrasound of the urinary tract (Table 3.3) forms part of the early screening of patients with hematuria, aimed at excluding renal cell carcinoma or tumors of the bladder and renal pelvis. The presence of a solid, heterogeneous renal mass with vascularity demonstrated on color flow Doppler is highly suggestive of a renal cell carcinoma. Thick or irregular calcifications may be visualized as highly echogenic foci.

Renal Masses

Renal cell carcinomas are typically very vascular, showing multiple collateral vessels or intratumoral arteriovenous shunting on Doppler ultrasonography. The widespread use of both CT and US has contributed to the increased detection of incidental space-occupying renal lesions in recent years. Thus more RCCs are being detected at an early, asymptomatic stage, which has contributed to improved survival (20,21). Ultrasound is used to diagnose and characterize a variety of renal lesions. Simple renal cysts are extremely common and when confidently diagnosed on US need no further follow-up unless they become symptomatic. Ultrasound can be used to characterize complex cystic lesions and highlight those that have features suspicious for malignancy and warrant consideration for surgical excision.

The Bosniak classification of cystic lesions (see Computed Tomography, below) is based on CT criteria but can be applied to US. The presence of multiple septations, particularly when thickened or nodular, soft tissue components, and thick or nodular calcification are features seen in cystic RCCs (22,23), and can be visualized with US. Septations may be more visible on US than on CT.

TABLE 3.3. Role of ultrasound in urologic oncology

Kidney
1. Investigation of hematuria
2. Detection of incidental renal cell carcinoma
3. Characterization of cystic renal lesions
4. Ultrasound guided intervention:
    Biopsy of suspected renal metastases or lymphoma
    Radiofrequency ablation of renal cell carcinoma
    Intraoperative ultrasound to aid nephron-sparing surgery
5. Tumor staging
    Perinephric and local invasion
    Venous invasion
    Characterization of liver lesions
6. Follow-up and surveillance
7. Assessment of suspected hydronephrosis in patients with pelvic malignancy

Adrenal
Incidental finding of adrenal mass lesion (space-occupying adrenal lesions not well seen with US unless very
    large)

Bladder
Investigation of hematuria

Prostate
Transrectal ultrasound (TRUS)-guided biopsy in patients with raised PSA

Testes
Investigation of palpable testicular mass

Ultrasound can be used to further characterize the very small (<1.5 cm) indeterminate cystic renal lesion detected on CT. Doppler US is highly sensitive for the detection of vascularity, the presence of which in soft tissue components of a cystic mass is suspicious for malignancy.

The presence of bilateral or multifocal RCCs clearly has an impact on the choice of patient management, and careful US examination of the remainder of the kidney and of the contralateral kidney should be made. This is particularly important in patients with von Hippel–Lindau (VHL) syndrome, where multiple RCCs may exist, often on a background of multicystic kidneys (see Chapter 14). Complex features of any cysts should be carefully evaluated. Renal cell carcinomas arising in small, complex cysts (<1.5 cm) in these patients are typically slow growing and are often followed up for some time.

Ultrasound may be used in conjunction with CT or MRI, although US is less accurate than CT or MRI in RCC staging, and perinephric invasion is poorly demonstrated. It is helpful, however, in diagnosing tumor extension into the renal vein and IVC (Fig. 3.4), which can be diagnosed with up to 75% sensitivity (24), or higher when clinically important IVC thrombus is considered (25). Supradiaphragmatic extension is not well seen, and if suspected, echocardiography should help to exclude tumor extension into the right atrium.

Urothelial Tumors

Ultrasound is performed in conjunction with IVU in the workup of patients with hematuria. The renal pelvis, proximal ureter, and bladder usually can be visualized with US. The ureter, however, unless dilated, is not well visualized throughout its length. The bladder should be well filled for its optimal examination with US, as focal areas of wall thickening can be mimicked by a collapsed bladder.

In patients with hematuria, demonstration of an echogenic mass on US within the renal pelvis, proximal ureter, or bladder suggests the presence of malignancy, commonly TCC. Visualization of the upper tract collecting system is improved in the presence of obstruction where an echogenic mass may be seen outlined by hypoechoic urine. Differentiation of echogenic debris from tumor within the collecting system or bladder can be made following the detection of vascularity on Doppler scan. It therefore can aid in characterizing an extrinsic mass or collecting system filling defect demonstrated on IVU. It may demonstrate evidence of extension of tumor outside of the renal collecting system or bladder, but overall staging is achieved with a combination of cystoscopy, CT and MRI.

Adrenal Glands

Normal adult adrenal glands are not usually visualized with US given their small size and deep location. Incidental adrenal mass lesions occasionally may be detected with US. Ultrasound may be useful to localize a large suprarenal mass seen on axial CT, where origin from or involvement of the liver, kidney, tail of pancreas, or adrenal gland may not be obvious. A large, heterogeneous, vascular adrenal mass may suggest the presence of a neoplastic lesion, particularly if local invasion is detected on US, but CT and MRI are the investigations of choice for the characterization of adrenal masses and staging of adrenal carcinoma. Ultrasound is not usually indicated to guide biopsy of suprarenal masses, which require a posterior approach and are generally performed with the patient in the prone position under CT guidance.

Testis

Given its superficial location, the testis is well visualized with US, which is the first-line investigation of a patient with a scrotal mass. Benign lesions of the epididymis such as simple cysts are common, and when a lesion has been detected clinically, US is used to determine whether it lies within the testis or not. Benign solid lesions within the testis are extremely rare, and all such lesions, in the absence of clinical features to suggest infection, are presumed to be malignant. Testicular germ cell tumors are typically solid, heterogeneous masses that may be multiple, and are often highly vascular (Fig. 3.3). Careful US examination of the contralateral testis is essential.

If such a suspicious testicular tumor is detected with US, urgent urology referral should be made. Staging of testicular tumors is primarily centered on the detection of retroperitoneal lymphadenopathy and excluding distant metastases to the lungs, bone, or brain. Computed tomography is the imaging modality of choice for this staging (see Computed Tomography, below). Ultrasound may aid interpretation of CT-visualized lymphadenopathy.

Prostate

Prostate US is indicated in patients with elevated prostate- specific antigen (PSA) in whom prostate carcinoma is suspected. Locally advanced tumors may be visualized on US within the bladder, and hydronephrosis due to outflow obstruction by a large or invasive tumor can also be diagnosed.

Endocavity US with a transrectal transducer (transrectal ultrasound, TRUS) places the beam in close proximity to the prostate gland. This is performed with the empty bladder. Anatomical detail of the prostate gland can be appreciated with clear delineation between the central and peripheral zones. Tumors are rarely demonstrated as a well-defined hypoechoic nodule within the peripheral zone with increased vascularity on color flow Doppler. More commonly, ill-defined hypoechoic areas within the peripheral zone are not clearly differentiated from fibrosis or chronic prostatitis. Instead, US-guided targeted biopsy of multiple sites of the peripheral zone is the main indication derived from TRUS, in those suspected of prostate carcinoma. Local staging is best achieved with MRI in those considered for radical treatment, with CT reserved for staging of nodal disease and distant metastases. This is described in detail in Chapter 18.

Contrast-Enhanced Ultrasound

In recent years intravascular contrast agents have been developed that when administered enhance both gray-scale and Doppler US (26,27). The US contrast agents that have been developed consist of small (<7 μm), encapsulated microbubbles. They are small enough to pass through the pulmonary and capillary circulation and stable enough to withstand hydrostatic pressure within the vascular system and acoustic pressure from the US wave. When administered they remain in the vascular system. Specific properties of the microbubble capsule and gas within induce greater reflection of the acoustic wave, resulting in increased backscatter. This increases the echogenicity and enhances the gray scale or Doppler image. New US imaging parameters have been developed that increase the conspicuity of microbubble-enhanced backscatter. The images produced are greatly enhanced compared to standard gray scale and Doppler imaging, and may aid in the detection and characterization of small isoechoic renal lesions.

Computed Tomography

General Principles

The production of an image by CT is based on the differential absorption of an x-ray beam by tissues within the body in the same way as conventional radiography.

In CT the x-ray beam is collimated into a narrow beam that passes through a thin slice of the patient. The attenuated x-ray beam is absorbed by detectors, which are capable of differentiating very subtle differences in tissue density. Computed tomography, therefore, has a much greater contrast resolution than plain x-rays and eliminates problems of superimposition of overlying structures to a much greater extent. The information collected by the detectors is converted into an arbitrary scale (Hounsfield units, HU) based on the attenuation of the x-ray beam by the tissues it has passed through, which varies with differing densities of body tissues. Bone or calcification are the most attenuating and are given a value of +1000 HU, while air, the least attenuating, is given a value of −1000 HU. The values are converted to a gray-scale image and assigned a brightness level, with the highest numbers white and the lowest numbers black. The range (window width) and mean value (window level) of density units is selected to optimize visualization of different tissue densities of interest. Tissues of densities outside of the range selected will not be discernible and will be either totally black or totally white. Standard settings can be selected to display lung, bone, or soft tissue windows as required.

Types of Computed Tomography

Conventional Computed Tomography

Conventional CT involves a rotating x-ray tube through which the patient moves on a bed as individual collimated x-ray beams acquire axial information on a slice-by-slice basis. The process is continued until the whole area of interest is scanned. With each slice collimated to a preset thickness, the process is time-consuming. To eliminate problems of motion artifact induced by respiration, patients usually need to hold their breath for each individual slice, as the process is too long to be performed in a single breath-hold. To keep the radiation dose to an acceptable level, an interslice gap is introduced between slices. Image artifacts can arise as different tissue densities lying within the gap or slice imaged are averaged together as part of the data processing creating a partial volume effect.

Spiral Computed Tomography

Newer generation scanners utilize a method of volume rather than slice-by-slice acquisition. A continuous fan x-ray beam traces a spiral path as the patient is moved through the gantry of the machine. Data are continuously acquired through each 360-degree rotation. Thus a volume of tissue rather than a slice is imaged. The distance the patient is moved through one revolution of the tube is equal to the slice thickness. Increased scan acquisition time is a significant advantage of this technique, enabling imaging of a larger volume of the patient in a singe breath-hold. This eliminates problems with variation of respiration with each slice. Partial volume effects are also minimized.

Multidetector Computed Tomography

It is now possible to acquire data from more than one slice simultaneously using parallel banks of detectors. Spiral scanners are now available that are able to acquire up to 128 slices in one tube rotation. Data are thus acquired much faster than with a single-slice spiral scanner.

Much thinner slices can be acquired resulting in greatly improved spatial resolution and reduced partial volume effects. In addition, postprocessing of the large volume of thin slices acquired enables three-dimensional (3D) and multiplanar image reconstruction. Three-dimensional reconstruction applications include CT angiography, virtual endoscopy, and CT fluoroscopy. Multiplanar images enable the tumor and its relationship to surrounding structures to be delineated accurately. Combined with CT renal angiography it plays an important role in the preoperative surgical planning for renal cell carcinoma, particularly when nephron-sparing surgery is being considered (Figs. 3.5B,C).

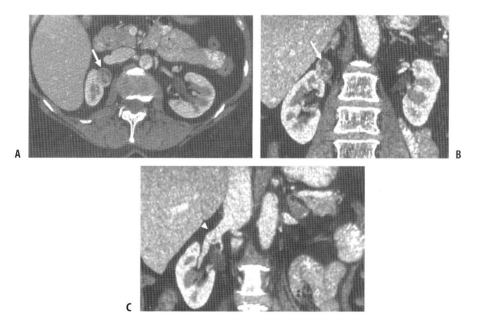

FIGURE 3.5. (A) Renal cell carcinoma (T3). CT obtained 30 seconds after administration of intravenous contrast medium showing enhancing exophytic tumor (arrow) arising from the upper pole of the right kidney with no perinephric invasion. (B,C) Coronal reformatted images showing relationship of tumor (arrow) to the remainder of the kidney and renal vein (arrowheads).

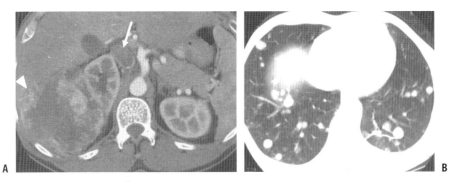

A   B

FIGURE 3.6. (A) Right renal cell carcinoma with local invasion. Contrast-enhanced CT scan showing large right renal cell carcinoma with local invasion of the right lobe of the liver indicated by loss of the normal fat plane between tumor and liver laterally (arrowhead). There is also evidence of thrombus within the IVC (arrow). (B) Same patient with pulmonary metastases.

Patient Preparation and Technique

Oral contrast medium or water is administered prior to the examination to optimize anatomical detail, particularly in the pelvis or retroperitoneum, where the presence of unopacified loops of bowel can be misinterpreted as soft tissue masses or lymph nodes. One liter of 2% solution containing iodinated contrast medium is administered orally at least 1 hour prior to the examination. For bladder and prostate tumors a moderately full bladder is preferable.

For characterizing space-occupying lesions of the kidney or an adrenal gland, initial unenhanced scans are obtained through the renal or adrenal area at a 5-mm slice thickness. The scan is obtained in a single breath-hold at either maximum inspiration or expiration. This allows for visualization of calcification within the lesion and enables the density of the lesion to be calculated. The scan is then repeated with intravenous contrast medium unless contraindicated (see Table 3.1). One hundred milliliters of nonionic iodinated contrast medium (300 to 350 mg iodine/mL) is administered via a pump injector at a rate of 2 to 3 mL/s. To optimize characterization of the liver, renal or adrenal lesions scans are obtained at times of different maximum vascular enhancement. For renal and adrenal lesions, scans are obtained at 40 seconds and 90 seconds following contrast infusion. In the kidney this equates to the corticomedullary and nephrographic phases of enhancement, respectively. While the nephrographic phase is more sensitive for the detection and characterization of small renal lesions, evaluation of the kidneys during both phases provides optimum information. In addition, images obtained during the corticomedullary phase allow for evaluation of the renal vein and the identification of accessory renal arteries. Images obtained at 3 to 10 minutes post–contrast infusion demonstrate contrast within the pelvicaliceal system (excretory phase), and can be used to delineate tumor within the renal pelvis or ureter.

For a full staging scan, axial 5-mm images are acquired through the whole abdomen from the level of the diaphragm to the pelvis. These are obtained with the 90-second scan when a renal protocol scan has been performed. Alternatively, scanning is timed to commence at approximately 60 seconds following contrast infusion so as to image the liver during maximum portal venous phase enhancement, the optimum time for the detection of most hepatic metastases. For tumors such as RCC and testicular carcinoma, which have a propensity to metastasize to the lung, images through the thorax are initially acquired at approximately 20 to 40 seconds after contrast infusion (Fig. 3.6B).

The Role of Computed Tomography in Urologic Oncology

Lesion Detection and Diagnosis (Table 3.4)

Computed tomography does not usually form part of the initial diagnosis of bladder, prostate, or testicular carcinomas, although the presence of a soft tissue filling defect within the contrast-filled renal collecting system or bladder may highlight the presence of a TCC. These carcinomas are best seen on delayed postcontrast images. Contrast enhancement of such a mass confirms the diagnosis and excludes the presence of debris or blood clot.

Occasionally testicular carcinoma might present as a large retroperitoneal lymph node mass, and in a young male patient the possibility of testicular germ cell tumor should be considered. Computed tomography has an established role

TABLE 3.4. Role of computed tomography in genitourinary cancers

Kidney
1. Detection of incidental renal cell carcinomas
2. Characterization of cystic renal mass lesions
3. Tumor staging
    Local: perinephric and organ invasion
    Nodal staging
    Venous invasion
    Distant metastases: lung, liver, bones, brain
4. 3D CT for surgical planning
5. Follow-up and surveillance

Adrenal
1. Detection and characterization of incidental adrenal mass lesions in oncology patients
2. Primary adrenal carcinoma staging: local and distant metastases: lungs, liver, bones

Bladder
1. Tumor staging: locally advanced disease; nodal: iliac and paraaortic lymph nodes
    Distant metastases: lung, brain, liver, bones
2. Radiotherapy planning

Prostate
1. Tumor staging: locally advanced disease; nodal: pelvic side wall and retroperitoneal
2. Radiotherapy planning

Testis
Tumor staging, nodal staging and follow-up and distant metastases: lungs, brain, liver, and bones

in the detection and characterization of indeterminate renal and adrenal lesions.

Renal Space-Occupying Lesions

Renal cell carcinomas are suspected on CT in the presence of a partially solid, enhancing, and often heterogeneous parenchymal renal mass, and are frequently detected incidentally (20,28). Cystic RCCs are well recognized and need to be differentiated from complicated benign cysts such as simple cysts that have become infected or bled.

Bosniak Grading

A system of grading the appearances of cystic renal masses with CT, according to the presence of features associated with malignancy, has been devised by Bosniak (22,23). Simple cysts with no suspicious features are within category I and those with increasingly complex features are graded up to category IV, which are frankly malignant (Figs. 3.6A). Suspicious features include the presence of thick punctate calcification, wall or septal thickening, and the presence of enhancing soft tissue components. Category III and IV lesions have some malignant features and should be surgically removed. Category II lesions have some complex features such as fine, linear calcification, and thin septa of increased density, but no enhancing soft tissue. These lesions do not need to be followed up. More recently, category IIF has been introduced and includes benign complicated cysts that require follow-up over time to confirm stability. Features in this group include those cysts with numerous but thin septa, and septal or wall enhancement, but no soft tissue component; hyperdense category II lesions that are totally intrarenal or greater than 3 cm (29) also fall into this category.

Adrenal Lesions

Adrenal mass lesions are detected incidentally in approximately 4% to 7% of the population (30). They are therefore not an infrequent incidental finding in patients with malignancy. The adrenal glands are also a site of hematogenous spread of other cancer. The principal concern when faced with a focal adrenal mass lesion is differentiating between a benign cortical adenoma, seen frequently in the adult population, and metastasis or a primary adrenal carcinoma. Lesions greater than 4 cm in maximum diameter are suspicious for malignancy, although adrenal metastasis in the absence of a known primary are exceedingly rare (31,32). However, 36% to 71% of incidental adrenal masses found in known oncology patients are metastases (33–35). Adrenal cortical carcinomas usually present as very large mass lesions that may or may not be functioning. Nonfunctioning carcinomas present later with symptoms related to mass effect. These tumors are usually heterogeneous with areas of enhancement. The differential diagnosis of a large adrenal mass includes adrenal metastasis or pheochromocytoma. Biochemical correlation will confirm the diagnosis in the latter.

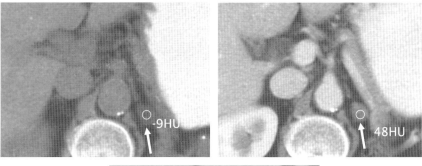

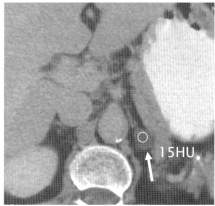

FIGURE 3.7. Left adrenal adenoma (arrows) with region of interest markers and CT density measurements in Hounsfield units (HUs) are shown. Images obtained (A) prior to administration of intravenous contrast medium and at (B) 60 seconds and (C) 15 minutes following intravenous injection of contrast medium. Calculation of the absolute contrast medium washout (see text for formula) shows this to be 58%. (Courtesy of Dr. A. Sahdev.)

Most adenomas contain an abundance of intracellular lipid and have relatively low density on unenhanced scans. An inverse relationship between percentage fat content and attenuation value on unenhanced CT has been shown (36), with lipid-rich adenomas characterized by density measurement of 20 HU or less.

Where a threshold of 20 HU or below is taken, diagnosis of a benign adrenal lesion is made with 88% sensitivity and 84% specificity (37). However, a subset of adenomas cannot be diagnosed on the basis of their unenhanced CT attenuation as they lack intracytoplasmic fat. The diagnosis of both lipid-poor and lipid-rich adrenal adenomas can be made with a high degree of certainty on CT based on their contrast medium enhancement and washout patterns (38,39). Adenomas typically enhance early with rapid contrast medium washout, compared with nonadenomas, which washout over a longer time period (Fig. 3.7).

By taking attenuation value measurements of the adrenal lesion 0 second (unenhanced), 60 seconds (initial enhancement), and 15 minutes (delayed

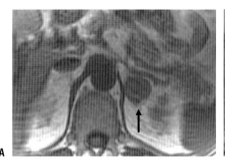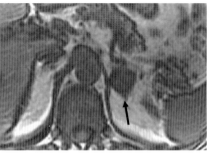

A   B

FIGURE 3.8. Left adrenal adenoma on chemical shift magnetic resonance imaging (MRI) (arrows). (A) In-phase (IP) T1-weighted MRI shows intermediate signal intensity left adrenal mass. (B) The out-of-phase (OP) sequence shows uniform signal loss of the adrenal lesion, indicating the presence of intracellular lipid, confirming the diagnosis of an adrenal adenoma.

enhancement) following contrast medium administration, the absolute and relative percentage contrast washout can be calculated:

$$\text{Absolute Percentage Washout} = ((\text{Initial} - \text{Delayed})/(\text{Initial} - \text{Unenhanced})) \times 100$$

$$\text{Relative Washout} = ((\text{Initial} - \text{Delayed})/\text{Initial}) \times 100$$

An absolute percentage washout of >60% and relative percentage washout >40% are used to make a diagnosis of adrenal adenoma with a sensitivity/specificity of 88%/96% and 96%/100%, respectively (38). Magnetic resonance imaging is used to characterize atypical, lipid-poor adenomas, which remain indeterminate by contrast medium washout criteria on CT (Fig. 3.8).

Tumor Staging by Computed Tomography

Tumor staging is vital to predict prognosis and for planning the treatment strategy. Staging of the primary tumor with reference to its size, evidence of invasion of local structures, nodal involvement, and distant metastases forms the basis of the internationally accepted tumor, node, metastasis (TNM) classification system. While not specifically a radiological classification system, CT is well placed to demonstrate these features. However, the sensitivity and specificity of the accuracy of CT varies with the tumor type and location.

Local Assessment of the Primary Tumor

Computed tomography is well suited to assess certain urologic tumors, in particular, renal cell, adrenal, and large bladder cancers. Superficial bladder tumors not invading the muscle layer, localized prostate carcinomas, and testicular tumors are best assessed with cystoscopy, MRI, or US, respectively. Local tumor invasion is diagnosed on CT where tumor is seen extending into surrounding fat or adjacent organs.

Loss of the fat plane between tumor and adjacent structures is not always a reliable indicator of invasion. This is particularly the case in the pelvis, where clear fat planes are not normally visible on CT between the posterior bladder wall, prostate, cervix, uterus, and rectum. Locally advanced bladder or prostate carcinoma is best diagnosed when enhancing soft tissue is seen directly invading adjacent structures. Other clues may be present that raise the suspicion of local tumor extension. For example, tumor involvement of the ureteric orifices in the bladder may be suspected in the presence of hydronephrosis. The good contrast resolution of CT enables visualization of abnormally placed pockets of gas, in the bladder or vagina, for example, which may raise the suspicion of vesicovaginal or colovesical fistulae secondary to tumor invasion.

Lymph Nodes

The detection of tumor extension to lymph nodes by CT is dependent on an assessment of lymph node size. A short axis diameter of above 1 cm is considered abnormal in the upper retroperitoneum, and above 8 mm within the pelvis.

These measurements are somewhat arbitrary, and normal or reactive nodes may frequently be larger. The limitations of using size criteria have been evaluated in RCC where nodes greater than 1 cm contain normal or hyperplastic lymphoid tissue in up to 43% of cases (40,41). The presence of enlarged reactive local nodes is increased further in the presence of tumor necrosis and venous invasion (42). Similarly, micrometastases within normal-sized lymph nodes account for false-negative rates of up to 4% in one series (42). Other features to suggest lymph node involvement include round rather than oval shape, irregular contour, attenuation, and contrast enhancement similar to the primary tumor, and necrosis.

Knowledge of the lymphatic drainage pathways of different tumor is essential in the CT evaluation for lymphadenopathy, and particular attention should be paid to the retroperitoneum in the case of testicular carcinoma and the pelvic side walls in the case of bladder and prostate carcinomas.

Distant Metastases

Unlike US and MRI, CT has the advantage of being able to image a large volume of the patient in a single scan. It is therefore the ideal imaging modality to detect distant metastases.

Scans of the thorax and liver are included as part of the standard staging for renal, adrenal, and testicular malignancies, and scan technique is optimized to demonstrate lesions in different sites, as discussed above. Bone metastasis will be diagnosed on CT if present in the areas covered in the scan and when the images are viewed on settings optimized for visualizing bone density (bone windows). They may be visible as sclerotic or lucent defects in the bone, which may or may not expand the bone contour. Attention should be paid to the bones, particularly vertebrae, in patients with renal cell, testicular, and prostate carcinomas. Computed tomography of the brain following intravenous injection of contrast medium may be performed acutely in patients presenting with neurological signs to exclude brain metastases, particularly those with testicular germ cell tumors. In this group, MRI is more sensitive but is reserved for those with clinical suspicion and is only performed routinely in those patients considered at high risk of developing brain metastases.

Tumor Staging: Disease-Specific Considerations

Renal Cell Carcinoma

The widespread use of cross-sectional imaging has resulted in the detection of earlier stage RCCs. Surgery remains the only chance of cure, and accurate preoperative staging is essential to plan an appropriate management strategy. The differentiation between tumors limited to the kidney (T1-2) and tumors with perinephric invasion (T3) (Figs. 3.9 and 3.10) can be difficult on imaging, although it is not clinically significant in patients treated with radical nephrectomy. However, since the introduction of nephron-sparing surgery for low-stage tumors, it is now essential that this distinction be made preoperatively. The most reliable indicator is the presence of focal soft tissue within the perinephric fat; if it measures up to 1 cm, it is 98% specific for diagnosing stage II disease. However this sign is not often seen (40). The presence of soft tissue stranding extending into the perinephric fat is suggestive of tumor invasion, or it can also be due to tumor-induced fibrosis, edema, and inflammation. This finding is present in up to 50% of those with stage I tumor confined to the kidney (40).

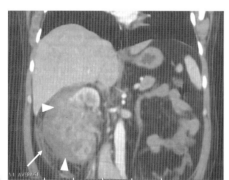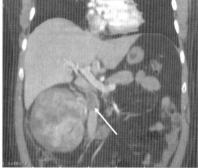

A   B

FIGURE 3.9. (A) Right renal cell carcinoma with perinephric invasion. Coronal reformatted CT images. Large right renal cell carcinoma extending into the perinephric fat (arrowheads) and involvement of the pararenal fascia, which is thickened (arrow). (B) Infrahepatic IVC tumor extension seen as low density filling defect.

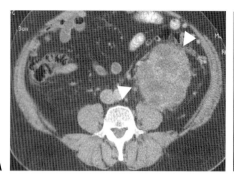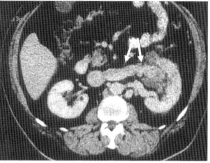

A   B

FIGURE 3.10. CT and MRI correlation. Left RCC renal vein and IVC extension. (A) Contrast-enhanced CT showing large left renal tumor with perinephric invasion (arrowheads). (B) Expansion of left renal vein with enhancing thrombus (arrow).

Gerota's fascia is well visualized on CT in most patients and tumor extension beyond is diagnostic of stage 4 disease (Figs. 3.6 and 3.9).

The presence of tumor invasion into the renal vein occurs in up to 25% of patients with renal cell carcinoma and into the IVC in up to 10% (43,44).

Estimation of the upper extent of intracaval tumor is essential for appropriate surgical planning. Indirect signs of IVC invasion include vessel enlargement and the presence of collateral vessels (Fig. 3.10). The most reliable sign is visualization of a persistent filling defect on contrast-enhanced images (Figs. 3.6A and 3.9B). Images must be obtained during peak enhancement of the renal vein and IVC and are acquired at 60 seconds post–intravenous contrast medium administration. Computed tomography has been reported to detect intracaval tumor with a sensitivity of 78% and specificity of 96% (40) and up to 100% accuracy has been reported with newer MDCT techniques (45). Venous invasion is also commonly seen in adrenal carcinomas, with the same implications for surgical planning when there is extension in the IVC. Suprahepatic caval tumor extension can be difficult to distinguish on CT, and if suspected an MRI should be performed (Fig. 3.4). A transesophageal echocardiogram can help to asses the tumor extension into the right atrium.

Transitional Cell Carcinoma

Imaging of the bladder with CT is ideally achieved with the patient's bladder being full and with intravenous contrast medium. Tumor within the bladder enhances to the same degree or greater than that of normal bladder wall. Tumors may be multifocal and are visualized as either plaque-like thickening of the bladder wall or mass-like soft tissue protruding into the bladder lumen. The important role of CT in bladder cancer staging is distinguishing between tumor confined to the bladder wall and those that have invaded thorough the wall, into the perivesical fat (stage T3b). Full-thickness bladder wall invasion is indicated by an irregular outer contour of the tumor and stranding of the adjacent

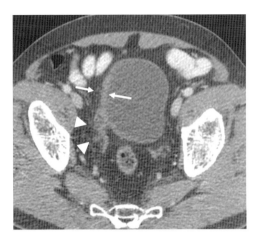

FIGURE 3.11. Transitional cell carcinoma (TCC) of bladder. Contrast-enhanced CT showing focal plaque-like thickening of the right lateral wall of the bladder with an irregular outer contour (arrows) and perivesical stranding (arrowheads) in keeping with stage T3 disease.

perivesical fat (Fig. 3.11). Invasion into adjacent structures indicates stage T4 disease.

Upper tract TCC can be visualized with CT using the same triple-phase technique as described for renal mass lesions. Focal TCCs may be seen as soft tissue filling defects within a dilated renal pelvis or calyces. Three-dimensional reformatted CT urogram (CTU) images akin to the IVU can also be achieved (Fig. 3.2). Stage T1 and T2 tumors invading the subepithelial connective tissue and muscularis layer, respectively, cannot be differentiated from each other with CT. Tumor invasion into the peripelvic or periureteric fat indicated stage T3 disease and is visualized as stranding or nodular projections. Abnormal areas of parenchymal enhancement suggest tumor invasion into the renal parenchyma (also stage T3), which typically enlarge the kidney while maintaining the normal renal contour (Fig. 3.12A).

Tumor invasion through the renal parenchyma and into the perinephric fat indicates stage T4 disease (Fig. 3.12B). As with bladder TCC, the importance in radiology is in detecting multifocal disease, and careful attention is paid to the contralateral kidney, ureter, and bladder.

Testicular Cancer

The role of CT in the management of malignant testicular tumors is to stage nodal disease accurately and to detect the presence of distant metastases in lungs, liver, bone, and brain. Ninety-five percent of testicular tumors are germ cell tumors, and these have a predictable pattern of lymphatic spread. Right-sided tumors spread to right-sided retroperitoneal nodes, such as pre-, para-, retro-, and aortocaval nodes and right renal hilar nodes, while left-sided tumors spread to the left retroperitoneum, such as preaortic, left paraaortic and left renal hilum (46). The pattern is so consistent that enlarged contralateral nodes in the absence of ipsilateral nodal enlargement are unlikely to be due to tumor. Extension to contralateral nodal groups can be seen in the presence of bulky ipsilateral nodes, greater than 2 cm, and crossover is seen more commonly from right- to left-sided adenopathy (47). Extension to lateral nodal groups anterior to the psoas muscle (echelon nodes) is uncommon but well recognized in testicular carcinoma (48). Retroperitoneal lymphadenopathy can be mimicked by the presence of unopacified bowel loops or variations in normal vascular anatomy, such as a retroaortic renal vein or double IVC and can be a potential diagnostic pitfall, particularly if good oral and intravenous contrast enhancement is not achieved. Nodal extension to pelvic nodes is only seen in the presence of massive retroperitoneal lymphadenopathy. Supradiaphragmatic extension can occur directly from the retroperitoneum via retrocrural extension and into the posterior mediastinum, or via the thoracic duct to the supraclavicular fossa. These areas should be included in the scan when retroperitoneal lymphadenopathy is present. The lungs are the commonest site of hematogenous disseminated and nodules as small as 3 mm are easily visualized with CT. Disease surveillance, however, is usually with chest x-ray.

Computed Tomography-Guided Intervention

The good spatial resolution of CT facilitates its use for a variety of image-guided procedures including FNA, biopsy, and drain insertion. These procedures can usually be performed under local anesthesia and with minimal distress to the patient.

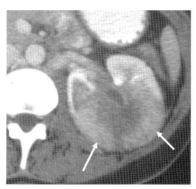 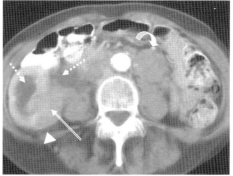

A   B

FIGURE 3.12. Advanced upper tract TCC on post–contrast-enhanced CT. (A) Infiltrative tumor within the renal parenchyma (arrows) causing abnormal enhancement pattern. (B) Advanced-stage T4 renal TCC in a different patient causing obstruction of the renal pelvis and calyces (broken arrows), parenchymal infiltration (open arrow), perinephric invasion (arrowhead), and paraaortic lymphadenopathy (curved arrow).

Technique

Patient positioning on the scan table is critical and should be both optimal for the procedure and comfortable for the patient, as it must be maintained throughout the procedure.

A scan through the relevant area is performed initially, and oral or intravenous contrast may be used when it is necessary to highlight neighboring vessels or bowel. A reference image is selected from which a direct and safe needle pathway from the skin to the lesion can be identified. Using the guide laser on the CT scanner, the selected point can be identified on the patient and marked on the skin. During needle insertion repeated scans through the area can be obtained to establish the exact position of the needle tip and ensure correct pathway. Computed tomography can be used to guide procedures in areas that are difficult to visualize with US, particularly the retroperitoneum, chest, and deep pelvis.

Surgical Planning

Knowledge of the spatial relationships of the tumor to other structures, particularly vessels, is an important consideration for surgical planning. It is important to document the presence of accessory renal arteries or normal variations in the location of the renal vein prior to surgery. Multidetector CT (MDCT) enables accurate CT angiographic images of the renal vascular supply to be generated via a variety of techniques. Maximum-intensity projection (MIP) images are commonly used to reconstruct angiographic images from pixels with the maximum attenuation value. Three-dimensional (3D) images can be generated, which allow the image to be viewed in multiple planes (Figs. 3.5 and 3.13). Three-dimensional volume-rendered imaging creates a 3D image from the entire data set without preliminary editing, and enables the spatial relationship

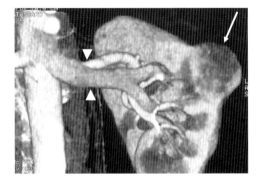

FIGURE 3.13. Left renal cell carcinoma. Surgical planning multidetector computed tomography (MDCT). Volume rendered three–dimensional reformatted images showing the relationship of the tumor (arrow) to the renal arteries and veins (arrowheads).

of the tumor to surrounding structures to be displayed (Fig. 3.13). Overlapping structures can be separated out to improve visualization. Three-dimensional volume-rendered angiography has been shown to be as accurate as conventional angiography in depicting renal vascularity (49). Three-dimensional images display anatomical detail in a format comparable to surgical appearances compared to conventional axial imaging.

Accurate staging information is essential for the selection of appropriate patients for nephron-sparing surgery. It is important to identify patients with bilateral or multifocal tumors, those with stage I disease confined to the kidney, and those without invasion of the collecting system or vascular structures. Lesions most suitable for nephron-sparing surgery are small (usually <4 cm), peripherally located, preferably exophytic, and away from the collecting system and renal hilum. These features are well demonstrated with 3D CT (50–52).

Imaging in the Postoperative Period

Computed tomography is useful in the evaluation of the postoperative patient. A degree of free fluid and inflammatory change is present in the abdomen or retroperitoneum in the immediate postoperative period, along with pockets of gas, particularly following laparoscopic surgery. However, increasing or new intraabdominal gas and fluid might suggest the presence of anastomotic dehiscence, for example, following cystectomy and ileal conduit formation. The detection of an anastomotic leak can be improved with the introduction of 20 to 50 mL of dilute (2%) water-soluble contrast medium via the stoma or rectum, where appropriate, prior to CT scanning.

Limitations of visualizing deeper portions of the abdomen with US make CT the more appropriate imaging modality when infected collections are suspected clinically. An abscess can be identified by the presence of a focal collection of fluid with an enhancing rim or pockets of gas within. Computed tomography can also be used to guide drain insertion into a collection, or plan US-guided or surgical drainage where most appropriate.

Tumor Volume Measurements

The aim of radiotherapy is to maximally irradiate the tumor while keeping the dose to surrounding normal tissues at a minimum. Advances in radiotherapy technology have made it possible to more accurately irradiate smaller volumes of tumor with higher doses. Conformal radiotherapy uses multiple collimators to shape the radiation beam much more closely to the contours of the tumor volume while reducing the dose to the surrounding area (53). Intensity-modulated radiotherapy (IMRT) is a more recent form of conformal radiotherapy in which the quantity of radiation across the beam is varied, enabling greater control of the shape of the radiation beam. The radiation beam can be varied to allow higher doses to different areas within the tumor volume (53). These techniques are currently being used in the treatment of pelvic malignancy including prostate and bladder carcinomas and require accurate localization of the tumor margin in order to map out the specific treatment area. Computed tomography is principally used, although techniques are being developed using MRI image fusion with radiotherapy for planning CT for accurate tumor volume co-location. It is important that the CT performed for radiotherapy planning be performed with the same technique and conditions as those later used to administer treatment. Differences in equipment, respiration, oral contrast administered, and degree of bladder filling can result in variations in tumor position and volume of tissue within the radiation field.

Magnetic Resonance Imaging

Basic Principles

Magnetic resonance imaging (MRI) is a nonionizing radiation method utilizing magnetic fields and radiofrequency (RF) waves to induce and detect a signal from different body tissues that is then converted into a gray-scale image. An MRI scanner consists of a large-bore circular magnet. When a patient is placed within it, spinning (precessing) hydrogen ions (protons) in water and lipid molecules of the body tissues are aligned, producing a net longitudinal magnetization along the line of the magnet field. An RF pulse at a specific frequency is applied, which induces a proportion of precessing protons to change alignment and flip through an angle, the size of which is determined by the strength and duration of the RF pulse. The net magnetization is tipped into a direction in the transverse plane and induces a small voltage or signal that can be detected by a receiver coil placed around the patient. This signal is amplified and processed into the pixel gray-scale level of the MRI image.

The strength of the signal partly depends on the proton density of the tissue but more significantly on the time for the transverse magnetization to decay and the longitudinal magnetization to regrow, which is dependent on two methods of energy loss or relaxation: T1 relaxation represents recovery of the longitudinal magnetization and depends on the time taken for the excited protons to give up energy and realign themselves along the line of the magnetic field. T1 relaxation is increased by the rapid jostling of heavy molecules within tissues removing energy from the excited protons. Tissues with protons attached to heavy molecules such as proteins or fat have a shorter T1 than lightweight molecules containing a high proportion of free water. T2 relaxation represents decay of the transverse magnetization and relies on the progressive dephasing of the excited protons once the RF pulse is switched off. This depends on the variation of local magnetic fields in different tissues, which is greatest in solids and rigid large molecules that have a very short T2 compared with free water. Rigid or fixed macromolecules such as those in bone, calculi, and metallic clips are relatively immobile and do not generate a signal. By varying the time between RF pulses and the time to collect the signal, images are produced when the difference of the signal produced by different tissues is greatest. Images are generated with either more T1 or T2 effects or weighting.

Advantages and Disadvantages of Magnetic Resonance Imaging Over Computed Tomography

Compared with CT, MRI produces images that reflect molecular differences between tissues rather than just tissue density, and therefore generates a much greater gray-scale range of soft tissue contrast. Images can also be generated in any plane and at any angle. Magnetic resonance imaging is particularly useful for imaging the pelvis where contrast and spatial resolution of organs is generally limited with CT. With MRI, molecular differences in the zonal architecture of the prostate can be delineated, for example, and a clear distinction between the central and peripheral zones of the gland can be demonstrated (Fig. 3.18A). The development of local pelvic RF transmit/receiver coils has enabled imaging to be targeted at a much smaller field of view, resulting in improved signal-to-noise ratio and spatial resolution. This has greatly facilitated the use of MRI in the staging of pelvic malignancy.

Intracavity receiver coils have also been developed. They are placed into the rectum and produce images with a much greater signal-to-noise ratio. The imaged field of view is much smaller with an endorectal coil, but greater resolution can be achieved in the areas imaged. These coils are used particularly to visualize the anal sphincter and prostate zonal anatomy, and for rectal cancer staging. Endorectal coils are generally tolerated by the patient, although scan times may be increased as a greater number of sequences are obtained.

Magnetic resonance imaging does not use ionizing radiation, and at present poses no known risks to patients. This makes MRI of value where it is desirable to limit radiation exposure, in particular in children or young adults, and in patients who require follow-up surveillance imaging.

Magnetic resonance imaging involves obtaining multiple sequences and planes, which is much more time-consuming than CT. Image quality is degraded by patient movement and respiration, and is therefore more dependent on patient cooperation. Thus, the study may be limited in sick patients or those requiring continuous monitoring. Some patients are unable to tolerate MRI and find the enclosed confines of the scanner claustrophobic. This may be overcome by using an open-bore magnet, which is available in some specialist centers.

Technique and Patient Preparation

The patient should be informed that the scan may take up to 30 to 45 minutes to perform, during which time they will be required to lie still within the scanner. During the scan, loud knocking noises are heard as the radiofrequency pulses are switched on and off. Pelvic MRI for bladder and prostate imaging is best performed with the patient's bladder full, although overdistention can result in patient movement artifact. Ideally the patient is asked to void approximately 2 hours before the scan. Bowel peristalsis can also create movement artifact and degrade the images. For renal and adrenal MRI, an antispasmodic agent such as buscopan or glucagon is administered immediately prior to the scan (54).

The diagnostic ability of MRI has been enhanced with the now-standard use of gadolinium, a chelate-based intravenous contrast agent. Like iodinated contrast medium used in CT, gadolinium, once injected, circulates within the vascular system and is taken up in vascularized tissue and tumors. Within the magnetic field of the MRI scanner, gadolinium has a paramagnetic effect, causing shortening of the T1 and T2 relaxation times. This is best appreciated on sequences weighted for T1 effects where the signal is increased. Thus, on T1-weighted imaging, vascularized tissue increases in signal intensity following gadolinium administration. Unlike iodinated contrast agents, the incidence of allergic reactions is extremely rare, and there are no other specific contraindications to its usage.

Safety Considerations

Ferromagnetic objects placed in or near the magnetic field are attracted to the magnet and can move. This may convert unfixed external objects into potentially hazardous projectiles. Objects within the body, such as aneurysm clips or other surgical clips, might be displaced or rotated in body tissues. The current practice is to use MRI-compatible nonmagnetic surgical objects where possible. It is important for the MR operator to check the compatibility of surgically inserted materials, particularly those inserted more recently. Joint prostheses are firmly fixed and don't generally cause a problem, although the susceptibility artifact induced by metallic hip prostheses may degrade images of the pelvis. Magnetic resonance imaging is contraindicated in patients with implantable cardiac pacemakers, neurostimulator devices, cochlear implants, certain types of aneurysm clips, and intraocular metallic foreign bodies.

Magnetic Resonance Imaging in Urologic Cancers

The main indications for the use of MRI in urologic oncology are summarized in Table 3.5. Because of resource and time implications, MRI is often reserved for specific problem solving, such as the characterization of lesions detected by other imaging modalities. This is particularly the case for those renal and adrenal lesions that remain indeterminate on CT, or in whom CT is contraindicated. Magnetic resonance imaging may also be performed to exclude hepatic metastases in a patient with an indeterminate liver lesion who is being considered for surgery. Magnetic resonance imaging is recommended for local bladder and prostate carcinoma staging in patients being considered for radical treatment. Magnetic resonance imaging is sensitive for the detection of pelvic fistu-

TABLE 3.5. Role of magnetic resonance imaging in urologic malignancy

Kidney
1. Characterization of focal renal lesions
2. Tumor staging
    Patients where CT is contraindicated
    Specific problem solving
        Perinephric invasion
        Local organ invasion
        Venous invasion
3. Follow-up/surveillance: to reduce radiation burden in high risk groups, e.g., von Hippel–Lindau syndrome

Adrenal
1. Characterization of adrenal mass lesion: adenoma versus metastasis/primary adrenal adenocarcinoma
2. Characterization of functional adrenal mass: adenoma versus adrenal adenocarcinoma
3. Local staging of primary adrenal carcinoma

Bladder
1. Local staging: bladder wall invasion
2. Identification of suspected vaginovesical, rectovesical or other fistulae
3. Radiotherapy planning

Prostate
1. Local staging
    Extracapsular invasion
    Seminal vesicle invasion
    Nodal staging
2. Spine MRI: suspected cord compression in patients with bone metastases

Testes
No role in assessment of local tumor
Brain and spine MRI for detection of metastases

lae that may arise as a complication of a pelvic tumor, surgery, or radiotherapy, and MRI is the imaging investigation of choice for this purpose.

Lesion Characterization

Renal Lesions

Solid renal mass lesions are frequently isointense to renal parenchyma on T1- and T2-weighted MRI and therefore not well seen. However, following the administration of gadolinium they enhance less than renal parenchyma and become more conspicuous (55). This is particularly important for the detection of small (<3 cm) RCCs, which are usually solid. Magnetic resonance imaging is useful for surveillance imaging in high-risk patients. In particular, patients with VHL syndrome, for example, have a propensity to develop RCCs, often from a relatively young age and on a background of multiple renal cysts. They frequently develop small (<3 cm) early RCCs that are slow growing. Magnetic resonance imaging is often the imaging method of choice for follow-up in these patients.

The Bosniak CT criteria for grading cystic renal masses (see Computed Tomography, above) can be applied to MRI, which may be used for lesion characterization in patients in whom iodinated contrast medium is contraindicated. Calcification within a lesion, however, cannot be easily detected with MRI, as it produces a signal void or absence of signal. Magnetic resonance imaging may detect subtle enhancement compared with CT and raise the suspicion of malignancy.

Adrenal Lesions

Magnetic resonance imaging techniques have been developed to aid in the characterization of adrenal lesions. Differentiation of benign from malignant lesions relies on the detection of intracellular lipid, seen almost exclusively within adenomas (36). This can be reliably detected on MRI with the use of a chemical shift imaging technique. This exploits the normal difference in precessional frequency between fat and water protons within a given voxel. The protons can be made to precess, or spin, at the same frequency and are in phase with each other, and an additive signal is produced. When they are made to precess out of phase, the signal is reduced in those voxels that contain both fat and water protons. In the case of adrenal adenomas, the lesion loses signal on the out-of-phase images compared with the in-phase images (Fig. 3.8). Adenomas can be diagnosed with up to 100% specificity and sensitivity (56) and thus can be distinguished from metastases and primary adrenal carcinoma. Primary adrenocortical carcinomas are usually large at presentation, heterogeneous, and enhance post–gadolinium administration (Fig. 3.14).

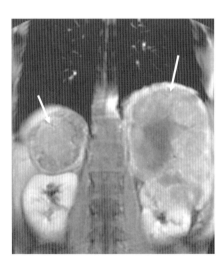

FIGURE 3.14. Bilateral adrenocortical carcinoma. Coronal T1 weighted MRI post–intravenous gadolinium. Large, bilateral, enhancing suprarenal masses (arrows) clearly arise separately from the kidneys, and no remaining normal adrenal gland could be identified.

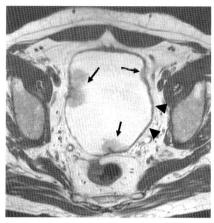
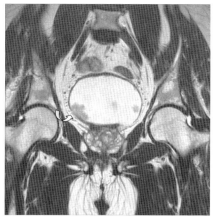

A   B

FIGURE 3.15. Multifocal bladder carcinoma. (A) Axial T2-weighted MRI. (B) Coronal T2-weighted MRI through the bladder showing multiple tumor deposits (arrows) arising from the bladder wall. The low signal muscle layer of the bladder (arrowheads) is indistinct at one point (curved arrow) in keeping with tumor invasion (stage T3). (Courtesy of Dr. S.A.A Sohaib.)

Tumor Staging

Bladder

Magnetic resonance imaging has an advantage over CT for staging of bladder carcinoma in that it can identify invasion of the deep muscle (54). It cannot, however, differentiate superficial muscle invasion from submucosal invasion. The bladder wall muscle is seen as low signal intensity on T2-weighted images, and disruption of this line indicates muscle invasion (Figs. 3.15 and 3.16). Magnetic resonance imaging also has better sensitivity for the detection of

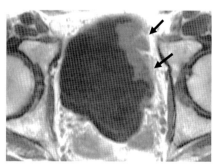
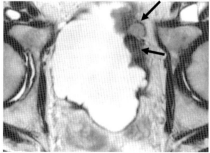

A   B

FIGURE 3.16. Transitional cell carcinoma (TCC) of the bladder, stage T3b. (A) T1-weighted MRI. (B) T2-weighted axial MRI showing large tumor arising from the left lateral wall of the bladder with clear invasion into the perivesical fat (arrows).

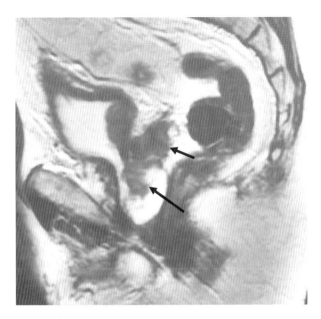

FIGURE 3.17. Locally advanced bladder cancer. Sagittal T2-weighted MRI showing tumor arising from the posterior wall of the bladder with invasion of the prostate and seminal vesicles (arrows)

perivesical fat and surrounding organ invasion, compared with CT. Involvement of the seminal vesicles is suspected when there is loss of their normal high signal intensity appearance (Fig. 3.17). The overall accuracy of MRI in staging bladder cancer is 75% to 85% (57).

Patients with pathological T2 stage disease on MRI are at risk of lymphatic and hematogenous extension, and full staging requires CT of the lungs and liver.

Prostate

High-resolution T2-weighted imaging of the prostate gland in multiple planes enables the zonal anatomy of the prostate gland to be well demonstrated (57–59). The peripheral zone is usually thinner and of higher signal intensity compared with the heterogeneous, lower signal intensity central zone (Fig. 3.18A). Prostate carcinoma can be identified as low signal intensity within the peripheral zone (Fig. 3.18B). However, this appearance is not specific and can also be seen with chronic inflammation and fibrosis, making detection and delineation of the tumor difficult (Fig. 3.18C). Low signal change can also be seen in the peripheral zone due to postbiopsy hemorrhage and is confirmed on T1-weighted imaging as high signal foci (Fig. 3.18D,E). The presence of hemorrhage makes it difficult to localize the tumor and reduces staging accuracy when MRI is performed less than 3 weeks postbiopsy (60). Tumors arising within the central zone cannot be differentiated from the markedly heterogeneous

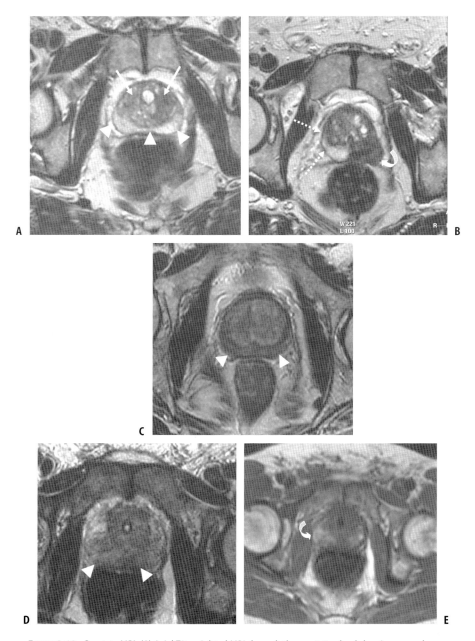

Figure 3.18. Prostate MRI. (A) Axial T2-weighted MRI through the prostate gland showing normal prostate zonal anatomy. Note the larger, heterogeneous central zone (arrows) in keeping with benign prostatic hypertrophy and high signal intensity peripheral zone (arrowheads). (B) The normal peripheral zone is replaced by low signal intensity tumor on the left side of the gland (curved arrow) in this second patient. The normal low signal intensity line of the prostatic capsule on the right (broken arrows) is disrupted, and there is a bulging tumor contour and loss of the normal rectoprostatic angle, all features in keeping with extracapsular tumor invasion. (C) Diffuse low signal is seen throughout the peripheral zone (arrowheads) in this third patient. This appearance is difficult to differentiate from chronic prostatitis, but was confirmed as bilateral prostate adenocarcinoma on biopsy. (D) Axial T2-weighted image. (E) T1-weighted MRI through the prostate in a different patient. Diffuse low signal in the peripheral zone (white arrowheads) on the T2-weighted MRI. However, patchy high signal change on the T1-weighted MRI (curved arrow), indicating postbiopsy hemorrhage make it difficult to delineate the tumor. (Courtesy of Dr. A. Sahdev.)

appearance of the central zone in coexistent benign prostatic hypertrophy. Tumor localization by MRI is reserved for patients with elevated PSA but previous negative biopsy, and in selected patients MRI has been shown to have a sensitivity and positive predictive value of 83% and 50%, respectively (61).

The principal role of MRI in the prostate, however, is in local tumor staging in patients with histologically proven carcinoma who are being considered for radical surgery or radiotherapy. The accuracy of prostate cancer staging varies but may be up to 88% with endorectal coil MRI (62). The detection of extracapsular extension and seminal vesicle invasion is of particular importance for treatment planning because of their prognostic implications (63). Features suggesting extracapsular invasion include interruption of the low signal peripheral capsule with a bulging tumor contour, but the most predictive features of invasion are asymmetry of the neurovascular bundles and obliteration of the rectoprostatic angle, with specificity of up to 95% but poor sensitivity of 38% (64). The location of the neurovascular bundles are an important site of invasion and can be seen posterolaterally in the 5 and 7 o'clock positions. Loss of the normal rectoprostatic angle at this point is suspicious for tumor extension (Fig. 3.18B). Seminal vesicle invasion is suggested when replacement of their normal high signal intensity with low signal intensity tumor is seen. Previous pelvic irradiation, however, may render the seminal vesicles fibrotic and of low signal intensity. Magnetic resonance imaging is also important in detection of local tumor invasion into the bladder or rectum.

Magnetic Resonance Spectroscopy in Prostate Cancer Staging

Magnetic resonance spectroscopy is a 3D technique for plotting relative concentrations of chemical compounds within the prostate gland by mapping signal intensities of chemicals resonating at different frequencies (59). In the normal peripheral zone a relatively high peak of the chemical citrate is seen compared to that of choline. Choline is a normal constituent of cell membranes, and in areas of tumor high cell turnover leads to a relative increase in the concentration of choline, with reversal of the normal choline/citrate ratio. Spatial mapping of such peaks within the prostate gland are used to plot the location and estimate the extent of tumor. When used in conjunction with standard endorectal or pelvic phased array prostate MR, this technique has been shown to improve tumor localization (65), increase staging accuracy, and reduce interobserver variability (66).

Specific Problem Solving in Renal and Adrenal Carcinoma Staging

In the case of renal and adrenal staging, MRI is usually reserved for resolving specific problems not answered with CT. The multiplanar imaging ability of MRI can help delineate the organ of origin of a large suprarenal or renal angle mass. Similarly, local organ invasion may be better differentiated with

MRI where accuracy rates of up to 100% have been reported (67) for RCC. The main role of MRI in renal and adrenal staging is in the diagnosis of venous tumor thrombosis and the delineation the uppermost level of extension. The suprahepatic IVC and right atrium, which may be difficult to visualize on CT, are well seen with MRI (Figs. 3.4C,D and 3.19A,B). Enhancement of thrombus

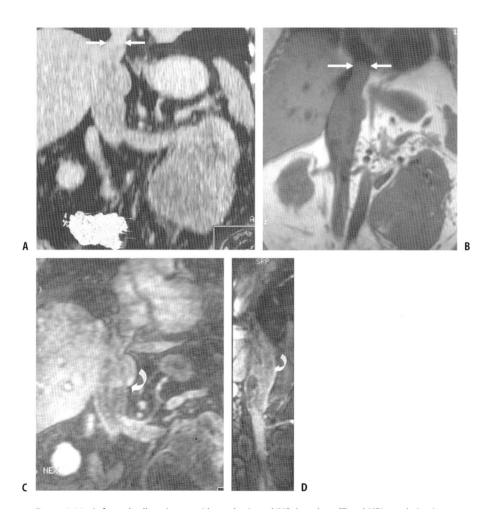

Figure 3.19. Left renal cell carcinoma with renal vein and IVC thrombus; CT and MRI correlation (*same patient as in figure 3.10*). (A) Coronal reformatted CT image showing extension of thrombus into the IVC. The upper level of thrombus (white arrows) does not extend above the level of the hepatic veins. (B) Corresponding image on T1 weighted coronal MRI. The upper level of thrombus is well visualised. (C, D) Coronal T1 weighted MRI post contrast medium administration showing non-enhancing bland thrombus within the IVC (curved arrows).

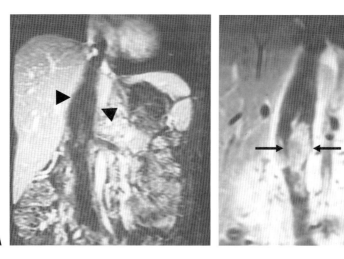

FIGURE 3.20. Inferior vena cava (IVC) thrombus extension from renal cell carcinoma. Coronal fat-suppressed T1-weighted MRI. (A) Non–contrast-enhanced images shows signal void within the IVC (arrows), which is expanded by thrombus. (B) Contrast-enhanced images show enhancing tumor thrombus (arrowheads) within the thrombosed IVC.

following gadolinium administration enables distinguishing between bland and tumor thrombus (68) (Figs. 3.19C,D and 3.20). Direct tumor thrombus invasion of the caval wall can also be diagnosed with 92% to 94% accuracy (68,69), with contrast-enhanced MRI (Fig. 3.21). Gadolinium-enhanced 3D MRI studies

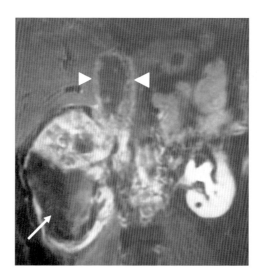

FIGURE 3.21. IVC thrombus invasion. Coronal fat-suppressed T1-weighted MRI with contrast enhancement. Right renal cell carcinoma (arrow) and thrombus within the IVC (arrowheads). Central nonenhancing (bland) thrombus with an enhancing rim of tumor thrombus extends up and invades the IVC wall.

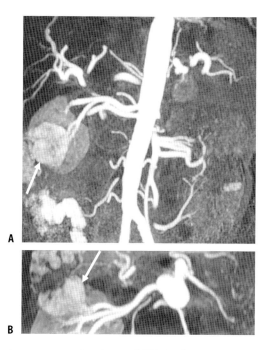

FIGURE **3.22.** Magnetic resonance renal angiogram (MRA). Small stage I renal cell carcinoma (arrows). Coronal (A) and axial (B) volume acquisition 3D gradient-echo MRI shows the relationship of the tumor to its arterial supply.

can be used to generate renal angiographic images and provide a preoperative vascular roadmap for potentially respectable tumors (Fig. 3.22).

References

1. Dalla PL. What is left of i.v. urography? Eur Radiol 2001;11(6):931–939.
2. Chalmers N, Jackson RW. Comparison of iodixanol and iohexol in renal impairment. Br J Radiol 1999;72(859):701–703.
3. Yousem DM, Gatewood OM, Goldman SM, Marshall FF. Synchronous and metachronous transitional cell carcinoma of the urinary tract: prevalence, incidence, and radiographic detection. Radiology 1988;167(3):613–618.
4. Kang CH, Yu TJ, Hsieh HH, et al. The development of bladder tumors and contralateral upper urinary tract tumors after primary transitional cell carcinoma of the upper urinary tract. Cancer 2003;98(8):1620–1626.
5. Joffe SA, Servaes S, Okon S, Horowitz M. Multi-detector row CT urography in the evaluation of hematuria. Radiographics 2003;23(6):1441–1455.
6. McNicholas MM, Raptopoulos VD, Schwartz RK, et al. Excretory phase CT urography for opacification of the urinary collecting system. AJR 1998;170:1261–1267.
7. Caoili EM, Cohan RH, Korobkin M, et al. Urinary tract abnormalities: initial experience with multi-detector row CT urography. Radiology 2002;222(2):353–360.

8. Kawashima A, Glockner JF, King BF Jr. CT urography and MR urography. Radiol Clin North Am 2003;41(5):945–961.

9. Roy C, Tuchmann C, Morel M, et al. Is there still a place for angiography in the management of renal mass lesions? Eur Radiol 1999;9(2):329–335.

10. Lin PH, Terramani TT, Bush RL, et al. Concomitant intraoperative renal artery embolization and resection of complex renal carcinoma. J Vasc Surg 2003;38:446–450.

11. Wunderlich H, Schumann S, Jantitzky V, et al. Increase of renal cell carcinoma incidence in central Europe. Eur Urol 1998;33(6):538–541.

12. Lui KW, Gervais DA, Arellano RA, Mueller PR. Radiofrequency ablation of renal cell carcinoma. Clin Radiol 2003;58(12):905–913.

13. Zagoria RJ. Imaging-guided radiofrequency ablation of renal masses. Radiographics 2004;24(suppl 1):S59–S71.

14. Goldberg SN, Gazelle GS, Mueller PR. Thermal ablation therapy for focal malignancy: a unified approach to underlying principles, techniques, and diagnostic imaging guidance. AJR 2000;174(2):323–331.

15. Gazelle GS, Goldberg SN, Solbiati L, Livraghi T. Tumor ablation with radiofrequency energy. Radiology 2000;217(3):633–646.

16. Pavlovich CP, Walther MM, Choyke PL, et al. Percutaneous radio frequency ablation of small renal tumors: initial results. J Urol 2002;167(1):10–15.

17. Farrell MA, Charboneau WJ, DiMarco DS, et al. Imaging-guided radiofrequency ablation of solid renal tumors. AJR 2003;180(6):1509–1513.

18. Veltri A, De Fazio G, Malfitana V, et al. Percutaneous US-guided RF thermal ablation for malignant renal tumors: preliminary results in 13 patients. Eur Radiol 2004; 14:2303–2310.

19. Wah TM, Arellano RS, Gervais DA, et al. Image-guided percutaneous radiofrequency ablation and incidence of post-radiofrequency ablation syndrome: prospective survey. Radiology 2005;237:1097–1102.

20. Thompson IM, Peek M. Improvement in survival of patients with renal cell carcinoma—the role of the serendipitously detected tumor. J Urol 1988;140(3):487–490.

21. Pantuck AJ, Zisman A, Belldegrun AS. The changing natural history of renal cell carcinoma. J Urol 2001;166(5):1611–1623.

22. Bosniak MA. The current radiological approach to renal cysts. Radiology 1986; 158:1–10.

23. Bosniak MA. The small (less than or equal to 3.0 cm) renal parenchymal tumor: detection, diagnosis, and controversies. Radiology 1991;179(2):307–317.

24. Habboub HK, Abu-Yousef MM, Williams RD, et al. Accuracy of color Doppler sonography in assessing venous thrombus extension in renal cell carcinoma. AJR 1997; 168(1):267–271.

25. Kallman DA, King BF, Hattery RR, et al. Renal vein and inferior vena cava tumor thrombus in renal cell carcinoma: CT, US, MRI and venacavography. J Comput Assist Tomogr 1992;16(2):240–247.

26. Robbin ML. Ultrasound contrast agents: a promising future. Radiol Clin North Am 2001;39:399–414.

27. Jakobsen JA. Ultrasound contrast agents: clinical applications. Eur Radiol 2001; 11(8):1329–1337.

28. Jayson M, Sanders H. Increased incidence of serendipitously discovered renal cell carcinoma. Urology 1998;51(2):203–205.

29. Israel GM, Bosniak MA. Follow-up CT of moderately complex cystic lesions of the kidney (Bosniak category IIF). AJR 2003;181(3):627–633.

30. Abecassis M, McLoughlin MJ, Langer B, Kudlow JE. Serendipitous adrenal masses: prevalence, significance, and management. Am J Surg 1985;149(6):783–788.
31. Glazer HS, Weyman PJ, Sagel SS, et al. Nonfunctioning adrenal masses: incidental discovery on computed tomography. AJR 1982;139(1):81–85.
32. Mitnick JS, Bosniak MA, Megibow AJ, Naidich DP. Non-functioning adrenal adenomas discovered incidentally on computed tomography. Radiology 1983;148: 495–499.
33. Francis IR, Smid A, Gross MD, et al. Adrenal masses in oncologic patients: functional and morphologic evaluation. Radiology 1988;166(2):353–356.
34. Krestin GP, Freidmann G, Fishbach R, et al. Evaluation of adrenal masses in oncologic patients: dynamic contrast-enhanced MR vs CT. J Comput Assist Tomogr 1991; 15(1):104–110.
35. Frilling A, Tecklenborg K, Weber F, et al. Importance of adrenal incidentaloma in patients with a history of malignancy. Surgery 2004;136(6):1289–1296.
36. Korobkin M, Giordano TJ, Brodeur FJ, et al. Adrenal adenomas: relationship between histologic lipid and CT and MR findings. Radiology 1996;200(3):743–747.
37. Boland GW, Lee MJ, Gazelle GS, et al. Characterization of adrenal masses using unenhanced CT: an analysis of the CT literature. AJR 1998;171:201–204.
38. Korobkin M, Brodeur FJ, Francis IR, et al. CT time-attenuation washout curves of adrenal adenomas and nonadenomas. AJR 1998;170(3):747–752.
39. Pena CS, Boland GW, Hahn PF, et al. Characterization of indeterminate (lipid-poor) adrenal masses: use of washout characteristics at contrast-enhanced CT. Radiology 2000;217(3):798–802.
40. Johnson CD, Dunnick NR, Cohan RH, Illescas FF. Renal adenocarcinoma: CT staging of 100 tumors. AJR 1987;148(1):59–63.
41. Fein AB, Lee JK, Balfe DM, et al. Diagnosis and staging of renal cell carcinoma: a comparison of MR imaging and CT. AJR 1987;148(4):749–753.
42. Studer UE, Scherz S, Scheidegger J, et al. Enlargement of regional lymph nodes in renal cell carcinoma is often not due to metastases. J Urol 1990;144(2 pt 1):243–245.
43. Clayman RV Jr, Gonzalez R, Fraley EE. Renal cancer invading the inferior vena cava: clinical review and anatomical approach. J Urol 1980;123(2):157–163.
44. Hatcher PA, Anderson EE, Paulson DF, et al. Surgical management and prognosis of renal cell carcinoma invading the vena cava. J Urol 1991;145(1):20–23.
45. Catalano C, Fraioli F, Laghi A, et al. High-resolution multidetector CT in the preoperative evaluation of patients with renal cell carcinoma. AJR 2003;180(5):1271–1277.
46. MacVicar D. Staging of testicular germ cell tumours. Clin Radiol 1993;47:149–158.
47. Dixon AK, Ellis M, Sikora K. Computed tomography of testicular tumours: distribution of abdominal lymphadenopathy. Clin Radiol 1986;37(6):519–523.
48. Williams MP, Cook JV, Duchesne GM. Psoas nodes-an overlooked site of metastasis from testicular tumours. Clin Radiol 1989;40(6):607–609.
49. Coll DM, Uzzo RG, Herts BR, et al. 3–dimensional volume rendered computerized tomography for preoperative evaluation and intraoperative treatment of patients undergoing nephron sparing surgery. J Urol 1999;161(4):1097–1102.
50. Smith PA, Marshall FF, Corl FM, Fishman EK. Planning nephron-sparing renal surgery using 3D helical CT angiography. J Comput Assist Tomogr 1999;23(5): 649–654.
51. Coll DM, Herts BR, Davros WJ, Uzzo RG, Novick AC. Preoperative use of 3D volume rendering to demonstrate renal tumors and renal anatomy. Radiographics 2000; 20(2):431–438.

52. Sheth S, Scatarige JC, Horton KM, Corl FM, Fishman EK. Current concepts in the diagnosis and management of renal cell carcinoma: role of multidetector CT and three-dimensional CT. Radiographics 2001;21(spec. No.):S237–S254.

53. Mangar SA, Huddart RA, Parker CC, et al. Technological advances in radiotherapy for the treatment of localised prostate cancer. Eur J Cancer 2005;41(6):908–921.

54. Mallampati GK, Siegelman ES. MR imaging of the bladder. Magn Reson Imaging Clin North Am 2004;12:545–555.

55. Rominger MB, Kenney PJ, Morgan DE, et al. Gadolinium-enhanced MR imaging of renal masses. Radiographics 1992;12(6):1097–1116.

56. Korobkin M, Lombardi TJ, Aisen AM, et al. Characterization of adrenal masses with chemical shift and gadolinium-enhanced MR imaging. Radiology 1995;197(2):411–418.

57. Heiken JP, Forman HP, Brown JJ. Neoplasms of the bladder, prostate, and testis. Radiol Clin North Am 1994;32(1):81–98.

58. Claus FG, Hricak H, Hattery RR. Pretreatment evaluation of prostate cancer: role of MR imaging and 1H MR spectroscopy. Radiographics 2004;24(suppl 1):S167–S180.

59. Rajesh A, Coakley FV. MR imaging and MR spectroscopic imaging of prostate cancer. Magn Reson Imaging Clin North Am 2004;12(3):557–579.

60. White S, Hricak H, Forstner R, et al. Prostate cancer: effect of postbiopsy hemorrhage on interpretation of MR images. Radiology 1995;195(2):385–390.

61. Beyersdorff D, Taupitz M, Winkelmann B, et al. Patients with a history of elevated prostate-specific antigen levels and negative transrectal US-guided quadrant or sextant biopsy results: value of MR imaging. Radiology 2002;224(3):701–706.

62. Huch Boni RA, Boner JA, Debatin JF, et al. Optimization of prostate carcinoma staging: comparison of imaging and clinical methods. Clin Radiol 1995;50(9):593–600.

63. Hull GW, Rabbani F, Abbas F, et al. Cancer control with radical prostatectomy alone in 1,000 consecutive patients. J Urol 2002;167(2 pt 1):528–534.

64. Yu KK, Hricak H, Alagappan R, et al. Detection of extracapsular extension of prostate carcinoma with endorectal and phased-array coil MR imaging: multivariate feature analysis. Radiology 1997;202(3):697–702.

65. Scheidler J, Hricak H, Vigneron DB, et al. Prostate cancer: localization with three-dimensional proton MR spectroscopic imaging—clinicopathologic study. Radiology 1999;213(2):473–480.

66. Yu KK, Scheidler J, Hricak H, et al. Prostate cancer: prediction of extracapsular extension with endorectal MR imaging and three-dimensional proton MR spectroscopic imaging. Radiology 1999;213(2):481–488.

67. Hricak H, Thoeni RF, Carroll PR, et al. Detection and staging of renal neoplasms: a reassessment of MR imaging. Radiology 1988;166(3):643–649.

68. Aslam Sohaib SA, Teh J, Nargund VH, et al. Assessment of tumor invasion of the vena caval wall in renal cell carcinoma cases by magnetic resonance imaging. J Urol 2002;167(3):1271–1275.

69. Myneni L, Hricak H, Carroll PR. Magnetic resonance imaging of renal carcinoma with extension into the vena cava: staging accuracy and recent advances. Br J Urol 1991;68(6):571–578.

4
Hematuria and Hematospermia: Clinical Evaluation and Principles of Management

Khurshid R. Ghani and Vinod H. Nargund

Hematuria

Hematuria is defined as the presence of blood in the urine on visual inspection or quantified on urine analysis. Regardless of the quantity of blood in the urine, hematuria is malignancy until proven otherwise in high-risk patients.

Types of Hematuria

Microscopic Hematuria

Microscopic hematuria is the presence of nonvisible amounts of blood detected in the urine with or without accompanying symptoms. The most commonly accepted normal upper limit of urinary red cells is 2 to 3 intact red blood cells (RBCs) per high power field (HPF) on microscopic evaluation of a centrifuged urine sample (1).

Asymptomatic Microscopic Hematuria

This is microscopic hematuria without symptoms and proteinuria and an incidental finding during a health checkup. Variables that affect the incidence of asymptomatic microscopic hematuria (AMH) include patient age, method of urinalysis (microscopy vs. dipstick), and the cutoff level of RBCs chosen for microscopy. Serious disease is rare under the age of 40 years.

Dipstick Hematuria

In the vast majority of patients microscopic hematuria is detected by dipstick testing (see later). Different dipstick kits vary in their sensitivity to detect blood, but most dipsticks detect 8 RBCs/HPF. Dipstick hematuria of 3+ equates to approximately 500 RBCs/mL. As dipstick testing is less sensitive compared to urine microscopy, a positive test should be confirmed with a second test and followed by urine microscopy.

Transient Microscopic Hematuria

Transient microscopic hematuria is diagnosed when hematuria is intermittent and caused by exercise, sexual intercourse, or mild trauma.

Idiopathic Hematuria

This is the term applied to microscopic hematuria that has been investigated and no cause has been found. Nearly 10% to 20% of patients with microscopic hematuria have no source identified.

Gross Hematuria

Gross (or frank) hematuria is blood in the urine in sufficient quantity to be visible to the naked eye. Gross hematuria has a community prevalence of 2.5% and it accounts for 4% to 20% of all urological consults (2). It indicates the risk of significant underlying disease such as urothelial cancer.

Exercise Hematuria

Microscopic or gross hematuria may occur immediately following noncontact strenuous exercise such as running, cycling, or swimming. It resolves within 2 to 3 days and may be a result of mucosal microcontusions due to blunt trauma from repeated impact of the posterior bladder wall against the trigone in a partially filled bladder.

Pseudohematuria

This is usually a red/brown discoloration of urine that mimics the appearance of gross hematuria. It can occur following ingestion of certain foods (carrots, beets, blackberries, riboflavin, vitamin A), drugs (chloroquine, phenacetin, sulfonamides, phenazopyridine, sulfasalazine, rifampin, laxatives containing phenolphthalein).

Factitious Hematuria

Very rarely, hematuria may be self-induced by contaminating urine samples with blood by patients who have a pathological desire to seek ill health and undergo investigation (Munchausen syndrome). Opiate addicts may try to seek drugs by mimicking renal colic and provide urine contaminated with venous blood.

Postcoital (Postejaculatory) Hematuria

This is extremely rare painless hematuria occurring in men immediately after sexual intercourse and may be associated with hematospermia. It is usually associated with a vascular anomaly such as a urethral hemangioma that bleeds during ejaculation.

Causes of Hematuria

Urological

Table 4.1 lists the causes of hematuria in the urinary tract classified by anatomical site of origin.

Systemic Disorders

Systemic disorders include Systemic lupus erythematosus (SLE), Henoch-Schönlein purpura (HSP), malaria, sickle cell disease, coagulopathies, endometriosis and alcohol abuse (papillary necrosis).

Drugs

Interstitial nephritis can be caused by penicillin, nonsteroidal antiinflammatory drugs (NSAIDs), cephalosporins, and frusemide. Nephrotoxic drugs include aminoglycosides and cyclosporine. Drug-induced hemorrhagic cystitis can be caused by cyclophosphamide and methicillin.

Anticoagulant-Associated Hematuria

Anticoagulation should not be discounted as the source of bleeding, as significant urinary tract disease may be present in up to 30% of patients (3). The majority of patients have no diagnosis found after thorough evaluation.

TABLE 4.1. Urological causes of hematuria in the urinary tract

Renal	Congenital: Pelvi-ureteric junction (PUJ) obstruction, arteriovenous (AV) malformations, cystic renal disease (adult polycystic kidney disease, APKD), medullary sponge kidney, renal cysts
	Genetic: renal tubular acidosis type I, cystinuria, von Hippel–Lindau disease, Alport disease, thin basement membrane disease
	Trauma: iatrogenic (nephrostomy)
	Neoplastic: Renal cell carcinoma, transitional cell carcinoma, angiomyolipoma
	Metabolic: calculi
	Infection: pyelonephritis, genitourinary tuberculosis
	Inflammatory diseases: interstitial nephritis, poststreptococcal glomerulonephritis, IgA nephropathy, Goodpasture's syndrome
	Radiation: nephritis
	Vascular: renovascular arterial disease, renal vein thrombosis, left renal vein hypertension due to nutcracker syndrome: compression of left renal vein between superior mesenteric artery and aorta, hemangiomas, renal papillary necrosis
	Foreign bodies: stent, nephrostomy
Ureteral	Calculi, neoplastic (transitional cell carcinoma, TCC), trauma (including iatrogenic), foreign bodies (stent)
Bladder	Neoplastic (TCC, squamous cell, adenocarcinoma, neuroendocrine tumors); anatomic (diverticulae, vesicoureteric reflux); infection (hemorrhagic cystitis, schistosomiasis); metabolic (calculi), post–acute urinary retention (decompression bleeding), trauma
Prostate	Benign prostatic hyperplasia, carcinoma, infection (prostatitis), metabolic (calculi)
Urethra	Hemangioma, tumor, stone, stricture, trauma, foreign bodies (catheter, stents, inserted bodies), iatrogenic (instrumentation)

Clinical Evaluation

Patients 40 years of age or older have a higher risk of urological malignancy. The incidence of significant pathology is lower in women. It is important to differentiate rectal and vaginal bleeding from hematuria. Gross hematuria with clots demonstrates significant bleeding and increases the likelihood of malignancy.

The timing of hematuria can give a clue to the anatomical site of bleeding: hematuria at the start of micturition (initial) indicates urethral bleeding; hematuria occurring throughout micturition (total) comes from the bladder or upper tracts; and hematuria at the end of micturition (terminal) indicates that the bleeding is in the prostatic urethra or bladder neck.

Hematuria associated with colicky abdominal flank pain and passage of stringy clots is indicative of upper tract bleeding. Constant severe lower abdominal pain may be due to clot retention. Prostatic bleeding due to benign prostatic hypertrophy (BPH) or urethral stricture is usually associated with lower urinary tract symptoms (LUTS). Dysuria, urgency, and incontinence may be due to prostatitis or urinary tract infection.

Systemic Symptoms

Loss of appetite, weight loss, and night sweats could be due to underlying carcinoma. Recent history of an upper respiratory tract infection is associated with nephrological causes of hematuria such as poststreptococcal glomerulonephritis. A viral illness with hemoptysis and abnormal renal function is typical of Goodpasture's syndrome. Timing of the menstrual period must be noted along with any history of endometriosis. Unprotected sexual intercourse increases the likelihood of acquiring sexually transmitted infections.

A history of previous instrumentation may lead to a history of urethral stricture. Pelvic radiotherapy could cause radiation cystitis. Chronic atrial fibrillation or recent myocardial infarct may result in renal emboli and hematuria. In endemic regions a history of tuberculosis may indicate genitourinary tuberculosis. Urological cancer may be prevalent in first-degree relatives (prostate, renal cancer—von Hippel-Lindau disease). A family history of urolithiasis may point toward calculi as the cause of hematuria.

Clinical assessment of hemodynamic status is essential against a background of significant gross hematuria.

Other features such as fever, sepsis, lymphadenopathy, hypertension (due to glomerulonephritis, renal parenchymal disease, renal failure, renal cystic disease, or vascular disease) and pulse rhythm (atrial fibrillation) will give clues to the diagnosis. Generalized edema may be due to glomerular disease.

Abdominal examination is done to rule out renal and bladder masses. Rectal examination helps in assessing the size, consistency, nodules, and tenderness of the prostate gland and finding rectal bleeding. The genitalia should be examined for signs of infection, bleeding, or discharge. In men, the penis is examined for growths, meatal stenosis, and phimosis.

Investigations

Laboratory

Midstream Urine

For optimal analysis, a clean-catch midstream urine specimen non-contaminated from external genitalia should be obtained and examined within 1 hour or refrigerated at 4°C. False-negative results arise when urine is stored at room temperature for longer than an hour due to changes in pH and disintegration of white or red cells.

Dipstix (Dipstick) Testing. The dipstick test is based on the liberation of oxygen from peroxide in the reagent strip because of the peroxidase-like activity of heme from erythrocytes, free hemoglobin, and myoglobin. The reaction causes the reagent strip to change color and turn green. The degree of color change is related to the amount of heme, hemoglobin, and myoglobin in the urine. Intact red cells cause a punctate color change on the strip, whereas free hemoglobin leads to uniform staining. When >250 RBCs/mL is present in the urine, the number of punctate dots increases to become uniform.

The overall sensitivity for the dipstick compared to phase contrast microscopy is over 90%, with specificity ranging from 65% to 90% (4). False-negative results occur in the presence of acidic urine (pH <5), high levels of ascorbic acid or certain drugs (captopril, rifampicin, phenolphthalein).

As well as free myoglobin and hemoglobin, povidone and microbial peroxidase from bacterial infection can lead to false-positive readings. False-positive readings are much less common than false-negative results, and up to 40% of patients with dipstick hematuria may not have hematuria confirmed on bright-field urine microscopy (4). A positive dipstick result in the presence of a negative urine microscopy or repeated dipstick test should not be discounted. The ideal standard for urine microscopy is phase-contrast microscopy, which is often not the standard investigation in most centers. One positive dipstick result, even if intermittent, should be considered worthy of full investigation, especially if risk factors for malignancy are present (see later). The presence of proteinuria indicates a likely glomerular origin for the hematuria.

Microscopy. The two main methods of microscopic examination of urine are bright field microscopy and phase contrast microscopy.

Red Blood Cells. *Bright-field microscopy* is the direct examination of centrifuged urinary sediment under a coverslip (sediment count), which is reported as the number of RBCs per HPF. The upper limit of normal of RBC excretion in the urine is approximately equal to 2 RBCs/HPF. Khadra et al. (2), using cutoffs of 10, 5, and 3 RBCs/HPF, would have missed 20%, 15%, and 10% of cancers of the urinary tract, respectively.

The speed of centrifugation, its timing, the volume in which sediment is resuspended, and the power of the HPF vary from laboratory to laboratory.

Another method of analyzing RBCs in the urine is by using counting chambers in the microscope, which determine the number of RBCs per milliliter of urine. The chamber count has greater sensitivity and precision than the sediment count, but the sediment count is easier to perform, less time-consuming, and more cost-effective.

Phase-contrast microscopy is regarded as the gold-standard microscopic examination. It is able to show components in a cell or bacteria that would be difficult to see in an ordinary light microscope. Not only are RBCs detected better, their morphology can be better determined with the phase contrast microscopy.

Circular isomorphic erythrocytes are characteristic of nonglomerular bleeding, while glomerular bleeding results in dysmorphic erythrocytes associated with proteinuria and RBC casts.

White Blood Cells. Greater than 10 white blood cells (WBCs) per HPF is seen in significant inflammation. Persistent pyuria with a negative culture may be indicative of urolithiasis, tuberculosis, or tumor.

Casts. A cast is a protein coagulum that is formed in the renal tubule and traps any tubular luminal contents within the matrix. Hematuria of glomerular origin is associated with casts. Red blood cell casts are diagnostic of glomerular bleeding. White blood cell casts may also be found in acute glomerulonephritis, pyelonephritis, and tubulointerstitial nephritis.

Crystals. Crystals of urate, calcium oxalate, or triple phosphate may be seen in those with urinary tract stones.

Culture. Urine specimens should be cultured within 24 hours of collection. Urinary tract infection is present when $>10^5$ colony-forming units (CFUs)/mL is detected in a midstream specimen of urine.

Cytology. Cytological analysis of urine may detect transitional cell carcinoma (TCC) but is highly operator dependent. Sensitivity is much higher for high-grade lesions and carcinoma in situ (CIS). Voided urine sensitivity may be improved if the first and second voided morning specimens over three consecutive days are analyzed. Barbotage cytology at cystoscopy also increases sensitivity.

Cytology does not add much in the diagnostic workup of transitional cell carcinomas, as most lesions are picked up on imaging or endoscopy. However, the real value of cytology lies in its ability to diagnose CIS, which can be easily missed during white light cystoscopy.

Cancer-Related Proteins. Various cancer-related proteins may be detected on urine analysis. Compared to cytology, it has a better sensitivity but low specificity. Extensively studied tests include nuclear matrix protein 22 (NMP-22) and bladder tumor antigen (BTA) stat test. NMP-22 can be increased 25-fold in patients with bladder cancer, and is detected in the urine by immunoassay with an NMP-22 detection kit (5). The BTA stat test detects basement membrane protein antigen released into the urine of patients with bladder cancer. Other tests include telomerase, quanticyt, immunocyte, and fibrin degradation products. Currently, urine cytology remains the standard urine test for cancer detection with no clear leader in this area.

Serum Analyses

Screening laboratory tests typically consist of coagulation studies, a complete blood count, serum chemistries, and serologic studies for glomerular causes of hematuria as directed by the medical history. Serum glucose should be checked to exclude diabetes (papillary necrosis). The prostate-specific antigen (PSA) in men should be checked to exclude prostate cancer.

Role of Imaging in Hematuria

Different imaging modalities vary in sensitivity for detecting different pathology and are described in detail in Chapter 3. The modality chosen is based on its diagnostic strengths balanced against the risks of the investigation (for example, radiation, contrast reaction), availability of equipment, and expertise to interpret image findings. The primary goal of imaging should be to exclude neoplastic disease of the urinary tract.

Intravenous Urography

Compared to ultrasound, intravenous urography (IVU) is better at detecting TCC, which usually manifests as a filling defect, in the intrarenal collecting system, pelvis, and ureter. It has limited sensitivity in detecting small renal masses 2 to 3 cm and <2 cm in diameter (sensitivity 52% and 21%, respectively) (6). It cannot distinguish solid from cystic masses, which require further evaluation with ultrasound, computed tomography (CT), or magnetic resonance imaging (MRI).

Ultrasound or IVU on its own is likely to miss upper urinary tract tumors (2). The detection rate is highest when both investigations are performed.

The IVU has a lower cost and radiation dose compared to CT. However the radiation dose is significant (3 to 4.5 mSv, equivalent to 80 chest x-rays!). It takes longer to perform than CT or ultrasound. Adverse reaction due to contrast media such as vomiting or urticaria may occur in up to 4% of patients, with a smaller proportion developing anaphylactic reaction, which can be fatal. Diabetic patients on metformin require cessation of metformin before and 48 hours after the investigation in order to avoid renal failure and lactic acidosis.

Ultrasound

Ultrasound is excellent at detecting and characterizing renal cystic masses. It is also excellent at assessing renal morphology, structure, and vasculature, and detecting hydronephrosis. It can assess bladder wall morphology, detect large bladder tumors, and assess bladder emptying. Nevertheless, ultrasound is less sensitive than IVU in diagnosing urothelial tumors.

Ultrasound has a lower sensitivity for detecting renal tumors less than 3 cm in size. Compared to CT, the sensitivity and specificity of ultrasound for detecting renal masses between 2 and 3 cm is 82% and 91%, respectively (6). The study by Khadra et al. (2) showed that if only ultrasound had been used, 43% of tumors would have been missed. The sensitivity for detecting calculi is also low, ranging from 37% to 64%, which is even poorer when compared with noncontrast helical CT (NCHCT) as the reference standard, with a sensitivity of 24% and a specificity of 90%. Stones in the pelvicaliceal system can be reliably identified only if they are larger than 5 mm (7).

The advantages of ultrasound include it being nonionizing, safe, easy to use, cheap, portable, and widely available. Therefore, in pregnant women it is the investigation of choice. The drawback of ultrasound is that it is very much operator dependent, and the spatial resolution of images is poor compared to CT.

Computed Tomography

Computed tomography is more sensitive than IVU or ultrasound in detecting small renal lesions. Noncontrast helical CT has overtaken the IVU as the investigation of choice for diagnosing urinary tract calculi. Its other advantage is its ability to detect radiolucent stones. Traditionally, CT has had a higher radiation dose compared to IVU, which discouraged its greater use. However, modern NCHCT protocols can achieve radiation doses that approach the dose of the IVU. Apart from the radiation burden and cost, disadvantages of CT include its limited availability, especially in an acute setting, and the need for specialists to interpret the images.

Magnetic Resonance Imaging

The detection rate of MRI for renal masses is comparable to CT. The slightly poorer resolution of the urinary tract on MRI compared to CT has meant that CT is more widely used. However, MRI has certain advantages over CT. Magnetic resonance (MR) urography does not require potentially nephrotoxic contrast media and therefore can be used in patients irrespective of renal function. Similar to CT, it can also combine angiography and urography in the same examination. The disadvantages of MRI are its high capital cost and limited availability. Patients with claustrophobia or metal implants are not suitable for scanning.

Arteriography

Arteriography has now been largely superseded by CT or MR angiography. It is mainly done prior to embolization (see Chapter 3).

Virtual Endoscopy

Volume-rendered three-dimensional (3D) reconstruction of CT and MR data can be explored with the technique of perspective rendering in which the computer simulates an endoscopic view of a hollow viscus or body cavity—the so-called virtual endoscopy. Virtual endoscopy has inherent advantages in that it is noninvasive and therefore avoids the risk of perforation, stricture formation, or infection.

The role of virtual ureterorenoscopy and cystoscopy in the evaluation of the urinary tract is still being defined, but it is likely that it will be useful in evaluating patients where endoscopy is difficult due to either anatomy or disease (e.g., strictures) (8).

Endoscopy

Endoscopy is ideal if the results of upper tract imaging are available before endoscopy.

Cystoscopy (Lower Tract Endoscopy)

Flexible Endoscopy. The diagnostic accuracy of flexible cystoscopy is equivalent to that of rigid cystoscopy if the urine is clear. For lesions at the anterior bladder neck, it may be superior to rigid cystoscopy. Flexible cystoscopy is a well-tolerated procedure, does not require general anesthesia, and causes less pain and complications. It can be performed in an office setting by a doctor or nurse, thus allowing rapid evaluation of the lower tract.

Rigid Endoscopy. For the vast majority of patients flexible cystoscopy should be the preferred investigation. The indications for rigid cystoscopy include persistent gross hematuria, diagnostic uncertainty at flexible cystoscopy, and in cases where access to the bladder is restricted due to disease (urethral stricture, large prostate).

Upper Tract Endoscopy/Retrograde Radiography

Ureterorenoscopy. Evidence of upper tract abnormality on imaging may warrant further evaluation by diagnostic upper tract endoscopy or retrograde ureteropyelography. Diagnostic ureterorenoscopy is then indicated for diagnosis and in suspected upper tract TCC, and for biopsy confirmation and cellular staging.

Frank hematuria that is unilateral and supravesical in origin that cannot be diagnosed by routine radiological, cytological, or hematological investigations is known as benign lateralizing hematuria (BLH). It is an indication for upper tract endoscopy, and its management is described later.

Retrograde Ureteropyelography. Retrograde ureteropyelography at the time of cystoscopy can confirm the presence of a known or suspected filling defect on IVU or discover further abnormalities.

Upper Tract Urine Cytology. The diagnostic yield of cytology can be significantly increased if selective upper tract urine cytology is performed using a ureteric catheter (aspiration or saline barbotage cytology). Retrograde brushings can also increase the sensitivity and specificity of cytological analysis.

Renal Biopsy

Microscopic hematuria in the presence of proteinuria (>500 mg of protein in the urine/24 hour collection), dysmorphic RBCs, RBC casts, or an elevated serum creatinine level should be evaluated by a nephrologist for renal parenchymal disease. The limit of detection of standard urine dipsticks for proteinuria is 300 mg/L (0.3 mg/mL). Hematuria of urological origin does not elevate protein concentration greater than 200 to 300 mg/dL (+2 to +3 on dipstick).

Management

Delaying Immediate Investigation

Referral to an urologist may be delayed in the following situations:

1. Hematuria in the presence of a positive urine culture: Although men should be investigated after a single episode, women should be treated with culture-specific antibiotics. Persistent hematuria after treatment with no evidence of urine infection warrants investigation. Microscopic hematuria in women who have repeated urinary tract infections should be investigated.
2. Exercise hematuria: Persistent hematuria after 48 to 72 hours of rest requires investigation.
3. Menstruation-associated hematuria: Hematuria during menses should be confirmed with a midcycle urine analysis before investigation.

Asymptomatic Microscopic Hematuria

Urological cancer has been detected in between 0.5% and 8.3% of patients with AMH (4). The risk of cancer increases with age and where there is a history of exposure to carcinogens.

American Urological Association Guidelines

The American Urological Association (AUA) best practice policy on the evaluation of AMH has divided patients with AMH into high- and low-risk groups (1). Patient risk factors for developing urological cancer are listed in Table 4.2. A single episode of either dipstick or urine microscopy hematuria in a patient with any of these risk factors should prompt thorough first-line evaluation consisting of urine cytology, upper tract imaging, and lower tract endoscopy. Patients with AMH and a low risk of malignancy do not necessarily require all of these investigations. In these patients, imaging of the upper tract is the primary investigation followed by cystoscopy if imaging is abnormal. If upper tract imaging is normal, urine cytology should be evaluated, followed by cystoscopy if cytology is abnormal or atypical.

For upper tract imaging, the choice remains between IVU, ultrasound, and CT. An ultrasound and plain abdominal radiograph may be sufficient in low-risk patients. High-risk patients should ideally undergo IVU and ultrasound, as

TABLE 4.2. Risk factors for developing urological cancer

1. Age >40 years
2. History of smoking
3. History of occupational exposure to chemicals (benzenes, aromatic amines, aniline dyes)
4. History of irritative voiding symptoms
5. History of cyclophosphamide treatment
6. History of analgesic abuse
7. History of pelvic irradiation
8. History of urinary tract infection
9. History of previous urological disorder or disease
10. History of gross hematuria
11. History of schistosomiasis infection

there is a risk, albeit small, of missing cancer if only one of these modalities is used (2). High-risk patients allergic to contrast medium are recommended to undergo retrograde ureteropyelography in replacement of IVU.

Gross Hematuria

The immediate consequences of gross hematuria are hemodynamic compromise and clot retention. Patients hemodynamically unstable or in urinary retention require emergency admission to hospital. The principles of immediate management are described in Chapter 11.

Significant hemodynamic compromise requires blood transfusion and close monitoring. This conservative approach is sufficient in managing the acute consequences of gross hematuria in the vast majority of patients.

Upper tract imaging and urine cytology may be carried out in the interim period while the hematuria is resolving. If the urine becomes clear, a flexible cystoscopy can be carried out under local anesthesia to assess the lower tract. Rigid cystoscopy under general anesthesia should be done where bleeding has not ceased.

Benign Lateralizing Hematuria

Benign lateralizing hematuria (BLH) is a diagnostic and therapeutic challenge. As first- and second-line investigations fail to identify a suitable cause for the bleeding, ureterorenoscopy (URS) assumes a pivotal role in diagnosis and therapy. Ureterorenoscopy usually identifies the bleeding to be emanating from a vascular lesion in the kidney, and through a combination of direct vision and biopsy, malignant lesions are ruled out.

Hemangiomas may appear as either as small red or bluish spots at the tip or base of a papilla, or as larger bulbous erythematous lesions on a papillary tip. Endoscopic treatment is the mainstay of the management for BLH. Patients with discrete lesions are more amenable to treatment. Up to 50% undergoing URS will have a discrete vascular lesion that can be treated. Diathermy fulguration and laser ablation are two effective treatments of discrete lesions that have a higher success rate (bleeding stops and does not return) compared to diffuse lesions.

Intractable Hematuria

Severe hematuria may occur as a result of radiation cystitis, bladder carcinoma, cyclophosphamide-induced cystitis, and severe infection.

Very rarely, fulguration of the bleeding lesion and subsequent irrigation on the ward through a three-way urethral catheter fails to stop bleeding. Such patients with massive uncontrollable hematuria will require other measures to stop bleeding.

Some of these methods can lead to significant morbidity and urological sequelae and are only employed when life is at risk or the patient is unable to tolerate a cystectomy. Management is discussed in Chapter 11.

Follow-Up

Urological

The concern with investigating hematuria is that malignancy may be missed. Data from studies following up patients with normal initial evaluation have demonstrated that the prevalence of malignancy is more or less nonexistent. In one study of 128 patients followed for 20 years with urine analysis, cytology, biennial cystoscopy, and IVU, malignancy was not detected (9). In the large study by Khadra et al. (2), subsequent follow-up of patients (range 2.5 to 4.2 years) with no abnormal findings revealed no neoplastic disease. This evidence provides reassurance to specialists who are able to discharge patients back to the family practitioner who should repeat urinalysis and urine cytology on an annual basis. A full evaluation including imaging and cystoscopy is required if the cytology is abnormal or symptoms develop.

Nephrological

The role of renal biopsy in patients with isolated hematuria has not been defined. Although many such patients may have structural glomerular abnormalities, they appear to have a low risk for progressive renal disease. The natural history of patients diagnosed with immunoglobulin A (IgA) nephropathy and isolated microscopic hematuria is usually benign. In up to half hematuria disappears, 20% have intermittent hematuria, and in the remainder hematuria persists. Some of these patients may develop hypertension and proteinuria over 5 to 10 years. The presence of proteinuria is the single biggest risk factor for progression of renal disease. Without proteinuria the risk of renal impairment is low and that of end-stage renal failure (ESRF) is extremely low. In the presence of significant proteinuria, hypertension, elevated serum creatinine, and additional abnormalities on renal biopsy, the risk of ESRF at 20 years may be as high as 30% (4). When the patient has persistent hematuria, either in the presence of a normal previous renal biopsy or where biopsy was not performed, follow-up should be with yearly evaluation by the primary care physician to exclude the development of hypertension, proteinuria, or renal insufficiency.

Hematospermia

Hematospermia is defined as the appearance of blood in the ejaculate. For hematospermia to occur, intact emission and ejaculation functions are necessary. Hematospermia is usually painless and self-limiting in most cases. Its exact incidence remains unknown as most ejaculates go unnoticed during intercourse. It may be indicative of a significant underlying genitourinary condition particularly in older patients where it may be a symptom of prostate cancer (10). Rarely bladder and testicular cancer can present with hematospermia.

Causes

Table 4.3 lists the causes of hematospermia (11). More recently an association between prostate cancer and hematospermia has been established. Nearly 14% of men presenting with hematospermia were found to have prostate cancer after investigation (10).

Clinical Evaluation

Clinical assessment is important in evaluating hematospermia. Most patients who notice hematospermia consult their doctor after the first episode. It is important, however, to make sure that the patient is actually describing hematospermia and not hematuria; in some cases both may coexist. If hematuria is present with hematospermia, hematuria is also investigated. Examination should include abdominal, genital, and rectal examination of prostate (11).

Investigations

The aims of investigation are to exclude neoplasia or a specific pathology that is treatable, thereby alleviating the patient's symptoms, and to reassure the patient if no causative factor is found.

Urinalysis and urine culture help to confirm the presence of urinary infection and hematuria, which if present require further radiological investigations where indicated. Semen analysis may show the presence of pus cells, which then warrants further investigation in search of an infectious etiology; this includes semen culture, urethral swabs, mycobacterial cultures, and viral serology.

Serum coagulation profile may reveal underlying bleeding disorders while the erythrocyte sedimentation rate (ESR) may be raised in tuberculosis. If sexually transmitted diseases are suspected, urethral cultures for gonorrhea and

TABLE 4.3. Causes of hematospermia

Congenital	Seminal vesicle (SV)/ejaculatory duct cysts
Inflammatory	Urethritis, prostatitis, epididymitis
	Genitourinary tuberculosis
	Cytomegalovirus, HIV
	Schistosomiasis, hydatid
	Condylomata of urethra and meatus
	Urinary tract infection
Obstruction	Prostatic and SV and ejaculatory duct calculi
	Postinflammatory SV cysts
	SV diverticula
	Urethral stricture
	Utricle cyst
	Benign prostatic enlargement
Tumors	Prostate, bladder, SV, urethra, testis, epididymis, melanoma
Vascular	Prostatic varices
	Prostatic telangiectasia
	Haemangioma
	Posterior urethral veins
	Excessive sexual intercourse, masturbation
Trauma/iatrogenic	Perineum
	Testicle
	Self-instrumentation
	Post–hemorrhoid injection, transrectal ultrasound (TRUS) biopsy
	Vasovenous fistula
Systemic	Hypertension, hemophilia, purpura, bleeding disorders, chronic liver disease, renovascular disease
	Leukemia, lymphoma
	Cirrhosis of the liver, amyloidosis

chlamydia are obtained. In patients who have a suspicious nodule on rectal examination or who are at risk of prostate cancer, a PSA test is required.

Transrectal ultrasonography (TRUS) may help in the diagnosis of prostatic and seminal vesicular pathology including calculi, cysts, müllerian duct remnants, varices, and inflammatory changes within the prostate. Any suspicious testicular swelling is investigated with an urgent testicular ultrasound examination. Magnetic resonance imaging, both conventional and endorectal coil, improves visualization of the anatomy of the pelvic organs.

Management (12)

The main aim is to exclude any underlying pathology, and if none is found after full evaluation, to reassure the patient. Although imaging may reveal the underlying cause of hematospermia, there is often little that can be offered in the form of conventional treatment.

Individuals with recurrent hematospermia and who are middle aged need specialist urological assessment and investigations. If infection is suspected, a course of 5-aminoquinolones or trimethoprim-sulfamethoxazole and doxycycline combination would be beneficial even if the urine cultures are negative. Systemic conditions are treated appropriately. Prostatic or seminal vesicular cysts can be aspirated under TRUS guidance. In recurrent hematospermia, cystourethroscopy may help to diagnose congested veins in the prostate and urethral abnormalities. Ejaculatory duct obstruction is managed by a transurethral resection (TUR) at the duct opening.

Persistent hematospermia presents difficulty from the management point of view, and a detailed radiological assessment may ascertain the exact cause. It is also important to keep these patients under follow-up for a limited period. In some patients persistent or recurrent hematospermia could be the only symptom of prostate cancer. In patients at high risk of prostate cancer, surveillance with PSA over a period of time is desirable.

References

1. Grossfeld GD, Litwin MS, Wolf JS, et al. Evaluation of asymptomatic microscopic hematuria in adults: the American Urological Association best practice policy-part I: definition, detection, prevalence, and etiology. Urology 2001;57:599–603.
2. Khadra MH, Pickard RS, Charlton M, et al. A prospective analysis of 1,930 patients with hematuria to evaluate current diagnostic practice. J Urol 2000;163:524–527.
3. Avidor Y, Nadu A, Matzkin H. Clinical significance of gross hematuria and its evaluation in patients receiving anticoagulant and aspirin treatment. Urology 2000; 5:22–24.
4. Tomson C, Porter T. Asymptomatic microscopic or dipstick haematuria in adults: which investigations for which patients? A review of the evidence. BJU Int 2002; 90:185–198.
5. Grossfeld GD, Litwin MS, Wolf JS Jr, et al. Evaluation of asymptomatic microscopic hematuria in adults: the American Urological Association best practice policy—part II: patient evaluation, cytology, voided markers, imaging, cystoscopy, nephrology evaluation, and follow-up. Urology 2001;57:604–610.
6. Brehmer M. Imaging for microscopic haematuria. Curr Opin Urol 2002;12:155–159.
7. Sandhu C, Anson KM, Patel U. Urinary tract stones—part I: role of radiological imaging in diagnosis and treatment planning. Clin Radiol 2003;58:415–421.
8. Ghani KR, Pilcher J, Patel U, Anson K. Three-dimensional imaging in urology. BJU Int 2004;94:769–773.
9. Howard RS, Golin AL. Long-term follow up of asymptomatic microhaematuria. J Urol 1991;145:335–336.
10. Han M, Brannigan R E, Antenor J-A V, et al. Association of hemospermia with prostate cancer. J Urol 2004;172:2189–2192.
11. Mulhall JP, Albertson PC. Haemospermia: diagnosis and management. Urology 1995;46:463–467.
12. Kumar P, Kapoor S, Nargund VH. Haematospermia—a systematic review. Ann R Coll Surg Engl 2006;88:339–342.

5
Nuclear Medicine in Urological Cancer

John Buscombe

In nuclear medicine the target organ is visualized by giving the patient oral or intravenous radioactive tracer material. The imaging is done with a gamma camera, which takes pictures of the radiation photons emitted by the radioactive tracer material. There are a wide range of applications of radiopharmaceutical agents in the investigation and management of urological cancers. Nuclear medicine techniques allow physiological processes to be followed in a noninvasive way, which can be done in its simplest form by using blood or urine sampling to show clearance of a radiotracer from the blood or appearance in the urine. Also processes can be imaged using scintillation devices such as the gamma camera.

The information provided is different from that obtained from other forms of radiology in that it is primarily physiological and not anatomical. Therefore, the results of nuclear medicine studies are complementary to other forms of radiology, and which type of test should be used depends on the clinical situation.

Atom Structure and Radioactivity

Every atom is made up of a nucleus and surrounding electrons. The number of positive charged protons in the nucleus matches the number of electrons in the atom in the uncharged elemental form of the atom. The number of protons determines the element to which the atom belongs and its chemical nature. However, there can be variation in the number of neutrons, which changes the atom mass of the atom but not its chemical nature; these variations are called isotopes. Some of them are unstable and spontaneously break apart, releasing energy as they do to; these are radioactive isotopes. The radioactive energy has three main forms. Alpha and beta particles are particulate and have mass and are not used in imaging. Gamma rays are pure electromagnetic energy and these are used in imaging as they can be detected by a gamma camera. The energy contained within these gamma rays is always the same for each radioisotope. A further complication is that some radioisotopes have a more unstable form (called metastable), and these are radionuclides of an individual isotope. Therefore, technetium 99m (^{99m}Tc) is the radionuclide that is the metastable form of the radioisotope of technetium, which has an atomic mass of 99.

The Tracer Principle

All nuclear medicine studies independent of their simplicity are based on de Heversey's tracer principle. In this study a small amount of a radioactive tracer is administered to the patient to track a specific physiological event, without having a pharmacological action, which may change the effect that is being observed. To do this, tiny amounts of a radioactive tracer are used, often less than a billionth of a gram. Then the radioactivity in a particular fluid in the body is measured or imaged with an external imaging device. These radioactive tracer substances are called radiopharmaceuticals.

Tracers Used in Nuclear Medicine

There is a range of radiopharmaceuticals used in the assessment of a patient's genitourinary system. These are divided into three groups:

1. Those with poor imaging characteristics that are used for in-vitro testing
2. Those that can be used for imaging using a single photon
3. Those using positron emission tomography technology

Most rely on gamma ray emission as they decay, to be detected either in a well counter or on an imaging device. When imaging the renal tract directly, most of the agents used are highly hydrophilic, allowing for rapid excretion through the kidneys. In the case of diethylenetriamine pentaacetic acid (DTPA), excretion is purely glomerular, with hippuran it is purely tubular, and mercaptoacetyltriglycine (MAG3) is mixed. In addition to the pharmaceutical there also needs to be an isotope. Together they make a specific radiopharmaceutical, which is designed to perform a specific task such as look at renal blood flow, uptake, and excretion, as in the case of DTPA.

Radionuclides

Iodine 131

The first isotopes that were used tended to be those that were produced as a by-product of the fission of uranium 238. The most common of these is iodine 131. On its own it is of little use, but it is added to hippuran to produce iodine 131 hippuran (written by convention as ^{131}I-hippuran). It is possible, using blood samples to measure the clearance of the agent from the blood, to give the effective renal plasma flow (ERPF). Using sodium iodide scintillation probes and later an Anger gamma camera, it is possible to draw uptake of the iodine 131 hippuran into the kidney and then its excretion. The images are of poor quality and the radiation dose is high, but this remains a valid test, though often a different isotope of iodine, ^{123}I, is now used as it gives slightly better images and at a lower radiation dose.

Technetium 99m

The most common isotope used in nuclear medicine is an artificial isotope of very short half-life of only 6.02 hours. This is a metastable form of technetium 99m conventionally written as ^{99m}Tc. This isotope is the decay product (called a daughter of another isotope molybdenum 99 (^{99}Mo). This too is a product of nuclear fission of ^{238}U (uranium).

However, to get sufficient quantities for medical use worldwide, special high neutron flux reactors are used because on any given day about 1 million ^{99m}Tc tests are performed for various different reasons worldwide. As the half-life is so short, it is best to have the equipment to separate ^{99m}Tc from the parent ^{99}Mo based as close to the patient as possible. Many hospitals have their own ^{99m}Tc/^{99}Mo generator on site, which can be used once or twice a day for up to 1 week.

The ^{99m}Tc is drawn off a column of insoluble molybdenum oxide and is oxidized to valency-7; therefore, it is chemically soluble sodium pertechnetate. Then using transitional metal chemistry it can be added to vials containing the required pharmaceutical with buffers and a reducing agent to allow for binding. Most of these radiopharmaceuticals take 10 to 30 minutes to prepare, depending on whether or not the product has to be boiled. Worldwide over 80% of all nuclear medicine tests use this isotope, and these techniques are widely used in developing countries.

Physical Characteristics

The ^{99m}Tc produces a single burst of radiation when it decays, called its characteristic radiation. This is measured in kiloelectron volts (keV), and for ^{99m}Tc it is 140 keV. This is ideal for the simple gamma cameras used based on a sodium-iodide scintillator. The range of radiopharmaceuticals that is available for use in urological cancers is listed in Table 5.1. Therefore, it can be seen that the same isotope can be used for a wide range of indications.

TABLE 5.1. Commonly used radiopharmaceuticals in urological cancer

Radiopharmaceutical	Indication
^{99m}Tc-diethylenetriamine-pentaacetic acid (DTPA)	Measurement of glomerular filtration rate (GFR), renography
^{99m}Tc-mercaptoacetylgly-cylglycylglycine (MAG3)	Clearance studies, renography
^{99m}Tc-dimercaptosuccinic acid (DMSA)	Divided renal function, characterization of renal space-occupying lesion
^{99m}Tc-methyldiphosphonate (MDP)	Assessment of bone metastases, renography
^{99m}Tc-labeled red cells	Assessment of cardiac function (pre- and postchemotherapy)

Measurement of Glomerular Filtration Rate

For in vitro testing of renal physiology, a long-lived isotope is preferable, attached to a product that is excreted via a single part of the nephron. For this purpose, chromium 51 (^{51}Cr) is ideal when attached to ethylenediaminetet-raacetic acid (EDTA), which is filtered by the glomerulus and not reabsorbed. The gamma irradiation is not good for imaging, but in small quantities, such as 3 to 4 MBq, it can be measured efficiently in a well counter and therefore can be used via the radioactivity in sequential blood specimens to calculate the glomerular filtration rate (GFR). This method is used in the assessment of renal function during chemotherapy, and in combination with ^{99m}Tc–dimercapto-succinic acid (DMSA) can be used to determine residual renal function after nephrectomy.

Positron Emitters

The second main class of imaging radiopharmaceuticals are positron emitters. Positrons are positively charged electrons emitted during decay of proton-rich nuclei. These are produced by bombarding a target element with positively charged particles, such as protons or alpha particles, at high speeds using a cyclotron. The resulting positron emitting isotopes tend to be of low atomic number such as oxygen nitrogen or fluorine. They have short half-lives, so they have to be used close to the site of production.

For example, the most commonly used of these positron emitters if fluorine 18 (^{18}F). It has a 2-hour half-life, and after production some time is taken to combine it with a physiologically useful organic molecule such as glucose, so it is generally considered practical if the images are performed within a 2-hour radius of the production site. This might mean, for example, 30 miles by motor vehicle or 600 miles by airplane.

Mechanism of Imaging by Positron Emitters

Positron emitters do not normally produce gamma rays per se, but the positron is essentially a form of antimatter; after it travels a short distance, normally 1 mm or so, it meets an electron and is annihilated. From Einstein's formula $E = mc^2$, we know that the tiny mass of both particles is released as a short burst of radiation, which, as the mass of the two particles is the same, is always 511 keV. These particles travel out at 180 degrees and can be detected by any paired detection system. Though traditional gamma cameras can be used, the energy is a little high for them to work efficiently, so a special crystal such as beryllium-germanium-oxide (BGO) is used. These crystals are set in a ring to collect the pairs of 511-keV photons, called co-incidence events. This type of machine is a PET camera.

Therapy Isotopes

The third type of radiopharmaceutical has a different form of emission, such as a beta or alpha particle. These particles destroy tissue but cannot be imaged, unless there is an accompanying gamma emission. However, these particles may be of use in targeting tumor tissue. In urological cancers their use until recently has been limited to pain relief from bone metastases; however, new agents that directly target cancer are entering phase II clinical trials.

Imaging Devices

To use these radiopharmaceuticals efficiently a range of imaging devices has been produced. They all rely on the same principle. They use a scintillator, which is a crystal that is temporarily energized by being hit by a gamma ray giving off light. This is picked up by a photomultiplier tube (PMT), which converts this signal to electrical energy that is amplified and passed to a computer. The simplest one of these devices has a scintillation crystal with a well in the center surrounded by a thick lead shield to prevent radiation from other sources being seen. A sample (for example, some plasma in a patient injected with ^{51}Cr-EDTA) is placed in the counter and the activity is measured over a period of time (e.g., counts/second).

The Anger Camera

A more complicated arrangement is to use a gamma camera. In this case the crystal is flat, and about 2 to 2.5 cm thick and up to 40 cm wide. About 30 to 70 PMTs are needed to cover the surface and are hexagonal to ensure that the surface is covered. To prevent scatter, which causes image degeneration, a focusing device called a collimator is affixed to the front of the machine, ensuring that only gamma rays perpendicular to the crystal face are seen. These collimators are made of lead, and the width of the septa are determined by the energy of the gamma rays and divided into low energy (0–180 keV), medium energy (181–300 keV), and high energy (>300 keV). The computer attached to the collimator determines where on the crystal a gamma ray arrived as well as its energy, as scattered photons that get past the collimator have lost energy and can be excluded.

These cameras can be mounted on gantries that can move along the patient to perform whole-body images and rotate around the patient, producing a three-dimensional image called single photon emission computed tomography (SPECT). The associated computer system can detect a series of images (every 0.5 seconds and upward) of a particular part of the body. This is called a dynamic image. Then the computer can calculate the activity of a radiopharmaceutical at any area of interest to construct a time activity curve as seen in renography.

Positron Emission Tomography Imaging

Positron emission tomography (PET) imaging does not need collimation, as a scattered gamma ray will be deflected much like a billiard ball hitting another ball. Therefore, it will not arrive at a 180-degree angle from its partner gamma ray released at the same time, and will not entail a coincidence event or be recorded. As no lead collimation is needed in PET, fewer gamma rays are stopped and the system is more efficient than a standard gamma camera.

Tomography

Both SPECT and PET are excellent methods to look at functional images of the body, and they play an increasing role in imaging of urological cancers. However, spatial resolution is limited to about 7 mm for SPECT and 3 mm for PET, although these figures are optimistic and describe the best attainable. Also, identifying the site of any abnormal uptake can be difficult due to the lack of anatomical markers. Therefore, both SPECT and PET machines have been added to CT scanners to allow for simultaneous SPECT/CT and PET/CT—a technique called image registration.

Radiation Dosimetry

The radiation burden for nuclear medicine tests tends to lie in the low to medium band. The unit of measurement is the sievert (Sv), which equals a joule of received energy per kilogram of tissue. Clearly as this is a lot of energy, normally a milli-sievert (mSv) is used.

Residents of London receive on average 2 to 5 mSv of radiation per year. Residents of Cornwall or Aberdeen who live on granite ground may receive 5 to 10 mSv due to radon gas seeping into their houses. Residents of the southern Caucasus could get 25 mSv per year, which would be enough to warrant a citation from a pollution inspector in the United Kingdom, but it seems to allow many resident there to live for over 100 years!

Unlike radiological tests, where the energy of the x-rays used may vary depending on the number of views taken, the energy of the beam and the exposure time in nuclear medicine are determined by the activity of radioisotope, which is itself governed by a statuary instrument and administered through the Administration of Radioactive Substances Advisory Committee (ARSAC) the Department of Health in the U.K., which publishes typical maximum activities and radiation doses received (Table 5.2) (1). A few radiological investigations are included for comparison. However, it can be seen that the excess radiation of a single nuclear medicine test is not great compared to background radiation.

TABLE 5.2. Radiation dose for investigations commonly used in urological cancer

Investigation	Radiation dose measured as effective dose equivalent (mSv)
3 MBq ^{51}Cr-EDTA for GFR	0.006
100 MBq ^{99m}Tc-MAG3 renogram	0.7
400 MBq ^{18}F-FDG PET scan	10
KUB plane x-ray	1–3
Spiral CT of kidneys with contrast	3–24
IVU-6 image	1–6

Assessment of Renal Function

The most commonly used isotopic test for the assessment of renal function is the measurement of the GFR with a radiopharmaceutical that is exclusively filtered in the glomerulus. There are several agents that can make this assessment, including ^{99m}Tc-DTPA and methyldiphosphate (MDP) (in the early postinjection stage). However, the short half-life of ^{99m}Tc of 6 hours means that counts must be decay corrected, and the timing of samples taken is vital.

Also in patients with impaired GFR (that is, below 30 mL/min) a 24-hour sample is needed, which is not practical with ^{99m}Tc-labeled pharmaceuticals. The method of choice, then, is ^{51}Cr-EDTA, which has a half-life of 27 days. This helps make counting simple with no real need to do decay correction, and samples may be counted 2 to 3 days after the test has been performed. In addition, taking late samples such as at 24 hours is simple.

The standard method is to take a background sample and then three samples 2, 3, and 4 hours after injection of 2 to 4 MBq of ^{51}Cr-EDTA. The activity in 1 mL of plasma is then plotted on a graph, and the rate of reduction of counts gives the GFR. However, a simpler method using one blood sample and some mathematical modeling by Martensson et al. (2) has shown that if the GFR is more than 50 mL/min, then it is just as accurate as a three-sample method. Likewise, if the GFR is less than 30 mL/min, a 24-hour sample should be added. As it may not be possible to predict the exact GFR before a test is done, more than one method may be needed. The creatinine clearance can be used as a guide, but it may be inaccurate if the patient is in a catabolic state from malnutrition (the anorexia of cancer or postchemotherapy) or has impaired renal function or a recent muscle injury, including an operation. Also the GFR is more accurate for sequential measurements, especially if treatment is given (3,4).

The main use of a GFR in urological cancer is to determine the correct dosing of nephrotoxic chemotherapy (especially platinum-based drugs) before and during therapy. The combination of the global GFR and the contribution to total renal function as determined on a DMSA scan facilitates predicting the residual renal function left after single kidney nephrectomy. The ERPF may be a better measure of early drug-induced renal toxicity than the GFR, but it has not been accepted into standard clinical practice.

Cardiac Assessment

Though not directly connected to the urological system, a well-functioning heart is required for efficient treatment of patients. Many nephrologists think the heart is there merely to perfuse the kidneys and there is some element of truth in that. However, there are two specific areas in which assessment of the heart using radionuclide techniques may be of particular value. The first is a general assessment of myocardial perfusion before any major surgery such as nephrectomy, as not only is cancer more common in the elderly but so is heart disease.

Therefore, the high negative predictive value of stress and rest myocardial perfusion scintigraphy using ^{99m}Tc-MIBI (methyliso butyliso nitrile), ^{99m}Tc-tetrofosmin, or thallium 201 chloride (^{201}TlCl) will determine, if no ischemia is identified, that a major operation can proceed without risk to the patient.

In addition, gated blood pool imaging using ^{99m}Tc-labeled red blood cells facilitates an accurate determination of left ventricular ejection fraction (LVEF), which is less dependent on left ventricular geometry than is stress echocardiography and may be more accurate in serial studies (5). It is used to assess the LVEF before and after chemotherapy with cardiotoxic drugs of the doxorubicin type, and it may be of particular value if the patient has coexistent hypertension or diabetes for which the commonly used nomograms for maximal tolerated drug may not apply.

Renography

Renography, acquired by dynamic gamma camera imaging normally with 300 MBq ^{99m}Tc-DTPA or preferably with 100 MBq ^{99m}Tc-MAG3, is not a primary method by which to assess urological cancers. However, it has two main roles. First, in combination with GFR, it may be used to determine the expected result of a nephrectomy in terms of residual renal function. For example, if a renogram demonstrates that each kidney contributes 50% of renal function and the total GFR is 80 mL/min, removal of one kidney will result in a residual GFR of 40 mL/min. Interestingly, as the most common agent used for bone imaging, ^{99m}Tc-MDP, is up to 80% excreted by kidneys during the first 20 minutes postinjection, it may be possible to combine a ^{99m}Tc-MDP renogram with a staging bone scan, which if also combined with a GFR may provide all the staging required for the patient. In nuclear medicine terms it is quick and efficient and reduces the cost and the radiation dose to the patient.

The second use of renography is to assess renal function if there is pelvic tumor that is suspected of blocking one or more ureters, in which case a high urine flow rate needs to be achieved to prevent false-positive studies due to ureteric dilatation from an old obstruction. Though frusemide can be given at any time during the renogram, if ureteric obstruction is suspected, giving the frusemide 15 minutes before the imaging agent (the Manchester protocol

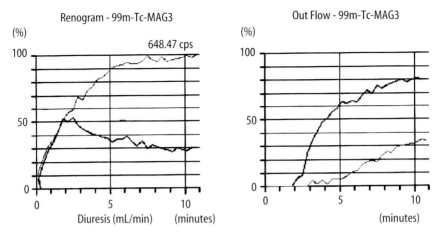

FIGURE 5.1. A flat or rising excretion phase curve suggests partial or complete obstruction of the ureter on that side.

or F-15 protocol) means that the maximum diuresis occurs when the imaging agent is injected (6). A flat or rising excretion phase curve suggests partial or complete obstruction of the ureter on that side (Fig. 5.2).

If the ureter is stented or a nephrostomy is placed, the F-15 renogram should be repeated about 48 hours later to determine if the kidney is now clearing. The divided function on the affected side will give some idea of how long the obstruction has been present, but if it is only a few days the function of the affected kidney will not be much affected; if it is more than 1 week, there can be significant reductions in divided function and recovery becomes less likely.

Ureteric Obstruction

In very acute complete obstruction, a renogram with ^{99m}Tc-MAG3 demonstrates an obstruction not in the renal pelvis but rather in the kidney parenchyma—a sort of "shock kidney" picture. The clues are that the divided function is normal, the other kidney drains, and ultrasound suggests a dilated collecting system. If this pattern is seen, early drainage procedures work well, often without any residual loss of function on the affected side.

Static Imaging of the Kidneys

Static imaging is performed in Europe using ^{99m}Tc-DMSA. This is filtered by the glomerulus and reabsorbed in the tubules and effectively maps working nephrons (Fig. 5.2). As such, it can be used to characterize space-occupying lesions seen on other imaging such as ultrasound or computed tomography (CT). A

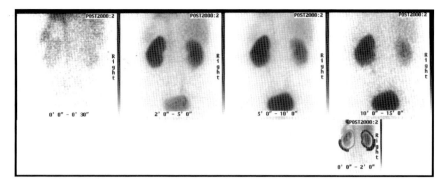

FIGURE 5.2. ^{99m}Tc-MAG3 scan showing better functioning left kidney.

study showing uptake of ^{99m}Tc-DMSA is useful in determining that cancer in unlikely. However, a defect may be due to cancer, a scar, an infarct, or a cyst. More commonly it may be used in combination with a GFR to calculate residual renal function after nephrectomy or renal call carcinoma. Imaging normally involves a series of static images including a posterior image and right and left posterior oblique images performed 2.5 to 3 hours after injection of about 150 MBq of ^{99m}Tc-DMSA.

Single photon emission computed tomography imaging can also be performed, producing three-dimensional images of the kidney (Fig. 5.3). It could be of additional use if patients suffer from congenital, recurrent, potentially bilateral, renal cell carcinomas, in which case an assessment of the residual working renal tissue can be made by the surgeons if they will attempt to maintain some working renal tissue.

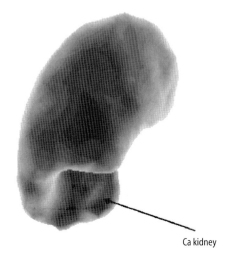

FIGURE 5.3. Single photon emission computed tomography (SPECT) image of kidney showing lower polar renal cell carcinoma (RCC).

Ca kidney

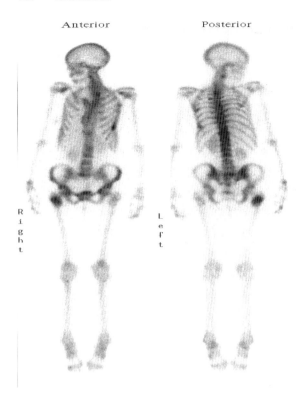

Anterior   Posterior

Right

Left

FIGURE 5.4. Bony metastasis in axial skeleton.

Bone Scanning

Bone scintigraphy is probably the test that most readers would associate with urological cancers. It is primarily used in prostate cancer, but also has a role in bladder and renal cell carcinoma as well.

The mechanism by which bone scintigraphy works is that the radiopharmaceutical, ^{99m}Tc-MDP (or one of its close associates), is injected into a vein. While dynamic imaging can be done, it is not needed for a metastatic survey. A renogram can be performed as described previously. About 3 hours after giving 550 MBq of ^{99m}Tc-MDP, a static bone scan is performed. This can be done as a series of "spot" views or as a whole-body run. In either technique it is essential that the parts of the skeleton that include the red bone marrow, namely the skull, spine, ribs, sternum, scapulae, pelvis, proximal humeri, and proximal femora, be covered (Fig. 5.4). The etiology of bone metastases being primarily hematogenous in spread, they therefore tend to be deposited in the red marrow–containing bones. The ^{99m}Tc-MDP does not attach directly to the metastases but is actually incorporated into new bone formation around the metastasis, as the bone tries vainly to repair the injury caused to itself by the metastatic cancer deposit. This laying down of new bone may be seen as increased density on x-ray and is therefore described as sclerotic type metastases. Purely lytic lesions very rarely result in uptake of ^{99m}Tc-MDP. Fortunately, in almost all cases urological cancer metastases are slow growing and tend to produce sclerotic lesions, which may be seen on radiology, but the radiological changes may lag behind the scintigraphic changes by 6 months. The actual target cell for the ^{99m}Tc-MDP is unclear and could be either the osteoblast, the fibroblast, or both.

Sensitivity and Specificity

Although the sensitivity and specificity are rarely formally tested, it has been assumed from clinical experience that bone scintigraphy is sensitive but not specific. This is generally the case, although methods that image bone marrow disease, such as magnetic resonance imaging (MRI), may be able to image metastases in the spine, pelvis, or long bones before bone scintigraphy, again by as much as 6 months. The main difficulty with bone scintigraphy has been the nonspecific uptake of the ^{99m}Tc-MDP to any injury, however trivial. Bone is slow to heal, and defects can be active for over 12 months. Typically the problem is in the ribs, where the patient might not remember trivial injuries such as walking into a door handle 9 months before. Also in older men who smoke spontaneous cough fractures are often seen in the winter and early spring. Other causes of false-positive uptake includes significant trauma such as falls, which if accompanied by a stroke or excessive alcohol intake might not be remembered; fortunately, these traumas produce linear uptake of equal intensity across several ribs (Fig. 5.5). If multiple such injuries are seen with different intensities, then frequent falls (from a cardiovascular cause or excessive alcohol intake) can be assumed.

If these causes are ruled out, then a more sinister nonaccidental injury may need to be considered, especially if the patient is incapacitated due to comorbidity and needs help from caregivers.

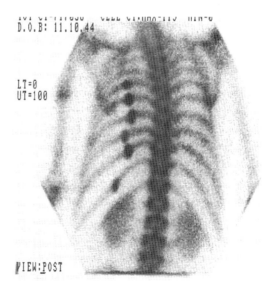

FIGURE 5.5. Isotope uptake in old rib fracture sites (left side).

The other area of nonspecific uptake is the spine. Metastases tend to favor the body of the vertebrae and the pedicles, producing areas of focal uptake within the vertebrae. Degenerative disease tends to affect the body of the vertebra adjacent to the disks, the facet joints, and anteriorly on the body if there is an active osteophyte. Correlative radiology confirming these areas and showing degenerative disease is sufficient. If, however, the x-ray or CT is normal, then metastases cannot be excluded and MRI or even bone biopsy may be needed. If there is uptake across the vertebral body with a smooth outline, a collapsed vertebra may need to be considered. It is often osteoporotic in nature, often affects more than one vertebra, and does so at different times. It then leads to a number of vertebrae having increased uptake at various intensities, often along with a cough and rib fractures. To the unwary observer it looks like multiple bone metastases but it is not.

Sometimes it is not possible to come to a definitive answer, but if antiandrogens are given, normally bone metastases respond and degenerative disease does not. Likewise, repeating the bone scan 6 or 12 hours later may provide and answer as long as curative surgery does not depend on a more rapid answer. Paget's disease commonly occurs in elderly men, and this is just the population that gets prostate cancer! The scintigraphic appearances are characteristic if one (mono-ostotic) or more than one (poly-ostotic) bone is involved (7).

In active disease uptake is intense throughout the bone, which is also expanded, and, in the case of the long bones, bowed. If the long bones are involved, then Paget's is the most likely explanation; however, in pelvic disease Paget's can look like very sclerotic metastases both scintigraphically and radiographically. This confusion can be increased if the patient has a high PSA, suggesting a high cancer load. A trial of antiandrogens may help, but it is possible for both diseases to coexist.

Diffusely increased uptake in the bones with little or no urinary activity but affecting the distal long bones equally to the axial skeleton may be due to a metabolic bone disease. Commonly this is due to hyperparathyroidism but also, surprisingly, a high proportion is due to osteomalacia.

Patterns of Abnormality

With prostate cancer the primary site for metastases beyond the locoregional area is bone. Therefore, sequential bone scintigraphies can help map the progress of the disease and the effect of any interventions. The disease load *at diagnosis* can also be predictive of outcome. Of the methods used to grade bone scans, the easiest and most robust is the one by Soloway et al. (8) (Table 5.3). The Soloway grade, along with the Gleason score, has been shown to be one of the best predictors of survival (Table 5.4) (9).

The pattern described as a "superscan" is an unusual variant in bone imaging of prostate cancer. In the case of the superscan, there is contiguous or almost contiguous metastases in the red marrow–containing bone (Fig. 5.6). All the

TABLE 5.3. Soloway grading of bone metastases at diagnosis

Grade	Appearance on bone scintigraphy
0	Normal, no metastases
1	1–5 lesions compatible with bone metastases
2	6–20 lesions compatible with bone metastases
3	More than 20 lesions but not a "superscan"
4	A "superscan" with more than 75% of axial skeleton, proximal humeri and femora involved

TABLE 5.4. Survival by Soloway grade (9)

Soloway grade	Survival at 3 years	Survival at 5 years
0	97%	96%
1	78%	68%
2–4	44%	21%

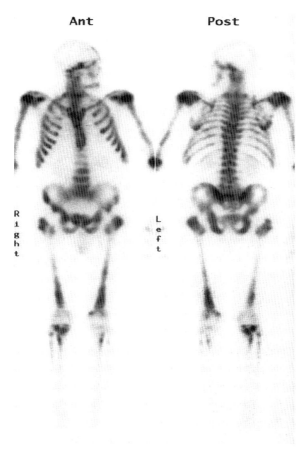

FIGURE 5.6. Anterior and posterior bone scintigraphy (Superscan in CaP [carcinoma of the prostate]): intense uptake of the isotope.

injected ^{99m}Tc-MDP is deposited in these bones, specifically the ribs, sternum, scapulae, spine, at least part of the skull, the pelvis, and the proximal humeri and femora, but not the distal long bones, which are often invisible. It is likely that such a patient would also have a PSA greater than 1000 and may have impaired bone marrow function.

Other Urological Cancers

Bladder and renal cell cancers seldom produce such a florid reaction in the bones. Often only two or three lesions are seen before death occurs from extensive soft tissue disease. However, renal cell metastases can be bizarre. There may be a single patellar metastasis and nothing else for years.

Often these metastases are painful, so any areas causing pain in these patients should always be imaged even if it is outside the normal area for metastases. In the 6 weeks following manipulation of androgens by drugs or surgery, there may be an increase or a start of bone pain accompanied by an apparent worsening of the bone scan; this is a "flare" reaction. Therefore, bone scanning should be avoided in this period, but if it is done and a flare reaction is suspected, then the scan should be repeated 3 months later when it should return to its normal activity.

A further rare appearance has been increased activity in the cortex of the tibiae, fibulae, and distal tibiae, sometimes called tram-lining. Though variously named it is known as hypertrophic pulmonary osteoarthropathy (HPOA) and may or may not be painful. Though normally associated with small cell lung cancer, it has been seen with pulmonary metastases from testicular and renal tumors.

Which Patients Should Have a Bone Scan?

Does every man with prostate cancer need a bone scintigraphy at diagnosis? The answer is plainly no. If the PSA is less than 10 and the Gleason score less than 3 + 3, the yield in a patient without bone pain does not justify a bone scan (10). However, if the patient has bone pain, a bone scintigram should be considered because if he has degenerative disease, this scan will provide a baseline for comparison, as new lesions tend to be metastatic. For a PSA greater than 20 and a Gleason score of 3 + 4, a bone scan at least at diagnosis should be performed. However, this is only a guideline, and bone scintigraphy is cheap and normally readily available; therefore, the threshold for its use should be low (11).

In renal, bladder, and testicular cancer, the case is less clear. For renal and bladder a bone scan may be useful before surgery with curative intent. If not, it should be directed by the patient's symptoms. However, presurgical screening of testicular and renal cancers may be done better by using PET rather than bone scintigraphy.

Therapy for Pain Relief

The same mechanism by which ^{99m}Tc-MDP is taken into the bone around metastases allows other radiopharmaceuticals with therapeutic isotopes also to be taken up in a similar fashion. There are three main groups: phosphorus, which is built into hydroxyapatite; analogues of calcium; and diphosphonates.

Radiophosphorus is cheap but the long penetrating beta particle of phosphorus 32 (^{32}P) means that it often results in significant bone marrow toxicity, and thus repeat treatments cannot be given. Strontium 89 (^{89}Sr) and samarium 153 lexidronate (^{153}Sm-lexidronate) produce good pain relief in 80% of patients, though the onset of pain relief is faster at 7 to 10 days after injection of ^{153}Sm-lexidronate, but retreatment is often needed after 3 months. ^{89}Sr has a longer onset of action related to its longer physical half-life, but retreatment is not normally needed for 6 months. In both agents a "flare" reaction may occur 24 to 48 hours before pain relief. Though these treatments are primarily directed toward pain relief, there is some evidence that repeat treatments can result in a delay in the advance of, or even a retreat in, bone metastases.

In continental Europe rhenium 186 diphosphonates (^{186}Re-HEDP) are used instead of ^{153}Sm-lexidronate. Interesting new research is suggesting that the use of low activities of the alpha emitter radium 232 (^{232}Ra) may prevent the development of new bone disease (12).

Sentinel Node

Since Cabanas (13) described the principle of sentinel node drainage 40 years ago in carcinoma of the penis, it has been widely used in many other cancers, such as melanoma and breast. The sentinel node principle states that every tumor has a logical lymph drainage to a particular first lymph node—the sentinel node. Other nodes and therefore other metastases are involved only after the sentinel node. Therefore, if this node is identified and removed, the possibility of cancer spreading beyond that node is very low. This node can be identified best by injecting a radiocolloid of about 100 nm such as ^{99m}Tc-nanocoll peritumorly in the subdermas. Using a combination of imaging and a hand-held gamma probe, the node can be identified and removed for histological assessment. This process may be aided by the addition of blue dye and accurate localizations of >98% have been obtained in other organs. Interest has therefore been rekindled in its use in penile, testicular, and prostate cancers.

Positron Emission Tomography

Positron emission tomography is normally performed with ^{18}F-fluorodeoxyglucose (FDG); FDG acts as a false substrate for glucose metabolism, which is increased in cancers compared to normal tissues, depending on the metabolic rate of the cancer being imaged. Unfortunately, the most common urological cancer from the prostate appears to have a low metabolic rate, and as a consequence ^{18}F-FDG is rarely positive in this disease and therefore is of little use.

Likewise, ^{18}F-FDG is excreted via the kidneys so that it may be difficult to differentiate a renal primary from background renal activity. However, in staging there is good evidence that ^{18}F-FDG PET is superior to CT in identifying lymph node disease in such a way that management was changed in 35% of patients. Overall accuracy in staging has been found to be 89% (14).

Testicular Cancer

As there are high levels of ^{18}F-FDG in the bladder, little work has been done in bladder cancer, although theoretically using catheters and bladder washout, bladder tumors could be better delineated. In testicular cancer, ^{18}F-FDG PET has been shown to have very high accuracy. In seminomas, multicenter trials have shown a sensitivity of 89% and specificity of 100% (15). One area in which PET has been found to be useful is looking for cancer in those patients with rising tumor markers but negative CT/MRI. Again the most likely area found to be abnormal is the lymph nodes, which appear on CT or MRI to be less than 1 cm and morphologically normal.

Other Positron Emission Tomography Tracers

To overcome the problem of carcinoma of the prostate having a low metabolic rate, researchers have looked at the increased uptake of amino acids in cancers, with promising results for ^{18}F-choline and ^{11}C-methionine, though the very short half-life of ^{11}C means that imaging can be done only in hospitals with their own cyclotron (16).

Antibody Imaging

After 30 years of false starts, antibodies have finally entered medicine for both imaging and therapy. In North America there has been an antibody used that is directed against prostate membrane–specific antigen (PSMA) in prostate cancer. This is labeled with indium 111 (^{111}In) and designated as CYT-356; it is commonly called Prostoscint (17). It has been shown to have a sensitivity of 86% in nodal disease but only 55% for bone disease. It has developed a role in characterizing the nature of pelvic lymph nodes that are equivocal on MRI. At present it is not available in the European Union on a routine basis.

Antibody Therapy

A final development has been the use of antibodies labeled with therapeutic isotopes that emit beta particles such as yttrium 90 (^{90}Y) and lutetium 177 (^{177}Lu) (18). These radiometals offer stable labeling of biomolecules via a linker molecule.

New antibodies have been developed, for example, J591, which is a genetically humanized antibody directed against prostate-specific prostate antigen, which is thought to be more specific of liver and growing prostate cancer than is prostate-specific antigen, which can remain expressed on dead tissue. After imaging with an indium 111–labeled version of the antibody to ensure localization on the tumor, a therapeutic dose can be given. In 29 patients treated with 300 to 1200 MBq of ^{90}Y-J591, at the higher activities there was a 40% to 90% reduction in measurable tumor and a 70% to 85% reduction in PSA. After a single treatment this was maintained for 6 months.

Nuclear medicine has an increasing role in both diagnosis and also treatment of urological cancers. Beyond the standard bone scan is an evolving role for PET and antibody-based imaging.

References

1. Notes For Guidance on the Clinical Administration of Radiopharmaceuticals and Use of Sealed Radioactive Sources Chilton, UK: ARSAC, NRBP, 1998.
2. Martensson J, Groth S, Rehling M, Gref M. Chromium-51-EDTA clearance in adults with a single-plasma sample. J Nucl Med 1998;39:2131–2137.
3. Daugaard G. Cisplatin nephrotoxicity: experimental and clinical studies. Dan Med Bull 1990;37:1–12.
4. Hjorth L, Wiebe T, Karpman D. Correct evaluation of renal glomerular filtration rate requires clearance assays. Pediatr Nephrol 2002;17:847–851.
5. Vorobiof DA, Iturralde M, Falkson G. Assessment of ventricular function by radionuclide angiography in patients receiving 4'-epidoxorubicin and mitoxantrone. Cancer Chemother Pharmacol 1985;15:253–257.
6. Upsdell SM, Testa HJ, Lawson RS. The F-15 diuresis renogram in suspected obstruction of the upper urinary tract. Br J Urol 1992;69:126–131.
7. Lentle BC, Russell AS, Heslip PG, Percy JS. The scintigraphic findings in Paget's disease of bone. Clin Radiol 1976;27:129–135.
8. Soloway MS, Hardeman SW, Hickey D, et al. Stratification of patients with metastatic prostate cancer based on extent of disease on initial bone scan. Cancer 1988;61: 195–202.
9. Richmond PJM, Dorman AM, Buscombe JR, et al. Extent of disease on initial isotope bone scan: an indicator of survival in prostate cancer patients. In: Taylor A, Nally JV, Thomsen H, eds. Radionuclides and Nephrology. Reston, VA: Society of Nuclear Medicine, 1997:211–215.
10. Cook GJ, Fogelman I. The role of nuclear medicine in monitoring treatment in skeletal malignancy. Semin Nucl Med 2001;31:206–211.
11. Oyen WJ, Witjes JA, Corstens FH. Nuclear medicine techniques for the diagnosis and therapy of prostate carcinoma. Eur Urol 2001;40:294–299.
12. Lewington VJ. Bone-seeking radionuclides for therapy. J Nucl Med 2005;46(suppl 1): 38S–47S.
13. Cabanas RM. An approach for the treatment of penile carcinoma. Cancer 1977;39; 456–466.
14. Schoder H, Larson SM. Positron emission tomography for prostate, bladder, and renal cancer. Semin Nucl Med 2004;34:274–292.
15. Hain SF, Maisey MN. Positron emission tomography for urological tumours. Br J Urol Int 2003;92;159–171.

16. Macapinlac HA, Humm JL, Akhurst T, et al. Differential metabolism and pharmacokinetics of L-(1–(11)C)-methionine and 2-((18)F) fluoro-2-deoxy-D-glucose (FDG) in androgen independent prostate cancer. Clin Positron Imaging 1999;2:173–181.
17. Feneley MR, Jan H, Granowska M, et al. Imaging with prostate-specific membrane antigen (PSMA) in prostate cancer. Prostate Cancer Prostatic Dis 2000;3:47–52.
18. Milowsky MI, Nanus DM, Kostakoglu L, et al. Phase I trial of yttrium-90–labeled anti-prostate-specific membrane antigen monoclonal antibody J591 for androgen-independent prostate cancer. J Clin Oncol 2004;22:2522–2531.

6
Anesthesic Considerations in Genitourinary Cancer Patients

Alistair F. McNarry and Heather Hackett

A successful outcome following major surgery in patients with malignant urological disease necessitates a multidisciplinary approach and close communication among the different disciplines involved in the patient's care. Surgical intervention in patients with urological malignancy must balance the benefits of early surgery, and the risks to patients, many of whom have preexisting conditions requiring investigation, treatment, and optimization.

Preoperative Assessment and Patient Optimization

Preoperative Assessment

This is a vital step in minimizing delays in scheduling surgery. Assessment allows existing medical conditions to be optimized and appropriate investigations to be carried out, preventing cancellation of patients on the day of surgery. Diseases such as ischemic heart disease, hypertension, chronic obstructive pulmonary disease, and diabetes mellitus are common in elderly patients. These conditions may be improved with simple measures such as the introduction of an inhaler, alteration of a drug dosage, or antibiotic therapy. Younger patients can also present for surgery with preexisting medical problems, the commonest being diabetes mellitus and asthma.

It is essential that underlying medical conditions are recorded at the earliest opportunity before surgery.

The Joint Anesthetic and Surgical Assessment Clinic

The ideal model for preassessment is a senior anesthetist and a junior surgeon reviewing patients in the light of the proposed surgery. This review facilitates:

- diagnosis of new ailments (e.g., hypertension)
- optimal management of existing diseases
- retrieval of notes from institutions involved in managing the patient's comorbidities

- information to be gathered from the family doctor about previous illnesses and current medications
- decision making regarding the appropriate location for a patient's post-operative care (whether that is a general ward or a specialized critical care area.)

Unfortunately, due to resource limitations, some clinics are run without any input from the anesthetic staff. This necessitates close liaison between the surgical team and the urological anesthetist.

Clinical Assessment

History

The preassessment clinic may be the first time the impact of multiple diseases can be considered. A full medical history should be taken, including a past medical history and previous hospital admissions.

Anesthetic History

It is inappropriate for a nonanesthetist to conduct an anesthetic assessment; however, two simple questions can alert staff to crucial anesthesia issues that should be reported to the anesthetist without delay:

"Have you had anesthesia before and were there any problems with it?"
"Have any family members ever had a problem with anesthesia?"

Patients' statements may have considerable significance. For example:

"They had to pass a telescope into my nose," which implies an awake fiberoptic intubation and difficult airway.
"I took a long time to wake up/breathe after surgery," which may imply suxamethonium apnea, a hereditary condition for which a diagnostic test exists.
"After my operation I woke up in the intensive care unit (ICU)." This can occur for any number of reasons, not all of them anesthesia related; however, if the surgery is not normally associated with ICU admission, then further details should be ascertained (from the notes or from the family doctor). An ICU admission may have been due to conditions such as malignant hyperpyrexia (also hereditary, diagnosed by muscle biopsy) or anaphylaxis (the precipitating agent can be found by patch testing and avoided). These rare conditions can be successfully managed, allowing surgery to proceed with early anesthesia team involvement.

Drug History

All medications including their dose and frequency must be documented. This list may differ from the list provided by a patient's family doctor. An accurate drug history facilitates therapy optimization if the medication is submaximal. Warfarin, clopidogrel, and ticlopidine can have an impact on surgery and should be discontinued. Appropriate instructions to discontinue anticoagulant therapy must be given at the preoperative visit, which may entail early hospital admission to provide an alternative anticoagulant regimen appropriate for the patient's underlying medical condition. Endocrine replacement therapy, cardiac medications, hypoglycemic agents, and immunosuppressant medications should all be recorded, as these may require specific management during the perioperative period. Other drugs may alert the clinician to previously unmentioned problems, for example, digoxin and atrial fibrillation. Eye drops, skin lotions, and nicotine patches must be documented; these drugs may not have an impact on the patient's hospital-stay but will affect their general well-being.

Allergies

Allergies and a description of the allergic response to all substances should be recorded.

Social History

Smoking. The patient's smoking history should be recorded, even for ex-smokers. The date of smoking cessation should be noted, and the extent of the patient's habit should be documented in *pack-years* by multiplying the number of packs smoked per day by the number of years. For example, smoking 20 cigarettes (one pack) a day for 10 years amounts to 10 pack-years; smoking 30 cigarettes ($1\frac{1}{2}$ packs) a day for 15 years amounts to 22.5 pack-years.

Alcohol. Ask patients for an honest estimate of their alcohol intake, which should be recorded in units. Patients who drink excessively or show signs of dependence may require an earlier admission date prior to surgery to undergo a detoxification regimen.

Recreational Drug Use and Herbal Remedies. Opioid and cocaine use both have an impact on anesthesia and should be documented. Herbal remedies may also have a signifficant effect in the perioperative period and their use should be documented.

Cardiovascular and Respiratory Systems Review

Functional status and exercise tolerance are most important, and can be measured in metabolic equivalent levels (METs) as follows:

<4 METs: poor
4 to 7 METs: moderate
>7 METs: excellent

Generally, 4 METs entails being able to walk up a hill or flight of stairs; swimming or taking part in strenuous exercise requires >10 METs (1,2). Sleeping in a chair in one's living room rather than climbing the stairs to one's bedroom may indicate severe cardiac or respiratory disease.

Other indicators of cardiac disease include the following:

- Crushing chest pain on exertion is likely to be angina, but not all presentations are typical, demanding a high index of suspicion. Chest pain at rest or on minimal exertion is always significant. Duration and frequency of attacks should be documented.

- Shortness of breath on lying flat (orthopnea) or waking up at night feeling breathless (paroxysmal nocturnal dyspnea) is a sign of heart failure. Patients may alleviate these symptoms by sleeping on several pillows. The interviewer should specifically address this issue.
- A cough may be drug induced, a sign of cardiac failure, a sign of acute infection (green sputum), or chronic bronchitis. The interviewer should ask, "Do you normally have this cough?"

Clinical Examination

Blood Pressure

A recent review suggested that it may be safe to anesthetize patients with a blood pressure of up to 180/110 mm Hg, but above this level invasive monitoring must be continued into the postoperative period in an appropriate critical care setting (3). Anesthetizing patients with preoperative hypertension must be considered in the light of the Anglo-Scandinavian Cardiac Outcomes Trial (ASCOT) study, showing benefit from amlodipine and perindopril when managing hypertension (4).

Heart Sounds

All patients with a heart murmur should have an echocardiogram to exclude valvular disease unless they have had recent review by a cardiologist. Similarly, for patients who are known to a cardiologist, the cardiologist should be consulted to ensure optimal perioperative management.

Auscultation of the Neck

Patients with an audible carotid bruit should have carotid Doppler studies performed.

Body Mass Index

Patients must be weighed in the preadmission clinic. A patient with a body mass index (BMI) of greater than 35 is a surgical and anesthetic challenge and more likely to have underlying ischemic heart disease, hypertension, and diabetes. Very heavy patients require special arrangements in the operating room to ensure, for example, that the operating table can support the extra weight.

An ICU bed may be required for obese patients, particularly those with symptoms of obstructive sleep apnea, such as daytime somnolence, headache on waking (CO_2 retention), or loud snoring (ask patient's partner).

Referral to Anesthesiologist

Anesthetists grade the patient's overall condition according to the American Society of Anesthesiologists (ASA) scheme originally devised in 1941 (5), with

TABLE 6.1. American Society of Anesthesiologists (ASA) Physical Status Classification (6)

ASA 1	A normal healthy patient
ASA 2	A patient with mild systemic disease
ASA 3	A patient with severe systemic disease
ASA 4	A patient with severe systemic disease that is a constant threat to life
ASA 5	A moribund patient who is not expected to survive without the operation
ASA 6	A declared brain-dead patient whose organs are being removed for donor purposes

Note: Emergency operation is designated by "E" after the appropriate classification.
The original scale did not have ASA 6.

the current version shown in Table 6.1 (6). Although the ASA scale does not correlate linearly with mortality, it is simple to apply.

Any patient seen in the preassessment clinic who is thought to be ASA 3 or above should be referred to the appropriate urological anesthetist for assessment as soon as possible.

Investigations

The investigations carried out should be determined by the history and examination. All investigations must be reviewed preoperatively.

Laboratory Investigations

The following laboratory tests should be done:

- Full blood count
- Grouping and cross-matching: Blood should be grouped and saved or cross-matched in accordance with hospital policy and the maximum surgical blood ordering schedule (Table 6.2) (if applicable). An allowance should be made for the invasion of vascular structures by renal tumors where appropriate.
- Creatinine, urea, and electrolytes
- Random blood sugar (may be included with electrolytes)
- Coagulation studies: Tests of hemostasis are unlikely to be abnormal unless the patient has been taking an anticoagulant or has deranged liver function. The effects of aspirin and the low molecular weight heparins will not be detected by standard clotting tests (LMWH requiring a factor Xa assay). Some anesthesiologists will require a clotting screen if they are planning a regional technique.

TABLE 6.2. Maximum surgical blood ordering schedule

Procedure	Number of units to be cross-matched
Cystectomy	6
Cystectomy and urethrectomy	8
Nephrectomy	2
Open prostatectomy (RPP)	2
TUR bladder tumour	Group and save only

RPP, retropubic prostatectomy; TUR, transurethral resection.

Patients on Anticoagulants

The following issues must be addressed:

1. What underlying condition is being treated? What investigations are required to establish its extent (e.g., arterial blood gases for a patient with pulmonary emboli)?

2. How soon before surgery should the anticoagulation be discontinued? This will require liaison between surgeons and hematologists. Patients with a mechanical heart valve may need their anticoagulation changed to a heparin infusion or its low-molecular-weight heparin (LMWH) equivalent. Liaison with the hematologist (and cardiologist) is essential.

3. How soon after surgery should anticoagulation be reintroduced?

4. Has an interim strategy to treat the underlying condition been considered?

When agreement has been reached to discontinue warfarin (generally 3 to 5 days before surgery), clotting studies (international normalized ratio, INR) should be repeated preoperatively. A multidisciplinary approach involving the surgeon, hematologist, and anesthetist is required.

Low-dose aspirin in isolation is not an anesthesia risk, although it may be stopped for surgical reasons. Multimodal antiplatelet therapy is a more complete issue and needs careful consideration.

Clopidogrel and ticlopidine are newer antiplatelet agents, and while results from the Clopidogrel in Unstable Angina to Prevent Recurrent Events (CURE) study (8) led some authors to suggest that where operative bleeding risks were high, discontinuation of clopidogrel 5 days prior to surgery would appear appropriate (9). The American Society of Regional Anesthesia suggested in 2003 that clopidogrel should be stopped 7 days prior to a regional anesthetic technique and ticlopidine should be stopped 14 days preceding it (10). In patients taking these agents, it is essential to establish why the agents were started. If their use is related to stenting of the coronary vasculature, the risks of stopping the drugs early to expedite surgery must be balanced with the potential for stent occlusion and myocardial infarction.

Anticoagulant guidelines are ever evolving and even the information in this chapter must not be considered up to date. Most recent guidelines should always be followed.

Liver Function Tests

Abnormal liver function tests (LFTs) may be due to medication or disease, but they are not normally requested without a clinical indication, unless used to establish a baseline in major surgery. Patients who consume, or are suspected of consuming, large quantities of alcohol should have a γ-glutamyltransferase (GGT) level recorded.

Tests for Sickle Cell Disease

Sickledex testing should be carried out on all Afro-Caribbean patients who do not know or who cannot provide evidence of their sickle status. A positive

Sickledex test does not differentiate heterozygous (sickle trait) or homozygous [sickle disease (HbSS)] patients. The disease state is associated with a lower hemoglobin.

Homozygous (HbS) patients should have their sickle-cell hemoglobin levels recorded. In liaison with the hematologists, the usual aim prior to surgery is to reduce HbS present in the blood to <30%. There are specific anesthetic considerations requiring early involvment of a senior anesthetist for sickle disease (HbSS) patients, early referral is paramount.

Arterial Blood Gasses

Arterial blood gas analysis and pulmonary function tests may be of benefit in certain cases, but should not be performed routinely without discussion with the anesthetist involved.

Radiological Investigations

Routine chest x-rays are unlikely to be beneficial but should be performed in the presence of cardiac or respiratory symptoms (*not* mild asthma) or where there is a suspicion of metastatic spread.

Electrocardiogram

A resting electrocardiogram (ECG) should be recorded on all male patients over 40 and all postmenopausal patients. Any other patients with signs or symptoms of cardiac disease should also have an ECG. Diabetics are at risk of silent myocardial ischemia and should have an ECG from the age of 35.

Other Cardiological Investigations

An echocardiogram should be performed in all patients with a cardiac murmur. It can estimate left ventricular function and give information on valvular disease. Exercise or pharmacological stress testing should be reserved for patients who demonstrate a poor physiological reserve or who are having a high-risk surgical procedure (advancing age, anticipated large blood loss/fluid shifts, prolonged surgery). If exercise testing is indicated, early consultation between the anesthetist and the cardiologist is mandatory, as some patients will need to proceed to angiography, a procedure not without risk.

Recently, the National Institute for Health and Clinical Excellence (in the United Kingdom) published guidelines (7) for appropriate preoperative testing (echocardiography or exercise testing were not included). The guidance above takes this document into account but does not follow it strictly.

All preoperative investigations should have a purpose, and the range of tests depends on the patient, the planned surgery, and the type of anesthesia.

Patients with Pacemakers

Pacemakers treat an underlying cardiac pathology. This pathology must be ascertained:

TABLE 6.3. The North American Society of Pacing and Electrophysiology/British Pacing and Electrophysiology Group generic pacemaker code (revised 2000) (11)

Position Category:	I Chamber(s) paced	II Chamber(s) sensed	III Response to sensing	IV Rate modulation	V Multisite pacing*
	0 = None	0 = None	0 = None	0 = None	0 = None
	A = Atrium	A = Atrium	T = Triggered	R = Rate	A = Atrium
	V = Ventricle	V = Ventricle	I = Inhibited	modulation	V = Ventricle
	D = Dual	D = Dual	D = Dual (T + I)		D = Dual
	(A + V)	(A + V)			(A + V)
Manufacturer	S = Single	S = Single			
designation only:	(A or V)	(A or V)			

*The original use of the 5th letter to indicate defibrillator function has been replaced by a letter that now describes multisite pacing.

- When was the pacemaker last tested? Pacemakers are usually tested yearly, but a test should be arranged preoperatively if one was not done recently; a liaison with the patient's local center can arrange it.
- What sort of device is it? Usually there is a five-letter code (Table 6.3) (11).

Bedside testing of pacemakers with a magnet is no longer appropriate.

Patients Having Periodic Transurethral Resections of a Bladder Tumor

This is one of the commonest operations performed in urology and warrants special mention. These patients have frequent surgical interventions, and thus are usually well known to the anesthesia and surgery teams. It is inappropriate to subject them to repeated tests that are always normal. It is equally inadvisable to expose them to the risks of anesthesia without doing the appropriate investigations first.

A balance must be struck on the investigations required based on clinical examination and evaluation at each presentation. This patient population tends to be older and it cannot be assumed that symptoms and signs will remain static. Questions such as, "Do you feel as well as you did when you had your last operation?" can be helpful. A full blood count, urea and electrolytes, and ECG need not be performed prior to every anesthetic (assuming the results are normal the patient's condition stable, and the time interval short). Patients on diurectics should always have their electrolytes checked and all patients should have their blood pressure and blood sugar measured on each visit. More complex investigations such as an echocardiogram should only be repeated if clinically indicated. Chest x-rays should only be performed if symptoms dictate.

Perioperative Management

Fasting

Fasting patients before surgery minimizes the risk of aspiration pneumonitis. Generally, no solid food should be taken 6 hours before surgery, but clear fluids are permitted until 2 hours preoperatively. Clear fluid is defined as fluid through which newspaper print can be read, not milky drinks. Most hospitals have a fasting policy that should be adhered to. Chewing gum appears to have a variable effect on gastric volume and pH, but to prevent confusion and complication it should be avoided for the six hours prior to surgery. Preoperative fasting should not prevent the administration of routine medications or a specified premedication.

Routine Medications

Most medications should be continued up to surgery (see above), particularly antihypertensive and diuretic drugs. For cardiac conditions, patients on beta-blockers with a heart rate <50 beats per minute may benefit from a dose reduction on the day prior to and the day of surgery, but this step should only be taken in discussion with the anesthetist. Simply stopping a beta-blocker may result in rebound hypertension. Some anesthetists omit angiotensin-converting enzyme (ACE) inhibitor drugs on the morning of surgery, but this practice is not universal.

If the patient is likely to be nil-by-mouth for a period postoperatively, consideration must be given as to how to administer drugs such as anticonvulsant medications. Intravenous dosing may be possible.

Endocrine Therapies (Excluding Management of Diabetes)

Patients who require bilateral adrenalectomy should have a perioperative plan that their endocrine team agrees to. Replacement therapy for hypothyroidism should be continued with the normal dose of thyroxine (T_4) up to surgery. Omitting a few doses postoperatively following surgery is not unsafe, as T_4 has a long half-life of 7 days. Patients taking steroid replacement for other diseases will need replacement if their steroid dose of prednisolone is >10 mg per day or has been in the preceding 3 months. They should continue their normal dose until surgery, when they should receive 25 mg hydrocortisone at induction and 100 mg/day for 48 to 72 hours postoperative (24 hours for TURBT [transurethral resections of a bladder tumor]) (12).

Medications for Patients with Transplant Organs

Patients with transplanted organs are a small faction of the population, but long-term survival continues to improve and patients can present with other diseases. They present problems for two reasons: (1) damage done to the rest of the body by the disease process prior to transplantation, and (2) the potentially complex and sometimes toxic immunosuppressant regimen required to protect the transplant. Early liaison with the transplant team to ensure optimal graft function perioperatively is advised, along with involvement of the pharmacist to ensure that appropriate immunosuppressants are available (intravenously if necessary).

Antibiotics

The best practice is to prescribe antibiotics preoperatively on the patient's drug chart. Different antibiotics (but with the same spectrum of cover) must be used if a patient is allergic to the usual combination. Recent antibiotic use may also necessitate a change.

Patients in the hospital for a prolonged period may require different antibiotics from those patients recently admitted. Patients with artificial or damaged heart valves should receive endocarditis prophylaxis in keeping with established guidelines, such as those of the British National Formulary (13). Clinicians should seek microbiological advice in difficult cases or where the appropriate therapy is unclear.

Bowel Preparation

Bowel preparation is potentially associated with the loss of large amounts of fluid and electrolytes, which should be replaced on the ward at the same time that bowel preparation is ongoing. One to 2 L of a crystalloid solution is appropriate in an otherwise healthy individual.

Diabetic Patients

Diabetes may be newly diagnosed at the preoperative assessment.

Patients with type 1 insulin-dependent diabetes are on insulin and generally have been diabetic since childhood. They are usually aware of their normal blood sugar range. They tend to understand how good their control is (HbA$_{1c}$, glycosylated hemoglobin). These patients are likely to be under yearly endocrine clinic review for various complications. Long-acting insulins should be omitted the night before surgery and shorter acting insulins from the morning of surgery.

Patients with type II non–insulin-dependent diabetes may control their blood sugar with insulin, oral hypoglycemics, or just diet alone. The diagnosis is usually made later in life. They may or may not regularly measure their blood sugar and may not be aware of their blood sugar range. Prior to major surgery insulin or oral hypoglycemics should be stopped in discussion with the anesthesiologist.

The key to the perioperative management of diabetes is the regular measurement of blood sugar. Fasting patients with an elevated blood sugar should be managed with a variable dose (sliding scale) of short-acting Actrapid insulin. Hypoglycemia should be avoided (cerebral damage) and patients should never routinely receive insulin infusions without a simultaneous dextrose infusion. All patients should have an easily administered emergency glycemic agent prescribed.

The results of the Van den Berghe et al. (14) study in critically ill patients may mean that postoperative normoglycemia will be the ideal, even in those nondiabetic patients who have an elevated blood sugar secondary to the stress of surgery. Type 2 diabetic patients requiring insulin tend to demonstrate a greater degree of insulin resistance; that is, they require more insulin to control their blood sugar than those with type 1 disease. However, the same care should be taken to avoid hypoglycemia.

Optimal control may be achieved by a feedback mechanism. The Actrapid dose is not dictated by an absolute blood sugar value, but it is controlled by the recent change in blood sugar. A rising blood sugar will trigger an increase in the sliding scale followed by more frequent blood sugar measurements until stability is restored. Usually local policies and protocols for the management of not-by-mouth diabetic patients been agreed in advance between the endocrine and anesthetic teams and should be followed. An endocrinologist and an anesthetist should be directly involved in the care of brittle diabetics and with those patients where a prolonged fast is envisaged.

Procedures like TURBT are frequent and usually of short duration. If the diabetic patient is scheduled for early surgery, the patient can return to the ward and eat and drink almost immediately, and then continue taking their antidiabetic medication, avoiding the need for the glucose/insulin sliding scale. Management of these patients is best arranged with the anesthetist and patient before surgery, and must again be dictated by regular blood sugar estimation.

Diabetics who present at preadmission with high blood sugar or whose blood sugar is poorly controlled require earlier hospital admission for management of their diabetes.

Deep Venous Thrombosis

Deep venous thrombosis (DVT) prophylaxis should be considered for every patient. Malignancy is one of many factors that increases the risk of venous thrombosis and consequently pulmonary embolism.

Simple preventative measures may include the use of Graduated Elastic Compression Stockings (e.g., TED-thromboembolism deterrent stockings). These must fit properly to have an effect. Intermittent compression devices which stimulate fibrinolysis can also be used. Pharmacological options include unfractionated and low molecular weight heparins. Individual surgeons and institutions will have there own policies, and these should be followed. However, all patients must have their risk of thromboembolic disease quantified, and they should be treated accordingly. Complex patients (e.g., previous DVT or PE) should be referred early for appropriate management, which may include an inferior vena cava filter in certain specific circumstances. Pharmacological measures must be timed to allow safe central neuraxial blockade—at least 6 hours preoperatively for heparin and 12 hours preoperatively for an LMWH. Similar caution is required when removing epidural catheter; anesthetic advice should be sought.

Choice of Anesthetic Technique

The decision on which type of anesthesia to use is based on the combination of the physiological status of the patient and the demands of the surgery. The choices are as follows:

- Local anesthesia, including individual peripheral nerve blockade
- Central neuraxial blockade
  - Spinal
  - Epidural
  - Combined spinal epidural technique
- General anesthesia

Local anesthesia infiltration may provide useful analgesia when administered into the wound as it is closed.

Spinal anesthesia (subarachnoid blockade) involves injection into the cerebrospinal fluid (CSF) (i.e., the dura is penetrated) of a small amount of local anesthetic usually mixed with a small dose of an opioid. This provides profound analgesia to a predetermined (although variable) dermatomal level for a limited time period. It is ideal for endoscopic procedures that will last around 60 minutes because the patient can remain awake, and any neurological deterioration that might be the first sign of hyponatremia is easily recognizable.

Patients who have had a spinal (or epidural) are unable to feel bladder distention until after the block has worn off, so careful attention must be paid to the catheter outflow channel to ensure that clot retention is not missed.

An epidural entails the placement of a catheter into the epidural space through which a local anesthetic (possibly with added opioid) is infused, which provides similar analgesia to a spinal but requires a higher dose of local anesthetic. Patients undergoing major surgery may have epidurals placed for postoperative pain relief; this may also serve to reduce intraoperative blood loss with improved circulation in the legs. Patients who have an epidural in situ must have an indwelling urethral catheter to prevent urinary retention. Patients with an epidural catheter in situ must be cared for only in wards or areas where the nursing staff are experienced with this type of patient. It is essential that an epidural be clearly labeled so that inadvertent administration of intravenous drugs into the epidural space does not occur, as this can cause catastrophic complications. In addition to clear labeling, some hospitals use different colored sets for intravenous and epidural infusions.

Patients with an epidural who complain of a headache in the postoperative period, particularly one made worse by sitting up or coughing, may have had an inadvertent dural puncture. The anesthetist should be alerted as soon as possible. Removal of epidural catheters must be done carefully to reduce the risk of epidural hematoma formation, as follows:

- 12 hours after or 2 hours before a dose of LMWH
- 6 hours after or 1 hour before a dose of unfractionated heparin

Patients who require systemic anticoagulation should be discussed with the anesthetist before or during surgery and a management plan established. In major cases most anesthetists use a combination of techniques.

TABLE 6.4. Levels of care, from the Intensive Care Society (15)

Level 0	Normal ward care in an acute hospital
Level 1	Care in an acute ward with additional support
Level 2	Care for a single organ failure or stepdown from a higher level of care
Level 3	Advanced respiratory support or support of two organ systems and including all complex patients with multiorgan failure

Postoperative Care

An important decision is whether the patient requires intensive, or level 3, care (Table 6.4) (15) following major surgery. Many countries throughout Europe report a shortage of intensive care beds (16), and patients requiring urgent cancer surgery may end up in level 2 or lower level care at the end of their procedure. This necessitates more medical input from the surgical team in order to correct any physiological deficit. Patients who are cared for in a ward environment with or without a specialist nurse will have to be entirely managed by the surgical team.

Invasive Monitoring in the Postoperative Period

Arterial Lines

Arterial lines principally provide beat-to-beat measurement of blood pressure and allow for easy blood sampling for routine postoperative bloods and blood gases. However, there are two major disadvantages: (1) The transducers need regular calibration and maintenance. Noninvasive blood pressure measurement should be carried out regularly to ensure agreement. (2) Arterial line disconnection can lead to rapid significant blood loss. For this reason arterial line use is limited to critical care areas where close monitoring is ensured.

Central Venous Catheters

Most patients undergoing major urological surgery will have a central line inserted in either the internal jugular or subclavian veins. When properly positioned it provides a guide to filling. All central lines should be x-rayed after the operation to ensure that the tip appropriately positioned (just above the right atrium) and that there are no complications such as a pneumothorax. Although central lines can be useful in the postoperative period, it is important to remember that fluid administration through a central venous (CVP) line is slower than that through a short wide (14-gauge) peripheral cannula. Regular CVP measurements can provide a guide to filling pressure; however, they are only part of the overall clinical assessment. Other simple observations such as peripheral temperature, conscious level, blood pressure, and urine output must also be considered. The CVP readings are influenced by patient and transducer position. If the readings are recorded manually, different staff may get different results. Central lines are also an infection hazard. They should be removed as soon as possible following surgery, and removed immediately if the skin around the insertion site becomes red or there are signs of an infection. They should not be left in situ to avoid peripheral cannulation.

Pain Relief

Postoperative pain relief is more than alleviating patient symptoms. Good pain relief allows for earlier mobilization and ensures the adequacy of the respiratory effort combatting pulmonary complications. It is usually provided in one of two ways:

1. Patient-controlled analgesia (PCA) device: This device delivers a set amount of an opioid (usually morphine or fentanyl) on patient demand after a safety "lock-out" period has been exceeded. Patients using a PCA must have regular observations of their pain score, respiratory rate, and consciousness level, with nursing staff empowered to discontinue the device if certain parameters exceed set limits. The disadvantages of PCA devices include the side effects of opioids, namely nausea and vomiting requiring regular antiemetic administration, and drowsiness.

Elderly patients may have difficulty using the PCA device button to administer the analgesia, and confused postoperative patients may not understand how to use the device effectively. Patients using a PCA device should have oxygen prescribed routinely because of the risk of hypoxemia secondary to hypoventilation.

2. Analgesia using an epidural: As discussed above, epidurals act by providing an infusion of local anesthetic around the spinal nerve roots. Due to reduced sympathetic tone when effective, the blood pressure is normally lower than in patients who do not have an epidural; urine output and conscious level are useful guides to organ perfusion in this situation. Patients receiving epidural infusions may develop a motor block in some areas of the distribution of the sensory loss causing significant leg weakness. This is an important consideration with early mobilization.

Complications Associated with Epidurals

A block above spine level T4 (sensory loss above the nipple line) may cause significant bradycardia and a secondary decrease in blood pressure. Should this occur the rate of epidural infusion should be reduced and help sought from the anesthetist supervising the epidural. If the epidural is inadequately controlling a patient's pain due to a low block, then the infusion rate can be increased to cause upward spread of the local anesthetic. This should be done only by staff members who have received appropriate training in epidural management. Help from the anesthetist should be sought early to ensure continuing analgesia. Epidurals may become dislodged or even be pulled out completely, causing the gradual return of pain and sensation. Should this occur, the epidural should be discontinued and substituted by a PCA device. Severe pruritus while an epidural is in situ is believed to be due to the added opioid. Small doses of intravenous naloxone can be used to treat pruritus.

Approximately 1% of patients who have had an epidural develop a postdural puncture headache characterized by occipital pain, or a nuchal headache that is worse on sitting up and resolves on lying down. The patient may be photophobic and display signs of meningism. The supervising anesthetist should be contacted promptly if this appears to be the case. If a postdural puncture headache is suspected, an infective cause should still be actively excluded. No epidural should be left in situ for more than 5 days, and it should be removed if the patients starts to complain of any symptoms or has signs of local or systemic infection.

Nonopioid Analgesics

No patient receiving PCA opioids or opioids as part of an epidural infusion should simultaneously receive opioids by another route. However, all patients following major surgery should receive multimodal pain control. Paracetamol is known to be opioid sparing and can now be given by IV, PO (by mouth), and PR (per rectum) routes. It should be administered regularly wherever possible to all patients. Nonsteroidal antiinflammatory drugs (NSAIDs) such as diclofenac sodium can be given IV, PO, or PR and are also opioid sparing. Some clinicians avoid NSAIDs in the immediate postoperative period because of concerns about the effect of this class of drugs on platelet function.

Other potential side effects of these drugs include renal dysfunction and gastrointestinal bleeding. Recently developed cyclooxygenase-2 (COX-2) selective NSAIDs should have a better side-effect profile in these areas; however, there have been concerns about their cardiac safety. The present clinical advice for their use in the acute setting remains unclear.

Oxygen Administration

Patients who have had major surgery are routinely prescribed oxygen in the postoperative period. Ideally this should be continued for three nights, because of the inherent risk of myocardial ischemia caused by the rapid eye movement (REM) rebound phenomenon. Myocardial ischemia may proceed to a silent postoperative myocardial infarction (MI), which has an associated high mortality. As stated previously, all patients with PCAs should also routinely have oxygen.

Blood Transfusion

Recent guidelines suggest that transfusion is strongly indicated if the hemoglobin is 7.0 g/dL or below, while it should not normally be considered if it is above 10.0 g/dL (17). The guidance suggests that a level between 8 and 10.0 g/dL is safe even for patients with significant cardiorespiratory disease.

TABLE 6.5. The patient-at-risk (PAR) score, an example of an early warning score (19)

	3	2	1	0	1	2	3
				Points scored			
TMP		<35.0	35.0–35.9	36.0–37.4	37.5–38.4	≥38.5	
HR	<40		40–49	50–99	100–114	115–129	≥130
SBP	<70	70–79	80–89	100–179		≥180	
RR		<10		10–19	20–29	30–39	≥40
SpO₂	<85%	85–89%	90–94%	≥95%			
CNS				A	C	V	P or U
UO	Nil	<0.5/k/h	Dialysis	0.5–3/k/h	>3/k/h		

TMP, temperature (° centigrade); HR, heart rate (beats per minute); SBP, systolic blood pressure (mm Hg); RR, respiratory rate (breaths per minute); SpO₂, oxygen saturation (%); CNS, central nervous system (neurological assessment): A, alert; C, confused; V, responds to voice; P. responds to pain; U, unresponsive (subjective assessment by scorer); UO, urine output (mL·kg⁻¹hour⁻¹); Dialysis, undergoing regular dialysis.

Points are scored depending on the degree of physiological abnormality, the total number of points are then summed to give the PAR (patient-at-risk) score.

A response is usually triggered if any category scores 3 points, or the total score is 5 or more.

Identifying the Critically Ill Patient

A patient's condition may deteriorate even after uneventful successful surgery, for example, due to a chest infection or acute on chronic renal failure. We know that patients with an increasing number of abnormal physiological measurements have an increased mortality (18). These patients can be identified by careful assessment and the use of early warning scores (Table 6.5) (19), which use easily recordable bedside parameters (heart rate, respiratory rate, conscious level, oxygen saturation, temperature, urine output, and blood pressure) to identify patients at risk. These patients should not be ignored, and rapid review by senior surgical staff should be arranged with input from critical care physicians if necessary. Early appropriate management may reduce intensive care (re)admissions and postoperative mortality.

References

1. Priebe H-J. The aged cardiovascular risk patient. Br J Anaesth 2000;85:763–778.
2. Eagle KA, Berger PB, et al. ACC/AHA guideline update for perioperative cardiovascular evaluation for noncardiac surgery—executive summary: a report of the American College of Cardiology/American Heart Association Task Force on Practice Guidelines (Committee to Update the 1996 Guidelines on Perioperative Cardiovascular Evaluation for Noncardiac Surgery). J Am Coll Cardiol 2002;39:542–553.
3. Howell SJ, Sear JW, Foëx P. Hypertension, hypertensive heart disease and perioperative cardiac risk. Br J Anaesth 2004;92:570–583.
4. Dahlöf B, Sever PS, et al., for the ASCOT investigators. Prevention of cardiovascular events with an antihypertensive regimen of amlodipine adding perindopril as required versus atenolol adding bendroflumethiazide as required, in the Anglo-Scandinavian Cardiac Outcomes Trial-Blood Pressure Lowering Arm (ASCOT-BPLA): a multicentre randomised controlled trial. Lancet 2005;366.

5. Saklad M. Grading of patients for surgical procedures. Anesthesiology 1941;2: 281–284.

6. http://www.asahq.org/clinical/physicalstatus.htm. Owned American Society of Anesthesiologists. Accessed on May 29, 2007.

7. http://www.nice.org.uk/pdf/Preop_Fullguideline.pdf. Site owned by National Institute for Health and Clinical Excellence (Formerly the National Institute for Clinical Excellence (NICE)). Accessed on May 29, 2007.

8. The Clopidogrel in Unstable Angina to Prevent Recurrent Events (CURE) trial investigators. Effects of clopidogrel in addition to aspirin in patients with acute coronary syndromes without ST segment elevation. N Engl J Med 2001;345:494–502.

9. Newby DE, Nimmo AF. Prevention of cardiac complications of non-cardiac surgery: stenosis and thrombosis. Br J Anaesth 2004;92:628–632.

10. Horlocker TT, Wedel DJ, et al. Regional anesthesia in the anticoagulated patient: defining the risks (the second ASRA consensus conference on neuraxial anesthesia and anticoagulation. Regional Anesth Pain Med 2003;28:172–197.

11. Bernstein AD, Daubert J-C, et al. The Revised NASPE/BPEG Generic Code for anti-bradycardia, adaptive-rate, and multisite pacing. PACE 2000;25:260–264.

12. Nicholson G, Burrin JM Hall GM. Peri-operative steroid supplementation. Anaesthesia 1998;53:1091–1104.

13. Joint Formulary Committee. British National Formulary, 49th ed. London: British Medical Association and Royal Pharmaceutical Society of Great Britain, 2005.

14. Van den Berghe G, Wouters P, et al. Intensive insulin therapy in the critically ill patients. N Engl J Med 2001;345:1359–1367.

15. Intensive Care Society. Levels of Critical Care for Adult Patients. London: ICDS, 2002.

16. Vincent JL. Forgoing life support in western European intensive care units: the results of an ethical questionnaire. Crit Care Med 1999;27:1626–1633.

17. Association of Anaesthetists of Great Britain and Ireland. Blood Transfusion and the Anaesthetist: Red Cell Transfusion. London: AAGBI, 2001.

18. Goldhill DR, McNarry AF. Physiological abnormalities in early warning scores are related to mortality in adult inpatients. Br J Anaesth 2004;92:882–884.

19. Goldhilll DR, McNarry AF, Mandersloot G, McGinley A. A physiologically based early warning score for ward patients: the association between score and outcome. Anaesthesia 2005;60:547–553.

7
Laparoscopy in Urological Oncology

Jose R. Colombo, Jr., Georges-Pascal Haber, and Inderbir S. Gill

The laparoscopic approach has evolved in the field of uro-oncology. In special-ized centers, the laparoscopic technique has been employed in the treatment of kidney, adrenal, prostate, bladder, urothelial, and testicular cancers. The minimally invasive approach reproduces open surgery with less morbidity, allowing quicker convalescence. This chapter presents the oncological outcomes of laparoscopic surgery and briefly discusses the technical aspects of each procedure.

Oncological Outcomes

Kidney Cancer

The laparoscopic approach to radical nephrectomy (LRN) is considered a stan-dard procedure for most patients with renal malignancy who are not eligible for a nephron-sparing procedure. Recent reports have indicated intermediate-term oncological data comparable to open radical nephrectomy. Since Clayman et al.'s (1) initial report of laparoscopic nephrectomy in 1991, laparoscopic nephrectomy has achieved a standard-of-care status for most patients with T_1 renal cancer. The major advantages of LRN over open radical nephrectomy include decreased perioperative morbidity, less blood loss, shorter hospital stay, and quicker convalescence (2,3). In a series at the authors' institution, with 63 patients with a mean follow-up of 65 months, the 7-year overall and cancer-specific survival was 72% and 90%, respectively (4). Survival data were evaluated according to clinical stage. For T_1 tumors (<7 cm), the 7-year oncological outcome was similar to that in a series of open radical nephrectomy as regards disease-free survival (97% vs. 96%, $p = .84$) and overall survival (64% vs. 80%). For pT_2 tumors, the disease-free survival was 66% and 87% ($p = .28$) and overall survival was 44% vs. 60%. In this study we also concluded that the overall renal function decreased significantly after radical nephrectomy, and is not affected by the surgical approach. Table 7.1 shows the largest recent series of laparo-scopic radical nephrectomy available in the literature.

TABLE 7.1. Laparoscopic radical nephrectomy oncological outcomes

Author	n	Follow-up (years)	Blood loss (mL)	Operative time (hour)	Hospital stay (days)	Projected 5-year cancer-specific survival
Dunn et al. 2000 (3)	44	2.1	NA	5.5	3.4	91%
Chan et al. 2001 (5)	66	2.9	280	4.2	3.8	95%
Ono et al. 2001 (6)	102	2.4	254	4.7	NA	95%
Portis et al. 2002 (7)	64	4.5	219	NA	4.8	98%
Saika et al. 2003 (8)	195	3.3	248	4.6	NA	87%
Permpongkosol et al. 2005 (9)	121	6	280	4.2	3.8	94%*
Colombo et al. 2006 (4)	48	5.4	179	2.8	1.4	91%*

*Actual 5-year survival.
NA, not available.

Although open partial nephrectomy was initially indicated for patients with compromised renal function, solitary kidney, and bilateral tumor, its use has expanded for patients with normal contralateral kidney. It offers long-term oncological outcomes equivalent to that of radical nephrectomy and long-term preservation of renal function in selected patients with small renal tumor (10).

Laparoscopic partial nephrectomy (LPN) has emerged as a viable alternative to open partial nephrectomy while minimizing patient morbidity (11). It was initially limited to patients with a small, superficial, solitary, peripheral, exophytic tumor. However, with increasing laparoscopic experience, the indications for LPN have been carefully expanded to include larger, central, hilar, and infiltrating tumors. In our experience with 100 patients, each with a minimum of 3 years of follow-up, overall survival was 86% and cancer-specific survival was 100% (12). Our data in 50 patients with 5 years of follow-up indicates overall and cancer-specific survival of 84% and 100%, respectively (13) (Table 7.2).

Adrenal Cancer

Laparoscopic adrenalectomy has become the gold standard for benign surgical adrenal disorders such as aldosteronoma, Cushing's disease, and

TABLE 7.2. Partial nephrectomy series: oncological outcomes

Authors	n	Approach	Follow-up (months)	Tumor size (cm)	Overall survival	Cancer-specific survival
Lerner et al. 1996 (14)	185	Open	44	4.1	77%	89%
Belldegrun et al. 1999 (15)	146	Open	57	3.6	86%	93%
Hafez et al. 1999 (16)	485	Open	47	2.7	81%	92%
Moinzadeh et al. 2006 (12)	100	Laparoscopic	42	3.1	86%	100%
Lane and Gill 2006 (13)	50	Laparoscopic	62	3.0	84%	100%

pheochromocytoma. In our institution we have performed more than 330 laparoscopic adrenalectomies. Our series with 31 patients with adrenal malignancy showed a 5-year survival estimate of 40%. In this study, local recurrence was noted in seven patients (23%), including three with metastatic renal cell carcinoma (RCC), two with metastatic colon cancer, and two with primary adrenal cortical carcinoma. Patients with local recurrence had significantly decreased 3-year survival compared to those without local recurrence (16.7% vs. 66%, $p = .016$). Survival was not associated with gender, age, tumor size, tumor side, estimated blood loss, specimen weight, operative time, or approach (transperitoneal vs. retroperitoneal). There was no survival difference in patients with solitary metastasis to the adrenal gland compared to those with primary adrenal malignancy. Five-year survival was similar in patients with an adrenal tumor of less than 5 cm vs. 5 cm or greater (36% vs. 46%, $p = .43$) (17).

These results compare favorably with those in a prior open series from Memorial Sloan-Kettering Cancer Center, in which 37 patients undergoing open adrenalectomy for nonprimary adrenal malignancy were found to have a 5-year actuarial survival of 24%, with a median survival of 21 months (18).

A contraindication to laparoscopic adrenalectomy is suspicion of periadrenal infiltration. For surgeons with advanced laparoscopic experience, size per se is a less important issue, although we generally limit laparoscopic adrenalectomy to tumors in the 10-cm range. Intraoperative concern regarding the adequacy of wide excision should prompt open conversion.

Bladder Cancer

Radical cystectomy is the gold-standard treatment for organ-confined, muscle-invasive, or high-grade superficial recurrent bladder cancer (19). The laparoscopic cystectomy is relatively new, and studies with surgical technique and feasibility are available in the literature with encouraging perioperative and short-term oncological data. The urinary diversion can be performed either intracorporeally or through a small incision. The oncological outcomes of laparoscopic radical cystectomy in our institution with 37 patients with a mean follow-up of 31 months (1–66 months) showed an estimated 5-year overall and cancer-specific survival of 58% and 68%, respectively. Both overall and cancer-specific survival were superior in organ-confined vs. non–organ-confined disease and node-negative vs. node-positive disease. Overall survival was superior when an extended lymphadenectomy was performed, but no benefit was noted in cancer-specific survival (20) (Table 7.3).

Prostate Cancer

Radical prostatectomy is the only tratment that has been shown to improve on cancer-specific survival in the context of a randomized trial (21). In a study by Guillonneau et al. (22) with 1000 laparoscopic radical prostatectomies, the rate

TABLE 7.3. Subgroup analysis of overall and cancer-specific survival in 37 patients undergoing laparo-scopic radical cystectomy

Final pathology	n	Mean follow-up (months)	Overall survival	Cancer specific survival
pT1	11	27	61%	100%
pT2	12	36	91%	100%
pT3	10	29	45%	85%
pT4	4	28	25%	66%
p-value			.08	.21
Organ-confined	23	32	77%	100%
Non–organ-confined	14	28	31%	76%
p-value			.01	.03
Concomitant CIS	8	25	41%	55%
No CIS	24	33	81%	100%
p-value			.03	.002
pN0	30	32	74%	100%
pN1	7	27	25%	33%
p-value			.02	.002

CIS, carcinoma in situ.
Source: Adapted from Haber and Gill (20).

of positive margins was 6.9%, 18.6%, 30%, and 34% for pT2a, pT2b, pT3a, and pT3b, respectively.

Overall biochemical progression-free survival was 90.5% at a follow-up of 3 years, with the range of 44% to 91% accordingly to the pathological stage. Rassweiler et al. (23) published their early experience with 180 cases with 16% positive margins, and biochemical progression-free survival of 95%. The early oncological results of laparoscopic radical prostatectomy are shown in Table 7.4.

The laparoscopic approach offers the advantage of magnification of the surgical field, allowing a better dissection of the neurovascular bundles and clear operative field for the urethrovesical anastomosis. Salomon et al. (25) reported a potency and continence rate after 12 months of 59% and 90%, respectively. In

TABLE 7.4. Laparoscopic radical prostatectomy series: oncological outcomes

Author	n	Gleason score	PSA (ng/mL)	Positive margins		Biochemical progression-free			
				pT2	pT3	pT2a	pT2b	pT3a	pT3b
Guillonneau et al. 2003 (22)	1000	NA	10	6–18%	30–34%	91.8%	88%	77%	44%
Rassweiler et al. 2005 (23)	500	6	11.7	7.4%	31.8%	95.9%	88%		
Solomon et al. 2002 (24)	137	5.7	11.6	21.9%	40.8%	90.4%	56.8%		

NA, not available.

a study by Guillonneau et al. (26) with 500 patients, the potency rate was 85%, and 82% of the patients were continients after a period of 12 months (Table 7.4). These results of laparoscopic radical prostatectomy are comparable to the open radical prostatectomy. Studies with long-term follow-up are needed to confirm the initial results of the minimally invasive technique.

Urothelial Cancer in the Upper Tract

A multicenter study enrolling 116 patients undergoing laparoscopic nephroure-terectomy for upper tract transitional cell carcinoma showed an overall 2-year survival accordingly to pathological grade: 88% for grade I, 90% for grade II, 80% for grade III, and 90% for grade IV. The 2-year cancer–specific survival was 89% for pT1, 86% for pT2, 77% for pT3, and 0% for pT4 (27).

Matin and Gill (28) reported different recurrence rates and survival related to the surgical technique employed to control the bladder cuff during laparoscopic nephroureterectomy. The results with cystoscopic detachment and ligation method were significantly better compared with the stapler technique.

Specific Considerations

Recurrence

The use of the laparoscopic approach in patients with urologic malignancies is increasing. Port-site metastasis, intraperitoneal dissemination, and local recur-rence represent a constant concern. Rassweiler et al. (29), in a study of over 1000 laparoscopic cases, found eight cases of local recurrence and two cases of port-site metastasis. Micali et al. (30), in a multicentric study with almost 11,000 laparoscopic surgeries for cancer, found 10 cases of port seeding, and three cases of peritoneal tumor spreading. Both studies concluded that the aggressiveness of tumor, the deficient immunological state of the oncological patient, and some surgical principles related to specimen extraction are responsible for these rare events.

Learning Curve

Laparoscopic surgery is relatively new in the urologic oncological field. It demands new surgical techniques, with a learning curve inherent to each surgi-cal procedure. The perioperative and oncological outcomes improve once tech-nical competence is achieved.

Follow-Up

The long-term oncological outcomes are not available for the majority of geni-tourinary malignancies treated by the laparoscopic approach. While intermedi-ate-term data are encouraging, multicentric studies with longer follow-up are necessary to validate this relatively new surgical approach.

Surgical Technique

Preoperative Preparation

Attention to the patient's cardiorespiratory status, bony or spinal abnormalities, coagulation studies, and history of prior surgery is imperative. Preoperative bowel preparation includes two bottles of magnesium citrate on the afternoon before surgery, with clear liquids allowed until midnight. Patients undergoing reconstructive procedures with bowel (neobladder and ileal conduit) need a more intense bowel preparation. A urinary catheter, compression stockings, and one dose of preoperative antibiotics are routine. An arterial line is mandatory in all patients with a pheochromocytoma.

All extremities must be placed in neutral positions and all pressure points meticulously padded with egg crate foam: head and neck, axilla, hip joint, knee, and ankle. We firmly secure the patient to the table with 6-inch adhesive cloth tape and a safety belt.

Both transperitoneal and retroperitoneal approaches can be used for the laparoscopic access.

Retroperitoneal Access

A horizontal 2-cm transverse skin incision is made just below the tip of the 12th rib. The retroperitoneum is accessed by piercing the dorsolumbar fascia with the index finger. Gentle dissection creates a space for placement of the balloon dilator. It is important that the finger dissection be performed between the psoas muscle and Gerota's fascia.

The anterior surface of the psoas muscle is our primary anatomic landmark, during both the initial finger palpation and the subsequent intraoperative laparoscopic viewing. If the blunt dissection is performed along the anterior surface of the psoas muscle and fascia, it automatically stays posterior to, and outside of, Gerota's fascia.

Additional working space in the retroperitoneum is created with a trocar-mounted balloon dilator (PDB; Origin Medsystems, Menlo Park, CA). The balloon device is distended with approximately 800 cc of air adjacent to the lower pole and midportion of the kidney. Then the balloon is deflated and manually advanced higher up along the psoas muscle into the retroperitoneum. The stiff shaft of the PDB balloon permits precise manual repositioning of the balloon dilator. This secondary cephalad balloon dilation of the upper retroperitoneum is performed in the vicinity of the adrenal gland and the undersurface of the diaphragm. Balloon dilation outside Gerota's fascia in the upper retroperitoneum effectively displaces the kidney anteromedially and opens up the potential retroperitoneal space, allowing access to the kidney and the adrenal, and exposes the entire anterior aspect of the psoas muscle, the primary anatomic landmark during retroperitoneoscopy. The balloon is then deflated and removed.

The dilation process can be monitored by inserting the laparoscope within the clear, transparent balloon to observe the following landmarks: psoas muscle, Gerota's fascia, and diaphragm.

A 10-mm blunt-tip trocar (Bluntip; Origin MedSystems) is placed as the primary port. This trocar has a doughnut-shaped, internal fascial retention balloon and an external adjustable foam cuff, which, when cinched down, creates an airtight seal at the primary port site.

Pneumoretroperitoneum with CO_2 is established (15 mm Hg), and the laparoscope is inserted. The anterior port is inserted near the anterior axillary line at least 3 cm cephalad to the iliac crest. The posterior port is inserted at the junction of the lateral border of the erector spinae muscle with the undersurface of the 12th rib. A fourth port (2 or 5 mm) may be required at the level of the primary port in the anterior axillary line for retraction of the adrenal gland and kidney anteriorly. This is sometimes required in the event of an inadvertent peritoneotomy, necessitating anteromedial retraction of the peritoneum.

Clear laparoscopic observation during port placement is imperative to guard against injury to the peritoneum (anterior port), great vessels (posterior port), or pleura (the occasional 4th port).

Transperitoneal Access

Initially, peritoneal insufflation is performed by inserting a Veress needle. The needle is located for the initial CO_2 insufflation, until a 12 to 15 mm Hg pneumoperitoneum is achieved. The Veress needle is replaced by a 12-mm laparoscopic port accordingly with the surgical procedure to be done. A total of four to six ports can be employed. Again, with the exception of the first one, all others are positioned under direct laparoscopic vision to prevent injuries.

Radical Nephrectomy

Retroperitoneal

Blunt dissection in this area of loose areolar tissue is performed to identify renal arterial pulsations. The renal artery is circumferentially mobilized, clipped, and divided. The renal vein is mobilized and controlled with a gastrointestinal anastomosis vascular stapler.

Suprahilar dissection is performed along the medial aspect of the upper pole of the kidney, and the adrenal vessels, including the main adrenal vein, are precisely controlled. Dissection is next redirected toward the superolateral aspect of the specimen, including the en bloc adrenal gland, which is readily mobilized from the underside of the diaphragm. In the areolar tissue in this location inferior phrenic vessels to the adrenal gland are often encountered and need to be controlled.

The anterior aspect of the specimen is mobilized from the undersurface of the peritoneal envelope. The ureter and gonadal vein are secured, and the specimen is completely freed by mobilizing the lower pole of the kidney. The entire dissection is performed outside Gerota's fascia, in keeping with standard onco-logical principles.

An Endocatch bag (U.S. Surgical, Norwalk, CT) is introduced through the right-hand port incision, and the specimen is entrapped. Intact specimen extrac-tion is performed through an appropriate muscle-splitting incision (Gibson or Pfannenstiel). Hemostasis is confirmed under lowered pneumoretroperitoneal pressure, and ports are removed under direct vision. Fascial closure is per-formed for all 10-mm or larger port sites using a 0 Vicryl suture.

Transperitoneal

The transperitoneal approach utilizes a four-port technique. Overlying bowel is reflected, and the colon-renal ligaments are released, as well as the ligaments with spleen and liver, in the left and right side, respectively, after exposing the Gerota's fascia and retracting the lower pole of the kidney to stretch the renal hilum.

The major hilar vessels are then exposed, ligated individually, and divided, initially the artery and posteriorly the vein. The Endocatch bag is used, and the entrapped specimen is extracted intact through a muscle-splitting, low Pfan-nenstiel incision without morcellation.

Partial Nephrectomy

Preoperative computed tomography with volume-rendered three-dimensional (3D) video reconstruction is performed to aid in surgical planning. Intraopera-tive flexible, contact renal ultrasonography is performed to precisely determine tumor size, depth of intraparenchymal extension, distance from the collecting system, proximity to major renal vessels, and further evaluation of any suspi-cious satellite renal. A ureteral catheter is placed cystoscopically to the renal pelvis. A syringe with dilute indigo carmine dye is attached to the catheter and used to inject retrogradely and check for entry in the collecting system. The ureteral catheter is kept for 1 to 2 days postoperatively if suture-repair of the collecting system was performed.

The patient is placed in the 90-degree flank position or in the 45-degree modi-fied flank position depending on whether the retroperitoneal or the transperito-neal approach is employed, respectively. Selection of the laparoscopic approach is based on tumor location to ensure adequate surgical exposure. The transperi-toneal approach is preferred for anterior, anterolateral, lateral, and apical tumors. The retroperitoneal approach is reserved for posterior or posterolateral tumors. The operative table is mildly flexed mainly during the retroperitoneal approach to increase the distance between the costal margin and the iliac crest.

Transperitoneal

The colon is mobilized medially to expose the renal hilum. On the right side, gentle mobilization of the duodenum may be needed, and the liver is retracted

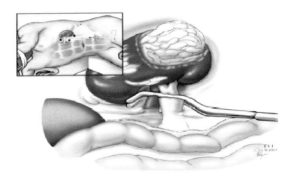

FIGURE **7.1.** Transperitoneal technique of laparoscopic partial nephrectomy. Laparoscopic Satinsky clamp is used to obtain en bloc control of renal hilum. Inset: Port arrangement. [Adapted from Fergany et al. (10), with permission of the Cleveland Clinic Foundation.]

cephalad above the renal upper pole. The ureter is identified and dissected off the psoas muscle to avoid inadvertent clamping along with the renal hilum. The renal artery and vein are not dissected individually, and the renal hilum is clamped en bloc using a Satinsky clamp. The port used to insert the Satinsky clamp is placed in the lower abdomen such that the Satinsky is applied parallel to the aorta and vena cava (Fig. 7.1).

Tissue surrounding the renal vessels should be dissected to avoid incomplete Satinsky occlusion. Gerota's fascia is incised and the kidney is mobilized to expose the tumor and surrounding normal renal parenchyma. Fatty tissue covering the tumor is maintained en bloc with the tumor. After adequate hydration and intravenous administration of mannitol (12.5 g), the renal hilum is clamped en bloc. Care is taken to ensure that any accessory vessels are clamped. If necessary, additional individual bulldog clamps can be employed.

The tumor is then excised, with a normal margin of renal parenchyma. Cold Endoshears are used to cut the renal parenchyma along the previously scored renal capsule. Pelvicaliceal integrity is tested by retrograde injection of dilute indigo carmine (Fig. 7.2). Any entry is identified and sutured in a watertight fashion.

Parenchymal hemostatic sutures are placed over a prepared Surgicel bolsters (Fig. 7.3). The biologic hemostatic agent Floseal (Baxter, Deerfield, IL) is layered directly onto the partial nephrectomy bed, deep to the bolster.

After hemostasis, the renal hilum is unclamped and warm ischemia time is noted. Hemostasis is rechecked after desufflating the abdomen to zero intraperitoneal pressure for 10 minutes. Occasionally, bleeding temporarily tamponated by pneumoperitoneal pressure can be unveiled and controlled.

The excised renal tumor is entrapped within an Endocatch bag and extracted intact from the lower port site. A Jackson-Pratt drain is placed if pelvicaliceal repair was performed. Ports are removed under vision after securing hemostasis.

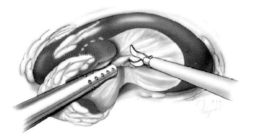

FIGURE 7.2. Tumor excision. Calyx adjacent to tumor is being deliberately entered sharply with shears to maintain a margin of healthy renal parenchyma. [Adapted from Fergany et al. (10), with permission of the Cleveland Clinic Foundation.]

Retroperitoneal

A three-port technique is usually employed. The first port is locate at the tip of the 12th rib, and under direct vision two secondary laparoscopic ports are placed. An anterior port is inserted 3 cm cephalad to the iliac crest along the anterior axillary line, and a posterior port is inserted at the junction of the lateral border of the erector spinae muscle with the undersurface of the 12th rib.

The renal hilum is put on stretch by anterolateral retraction of the kidney. The renal artery and vein are individually dissected in preparation for temporary clamping. The kidney is mobilized from within the Gerota's fascia in a fashion similar to the transperitoneal approach (Fig. 7.4).

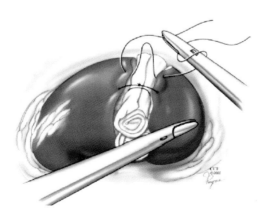

FIGURE 7.3. Renal parenchymal repair over bolsters. [Adapted from Fergany et al. (10), with permission of the Cleveland Clinic Foundation.]

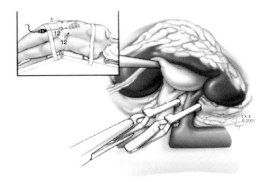

FIGURE 7.4. Retroperitoneal laparoscopic partial nephrectomy. Because of limited operative space, two laparoscopic bulldog clamps are used for individual control of the mobilized renal artery and vein, respectively. Inset: Three-port retroperitoneal approach. [Adapted from Fergany et al. (10), with permission of the Cleveland Clinic Foundation.]

Nevertheless, the retroperitoneal space is limited, adding difficulty to the procedure. Bulldog clamps are placed on the renal artery and vein separately during a retroperitoneal partial nephrectomy. Following hilar control, surgical steps including tumor excision, reconstruction of the renal parenchyma and collecting system, tumor extraction, and laparoscopic exit are similar to the transperitoneal approach.

Adrenalectomy

Retroperitoneal

The posterior aspect of Gerota's fascia is incised transversely at the level of the upper pole of the kidney. The aim of the ensuing dissection is to circumferentially mobilize the upper pole and midregion of the kidney and the covering Gerota's fascia. The upper pole is now dropped posteriorly onto the psoas muscle away from the adrenal gland. This dissection proceeds immediately adjacent to the parenchyma of the upper pole of the kidney. Care must be taken not to injure any accessory vessel entering the upper pole of the kidney. At this juncture, the unmobilized adrenal gland is still located in its normal position, attached anteriorly to the parietal peritoneum.

During the left adrenalectomy, careful blunt and sharp dissection is performed toward the renal hilum, between the upper pole of the kidney posterolaterally and the adrenal anteromedially. The caudal limit of this dissection is the renal hilar vessels, usually the superior branch of the renal artery.

Multiple small renal hilar vessels supplying the adrenal gland are encountered in this location, which are securely clipped and divided. Dissection is now transversely continued medially along the renal vein or artery, and the main left adrenal vein may be identified at this juncture and clipped (5-mm clips) and transected. If the main left adrenal vein cannot be identified at this stage, dissection is redirected toward the undersurface of the diaphragm. The adrenal gland is mobilized along its cephalad aspect, controlling the inferior phrenic branches. Multiple aortic branches to the adrenal gland may need to be controlled in this area. Continued dissection along the medial and inferomedial aspect of the adrenal gland will identify the main left adrenal vein as its sole remaining attachment.

The left adrenal vein is longer than the right, arises from the inferomedial aspect of the left adrenal gland, and courses obliquely to drain into the proximal left renal vein. The vein is then clipped and transected.

In the right side, the main adrenal vein is shorter, horizontally located along the superomedial edge of the adrenal gland, and drains directly into the inferior vena cava.

Dissection is carried cephalad along the lateral aspect of the inferior vena cava, between it and the adrenal gland, until the right adrenal vein is seen, circumferentially mobilized, clipped, and divided. The adrenal gland is then mobilized from the undersurface of the diaphragm. The main right adrenal vein usually arises from the superomedial aspect of the right adrenal gland. Although multiple small renal hilar arteries and veins enter the adrenal gland along its inferior and inferomedial edge, the larger, more well-defined main right adrenal vein usually resides in a more cephalad location, beneath and along the posterior edge of the right lobe of the liver.

After control of the adrenal vasculature has been secured, sequential blunt and sharp dissection of the remaining attachments frees up the adrenal gland. Inferior phrenic vessels are often encountered along the undersurface of the diaphragm. During specimen mobilization, one should be careful not to create an unintentional peritoneotomy. Although a peritoneotomy does not significantly compromise operative exposure during a retroperitoneoscopic radical nephrectomy, a peritoneotomy during retroperitoneoscopic adrenalectomy may decrease the operative field in the vicinity of the undersurface of the diaphragm. In this circumstance, placement of a fourth port may be necessary for anterior retraction. A 2-mm port suffices for this purpose.

The Endocatch bag is introduced through the right-hand port, and the excised specimen is entrapped and extracted intact through the primary port site. Hemostasis is confirmed and the ports are removed under laparoscopic vision. The larger (10–12 mm) port site(s) is (are) closed in fascial layers, and the smaller (5-mm) ports are closed with subcuticular sutures.

Transperitoneal

On the right side the liver is retracted anterior and the posterior peritoneum is transversely incised high along the under surface of the liver, extending from the line of Toldt laterally up to the inferior vena cava medial. Visualized without any need for mobilizing the hepatic flexure, the adrenal gland, which is surrounded by periadrenal fat, is retracted laterally. The main adrenal vein is dissected, clip ligated, and divided.

In contrast, on the left side of the spleen, the splenic flexure, the descending colon, and the tail of the pancreas require extensive mobilization to visualize the left adrenal gland. Recently a supragastric transperitoneal approach to the left adrenal gland was described, in which dissection is performed along the greater curvature of the stomach, cephalad to the body of the pancreas. This maneuver avoids mobilization of the descending colon and spleen, which is the primary advantage of this technique.

Radical Cystectomy

With the patient in the supine lithotomy position, a six-port transperitoneal approach is used. With the bladder retracted anteriorly and the sigmoid colon retracted posteriorly and cephalad, a wide horizontal incision is made in the posterior parietal peritoneum covering the rectovesical pouch, starting in the midline and extending up to the common iliac artery on either side. Both vasa deferentia are divided, and dissection is performed along the posterior aspect of the seminal vesicles toward the bladder base. The Denonvilliers fascia is incised, and the plane between the prostate and the rectum is developed. Generous ureteral mobilization is performed bilaterally from the retroperitoneum up to their entry into the urinary bladder. This allows definition of the lateral and posterior vascular pedicles of the bladder, which are controlled by serial applications of the Endo-GIA stapler (U.S. Surgical).

The bladder is distended with 200 mL, and an inverted-V incision is made in the anterior parietal peritoneum. The urachus is detached from the umbilicus, and the bladder is mobilized posteriorly.

The retropubic space is developed, and the endopelvic fascia is divided bilaterally. The puboprostatic ligaments are divided, and the dorsal vein complex is suture-ligated laparoscopically. The urethra is transected distal to the apex of the prostate, the rectourethralis muscle is divided, and the remaining attachments are released to completely free the radical cystoprostatectomy specimen (Fig. 7.5), which is immediately entrapped within an Endocatch bag. We elect to perform the pelvic lymphadenectomy after the cystectomy in order not to compromise tissue planes and avoid blood-staining in the pelvis.

Ileal Conduit

A 15-cm segment of ileum is identified approximately 15 cm proximal to the ileocecal junction. The Endo-GIA stapler is used to isolate the ileal loop and its mesentery. Complete hemostasis at the cut end of the mesentery is obtained by the additional selective application of metallic clips. Intestinal continuity is reestablished by creating a generous side-to-side ileo-ileal anastomosis with two sequential firings of the Endo-GIA stapler. The open ends of the bowel are closed with two transverse applications of the Endo-GIA stapler.

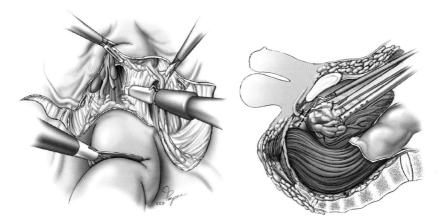

FIGURE 7.5. The urethra is transected distal to the apex of the prostate, the rectourethralis muscle is divided, and the remaining attachments are released to completely free the radical cystoprostatectomy specimen. (Courtesy of Section of Laparoscopic and Robotic Surgery, Cleveland Clinic Foundation, Cleveland, OH.)

The left ureter is delivered retroperitoneally to the right side of the abdomen under the sigmoid mesocolon. The distal end of the ileal loop is exteriorized through the preselected stoma site in the right rectus muscle followed by creation of stoma. A 90-cm, 7-French (F), single-J ileoureteral stent, grasped by a laparoscopic right-angle clamp, is inserted through the stoma into the conduit lumen, so as to tent the ileal loop within the abdomen at the desired site of ileoureteral anastomosis. Using a laparoscopic electrosurgical J-hook, a small ileotomy is created at that site, and the stent is delivered into the abdominal cavity.

The right ileoureteral anastomosis is performed initially. After spatulating the ureteral cut edge, the initial stitch is passed outside-in at the apex of the ureteral spatulation and anchored at the appropriate site (6-o'clock position) on the ileal conduit (4-0 Vicryl, RB-1 needle). After performing a continuous suture to approximate 80% of the posterior (far) wall of the ileoureteral anastomosis, the J-stent is passed into the ureter up to the renal pelvis. The remainder of the posterior wall is then completed. The anterior (near) wall of the anastomosis is completed with a separate running suture to preclude circumferential anastomotic narrowing. The left ileoureteral anastomosis is performed in a similar fashion. Laparoscopic free-hand suturing and in situ knot-tying techniques are used exclusively.

The bilateral pelvic lymphadenectomy is completed. Two 10-mm Jackson-Pratt drains are inserted through different port sites, and a Foley catheter pelvic drain is inserted per urethra. The entrapped specimen is extracted intact through a 3.5-cm extension of a port-site incision. Hemostasis is confirmed and laparoscopic exit performed.

Orthotopic Neobladder

An additional 5-mm port is inserted in the midline, midway between the symphysis pubis and umbilicus. The laparoscope is now repositioned in the left lateral port, pointing toward the liver, with the surgeon working through the midline infraumbilical and right pararectal ports. The ileocecal junction is identified, and a 65-cm segment of ileum is selected 15 to 20 cm away from the ileocecal junction. Precise measurement of bowel length is obtained by inserting a malleable foot ruler into the abdomen through a 12-mm port. The distal end of the selected ileal segment is transected with an Endo-GIA stapler using the 3.5-mm blue cartridge. Division of the ileal mesentery at this location is performed by two sequential firings of the Endo-GIA stapler using the 2.5-mm gray vascular cartridge.

During mesenteric transection, care is taken to avoid the primary mesenteric vessels by close laparoscopic inspection. Additionally, the line of mesenteric division remained perpendicular to the mesenteric border of the ileum to avoid risking bowel ischemia by veering too close to the bowel. In a similar manner, the proximal end of the 65-cm ileal segment is transected and the proximal mesenteric division is performed with only one firing of the stapler.

The excluded ileal segment is dropped posteriorly, and side-to-side ileo-ileal continuity is restored by two sequential firings of the Endo-GIA stapler (3.5-mm blue cartridge) along the respective antimesenteric borders of the two adjacent loops of ileum. Two to three transverse firings of the Endo-GIA stapler are performed to secure both open ileal ends, thereby completing the side-to-side anastomosis. For added security, the transected ends of the ileum are oversewn with running 2-0 polyglactin suture. The window in the ileal mesentery is closed with two to three interrupted stitches.

The proximal 10-cm length of the isolated ileal segment is maintained intact for the Studer limb. The remaining distal 55-cm length of the ileal segment is detubularized along its antimesenteric border using a combination of electrosurgical Endoshears and the harmonic scalpel. Before detubularization, the ileal segment is gently irrigated with the suction irrigator device inserted in the bowel lumen through a small ileotomy incision to preclude peritoneal soiling. The posterior plate of the neobladder is created by continuous intracorporeal suturing of the corresponding edges of the detubularized ileum using 2-0 polyglactin suture on a CT-1 needle. The ileal plate is delivered into the pelvis toward the urethral stump. Care is taken to ensure that the ileum is not under any undue tension and that the mesenteric pedicle is not twisted. The most dependent site along the apex of the ileal plate is selected for performing the running circumferential urethro-ileal anastomosis using 2-0 polyglactin suture on a UR-6 needle. A 22F silicone Foley catheter is inserted per urethra before completing the urethro-ileal anastomosis. In female patients a 90-cm single ileo-ureteral J-stent is inserted via the external urethral meatus alongside the Foley catheter and delivered into the neobladder. In the male patient the two ileo-ureteral stents are inserted through the right lateral port, which is then removed and reinserted alongside the stents. In this manner, although the ileo-ureteral stents are inserted through the port-site incision, they are not occupying the port itself. The anterior wall of the orthotopic neobladder is folded over and suture-approximated to achieve globular configuration of the neobladder. Before completion of the anterior wall, both ileo-ureteral stents are delivered into the Studer limb and retrieved into the peritoneal cavity through two separate, small (1 to 1.5 cm) ileotomy incisions, which are precisely created at the proposed site of the ileo-ureteral anastomoses. Bilateral ureteroileal anastomoses are performed sequentially, with the right ureteral anastomosis performed initially on the more distal ileotomy incision.

Each ureteroileal anastomosis is done in a continuous manner using two separate 3-0 polyglactin sutures on an RB-1 needle, with one suture each for the anterior and the posterior ureteral wall, respectively. Before completion of the anastomosis, the single ileo-ureteral J-stent is advanced up to the renal pelvis. The left ureteroileal anastomosis is completed in similar manner. All suturing and knot tying is performed intracorporeally using free-hand laparoscopic techniques exclusively. The constructed orthotopic neobladder is irrigated through the Foley catheter, and any obvious leakage site is precisely repaired by a figure-of-8 stitch. A suprapubic catheter is inserted into the neobladder through the midline port-site incision. Two Jackson-Pratt drains are inserted, one through each lateral port site, and the specimen is extracted through a 2- to 3-cm circumumbilical extension of the umbilical port incision. The laparoscopic exit is completed. An Indiana pouch and continent catheterizable ileal limb can be created extracorporeally through a minilaparotomy incision by standard open techniques, and the bowel is reinserted into the abdomen for the bilateral ureteroileal anastomoses to be created intracorporeally by free-hand laparoscopic techniques. A catheterizable, continent ileal stoma is then fashioned to the umbilicus. Postoperatively, the urethral Foley catheter is irrigated every 4 to 6 hours for the first 2 to 3 days and every 8 hours thereafter. The Jackson-Pratt drains are removed sequentially as drainage decreased appropriately. A cystogram is obtained at 4 to 6 weeks to confirm complete healing of the neobladder before removing the Foley catheter.

Radical Prostatectomy

A six-port transperitoneal or extraperitoneal laparoscopic approach can be employed. In our institution, we use the transrectal real-time ultrasound image guidance during the procedure.

In the transperitoneal access, the prevesical space is achieved through an incision in the peritoneum and subsequently blunt dissection between the bladder and abdominal wall. During the extraperitoneal access, after a finger-dissection of the Retzius' space, a balloon trocar is used to create the working space.

An anterior incision is made in the bladder neck and prolonged laterally to exposure the prostate posteriorly. The posterior wall is opened and the vas deferens are dissected, clamped, and divided, followed by the seminal vesicles bilaterally.

Care must be taken not to employ any source of energy along the tip and lateral surface of the seminal vesicle due to its proximity to the neurovascular bundles (NVBs). A Hem-o-lok clip (Weck Closure Systems, Research Triangle Park, NC) is placed to control the artery to the seminal vesicle, which is then transected with cold scissors. Denonvilliers' fascia is incised, entering the pre-rectal space along the posterior surface of the prostate.

The right lateral pedicle and NVB are addressed initially. Bilateral seminal vesicles and vas deferens, grasped by an atraumatic bowel clamp introduced through the 5-mm suprapubic port, are tautly retracted anterolaterally to the left side, placing the right lateral pedicle of the prostate on gentle stretch. A 25-mm, straight, atraumatic bulldog clamp is placed obliquely at a 45-degree angle across the right lateral pedicle close to the bladder neck, at some distance from the right posterolateral edge of the prostate (Fig. 7.6).

Using Endoshears, the lateral pedicle is carefully divided in small tissue bites, while leaving an approximately 1 to 2 mm edge of pedicle tissue protruding from the jaws of the bulldog clamp. Transrectal ultrasound imaging provides real-time guidance along the posterolateral edge of the prostate, thus minimizing inadvertent compromise of the prostate capsule (Fig. 7.6B). As the last few remaining attachments of the lateral pedicle are divided, the NVB begins to be visualized. At this point, a combination of scissor cuts and blunt teasing with a laparoscopic Kittner releases the NVB toward the apex. The prostate capsule must be maintained intact along the posterolateral and lateral edge. Because of this clear visualization, even a minute inadvertent prostate capsulotomy can be

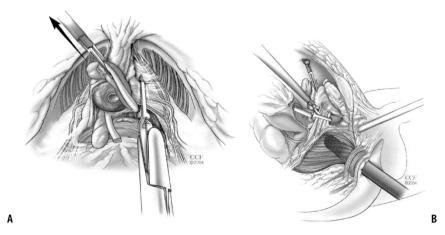

A   **B**

Figure 7.6. A 25-mm, straight, atraumatic bulldog clamp is placed obliquely at a 45-degree angle across the right lateral pedicle close to the bladder neck, at some distance from the right posterolateral edge of the prostate. (Courtesy of Section of Laparoscopic and Robotic Surgery, Cleveland Clinic Foundation, Cleveland, OH.)

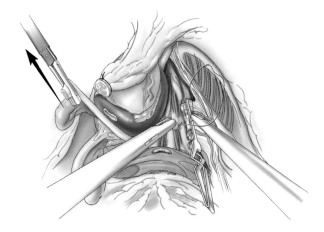

FIGURE 7.7. A 4-0 Vicryl suture is employed to superficially suture the transected lateral pedicle. (Courtesy of Section of Laparoscopic and Robotic Surgery, Cleveland Clinic Foundation, Cleveland, OH.)

identified and sharply corrected, thereby staying in the correct plane outside the prostatic fascia. At this time, a 4-0 Vicryl suture is employed to superficially suture the transected lateral pedicle (Fig. 7.7).

The initial stitch is placed at the proximal cut end of the lateral pedicle close to the bladder neck. One to two additional small suture bites are taken superficial to the jaws of the closed bulldog clamp in order to anchor the stitch. The bulldog clamp is removed, and any bleeding vessels meticulously sutured for hemostasis.

The dorsal vein complex is ligated and divided. This step can be performed using absorbable sutures stitches or employing an Endo-GIA stapler, accordingly with the surgeon's preference.

The prostate apex is then mobilized, and both NVBs are gently dissected away from the prostate apex. The urethra is sharply transected with cold Endoshears, the specimen is entrapped, NVB hemostasis is confirmed, and urethrovesical anastomosis is completed with a running suture.

Laparoscopic Radical Nephroureterectomy

Retroperitoneal

After the creation of the retroperitoneal workspace, the kidney is then retracted anterolaterally with a forceps, placing the renal hilum on traction. Gerota's fascia is incised longitudinally in the general area of the renal hilum, parallel and 1 to 2 cm anterior to the psoas muscle. Blunt dissection in this avascular area of loose areolar fatty tissue is performed to identify renal arterial pulsations. The renal artery is circumferentially mobilized, clip occluded, and divided. The renal vein is mobilized and controlled with a gastrointestinal anastomosis vascular stapler. Suprahilar dissection is performed along the medial aspect of the upper pole of the kidney, and the adrenal vessels, including the main adrenal vein, are precisely controlled.

Dissection is next redirected toward the superolateral aspect of the specimen, including the en bloc adrenal gland, which is readily mobilized from the underside of the diaphragm. In the avascular flimsy areolar tissue in this location, inferior phrenic vessels to the adrenal gland are often encountered and controlled. The anterior aspect of the specimen is mobilized from the underside of the peritoneal envelope. The ureter and gonadal vein are secured, and the specimen is completely freed by mobilizing the lower pole of the kidney. The entire dissection is performed outside Gerota's fascia, duplicating the oncological principles of open surgery. The specimen is entrapped in an Endocatch bag and extracted intact by enlarging the primary port-site incision appropriately. For larger specimens an intentional peritoneotomy is occasionally created, strictly for specimen entrapment. Hemostasis is confirmed under lowered pneumoretroperitoneum, and ports are removed in routine manner. Fascial closure is performed for all 10 mm or larger port sites.

Transperitoneal

The transperitoneal approach utilizes a four-port technique. Overlying bowel is reflected, the colon-renal ligaments are released, as well as the ligaments with the spleen and liver, in the left and right side, respectively, after exposing the Gerota's fascia and retracting the lower pole of the kidney to stretch the renal hilum. The major hilar vessels are then exposed, ligated individually, and divided, initially the artery and posteriorly the vein. The ureteral dissection, bladder cuff removal, and specimen extraction are similar to the retroperitoneal approach described above.

References

1. Clayman RV, Kavoussi LR, Soper NJ, et al. Laparoscopic nephrectomy: initial case report. J Urol 1991;146:278–282.
2. Saranchuk JW, Savage SJ. Laparoscopic radical nephrectomy: current status. BJU Int 2005;95(suppl 2):21–26.
3. Dunn MD, Portis AJ, Shalhav AL, et al. Laparoscopic versus open radical nephrectomy: a 9-year experience. J Urol 2000;164:1153–1159.
4. Colombo JR Jr, Haber GP, Lane B, et al. laparoscopic radical nephrectomy: oncological and functional outcomes. (Submitted)
5. Chan DY, Cadeddu JA, Jarrett TW, et al. Laparoscopic radical nephrectomy: cancer control for renal cell carcinoma. J Urol 2001;166:2095–2100.
6. Ono Y, Kinukawa T, Hattori R, et al. The long-term outcome of laparoscopic radical nephrectomy for small renal cell carcinoma. J Urol 2001;165:1867–1870.
7. Portis AJ, Yan Y, Landman J, et al. Long-term follow-up after laparoscopic radical nephrectomy. J Urol 2002;167:1257–1262.

8. Saika T, Ono Y, Hattori R, et al. Long-term outcome of laparoscopic radical nephrectomy for pathologic T1 renal cell carcinoma. Urology 2003;62:1018–1023.

9. Permpongkosol S, Chan DY, Link RE, et al. Long-term survival analysis after laparoscopic radical nephrectomy. J Urol 2005;174:1222–1225.

10. Fergany AF, Hafez KS, Novick AC. Long-term results of nephron sparing surgery for localized renal cell carcinoma: 10-year follow-up. J Urol 2000;163:442–445.

11. Gill IS, Matin SF, Desai MM, et al. Comparative analysis of laparoscopic versus open partial nephrectomy for renal tumors in 200 patients. J Urol 2003;170:64–68.

12. Moinzadeh A, Gill IS, Finelli A, Kaouk J, Desai M. Laparoscopic partial nephrectomy: 3-year follow-up. J Urol 2006;175:459–462.

13. Lane BR, Gill IS. Five year outcomes of laparoscopic partial nephrectomy. J Urol 2007;177:70–74.

14. Lerner SE, Hawkins CA, Blute ML, et al. Disease outcome in patients with low stage renal cell carcinoma treated with nephron sparing or radical surgery. J Urol 1996; 155:1868–1873.

15. Belldegrun A, Tsui KH, deKernion JB, Smith RB. Efficacy of nephron-sparing surgery for renal cell carcinoma: analysis based on the new 1997 tumor-node-metastasis staging system. J Clin Oncol 1999;17(9):2868–2875.

16. Hafez KS, Fergany AF, Novick AC. Nephron sparing surgery for localized renal cell carcinoma: impact of tumor size on patient survival, tumor recurrence and TNM staging. J Urol 1999;162:1930–1933.

17. Moinzadeh A, Gill IS. Laparoscopic radical adrenalectomy for malignancy in 31 patients. J Urol 2005;173:519–525.

18. Kim SH, Brennan MF, Russo P, Burt ME, Coit DG. The role of surgery in the treatment of clinically isolated adrenal metastasis. Cancer 1998;**82:**389–394.

19. Dalbagni G, Genega E, Hashibe M, et al. Cystectomy for bladder cancer: a contemporary series. J Urol 2001;165:1111–1116.

20. Haber GP, Gill IS. Laparoscopic radical cystectomy for cancer: 5–year oncologic outcomes. (Submitted)

21. Bill-Axelson A, Holmberg L, Ruutu M, et al. Scandinavian Prostate Cancer Group Study No. 4. Radical prostatectomy versus watchful waiting in early prostate cancer. N Engl J Med 2005;352:1977–1984.

22. Guillonneau B, El-Fettouh H, Baumert H, et al. laparoscopic radical prostatectomy: oncological evaluation after 1,000 cases at Montsouris Institute. J Urol 2003;169: 1261–1266.

23. Rassweiler J, Schulze M, Teber D, et al. Laparoscopic radical prostatectomy with the Heilbronn technique: oncological results in the first 500 patients. J Urol 2005;173: 761–764.

24. Eden CG, Cahill D, Vass JA, Adams TH, Dauleh MI. Laparoscopic radical prostatectomy: the initial UK series. BJU Int 2002;90:876–882.

25. Salomon L, Levrel O, de la Taille A, et al. Radical prostatectomy by the retropubic, perineal and laparoscopic approach: 12 years of experience in one center. Eur Urol 2002;42:104–110.

26. Guillonneau B, Cathelineau X, Doublet JD, et al. Laparoscopic radical prostatectomy: assessment after 550 procedures. Crit Rev Oncol Hematol 2002;43:123–133.

27. El Fettouh HA, Rassweiler JJ, Schulze M, et al. Laparoscopic radical nephroureterectomy: results of an international multicenter study. Eur Urol 2002;42:447.

28. Matin SF, Gill IS. Recurrence and survival following laparoscopic radical nephroureterectomy with various forms of bladder cuff control. J Urol 2005;173:395–400.

29. Rassweiler J, Tsivian A, Kumar AV, et al. Oncological safety of laparoscopic surgery for urological malignancy: experience with more than 1,000 operations. J Urol 2003; 169:2072–2075.

30. Micali S, Celia A, Bove P, De Stefani S, et al. Tumor seeding in urological laparoscopy: an international survey. J Urol 2004;171(6 pt 1):2151–2154.

8
Clinical Trials and Their Principles

Denise C. Babineau and Michael W. Kattan

Clinical trials are needed for the development and evaluation of any type of treatment used to detect, prevent, or treat genitourinary cancer. This chapter introduces clinical trials in this context. The discussion largely focuses on the design and implementation of a clinical trial in its various stages. Possible sources of bias in clinical trials and methods of minimizing or eliminating this bias are also discussed.

Phases of a Clinical Trial

A clinical trial is a research study that evaluates the safety and efficacy of a new treatment for a specific disease in human patients. Although this chapter focuses on clinical trials that are used to investigate newly discovered drugs, other forms of treatment, such as a new type of surgery or therapy regimen, can also be evaluated. Regardless of treatment, the design of a clinical trial must be carefully considered. This section presents the four possible phases of a clinical trial.

Phase I (Toxicity and Safety)

Once a new drug is tested in animals and is shown to have promise, a phase I clinical trial is carried out to evaluate the drug in human subjects. Its primary purpose is to estimate the dose range that is safely tolerated in patients by determining the maximum tolerated dose (MTD). Other secondary outcomes of interest are the drug's pharmacokinetics and any drug-related side effects. Patient selection is typically limited to those patients in an advanced diseased state for which no other treatment has been effective. The number of patients recruited to the trial is also kept to a minimum (less than 80) to ensure patients are not unnecessarily exposed to a drug that may be of little clinical use or that may have adverse side effects.

The design of a phase I trial generally follows a dose-escalation scheme that depends on the number of observed toxicities. There are many different designs to choose from, but a typical scheme is as follows. Three patients are treated

TABLE 8.1. Probability of dose escalation in phase I clinical trial

	True rate of toxicity						
	10%	20%	30%	40%	50%	60%	70%
Probability of escalation	0.91	0.71	0.49	0.31	0.17	0.08	0.03

using an initial dose of the drug under investigation. If more than one of these patients experiences an unacceptable toxicity (as predefined by the investigator), accrual stops and the next lower dose is accepted as the MTD.

If no unacceptable toxicities occur, the dosage is escalated to the next highest dose level. If one unacceptable toxicity occurs, three additional patients are entered at that dose level. The dosage is escalated to the next higher level if none of these three patients experiences unacceptable toxicity, but if one or more patients experience toxicity, accrual stops and the next lower dose is accepted as the MTD.

To evaluate this scheme (or a similar type scheme), it is also useful to estimate the probability of dose escalation under various toxicity rates. In general, the number of patients who experience toxicity is given by a binomial distribution so that the probability of dose escalation in the above design is given by

$$P \text{ (dose escalation)} = (1 - t)^3 + 3t(1 - t)^5,$$

where t represents the true rate of toxicity at the current dose level. Table 8.1 gives the probability of dose escalation for a variety of hypothesized toxicity rates. For example, there is a 91% chance or greater of dose escalation if the underlying toxicity rate is 10% or less.

As a simple example, suppose a phase I clinical trial is used to investigate intravesical gemcitabine therapy in superficial transitional cell bladder carcinoma. Toxicity of the gemcitabine dose is defined by any the Eastern Cooperative Oncology Group (ECOG) grade 3 or 4 hematologic toxicity or grade 3 or higher nonhematologic toxicity (1). The study begins by using an initial dose of 500 mg of gemcitabine in 100 mL 0.9% NaCl (normal saline). Using increasing doses of 100 mg and the previous dose escalation scheme, the MTD of intravesical gemcitabine therapy to be used in further studies is determined.

Phase II (Safety and Efficacy)

Phase II trials assess the safety and efficacy of a drug in a single patient cohort. Their design is fixed, staged, or sequential in nature. For a fixed design, a cohort of patients (typically of size less than 200) is given the MTD that was determined in a phase I clinical trial. Patient response, as defined by the investigator, is then measured after a predefined period of time. For instance, in the assessment of a drug to treat a tumor, the response can be classified as either partial (tumor has shrunk by some percentage) or complete (no measurable tumor). Secondary outcomes that may also be investigated are the duration of the response, side effects of the drug, ease of administration to patients, and cost. Depending on the observed response rate, the drug is either accepted for further testing in phase III trials or it is concluded that the drug is not clinically effective in improving patient response. This trial design was used to investigate the pain response in patients taking tesmilifene plus mitoxantrone for hormone refractory prostate cancer (2).

More commonly used designs are staged designs involving two or more patient cohorts. In staged designs, the response for the first cohort is assessed and, depending on the cohort's response rate, the trial is either terminated (due to strong evidence against or in favor of the efficacy of the drug) or continued to the next stage to evaluate the next cohort of patients. A detailed review of these designs is given in Fleming (3) and Simon (4), although a brief introduction to two-stage designs is also given below (see Sample Size Considerations). A related design that is less commonly used is termed sequential because each patient's response is assessed before the next patient is recruited to the trial.

Multiple-stage designs are preferred over a fixed or single-stage design because the trial is terminated early if sufficient evidence exists partway through the trial that indicates that the treatment is ineffective in improving patient response. Early termination increases the speed with which trial results are reported, reduces the cost of the trial, and minimizes the number of patients who are given an ineffective treatment.

However, multiple-stage designs are much harder to implement if the response to treatment takes a long period of time. In this case, the investigator must decide if accrual of patients should continue in between stages.

To accelerate the drug testing process, phase I/II clinical trials have also been considered where the first part of the trial establishes the safety of the drug and its MTD, and the second part of the trial assesses the safety and efficacy of the drug. This type of combined trial was used to evaluate the safety and efficacy in the administration of dendritic cells and prostate specific membrane antigen (PSMA) peptides in patients with advanced prostate cancer (5).

Phase III (Comparative)

Once phase I and II clinical trials have successfully demonstrated the safety and efficacy of a new treatment, phase III clinical trials are implemented to compare the efficacy of a new treatment to a control treatment. The control treatment may be the standard treatment that is currently being used for the disease, may involve the use of a placebo, or may involve no form of treatment at all. Patients are randomly assigned to the treatment or control arm, and patient response is assessed after a period of time. In this phase of trials, patient response is typically measured by the time to disease recurrence or death.

Another type of design that is occasionally used in phase III trials is called a crossover design and is only used if the administration of treatments and response measurement are of short duration. In a two-period crossover design, patients are first randomly assigned to one of the two possible treatments. Patient response is then assessed after a certain time period. After a washout period where the effects of the first treatment are considered to be absent in the patient, the patient is then given the second treatment. Patient response is assessed again after the same length of time that was used for the first treatment. Such a paired design requires fewer patients than the first parallel group design discussed previously. However, a washout period is unethical in some trials due to a patient's need for treatment at all times. In addition, there is a high likelihood of a carryover effect where the effects of the first treatment affect the response of the second treatment.

The size of phase III trials depends on the trial design and may range from a few hundred to several thousand patients. Because the number of patients is so large, patients are usually recruited from several medical centers to ensure that sample size requirements are met within a reasonable time frame. Multicenter trials also provide heterogeneous populations so that the clinical trial results can be generalized to a much broader population. However, this variability in patients also causes more difficulty in detecting treatment differences and requires a more organized and expensive effort on the part of all investigators involved in the planning and administration of the clinical trial.

An example of a phase III trial is a trial that was used to investigate the effect of finasteride on the development of prostate cancer in 18,882 men (6). Patients were randomly assigned to receive finasteride (5 mg per day) or placebo for 7 years. In this case, the response to treatment was the amount of time between drug administration and development of prostate cancer.

Phase IV (Postmarketing Surveillance)

After the successful completion of phase III trials, the new treatment will likely achieve regulatory approval and will be made available to the public. Phase IV trials then monitor the treatment for uncommon side effects not seen in phase III trials. Phase IV trials also assess the long-term effects of the treatment as well. Typically, thousands of patients with the disease are involved, and comparison of treatment side effects is done without randomization of patients to different treatment arms.

Design Considerations

The design of any phase in a clinical trial requires careful thought and consideration. A properly designed clinical trial minimizes the amount of bias present in the study while providing ethical treatment to all patients involved. This section briefly addresses these and other issues in the context of study objectives, primary and secondary end points, patient selection, treatment choice, randomization, blinding, and sample size requirements.

Study Objectives and End Points

The planning of a clinical trial begins with a clear definition of the study objectives. These objectives are defined by a precise explanation of the disease under study and the treatment(s) to be evaluated. Primary and secondary end points are also needed to define the quantitative measurements that can be measured accurately and precisely throughout the trial to assess patient response to treatment. In cancer trials, the primary end point of interest is often the overall or cancer specific survival rates following treatment.

Secondary end points, such as the change in a patient's quality of life as measured through the use of previously validated questionnaires, are also of interest. If the end point of interest cannot be measured directly due to resource limitations or inability, surrogate end points are often used. For instance, D'Amico et al. (7) state that it is generally agreed upon that a patient with a history of prostate cancer having a Gleason score of 8 or prostate-specific antigen (PSA) level greater than 20 has a high risk of relapse. This could be used as a surrogate end point to indicate recurrence of prostate cancer. However, the use of a surrogate end point depends heavily on the assumption that the surrogate end point is a good measure of the primary end point, which in some cases cannot be shown to be true.

Patient Selection and Recruitment

Careful selection of patients is critical to the success of any clinical trial. The selected group of patients must be somewhat homogeneous to ensure that the clinical trial results can be applied to a defined population. However, the guidelines must also be flexible enough to meet sample size requirements in a timely fashion and to ensure that the clinical trial results can be generalized to the broader population of patients that is of interest to a practicing physician. Striking a balance between these two populations can be quite difficult.

Patient selection is determined by inclusion and exclusion criteria such as a patient's age, sex, type and stage of disease, treatment, and medical history.

To determine appropriate criteria, the following guidelines have been suggested (8). A patient should be excluded in any of the following situations:

1. The treatment's known side effects may cause them harm.
2. A placebo is being used for comparison and a patient's disease state is severe enough to require some form of treatment at all times.
3. A patient is at a very low risk (or not at risk at all) of developing the primary outcome of interest.
4. A patient is taking an existing treatment(s) that may interfere with the new treatment or may affect his or her response to any treatments.
5. A patient's disease state will cause him or her to never respond to the new treatment.

6. A patient is unlikely to follow the trial protocol (may not follow treatment schedule, may move within the allotted follow-up time, etc.).
7. A patient does not consent to the clinical trial.

These guidelines also depend on the phase of the clinical trial. In phase I and some phase II clinical trials, patients with advanced disease who are receiving no known effective treatment are often chosen. These patients are easier to recruit for these types of preliminary studies, although it is quite likely that they do not form a representative population to which the treatment will be applied in the future. This is not the case in phase III trials, which apply very stringent guidelines to patient selection.

Once inclusion and exclusion criteria have been determined, it is also up to investigators to determine how and where to recruit patients. If patients volunteer or some type of financial incentive is used to recruit patients, differences between this population and the population that is not recruited must be carefully considered to ensure the study population is not biased. It is also common for patients to be recruited from institutions that are highly skilled in conducting clinical trials. This type of recruitment also introduces bias because these patients may represent challenging cases that have been referred to these institutions due to their expertise in the research area.

Treatment Choice

The treatments used in a clinical trial must be carefully considered. The investigator must have reason to believe that the new treatment has benefits (and comparably fewer risks) that are not seen in the control treatment. The administration of the treatments to the patients must also be determined; the method used to administer the drug, the dosage level, the frequency and duration, dose modifications in response to adverse events, interactions with other treatments, packaging, and distribution are just a few of the issues that must be reviewed. These issues may differ for each phase of trials as well. For instance, in a phase I trial, the initial dose is chosen by taking into account any prior knowledge the investigator may have regarding its toxicity. One commonly used initial dose is LD_{10}, so called because it is one tenth of the dose that causes 10% mortality in animals. In a phase II trial, the dose used is the MTD established in the phase I trial. Phase III trials have also been implemented that compare more than one treatment to the control treatment. For example, this is common when investigating treatments of various combinations (drugs, surgery, other types of therapy, etc.).

The control treatment that is used in a phase III clinical trial is also carefully selected. If there is no effective standard treatment that can be used for comparison, a placebo should be used in its place rather than the patient receiving no form of control treatment. This avoids the placebo effect, so called because if no treatment was given to patients, the psychological toll that this may have on a patient may result in a greater treatment effect than is actually present.

However, the use of a placebo may be unethical because patients assigned to receive placebo may need some type of treatment for their disease. This problem can be avoided by giving all patients some type of treatment in addition to the new treatment or placebo that they are given. This problem is also encountered in surgical studies because in most circumstances, it is unethical to give a patient that is assigned to the control arm a sham surgery.

Some studies have avoided the use of a control treatment altogether through the use of historical controls. A historical control group is a group of patients with the disease who have been treated in the past using the standard treatment for that time period. Unfortunately, the use of historical controls introduces a wealth of bias into the study. Due to the difference in time when patients receive their treatment and the fact that patients assigned to the new treatment are enrolled in a clinical trial, the standard of care may be much lower for historical controls. Data that are collected for patients assigned to the new treatment is also of much higher quality than historical control data because data quality is strictly monitored in a clinical trial. In addition, patient selection may differ between the two groups because specific factors that define inclusion/exclusion criteria may be unknown for historical controls. These issues may cause the two groups of patients to differ with respect to several factors that affect response. Some methods of statistical analysis (for instance, analysis of covariance) can be used to compensate for the lack of comparable treatment arms by taking into account any factors that differ between the two arms. However, bias will still be present in the study because the analysis cannot account for unknown factors that differ between the two patient cohorts.

Randomization

Once the treatments to be compared are selected in a phase III trial, patients must be properly randomized to receive one of the treatments. Randomization is needed to ensure that the investigators do not bias the results of the study by giving the new treatment to only those patients whom they believe will respond well to it. If such a subjective allocation scheme is used, both known and unknown factors that affect response will be unbalanced between the treatment arms, leaving it impossible to compare the treatment groups in an unbiased manner. In addition, if an investigator does have some prior knowledge regarding the benefits of one treatment over another, they are ethically obliged to offer that treatment (9) and forgo the trial altogether. On the other hand, Freedman (9) also states that if an investigator does have genuine uncertainty regarding the benefits or merits of each treatment under investigation, which Freedman defines as clinical equipoise, the ethical dilemma in randomly assigning patients to a treatment that may be inferior to the control treatment must also be carefully evaluated.

Historically, randomization of patients to treatment arms is associated with phase III trials. A more recent development is randomized phase II trials. These types of trials are used when several similar treatments must be compared in the same patient population. If nonrandomized phase II trials are carried out for each treatment and the results from each trial are compared with one another, the separate patient populations used in each trial may differ to such a large extent that the result of any comparison between trials is biased. This problem is avoided using a randomized phase II trial because patients are selected from the same patient population and simply randomized to one of the several treatments under investigation. The treatment with the best response rate is then chosen for further study in phase III trials. An example of a randomized phase II trial is a study that randomized 57 patients with recurrent or metastatic bladder cancer to either a cisplatin-containing regimen or a carboplatin-containing regimen (10). In this case, the two regimens were compared using several toxicity measures (ototoxicity, gastrointestinal, nephrotoxicity, neurotoxicity) and response to treatment.

There are several approaches that can be used to randomize a patient to a treatment arm. A simple randomization scheme can be used where each patient is randomized to a treatment arm with a probability of 0.5. More often than not, this scheme is not useful because the number of patients randomized to each group will not be equal. To prevent this, blocked randomization schemes are used. In these schemes, each block contains the same number of patients and its size is a multiple of the number of treatments. For example, suppose a trial has two treatments. Within each block, patients are randomized until exactly half of the patients are randomized to one treatment. The remaining patients are assigned to the other treatment.

Randomization schemes must also attempt to ensure that the distribution of any factor is similar in each of the arms. If the arms are imbalanced with regard to the number of patients or the distribution of factors, the credibility of the study is compromised. This can be avoided using stratified randomization schemes. In this case, the patients are divided into subgroups of patients, called strata, with similar distributions of factors. Within each strata, a blocked randomization scheme is used.

For instance, if it is known that patients who are younger than 45 years old have a lower response rate than older patients, a stratified randomization scheme can be used to ensure that randomization to treatments is evenly balanced in both groups of patients. This type of randomization is useful for smaller trials and does not typically use more than two or three stratification variables due to patient availability and cost.

The time at which randomization occurs is also important. Regulatory agencies typically want all data reported on any patient who is randomized to an arm of the trial, regardless of whether or not the patient complied with the treatment protocol. If patients are immediately randomized to a treatment arm once they are enrolled in the clinical trial, there may be a large delay between time of enrollment and the time a patient is given the treatment, during which the patient may decide to drop out of the study. Such a patient must still be followed throughout the trial, and any adverse events must be reported. On the one hand, this will not affect the per-protocol analysis of the data, which only includes patients that followed treatment protocol. However, patients who drop out of the study will be included in an intent-to-treat analysis that includes all patients who were randomized to any arm of the study. Randomizing patients too early may bias the results of this analysis.

Blinding

Blinding is also another design consideration that is used to minimize the amount of bias introduced into a study. A single blinded study is where either the physician or patient is unaware of the treatment the patient is receiving. A double-blinded study is where both the physician and patient are blinded to the treatment being received. There are also studies where all investigators (physicians, those who assess response, statisticians) and patients are blinded until after the trial is closed and the data analysis is complete. For physicians, blinding ensures that all patients, regardless of their treatment, receive the same standard of care. Patients who know their treatment assignment may also inadvertently affect their response to treatment based on their own belief in the treatment under investigation. There are also situations where blinding is not feasible. For instance, surgeons cannot be blinded to the type of surgery performed on a patient.

Blinding also may not be possible if there are complicated dose schedules, possible dose modifications, or obvious treatment side effects.

Sample Size Considerations

Sample size considerations begin with the formulation of a clearly defined hypothesis that is to be tested in the clinical trial. In phase I clinical trials, sample size requirements are unnecessary because of the exploratory nature of the trial. In phase II and III clinical trials, sample size calculations are required to ensure that the sample size is large enough to detect clinically meaningful response rates for a treatment (phase II) or differences in response rates between treatments (phase III). At the same time, the sample size must be small enough to meet budgetary constraints.

In any sample size calculation, the investigator must pre-specify acceptable probabilities of making incorrect decisions based on the trial results. For instance, suppose trial results indicate an effective treatment but in truth, the treatment does not have a clinically meaningful effect. This is called a type I error (or a false positive) and its probability is denoted by the Greek letter α. A type I error is undesirable because the ineffective treatment is further tested in other clinical trials, wasting time and money and possibly causing harm to future patients. To minimize the likelihood of such an error, α is typically set to .05 or lower. Another type of error is called a type II error (or a false negative) and its probability is denoted by the Greek letter β. In this case, trial results indicate an ineffective treatment even though the treatment truly has a clinically meaningful effect. Although this type of error is still of concern, it is typically larger than α and is set to .10 or .20. Traditionally, discussion of sample size involves the type I error rate and the power to detect a response, specified as the probability of not making a type II error. This is given by $1 - \beta$. By carefully defining a formal hypothesis and calculating an appropriate sample size based on it, the investigator ensures that the probability of a false positive is minimized and the power of the study to detect a clinically relevant response is maximized. The remainder of this section reviews basic sample size calculations for commonly used phase II and III clinical trials.

Sample Size Considerations for Phase II Clinical Trials

To determine the sample size requirements for commonly used designs in phase II clinical trials, investigators must decide how stringent they will be in concluding that the treatment under investigation is active or inactive. Suppose p represents the true, but unknown, response rate of the treatment. The investigator must decide the largest possible response rate, p_0 that indicates an inactive treatment and the smallest possible response rate, p_1 that indicates an active treatment. Using these pre-specified rates, the hypothesis that is commonly tested in phase II clinical trials is

$$H_o : p \leq p_0 \quad \text{versus} \quad H_a : p \geq p_1.$$

Using this hypothesis, the sample size requirements for single-stage (fixed sample size) and two-stage designs are now reviewed.

Single-Stage Designs

A single stage design of a phase II clinical trial requires a fixed sample size calculation. It is based on the decision rule that the drug is considered active if r or more patients respond to the treatment and inactive if fewer than r patients respond to the treatment. Fleming (3) showed that the required sample size, N, and decision rule for such a design is given by

$$N = \left(\left[Z_{1-\beta} \sqrt{p_1 (1 - p_1)} + Z_{1-\alpha} \sqrt{p_0 (1 - p_0)} \right] / \left[p_1 - p_0 \right] \right)^2 \quad \text{and}$$

$$r \geq N p_0 + Z_{1-\alpha} \sqrt{N p_0 (1 - p_0)},$$

where Z_q is the qth quantile of a normal distribution with mean 0 and variance 1. The qth quantile of a distribution is the value at which q percent of the distribution is below. Quantiles of a standard normal distribution can be found using a quantile table, although frequently used quantiles are given by

$$Z_{0.80} = 0.8416, \quad Z_{0.85} = 1.0364, \quad Z_{0.90} = 1.2816,$$
$$Z_{0.95} = 1.6449, \quad Z_{0.975} = 1.96, \quad Z_{0.99} = 2.3263.$$

Note that this sample size and decision rule is based on the assumption that the binomial distribution is well approximated by the standard normal distribution when $Np \geq 10$.

TABLE 8.2. Operating characteristics of a single-stage design in a phase II clinical trial

	Underlying response rate						
	0.25	0.30	0.35	0.40	0.45	0.50	0.55
Probability of inactive drug	0.99	0.93	0.76	0.49	0.23	0.08	0.02

If this assumption is not met, sample size requirements must be determined using exact probabilities based on the binomial distribution (11).

Of particular interest in any phase II trial are the design's operating characteristics. In a single stage, the operating characteristics are defined by the probability that the drug is declared inactive, given by

$$P \text{ (Inactive treatment)} = \sum_{x=0}^{r-1} \binom{N}{x} p^x (1-p)^{N-x}.$$

As an example, suppose an overall response rate (the proportion of complete and partial responses) of 50% or greater indicates an effective drug but a response rate of 30% or less indicates an ineffective drug. Suppose we set $\alpha = .05$ and $\beta = .10$. Using the above formulas, a one-stage phase II trial needs a total of 49 patients. Furthermore, if 20 or more patients have a treatment response (corresponding to a response rate of 40.8%), the drug is considered active. However, if fewer than 20 patients respond to the treatment, the drug is considered inactive and is not viable for future study.

Table 8.2 gives the operating characteristics for this design. In particular, the probability of declaring an inactive drug is 93% or greater if the underlying response rate is 30% or less. If the drug is truly active (as defined by a 50% or greater response rate), the probability of declaring it inactive is 8% or less.

Two-Stage Designs

A two-stage design is sometimes preferred over the previous one-stage design in a phase II clinical trial because it is possible for the trial to be terminated if sufficient evidence exists partway through the trial indicating an ineffective treatment. This may increase the speed with which trial results are reported, reduce the cost of the trial, and minimize the number of patients who are given an ineffective treatment.

The typical two-stage design is discussed in Simon (4) and is briefly introduced here. The first stage accrues n_1 patients. If more than r_1 responses are observed among these n_1 patients, an additional n_2 patients are entered into the study. If more than r_2 responses are observed among the $n_1 + n_2$ patients (corresponding to an observed response rate of at least $(r_2 + 1)/(n_1 + n_2)$, the drug under investigation is accepted for further testing in phase III trials. Alternatively, if r_1 or fewer responses are observed in patients entered in the first stage or if r_2 or fewer responses are observed in patients entered in the first and second stage, the drug is not accepted for further testing. This design could be further modified to allow the trial to stop early if significant activity was observed among the first n_1 patients (i.e., if more than r_2 responses were observed in the first stage of accrual). However, the previous design that accrues additional patients to the potentially active drug permits more precise estimates of response and other secondary outcomes of interest.

The choice of n_1, r_1, n_2, r_2 depends on the design parameters p_0, p_1, α, and β. Because there are a number of different designs that could satisfy all of the design parameters, the design having the smallest expected sample size under H_0 is determined using a search algorithm. This was done in Simon (4) who termed this type of design as optimal.

The operating characteristics for a two-stage design are defined by the probability of trial termination in the first and second stage under various response rates. The following probabilities are based on the previous two-stage design.

$$P\ (\text{trial termination in 1st stage}) = \sum_{x=0}^{r_1} \binom{n_1}{x} p^x \left(1-p\right)^{n_1-x}$$

$$P(\text{trial termination in 2nd stage}) = \sum_{x=r_1+1}^{r_2} \left[\binom{n_1}{x} p^x \left(1-p\right)^{n_1-x} \sum_{y=0}^{r_2-x} \binom{n_2}{y} p^y \left(1-p\right)^{n_2-y} \right]$$

Using the probability of termination in the first stage of accrual, the expected number of patients that must be accrued to the trial is given by

$$\text{Expected sample size} = n_1 + n_2 \left(1 - \sum_{x=0}^{r_1} \binom{n_1}{x} p^x \left(1-p\right)^{n_1-x} \right).$$

This is also useful to investigators to ensure that the required sample size is feasible.

As an example, the same design parameters used for the single-stage design are now considered. In particular, these are given by $p_0 = 0.3$, $p_1 = 0.5$, $\alpha = .05$, and $\beta = .10$. Simon (4) showed that the optimal two-stage design has $n_1 = 24$, $r_1 = 8$, $n_2 = 39$, and $r_2 = 24$. Table 8.3 gives the operating characteristics of this design. In particular, if the drug is not active (30% response or less), the overall probability of declaring the drug inactive is 96% or greater. Sample size will be

TABLE 8.3. Operating characteristics of a two-stage design in a phase II clinical trial

	Underlying response rate						
	0.25	0.30	0.35	0.40	0.45	0.50	0.55
Probability of stopping in 1st stage and rejecting drug	0.88	0.73	0.53	0.33	0.17	0.08	0.03
Probability of stopping in 2nd stage and rejecting drug	0.12	0.23	0.27	0.19	0.08	0.02	0.003
Overall probability of rejecting drug	1	0.96	0.80	0.52	0.25	0.10	0.033
Expected number of patients	28.7	34.7	42.5	50.2	56.3	60.0	61.9

35 patients on average. If the drug is active (50% response or greater), the overall probability of declaring the drug inactive is 10% or less. In this case, sample size will be 60 patients on average. Compared to the single-stage design, this particular two-stage design has a slightly higher probability of declaring an inactive drug. However, if the underlying response rate is less than 40%, the expected sample size is smaller than the single stage trial.

Sample Size Considerations for Phase III Trials

A phase III trial attempts to detect clinically relevant differences between treatments using the primary end point (outcome). In general, there are two types of primary outcomes, dichotomous and continuous, and each requires its own method of sample size calculation. Although other outcomes are certainly used (censored survival data), only these types are considered in this section to simplify the discussion.

Dichotomous Outcome

A dichotomous outcome measures whether or not a particular event occurred in a patient. An example is cancer recurrence 6 months after drug administration. In a trial that has a dichotomous primary outcome, the goal is to determine if there is a difference in event rates between the arms. To determine the number of patients in the trial, the investigator must first specify the rates of the event in the control and treatment arms, given by p_c and p_t respectively. The rate for the control arm must be based on prior knowledge. On the other hand, the rate for the treatment arm is determined by the largest difference between the rates that is of clinical interest. Using this notation, the required sample size is calculated based on testing the hypothesis

$$H_0 : p_c = p_t \quad \text{versus} \quad H_a : p_c \neq p_t$$

such that the probability of a false positive is α and the power to detect the largest clinically relevant difference in event rates is $1 - \beta$. Assuming that both the treatment and control arms consist of independent groups of patients, Pocock (12) suggests a chi-squared test without continuity correction be used to test the above hypothesis.

Based on this test, the required sample size for each arm is given by

$$N = \frac{\left(Z_{1-\alpha/2} + Z_{1-\beta}\right)^2 \left[p_c\left(1 - p_c\right) + p_t\left(1 - p_t\right)\right]}{\left(p_t - p_c\right)^2},$$

where Z_q is the qth quantile of a normal distribution with mean 0 and variance 1. Note that several other methods can be used to determine sample size in this situation, and the present formula is only presented as a general guideline.

As an example, suppose it is known that the control treatment has a 30% response rate and it is of clinical interest to detect a 50% response rate in the new treatment with 90% power. The investigator would also like to ensure that the probability of a false positive is 5%. Using the above formula, each arm of the study requires 121 patients.

Continuous Outcome

A continuous outcome is a value that ranges between $-\infty$ and ∞. An example is the change in PSA level 3 months after drug administration. In a trial that has a continuous primary outcome, the goal is to determine if there is a difference in outcome means between the arms. To determine the number of patients in the trial, the investigator must first specify the expected means in the control and treatment arms, given by μ_c and μ_t respectively. The standard deviation in the control group's outcome, σ, must also be specified. As before, the mean and standard deviation for the control arm must be based on prior knowledge, and the mean for the treatment arm is determined by the largest difference between the group means that is of clinical interest. Using this notation, the required sample size is calculated based on testing the hypothesis

$$H_0 : \mu_c = \mu_t \quad \text{versus} \quad H_a : \mu_c \neq \mu_t$$

such that the probability of a false positive is α and the power to detect the largest clinically relevant difference in means is $1 - \beta$. Assuming that both the treatment and control arms consist of independent groups of patients and the standard deviation in the control arm is similar to that in the treatment arm, a two-sample t-test without continuity correction is used to test the above hypothesis. Based on this test, the required sample size for each arm is given by

$$N = \frac{2 \left(Z_{1-\alpha/2} + Z_{1-\beta} \right)^2 \sigma^2}{\left(\mu_t - \mu_c \right)},$$

where Z_q is the qth quantile of a normal distribution with mean 0 and variance 1. Note that this is only an approximate formula that has been presented as a general guideline and is not suitable for small sample sizes.

As an example, suppose it is known that the outcome in the control arm has a mean of 30 units with a standard deviation of 20. It is of clinical interest to detect a mean outcome of 35 units in the new treatment with 90% power. The investigator would also like to ensure that the probability of a false positive is 5%. Using the above formula, each arm of the study requires 337 patients.

Other Sample Size Considerations

Investigators must also provide accurate estimates of the rate of patient withdrawal from the study, the rate at which patients deviate from the treatment protocol, and the rate at which patients are accrued. These rates will affect the time needed to carry out the trial because more patients must be recruited to meet the specified sample size requirements. The monetary cost of the trial per patient must also be considered to ensure that budgetary constraints are met.

Conclusion

Clinical trials have significantly improved the treatment of patients with any disease. However, results from a clinical trial can only be accepted by physicians and regulatory agencies alike if it is carefully designed and implemented. This discussion attempts to give a brief outline of the various issues that must be considered. A more thorough discussion is given by Pocock (12) and Piantadosi (13).

References

1. Laufer M, Ramalingam S, Schoenberg MP, et al. Intravesical gemcitabine therapy for superficial transitional cell carcinoma of the bladder: A phase I and pharmacokinetic study. J Clin Oncol 2003;21(4):697–703.
2. Raghavan D, Brandes LJ, Klapp K, et al. Phase II trial of tesmilifene plus mitoxantrone and prednisone for hormone refractory prostate cancer: high subjective and objective response in patients with symptomatic metastases. J Urol 2005;174(5): 1808–1813.
3. Fleming T. One-sample multiple testing procedure for phase II clinical trials. Biometrics 1982;38(1):143–151.
4. Simon R. Optimal two-stage designs for phase II clinical trials. Control Clin Trials 1989;10(1):1–10.
5. Tjoa BA, Simmons SJ, Bowes VA, et al. Evaluation of phase I/II clinical trials in prostate cancer with dendritic cells and PSMA peptides. Prostate 1998;36(1):39–44.
6. Thompson IM, Goodman PJ, Tangen CM, et al. The influence of finasteride on the development of prostate cancer. N Engl J Med 2003;349(3):215–224.
7. D'Amico AV, Renshaw AA, Cote K, et al. Impact of the percentage of positive prostate cores on prostate cancer-specific mortality for patients with low or favorable intermediate-risk disease. J Clin Oncol 2004;22(18):3726–3732.
8. Hulley SB, Cummings SR, Browner WS, et al. Designing Clinical Research, 2nd ed. Philadelphia: Lippincott Williams & Wilkins, 2001.
9. Freedman B. Equipoise and the ethics of clinical research. N Engl J Med 1987; 317(3):141–145.
10. Petrioli R, Frediani B, Manganelli A, et al. Comparison between a cisplatin-containing regimen and a carboplatin-containing regimen for recurrent or metastatic bladder cancer patients. A randomized phase II study. Cancer 1996;77:344–351.
11. A'Hern RP. Sample size tables for exact single-stage phase II designs. Stat Med 2001; 20(6):859–866.
12. Pocock SJ. Clinical Trials: A Practical Approach. New York: John Wiley, 1983.
13. Piantadosi S. Clinical Trials: A Methodologic Perspective. New York: John Wiley, 1997.

9
Principles of Chemotherapy for Genitourinary Cancer

Sujith Kalmadi and Derek Raghavan

Cytotoxic chemotherapy evolved from the concepts of Lissauer and Ehrlich early in the 20th century. The initial chemotherapy protocols were characterized by a lack of specificity, often with significant toxicity to the host. This has been subsequently improved due to a better understanding of tumor biology, the basis of the cell cycle and constituency of the human genome, and the biochemical basis of action of the chemotherapy regimens. In the past century, insight into the intracellular pathways that result in sensitivity and resistance of the neoplastic cells to drug treatment have led to significant refinement of our technology, leading to more effective and less toxic treatment regimens.

Tumor Cell Kinetics

The biological behavior and heterogeneity of tumors is explained by several factors, including heterogeneity of constituent cell populations, variable function of cell regulatory functions, nutritional factors, tumor volume/cell number, and cytokinetics (1). This can lead to wide variations in the expression of the cell cycles of different tumors, although we now have quite a clear understanding of the factors that control the growth cycle of cells (2).

Cells grow and divide via an ordered sequence, consisting of the following key stages (Fig. 9.1):

1. Resting phase (G0)
2. Cells that are committed to replication enter the interphase (G1) that is characterized by synthesis of ribonucleic acid (RNA) and protein, preparing the cell to enter the next phase
3. Deoxyribonucleic acid (DNA) synthetic (S) phase, in which the DNA content is doubled
4. Second resting (G2) phase prior to the cell undergoing mitosis
5. Mitotic phase (M), in which the chromosomes separate and divide, forming two daughter cells

Mitosis results in cells that consist of (1) nondividing, terminally differentiated cells; (2) resting cells (G0), which can be recruited into the cell cycle; and

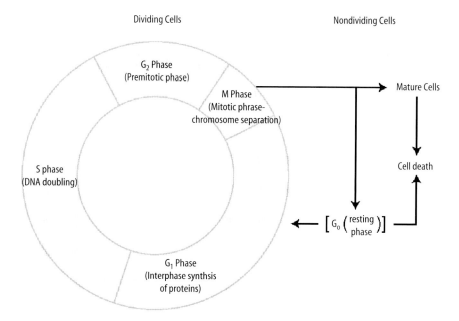

FIGURE 9.1. Cell cycle. [From Kalmadi and Raghavan (2005), with permission.]

(3) continually dividing cells, which enter into G1 phase again. Major checkpoints in the cell proliferation occur in G1 when cells must commit themselves to division and in G2 before undergoing mitosis. The cell cycle is under the control of numerous regulatory mechanisms, including cyclins, which are proteins that are positive regulators, and cyclin-dependent kinases (CDKs), which are present in all phases of the cell cycle and control the cascade of proliferative signals.

Regulation of these CDKs by the cyclin molecules causes their levels to fluctuate, leading to synchronization of the processes of cell division.

Chemotherapy and radiation are most effective in achieving cytotoxicity when the cells are in cycle. One approach to the categorization of cytotoxics is based on their activities relative to the cell cycle:

1. Phase-specific drugs are effective only if present in the tumor cell during a specific phase of the cell division. Increasing the drug level or dose will not result in more tumor kill, although exposure over a longer period of time will allow more cells to enter the specific lethal phase of the cycle, leading to higher cell kill. Examples include antimetabolites during the S phase, and taxanes and alkaloids during G2 and M phase.

2. Phase-nonspecific agents can be further divided into cycle-nonspecific drugs, which can kill nondividing cells (e.g., steroids, some antitumor antibiotics), and cycle-specific drugs, which can kill cells that enter into the cell cycle (e.g., alkylating agents). Phase-nonspecific agents have a linear dose-response

curve: the higher the dose administered, the greater the fraction of cells killed.

As a result of studies of the human genome, a clearer understanding of the level of molecular checks and balances involved in the regulation of the cell cycle is emerging. However, a detailed discussion of this topic is beyond the scope of this overview, apart from details that relate to targeted therapeutics (see below).

Tumor Kinetic Modeling

The growth of a tumor can be simplistically visualized as being dependent on several variables, which include rate of cell loss, growth fraction (proportion of cells in proliferative phase), and cell doubling time. Numerous models have been devised that explain the impact of therapeutic regimens on the tumor cell cycle (3). We will review these proposed models and our understanding of current chemotherapy/radiotherapy models in a historical fashion, sketching out their evolution.

The log kill model originally proposed by Skipper and colleagues (4) was based on the behavior of L1210 leukemia cell lines in rodents (5). They postulated that the increase in life span of the host after chemotherapy was due to the cytocidal effects on the cancer cells and that tumor growth and tumor regression in response to chemotherapy were exponential in nature. In this model, a drug that would cause the tumor burden to decrease from 10^{12} to 10^{11}, if given in the same dose, would decrease the burden from 10^6 to 10^5 (each reflecting a 90% tumor cell kill). This formed the basis for the use of repeated cycles of chemotherapy to achieve maximal tumor eradication. However, it has become clear that exposure to the same regimen for more than four to six doses has not improved outcomes. We now understand the growth models of tumor have also a mixed nature with respect to different cancer cells in vivo (6). The Gompertzian sigmoid-shaped growth is characteristic of many solid tumors. Tumors grow most rapidly at smaller sizes and then the growth rate slows, secondary to problems with vascularity, hypoxia, and interaction with the other cells in their microenvironment (7–10).

Concepts derived from resistance in antibacterial therapy were applied to the study of antimetabolites in the treatment of L1210 cells, and it was shown that resistance is acquired at various points during the growth of the tumor. These concepts can be shown in human tumor cells, and it has been postulated that larger tumors have more cells and thus have a greater chance of sustaining spontaneous mutation (11). These mutations may confer resistance to chemotherapy.

Based on these concepts, it has been suggested that tumors are better treated at a smaller size, before they have the ability to develop mutations and resistance. This has also led to the concept that non–cross-resistant multiple-agent chemotherapy would have a greater tumor kill and could prevent development of resistance.

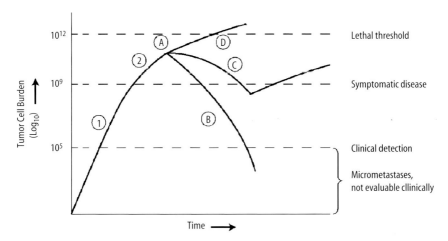

FIGURE 9.2. Gompertzian model of tumor growth. Relation among tumor mass, diagnosis, and treatment regimens. Growth phases: 1, exponential growth; 2, plateau phase with slower growth due to cells outgrowing vascular supply and nutritional resources, and possible other regulatory mechanisms. Treatment responses: A, initiation of treatment; B, curative therapy; C, initial response with secondary resistance; D, primary resistance. [From Kalmadi and Raghavan (2005), with permission.]

Another fundamental concept of cell cycle kinetics is the so-called Norton-Simon regression hypothesis (12). This postulates that delivering chemotherapy at shorter time intervals (dose-intense chemotherapy) will maximize tumor cell kill. As noted above (Fig. 9.2), some tumors do not grow in a simple exponential manner but rather follow a Gompertzian growth pattern (13). Norton and Simon have also proposed that less time available for tumor regrowth between treatments will improve the likelihood of cure.

These investigators have also proposed that sequential dose-dense, non–cross-resistant regimens will minimize drug resistance by destroying the dominant tumor population initially via the first component of treatment, with different agents addressing the residual resistant cells.

The Goldie-Coldman and Norton-Simon hypotheses have rationalized the empirical approach to adjuvant chemotherapy after definitive local therapy, which has resulted in improved cure rates, perhaps due to increased cytotoxicity and a reduced chance for the emergence of drug resistance (13–15).

Pharmacology of Antineoplastic Agents

The clinical pharmacology of antineoplastic agents has been an evolving field for the past century, with the most progress having been made in the past decade through the advent of analytical tools such as liquid chromatography and mass spectroscopy. Most cytotoxic agents offer a very narrow therapeutic index compared with most drugs (16).

Pharmacokinetic Principles

Pharmacokinetics involves the study of the fate of administered medications, including absorption, distribution, metabolism, and excretion. Absorption has historically not been a major issue for oncologists, because (until recently) most drugs were administered intravenously. With the advances in drug delivery involving orally administered targeted agents and prodrugs, this has become an issue with oral and cutaneously absorbed drugs. The level of bioavailability is calculated by comparing the area under the curve (AUC) of an oral drug to the same dose given intravenously.

Clearance of the drug is the most critical aspect and can be conceptualized as being a function of drug distribution, metabolism, and elimination. Although drug distribution can be viewed most simply as being two-compartmental (extracellular and intracellular), it is actually more complex. It should more properly by considered as a multicompartment model with frequent redistribution within. The presence of sanctuary sites with poor penetration of the drug may result in apparent resistance of tumors that would otherwise be responsive to chemotherapy.

Distribution can also be affected by disease states such as cardiac failure, resulting in pleural effusions and ascites, thus creating pathological compartments.

When third spaces are present (such as pleural effusions or ascites), some agents (e.g. methotrexate) can cause excessive toxicity due to prolonged exposure as they accumulate within these spaces, causing prolonged drug exposure. Elimination is studied along two different models: linear versus nonlinear. The linear kinetic model is based on the assumption that the half-life of the drug is constant. Nonlinear kinetics assumes that the elimination of the drug is saturable, resulting in different rates of excretion at different concentrations, leading to variable half-lives.

The metabolism of these agents is determined by the amount of resemblance that they show to physiological substrate. Drugs (e.g., purine and pyrimidine analogues) that are similar to normal metabolites are processed by the same mechanisms as the normal metabolites intracellularly. Those that are less similar are degraded in the liver, in reactions involving oxidation (controlled by the cytochrome P-450 enzymes) and conjugation. The ultimate excretion of the drug from the body is via the hepatobiliary system or the kidney. Creatinine clearance, often used as a surrogate marker of renal function, assesses the glomerular function rate. However, tubular secretion and reabsorption may also play a role in drug excretion. These changes in the renal excretion of the drugs can alter their efficacy and toxicity profile.

Hepatic excretion involves a number of transport systems including P-glycoprotein and canalicular multispecific organic anion transporter (cMOAT). Enterohepatic recirculation also plays a major role, especially in the drugs metabolized by the glucuronide pathway. Changes in the regulation of the cytochrome system by other medications being used may cause changes in the bioavailable levels of chemotherapeutic agents metabolized by this system. The use of liver function tests to modify the dosage of these drugs is thus fraught with numerous pitfalls, since it does not always accurately predict the toxicity risk due to the fact that they do not accurately estimate the level of dysfunction (17).

Another important component of the system is interpatient pharmacokinetic variability (18). Pharmacogenetic variation explains some of the variability in the response and toxicity of patient groups to agents like 5-fluorouracil (5-FU) and irinotecan (19).

Deficiency of dihydropyrimidine dehydrogenase, reflecting different polymorphisms of the DPD gene, which inactivates 5-FU, will lead to increased toxicity from this cytotoxic. The active form of irinotecan, SN38, is inactivated via glucuronidation. Reduced activity of UGT1A1, which is involved in this glucuronidation, leads to dose-limiting diarrhea and neutropenia. Of note, this genetic anomaly is a sine qua non of Gilbert's syndrome.

Other factors may also cause interpatient variation in pharmacokinetics. The variability in absorption of oral drugs secondary to chemotherapy-induced damage to the mucosa can alter efficacy and toxicity of these agents. Most chemotherapy regimens are dosed based on body surface area, which is calculated by using body weight and height. Obesity, which causes an increase in the lipophilic compartment, is not well addressed by this calculation of drug dosing. The amount of lipid solubility of a drug can cause changes in the drug levels in the obese. Hypoalbuminemia causing decreased binding and increased free concentration of the drug can increase side effects. This may be quite important in a pretreated patient with advanced cancer and cachexia, which is commonly associated with hypoalbuminemia.

Pharmacodynamics

The fundamental objective of pharmacodynamics is to understand dose-response relationships, usually predicated on the assessment of drug levels in different tissues (20), as well as the pharmacogenomic considerations noted above. Phase I clinical trials attempt to define the maximally tolerated dose and the dose limiting toxicities as a function of dose. Initial pharmacodynamic principles were based on the concept that all drugs have a sigmoidal shape in their drug effect, based on the theory that drugs require a receptor interaction for their effect. However, this rule is not valid for phase-specific antineoplastic agents. When cells are not in the specific phase, increasing the dose does not increase the sensitivity, but increasing the time of exposure may have the desired effect.

The prediction of toxicity and response in an individual patient should be based on both pharmacokinetic and pharmacodynamic principles. Reducing drug dose for excessive toxicities may seem to be logical in the case of altered excretory function, but may not be effective in the case of reduced hematological reserve after prior treatment, resulting simply in underdosing.

Monitoring of drugs with a narrow therapeutic index (for example, digoxin) is usually done by monitoring drug levels in the body, in most other areas of medicine. This is more complicated in cancer treatment because of the frequent use of combination chemotherapy. Techniques such as weekly dosing (e.g., taxanes) and AUC dosing based on creatinine clearance (carboplatin) are being used to limit toxicity without compromising efficacy.

Patterns of Drug Response and Resistance

Response of tumors can be divided generally into three groups (21,22): (1) drug-sensitive tumors, with treatment resulting in cure; (2) highly responsive tumors, but with eventual refractoriness to cytotoxic treatment; and (3) tumors with little responsiveness to chemotherapy (Table 9.1).

Drug resistance has been studied both in vivo and in vitro in a range of models. Multiple reasons involving anatomical, pharmacological, and bio-chemical mechanisms explain various aspects of tumor resistance to cytotoxic chemotherapy:

- Reduced intracellular levels secondary to transport system inhibition (e.g., the folate transport mechanism leading to methotrexate resistance), and reduced diffusion across the cell membrane or increased efflux (P-glycoprotein MDR1 drug efflux pump): Classical multidrug resistance (MDR) is associated with the overexpression of P-glycoprotein (MDR1, P-170) (23,24). This causes increased efflux of various antineoplastic agents from the cell leading to decreased accumulation intracellularly. This has been implicated in the cross-resistance patterns between anthracyclines (e.g., doxorubicin), taxanes (e.g.,

TABLE 9.1. Responsiveness of genitourinary tumors to chemotherapy

1. Highly sensitive
   A. Childhood cancers, such as Wilms' tumor, Ewing tumor, and rhabdomyosarcoma
   B. Germ cell tumors, e.g., of testis, retroperitoneum
   C. Lymphoma (extranodal): Hodgkin's disease; Burkitt's lymphoma
2. Moderately sensitive
   A. Adenocarcinoma of the prostate
   B. Transitional cell carcinoma of bladder and urothelial tract
   C. Squamous cell carcinoma of penis or urethra
   D. Some non-Hodgkin's lymphomas involving genitourinary tract
   E. Small cell anaplastic carcinoma: prostate, bladder
   F. Sarcomas of bladder or prostate in adults
3. Minimally sensitive
   A. Adrenal gland cancers
   B. Renal carcinoma*
   C. Adenocarcinoma of bladder

*Note: emerging changes with recent development of targeted therapies.

paclitaxel), vinca alkaloids (e.g., vincristine), and the topoisomerase inhibitors (e.g., etoposide). Tumors that overexpress this gene have sometimes demonstrated increased resistance and poor response to chemotherapy.

- Defects in cellular death mechanisms: Alkylating agents cause cell death by intrastrand DNA linkages. This results in defective cell repair systems that should lead to cell death. However, if this system does not recognize the DNA defects, this will prevent tumor cell death, resulting in resistance (16,25). Defects in the apoptotic pathway can also involve the Bcl-2 family of proteins and other regulatory mechanisms, such as p53. Bcl-2 family proteins include both up- and downregulators of apoptosis. Chemotherapy-induced damage to cells is perceived by p53, which can then initiate either apoptosis or cell repair. Altered p53 is one of the most common genetic abnormalities seen in solid tumors. Expression of wild-type p53 and changes in Bcl-2 family members can result in altered sensitivity of the tumor cell to chemotherapy agents (26,27).
- Alteration of drug targets, including receptors or enzymes (e.g., thymidylate synthetase in 5-FU resistance) (28): Increased levels of cell protective agents (e.g., glutathione in cisplatin resistance), which prevent oxidative damage and death of the cell via cell scavenging functions, have been implicated in preclinical models of bladder cancer (29).
- Modification of drug metabolism: Modification can be catastrophic to antineoplastics that are designed as prodrugs (e.g., cyclophosphamide must be activated in the liver; irinotecan must be converted to SN-38, its active moiety).
- Tumor cell heterogeneity: Heterogeneity with spontaneous genetic mutations occurs even before exposure to treatment (27,30). After chemotherapy eliminates the sensitive cells, these resistant cells may grow to become the predominant cell population.

Approaches to circumvent drug resistance have involved the use of multidrug combinations, dose escalation, agents that reverse increased efflux, cofactors that amplify drug efficacy, and inhibition of drug inactivation. Liposomal and nanoparticle albumin-stabilized formulations have been applied to overcome drug resistance (31). These increase the delivery of chemotherapy to the tumor cell while minimizing toxicity.

Combination Chemotherapy Principles

Single-agent regimens, with few exceptions (e.g., gestational choriocarcinoma), are rarely able to achieve cure. In view of this and the observations above, combination chemotherapy regimens have been devised to accomplish the major objectives of attaining maximum tumor kill with minimal toxicity and to prevent drug resistance (16,32). The era began when numerous active drugs became available simultaneously and were applied to curative management of leukemias and lymphomas in the late 1970s. Fundamental principles used in the selection of the drugs for combination regimens include the following (32):

- Drugs with activity against the tumor
- Different patterns of resistance
- Varying mechanism of action with potential synergy
- Nonoverlapping dose-limiting toxicities
- Optimal dosing and timing in combination to make the treatment-free interval be the shortest

The relation between doses and combination of these agents is complex (32,33). The maintenance of dose intensity has proved to be important in the success of many of these regimens. Reduction of dose can result in significantly decreased cure rates, especially in the more responsive tumors such as germ cell cancer. Thus, although responses continue to be observed with dose reduction, residual tumor cells often persist, leading to eventual relapse and decreased survival. The concept of relative dose intensity (amount of drug delivered in a given time frame) has evolved over the past two decades, but it remains controversial as to whether this is a major factor in cure (34). Ideally drugs should be used in their optimal schedule and dosage even when being combined with other agents. In general, the interval of drug delivery also needs to be consistent, keeping the treatment-free interval the shortest time necessary for resolution of any dose-limiting toxicity (usually bone marrow toxicity) to maintain dose intensity (32,33,35).

The selection of patients to receive combination chemotherapy has also undergone refinement. In the present era, we are more cautious than in the past, and many oncologists believe that it may not be appropriate for a patient with a poor performance score [e.g., Eastern Cooperative Oncology Group (ECOG) level 3 to 4] to be given a toxic regimen, unless there is substantial evidence that his disease is likely to be highly responsive to the treatment sensitive. By contrast, with better understanding of age-related changes in drug pharmacology and the importance of performance status, more venturesome approaches are now being explored in the chemotherapy of the fit elderly with advanced cancer (36,37).

High-Dose Chemotherapy and Stem Cell Transplantation

High-dose chemotherapy involves the use of dose-intensive chemotherapy with or without radiation, followed by rescue with hematopoietic stem cells obtained from the blood or by marrow harvest and storage (38–41). This is predicated on the concepts that (1) there is a dose-response relationship for a specific regimen in certain tumors; (2) there is benefit to dosing at a higher level than can be survived by normal tissues (e.g., bone marrow), provided that re-infusion of bone marrow can avoid the death of the host. This modality, which is predominantly used in hematological malignancies, has been applied to the management of relapsed or poor-risk metastatic germ cell tumors (38). To date, despite evidence of anticancer activity, randomized trial data have not shown a survival benefit from this approach to the management of advanced germ cell tumors, compared to standard dose poor-risk or salvage regimens (38).

Allogeneic bone marrow transplantation involves obtaining the stem cells from a donor who has some human leukocyte antigen (HLA) match with the patient (39–41). This can include matched related donor, matched unrelated donor (e.g., HLA matched donor from the bone marrow registry), stored cord blood, or syngeneic (identical twin) or haploidentical transplantation (e.g., sibling/parent who is half matched to the patient). Complexities of allogeneic bone marrow transplantation involve immunosuppression after the transplant to prevent rejection of the donor cells by the host. This milieu of intense cytotoxic damage to the bone marrow and immunosuppression allows the donor graft cells to launch a response against the recipient termed as graft-versus-host disease (GVHD). Graft-versus-host disease can also have a positive effect on the tumor by having a graft versus tumor effect, which can be curative in some malignancies like chronic myelogenous leukemia. Advantages of allogeneic bone marrow transplantation include the graft versus tumor effect, a curative option in patients with tumor involvement of the bone marrow and no tumor contamination of the graft cells.

Disadvantages include GVHD, higher treatment related mortality, higher infectious complications secondary to immunosuppression needed after transplant, and the need to locate a suitable donor. In addition, increasing evidence is available regarding late complications, including the development of second malignancies (40,41).

Autologous bone marrow transplantation uses the patient's own hematopoietic stem cells, which are harvested and cryopreserved prior to initiation of treatment (38). After the completion of high-dose chemotherapy or radiation, the harvested marrow is re-infused. Advantages include the following: no immunosuppressive therapy is needed after infusion of stem cells; GVHD does not occur; transplantation can be used for older patients; no donor is needed; and there is a lower treatment-related mortality of about 2% to 5%. Some of the disadvantages of this approach include the absence of graft versus tumor effect, and the risk of re-seeding tumor cells if there is marrow involvement by the malignancy.

Brief Overview of Cytotoxic Agents

Alkylating Agents

These agents form the backbone of numerous regimens. They impair cell function by transferring alkyl groups to amino, carboxyl, phosphate, or sulfhydryl groups of nucleic acids (DNA and RNA). The most actively alkylated site is the

N-7 position of guanine. This results in cross-linked DNA strands that cannot replicate, impaired transcription of RNA, and other damage to the genetic material. These agents are cell cycle specific, but not phase specific. They have traditionally been divided into five classes, although the platinum complexes (with similar, bifunctional alkylating action) have been included as a sixth class. Nausea, vomiting, alopecia, and myelosuppression are common acute side effects. These agents can also cause secondary acute leukemia or other solid tumors several years after the initiation of treatment. This iatrogenic leukemia, typically preceded by a myelodysplastic phase of variable duration, is associated with abnormalities of chromosome 5, 7, or 8. The features of the common alkylating agents are summarized in Table 9.2 (43).

TABLE 9.2. Major alkylating agents in clinical genitourinary cancer practice

Drug	Pharmacology	Uses	Toxicity
Carboplatin	Second-generation platinum compound similar to cisplatin with different toxicity; half-life is shorter than cisplatin	Modest activity against germ cell tumors and perhaps prostate cancer	DLT = myelosuppression especially thrombocytopenia; dosage typically done by AUC with Calvert's formula
Cisplatin	First heavy metal antineoplastic; long half-life, may remain in tissues for months; poor CNS penetration; primarily excreted in the urine; clinical cross-resistance with carboplatin	Active against germ cell tumors and bladder cancer; some activity against prostate and adrenal cancers	DLT = cumulative nephropathy which can be reduced to <5% with vigorous hydration; cumulative peripheral sensory neuropathy; ototoxicity with tinnitus and high-frequency hearing loss
Cyclophosphamide	Both oral and IV forms; requires activation in the liver to form acrolein and an alkylating metabolite; drugs affecting microsomal enzymes will affect efficacy	Activity against prostate cancer; some activity against germ cell tumors; modest activity against TCC	DLT = myelosuppression; high dose as preparation for BMT can cause cardiac necrosis; hemorrhagic cystitis is secondary to a metabolite and can be prevented by hydration and Mesna
Ifosfamide	IV formulation; requires activation in the liver similar to cyclophosphamide	Bladder TCC, sarcomas, germ cell tumors	DLT = myelosuppression; hemorrhagic cystitis; high doses can lead to encephalopathy
Nitrosureas	Highly lipid soluble; rapidly biotransformed	Modest activity in hormone refractory prostate cancer	DLT = myelosuppression can be prolonged and cumulative; nausea and vomiting can last up to 24 hours
Temozolamide	Oral medication that is activated spontaneously to the same active metabolite as DTIC	Being tested in hormone refractory prostate cancer	DLT = myelosuppression especially thrombocytopenia; moderate gastrointestinal side effects

AUC, area under the curve; BMT, bone marrow transplantation; CNS, central nervous system; DLT, dose-limiting toxicity; DTIC, diethyl triazeno imidazole carboximide.

TABLE 9.3. Antimetabolites in clinical genitourinary cancer practice

Drug	Pharmacology	Uses	Toxicity
Capecitabine	Prodrug of 5-FU that can be given orally	Possible activity against bladder adenocarcinoma	DLT = diarrhea; hand-foot syndrome is common and can be dose limiting
5-Fluorouracil	Inhibition of thymidylate synthetase by inhibits DNA synthesis; other metabolites may interfere with RNA function; differs from other antimetabolites in having a log linear cell kill; leucovorin enhances the action by acting at thymidylate synthetase	Modest activity against bladder adenocarcin oma and minor activity against prostate cancer	DLT = myelosuppression (more common with bolus regimens), mucositis and diarrhea (more common with infusion regimens); other toxicities include cardiac, excessive lacrimation, nasal discharge, and cerebellar toxicity
Methotrexate	Synthetic analogue of folic acid, which blocks the enzyme; dihydrofolate reductase preventing formation of reduced folic acid that interferes with vital cellular enzymes	Active against germ cell tumors and bladder cancer; minor activity against prostate cancer and penile cancer	DLT = myelosuppression, stomatitis, renal dysfunction, neurotoxicity, depending on dose and duration of use; leucovorin rescues normal tissues from toxicity and is used in high-dose regimens

Antimetabolites (Table 9.3)

Antimetabolites have been used since 1948, when they first produced temporary remission in children with acute lymphatic leukemia. Subsequently, methotrexate proved that chemotherapy could cure cancer as a single agent in gestational trophoblastic neoplasia. These antimetabolites constitute a large group of drugs that interfere with the building blocks of DNA/RNA synthesis. They can be structural analogues of normal molecules needed for cell growth or inhibit enzymes needed for the synthesis of essential compounds. Therefore, their activity is greatest in the S phase of the cell cycle. Pharmacokinetics is characterized by their nonlinear dose-response curve (an exception being 5-FU). After a certain dose, there is no more cell death; however, increasing the length of time that the cells are exposed will increase the cell killing potential.

Antitumor Antibiotics (Table 9.4)

Antitumor antibiotics are generally derived from microorganisms. They interfere with DNA by intercalation, where the drug inserts between DNA base pairs. This interferes with DNA replication and messenger RNA production. They also interfere with topoisomerase function. They are cell cycle nonspecific drugs and are an important component against slowly growing tumors with a low growth

TABLE 9.4. Antitumor antibiotics in clinical genitourinary cancer practice

Drug	Pharmacology	Uses	Toxicity
Actinomycin D (dactinomycin)	Extensively tissue bound with long half-life (36 hours)	Active against Wilms' tumor, sarcoma, germ cell tumor	DLT = myelosuppression; may cause severe nausea and vomiting and allergic reactions
Bleomycin	Activated by microsomal reduction; radiation sensitizer	Active against germ cell tumors; modest activity against penile cancer	Chills and febrile reactions that are infusion related; pneumonitis can occur 4–10 weeks after initiation; skin pigmentation
Doxorubicin	Extensively plasma protein bound with long half-life; liposomal formulation (Doxil) is undergoing trials in various tumors	Activity against small cell anaplastic cancers, prostate cancer, bladder cancer	DLT = myelosuppression, commonly leukopenia; cardiomyopathy with congestive heart failure (CHF) is more frequent after a cumulative dose of 550 mg/m^2 (400 mg/m^2 with previous mediastinal irradiation)
Epirubicin			
Mitomycin	Also functions as an alkylating agent	Active against bladder cancer; modest activity against prostate cancer	DLT = myelosuppression, which can be cumulative and prolonged; thrombocytopenia may occur up to 8 weeks

fraction. As a class they tend to be vesicants, and extravasation may cause skin necrosis and ulceration. Common side effects include nausea, vomiting, alopecia, and myelosuppression.

Tubulin Targeting Agents (Table 9.5)

The class of antitubulin drugs includes the vinca alkaloids and taxanes. The primary target of these drugs is the mitotic spindle.

The vinca alkaloids bind to microtubular proteins, inhibiting their assembly and leading to mitotic spindle dysfunction, mitotic arrest, and eventually cell death from apoptosis. The taxanes bind to tubulin polymers, promoting their assembly but making them resistant to depolymerization, resulting in nonfunctional microtubules. Each of this class of cytotoxics may be exported from the cancer cell by the function of p-glycoprotein.

Topoisomerase Inhibitors (Table 9.6)

Semisynthetic glycosides of the naturally occurring podophyllotoxins, the epipodophyllotoxins (etoposide and teniposide), have been in clinical use for 30 years, because of efficacy and modest toxicity.

TABLE 9.5. Tubulin targeting agents in clinical genitourinary cancer practice

Drugs	Uses	Pharmacology	Toxicity
Docetaxel	Activity against hormone refractory prostate cancer, bladder cancer, germ cell tumors, and squamous cancers	Semisynthetic and thus more soluble; does not require Cremophor; triphasic decline; degradation via metabolism, rather than excretion	DLT = myelosuppression; fluid retention is dose dependent, secondary to increased capillary permeability and is reversible; hypersensitivity reactions similar to paclitaxel (despite not being formulated in Cremophor) can occur
Paclitaxel	Activity against hormone refractory prostate cancer, bladder cancer, germ cell tumors, and squamous cancers	Requires Cremophor for dissolution, adding toxicity; recent nano-engineered preparation may improve cellular uptake and reduce toxicity; altered disposition with increasing age; biphasic or triphasic decline of levels; metabolic clearance	DLT = myelosuppression; hypersensitivity (3%) to Cremophor (carrier vehicle) occurs usually within 20 minutes of initiating treatment, 90% of which happen within the first two doses; premedication with steroids and histamine blockers is routinely recommended; peripheral neuropathy is dose dependent
Vincristine Vinblastine	Activity against bladder cancer and germ cell tumors	Hepatic clearance; triphasic decline; these agents are vesicants	DLT = dose dependent peripheral neuropathy universally develops; it is reversible, however, it can take several months; this can result in cranial nerve palsies, abdominal pain, obstipation, ataxia, footdrop, cortical blindness, seizures

TABLE 9.6. Topoisomerase inhibitors in clinical genitourinary cancer practice

Drugs	Pharmacology	Uses	Toxicities
Etoposide (VP-16)	Can be used orally and IV; bioavailability is 50%, however, it is nonlinear and decreases with doses higher than 200 mg	Activity in germ cell tumors	DLT = neutropenia; gastrointestinal toxicities common with oral drug
Irinotecan (CPT-11, Camptosar)	Needs to be activated to SN-38; this conversion occurs primarily in the liver, but can also occur in the plasma and in the intestinal mucosa	Undergoing phase II trials in bladder cancer	Early diarrhea within 24 hours of the infusion is cholinergic and is controlled with atropine; late diarrhea is due to SN-38 and needs to be controlled with antibiotics and Loperamide

More recently, camptothecin derivatives (irinotecan and topotecan) have been introduced into clinical practice. DNA attachment to the nuclear matrix occurs at areas called "domains." Topoisomerases bind to these areas, forming a complex allowing DNA to unwind for cell division. Topoisomerase I helps in the relaxation of supercoiled DNA, while topoisomerase II catalyzes the breaking and resealing of DNA. These enzymes are crucial in several critical steps of the cell cycle. Epipodophyllotoxins inhibit topoisomerase I and camptothecins inhibit topoisomerase II. Anthracyclines also exhibit topoisomerase inhibition. Topoisomerase II inhibitors can cause secondary leukemia with a shorter latency period than with alkylating agents and not typically preceded by a myelodysplastic phase. These are associated with a balanced translocation involving chromosome 11 (11q23) or 21 (21q22).

Principles of Targeted Therapies

Since Paul Ehrlich proposed the concept of the "magic bullet" to cure each infection with a specific targeted drug, there has been a search for similar applications in cancer. The discovery of drugs with targets that are variably expressed in neoplastic cells would theoretically result in an increased anticancer effect and reduced toxicity. Recently, with the unraveling of the human genome and of the molecular pathways in cancer biology, functional targeted therapies have been discovered (44,45).

The prototype compound has been imatinib mesylate ("Gleevec"), a signal transduction inhibitor that targets the BCR-ABL protein and related tyrosine kinases (the constitutive abnormality created by the Philadelphia chromosome in chronic myeloid leukemia). This agent has had application in gastrointestinal stromal tumors and some sarcomas. The agent inhibits differentiation and proliferation, and induces apoptosis in BCR-ABL positive cells.

HER Family of Membrane Receptors

This family is composed of four members: HER1 (also called epidermal growth factor receptor, EGFR), HER 2 (ErbB2 or HER2/Neu), HER3, and HER4. They have a similar structure with an extracellular ligand-binding domain, a transmembrane domain, and an intracellular domain with tyrosine kinase (TK) activity. Binding of ligands to the receptor can initiate signal transduction cascades, which influence numerous pathways in the cell cycle. These receptors are overexpressed in many malignancies:

- HER1 (EGFR) receptor has been targeted using monoclonal antibodies against the external domain and TK inhibitors, which compete with adenosine triphosphate (ATP) to bind to the kinase pocket of the receptor. Cetuximab (C225) is a chimeric human-mouse monoclonal antibody that has recently been approved for use in metastatic colon cancer. Gefitinib (Iressa) is an oral

TK inhibitor that is being used in non–small-cell lung cancer. This may have increased anticancer efficacy in female nonsmokers with lung cancer and in bronchoalveolar carcinoma of the lung. Side effects of these agents include diarrhea, skin rash, and acne, and there has been controversy as to whether cardiopulmonary toxicity is a widespread problem. Having demonstrated antitumor activity against preclinical models of prostate cancer, gefitinib has been tested in combination with docetaxel and estramustine in phase I clinical trials for patients with prostate cancer, but its true utility has not yet been defined (46).

- HER2 has been shown to be dramatically overamplified in breast cancer tumors (30%). Trastuzumab (Herceptin) is a monoclonal antibody that targets the extracellular domain of HER2. Combined with chemotherapy, it has improved the progression and overall survival in metastatic breast cancer, which overexpresses HER2. It represents the first successful HER targeted therapy. Cardiotoxicity leading to congestive heart failure can occur with this agent. In view of this, it is not being used concurrently with anthracyclines. Infusion-related hypersensitivity reactions also occur in half the patients, usually with the first infusion.

Vascular Endothelial Growth Factor Pathway

Angiogenesis is crucial for tumor growth, and it is promoted by oncogene-driven expression of vascular endothelial growth factor (VEGF), interleukins, and other growth factors (44,45,47). In tumors VEGF is constitutively overexpressed as compared to normal tissue, and is further increased by hypoxia (47). It has been targeted with monoclonal antibodies and TK inhibitors similar to the approach in the HER family. Bevacizumab (Avastin) is a recombinant humanized monoclonal antibody against VEGF that has been recently approved in metastatic colorectal cancer (44,45). It is now being actively studied in combination with chemotherapy and other targeted therapies in other cancers, and appears to have activity against renal cell carcinoma. Toxicities include gastrointestinal perforation, poor wound healing, hypertension, and nephrotic syndrome.

Summary

The nature and scope of chemotherapy has changed dramatically in the past 50 years. Therapeutic strategies that were initially empirical, highly toxic, and broadly based have given way to rationally predicated, specifically targeted approaches. The emphasis of drug design has been to apply our knowledge of the human genome to identify useful therapeutic targets, and to create new compounds or analogues of old agents that have reduced toxicity profiles. The concepts of dose density and dose intensity remain controversial, but offer other potential options for increasing the cure rate of the few remaining resistant cancers.

References

1. Tannock IF. Cell kinetics and chemotherapy. A critical review. Cancer Treat Rep 1978;62:1117–1133.
2. Young RC, De Vita VT. Cell cycle characteristics of human solid tumors in vivo. Cell Tissue Kinet 1970;3:285–290.
3. Alberts DS. A unifying vision of cancer therapy for the 21st century. J Clin Oncol 1999;17(11 suppl);13–21.
4. Skipper HE, Schabel FM Jr, Wilcox WS. Experimental evaluation of potential anticancer agents XII: on the criteria and kinetics associated with "curability of leukemia." Cancer Chemother Rep 1964;35:1–111.
5. Yankee RA, De Vita VT, Perry S. The cell cycle of leukemia L 1210 cells in vivo. Cancer Res 1968;27:2381–2385.
6. Schnipper L. Clinical implications of tumor-cell heterogeneity. N Engl J Med 1986; 314:1423–1431.
7. Hanahan D, Weinberg RA. The hallmarks of cancer. Cell 2000;100:57–70.
8. Tubiana M. Tumor cell proliferation kinetics and tumor growth rate. Acta Oncol 1989;28:113–121.
9. Brown JM, Giaccia AJ. The unique physiology of solid tumors: opportunities (and problems) for cancer therapy. Cancer Res 1998;58:1408–1416.
10. Nowell PC. The clonal evolution of tumor progression. Science 1976;194:23–28.
11. Nowell P. Mechanisms of tumor progression. Cancer Res 1986;46:2203–2207.
12. Coldman AJ, Goldie JH. Impact of dose-intense chemotherapy on the development of permanent drug resistance. Semin Oncol 1987;14(suppl):29–33.
13. Norton L, Simon R. The Norton-Simon hypothesis revisited. Cancer Treat Rep 1986;70:163–169.
14. Norton LA. A gompertzian model of human breast cancer growth. Cancer Res 1988; 48:7067–7071.
15. Newell DR, McLeod HL, Schellens JHM. The pharmacology of anticancer drugs. In: Souhami RL, Tannock I, Hohenberger PF, Horiot J-C, eds. Oxford Textbook of Oncology, 2nd ed. London: Oxford University Press, 2002:623–637.
16. Gurney H. Dose calculation of anticancer drugs: a review of the current practice and introduction of an alternative. J Clin Oncol 1996;14:2590–2611.
17. Canal P, Chatelut E, Guichard S. Practical treatment guide for dose individualization in cancer chemotherapy. Drugs 1998;56:1019–1036.
18. Iyer L, Ratain MJ. Pharmacogenetics and cancer chemotherapy. Eur J Cancer 1998; 34:1493–1499.
19. Ratain MJ, Schilisky RL, Conley BA, Egorin MJ. Pharmacodynamics in cancer therapy. J Clin Oncol 1990;8:1739–1753.
20. Frei E III. Curative cancer chemotherapy. Cancer Res 1985;45:6523–6537.
21. Krakoff IH. Systemic treatment of cancer. CA Cancer J Clin 1996;46:134–141.
22. Endicott JA, Ling V. The biochemistry of P-glycoprotein mediated multidrug resistance. Annu Rev Biochem 1989;58:137–171.
23. Goldstein LJ, Galski H, Fojo A, et al. Expression of multidrug resistance gene in human tumors. J Natl Cancer Inst 1989;81:116–124.

24. Hickman JA. Apoptosis and chemotherapy resistance. Eur J Cancer 1996;32A: 921–926.
25. Schmitt CA, Lowe SW. Apoptosis and therapy. J Pathol 1999;187:127–137.
26. Moolgavkar SH, Knudsen AG. Mutation and cancer: a model for human carcinogenesis. J Natl Cancer Inst 1981;66:1037–1052.
27. Stoehlmacher J, Park DJ, Zhang W et al. A multivariate analysis of genomic polymorphisms: prediction of clinical outcome to 5–FU/oxaliplatin combination chemotherapy in refractory colorectal cancer. Br J Cancer 2004;91:344–354.
28. Pendyala L, Velagapudi S, Toth L, et al. Translational studies of glutathione in bladder cancer cell lines and human specimens. Clin Cancer Res 1997;3:793–798.
29. Fearon EC. Human cancer syndromes: clues to the origin and nature of cancer. Science 1997;278:1043–1058.
30. Sikic BL. Modulation of multidrug resistance: at the threshold. J Clin Oncol 1993; 11:1629–1635.
31. De Vita VT, Schein PS. The use of drugs in combination for the treatment of cancer: rationale and results. N Engl J Med 1973;228:998–1006.
32. Skipper HE. Critical variables in the design of combination chemotherapy regimens to be used alone or in adjuvant settings. Colloque INSERM 1986;137:11.
33. Hyrniuk WM. Average relative dose intensity and the impact on design of clinical trials. Semin Oncol 1987;14:65–74.
34. Day RS Treatment sequencing, asymmetry and uncertainty: protocol strategies for combination chemotherapy. Cancer Res 1986;46:3876–3880.
35. Raghavan D, Weiner JS, Lipson L. Cancer in the elderly. In: Souhami RL, Tannock I, Hohenberger PF, Horiot J-C, eds. Oxford Textbook of Oncology, 2nd ed. London: Oxford University Press, 2002:863–874.
36. Raghavan D, Brandes LJ, Klapp K, et al. Phase II trial of tesmilifene plus mitoxantrone and prednisone for hormone refractory prostate cancer: high subjective and objective response in patients with symptomatic metastases. J Urol 2005;174: 1808–1813.
37. Bolwell BJ. Factors predicting success or failure associated with common types of transplants. Pediatr Transplant 2005;9:2–11.
38. Margolin K. High dose chemotherapy and stem cell support in the treatment of poor-risk germ cell cancer. In: Raghavan D, ed. American Cancer Society Atlas of Clinical Oncology—Germ Cell Tumors. London: BC Decker, 2003:168–181.
39. Socie G, Stone JV, Wingard JR, et al. Long term survival and late deaths after allogeneic bone marrow transplantation. N Engl J Med 1999;341:14–21.
40. Brown JR, Yeckes H, Friedberg JW, et al. Increasing incidence of late second malignancies after conditioning with cyclophosphamide and total body irradiation and autologous bone marrow transplantation for non-Hodgkin's lymphoma. J Clin Oncol 2005;23:2208–2214.
41. Perry MC, ed. The Chemotherapy Sourcebook, 3rd ed. Baltimore: Williams & Wilkins, 2001.
42. Kalmadi S, Raghavan D. Fundamentals of cancer treatment—effects of chemotherapy on neoplastic cells. In: McLain R, ed. Current Clinical Oncology: Cancer in the Spine—Comprehensive Care. Totowa, NJ: Humana Press, 2005:31–42.
43. Schwartz GK, Shah MA. Targeting the cell cycle: a new approach to cancer therapy. J Clin Oncol 2005;23:9408–9421.
44. Bergsland EK. When does the presence of the target predict response to the targeted agent? J Clin Oncol 2006;24:213–215.

45. Wilding G, Soulie P, Trump D, Das-Gupta A, Small E. Results from a pilot phase I trial of gefitinib combined with docetaxel and estramustine in patients with hormone-refractory prostate cancer. Cancer 2006;106:1917–1924.

46. Ferrara N. VEGF and the quest for tumor angiogenesis factors. Nat Rev Cancer 2002; 2:795–803.

47. Wedge SR, Kendrew J, Hennequin LF, et al. AZD2171: a highly potent, orally bioavailable, vascular endothelial growth factor receptor-2 tyrosine kinase inhibitor for the treatment of cancer. Cancer Res 2005;65:4389–4400.

10
Principles of Radiotherapy in Urologic Tumors

Irwin H. Lee and Howard M. Sandler

Practical Considerations

Attempts at using radiation for treating human malignancies began soon after the discovery of x-rays by Wilhelm Roentgen in 1895. Radiotherapy is a local treatment-modality in which ionizing radiation is delivered to areas either with gross tumor or with a high-risk of harboring microscopic disease. It is essentially noninvasive when delivered from an external source (teletherapy) or minimally invasive when using implanted radioactive sources (brachytherapy). Over the past century, advances in the understanding of the physics and biology of radiotherapy, as well as developments in imaging and radiation sources, have led to improved efficacy of radiation in controlling cancers while decreasing toxicity. Currently, radiotherapy plays a central role in the management of many genitourinary malignancies, for both definitive management of localized disease and palliation of metastatic disease.

Radiotherapy uses *ionizing* radiation, which refers to any radiation with sufficient energy to generate ionized species by freeing electrons from their orbits. Ionizing radiation may consist of either electromagnetic waves (e.g., x-rays) or small particles (e.g., electrons, protons, or neutrons). In the case of x-rays, the energy is carried in the form of photons, which are small packets of energy. As the radiation passes through matter, energy is deposited along its path; the amount of energy absorbed is the *dose* of radiation and is measured in gray (Gy), with $1\,\text{Gy} = 1\,\text{J/kg}$. The total amount of energy deposited during therapeutic radiation is low, so that there is essentially no increase in temperature; however, the deposition of energy is very discrete and locally is intense enough to cause ionization and breakage of molecular bonds. The dose of radiation within a radiation field can vary widely from one point to another, depending on (among other things) the type of radiation, the energy of the beam, the distance from the radiation source, and the depth of the point in question. In general, the goal of radiotherapy is to maximize dose to the target while minimizing dose to normal tissues.

Megavoltage Radiation and Skin-Sparing

Modern radiotherapy became possible only with the development of relatively high-energy radiation sources, which permit safe delivery of a high-dose radiation to deep tissues. With early radiation sources, which consisted of relatively low-energy x-rays, dose was highest at the surface and decreased as the radiation moved deeper into tissue. As a result, to treat a deep target to a given dose, more superficial structures would necessarily be treated to a much higher dose than the target itself. Skin toxicity thus represented a major limiting factor when attempting to treat deeper structures, such as the prostate or bladder. In the 1950s, however, higher-energy megavoltage radiation sources became available using cobalt-60. Radiation with energy in excess of 1 megavolt has the important property of *skin-sparing*, meaning that the depth of maximal energy (D_{max}) deposition is not right at the surface. In the case of cobalt-60, which emits two photons of similar energy that average 1.25 MeV, the D_{max} is ~0.5 cm. More recently, linear accelerators capable of delivering even higher energy photons (in the range of 10 to 20 MV) have become available. At these energies, the D_{max} increases to ~2.5 cm, making it feasible to treat deep targets, often with minimal skin reaction.

Logistics and Simulation

To minimize toxicity, it is important not only to use appropriate beam energy but also to exclude normal structures as much as possible from the radiation field. *Simulation* and subsequent planning are the essential steps in accomplishing this goal. In the simulation process, the patient is marked either with temporary skin indices or small, ~1 mm permanent tattoos to facilitate accurate repositioning of the patient at the time of treatment; any needed immobilization devices are customized to the patient; and imaging is obtained, usually with high-resolution axial computed tomography (CT), to delineate treatment targets and normal structures to be avoided when delivering the radiation. With more reliable patient setup, toxicity is reduced because during the treatment planning process, one must always create a margin for uncertainty in target location. As this uncertainty is decreased, the field may be more tightly focused on the target, reducing the exposure of normal tissues to radiation.

Mechanism of Action

Deoxyribonucleic Acid Damage and Repair

Although many of the details on how radiation leads to cell death are unknown, it is clear that radiation-induced damage of deoxyribonucleic acid (DNA) plays a central role. DNA damage may result from a *direct* interaction between the ionizing radiation and DNA molecules, or it may occur through *indirect* action as free radicals are generated when radiation interacts with other molecules, particularly water, in the neighborhood of the DNA. The result, in either case, may be single- or double-stranded DNA breaks. Although there exists mechanisms for DNA repair, the latter type of damage is particularly challenging to reverse and is thought to be the type of damage most important in radiation-induced killing. The two main mechanisms of repairing double-stranded breaks are homologous recombination, which depends on the presence of an undamaged template that is copied to damaged DNA, and nonhomologous end-joining, which simply reconnects two broken DNA fragments in a somewhat haphazard fashion. The latter mechanism is clearly error-/mutation-prone. Cells that inadequately repair radiation-induced DNA damage will most often die or at least become unable to divide further. In general, normal tissues are more likely to be successful in repairing radiation damage than rapidly dividing cancer cells, and this difference in the capacity for repair is an essential component of the therapeutic index of radiotherapy.

Cell-Cycle Regulation

It is important to recognize that at a minimum, successful DNA repair requires adequate time for these mechanisms to occur. Normally dividing cells progress through the cell cycle, which consists of four phases (M-mitosis, G1, S-synthesis of DNA, and G2), with molecular checkpoints at each transition. These checkpoints ensure that the cell has enough time to complete any repairs that may be necessary before proceeding to the next phase of the cell cycle. One of the best characterized molecules involved in cell-cycle regulation is p53, which causes delays in G1 and G2 when activated (1). p53 is regulated by phosphorylation by many different kinases, among them ataxia telangiectasia mutated (ATM), a DNA damage "sensor" that is activated specifically after radiation-induced DNA damage.

Following exposure to radiation, it is likely that multiple cell cycle "brakes" are activated in order to allow for attempts at repairing radiation-induced damage. Of course, most malignant cells have defects in their cell-cycle regulation, including mutations in p53, and might therefore be more prone to advancing to the next phase of the cell cycle despite DNA damage from radiation.

Cell Death

If repair fails, either because of excessive DNA damage or because of a failure in cell-cycle regulation, cell death may occur through two fundamentally different mechanisms: apoptosis or necrosis. Apoptosis (programmed cell death) occurs through activation of pathways that are a normal part of tissue development and homeostasis. In cells with intact apoptotic pathways, radiation-induced DNA damage may provide a trigger for them to undergo apoptosis either immediately or after a failed attempt at repair. For example, p53 is known to be important in promoting apoptosis in addition to regulating the cell-cycle following exposure to radiation. Unlike apoptosis, necrosis is a pathological process that does not require the presence of any specific pathways. It may occur after vascular damage or in damaged cells that are unable to undergo apoptosis. Cells dying by necrosis are more likely to generate an inflammatory response as cellular contents are spilled in an uncontrolled fashion.

Radiation-induced cell death may also be classified based on its timing. While the majority of radiation-induced cell-death occurs as cells are dividing (mitotic death), some cells may die a rapid interphase death. The latter phenomenon occurs on the time scale of hours, requires relatively low doses of radiation, and is dependent on apoptosis. It is therefore found mainly in cell populations that are more prone to undergo apoptosis and that are clinically observed to be radiosensitive. In contrast, mitotic death may occur in any cell that attempts to divide following radiation exposure. Death may be apoptotic or necrotic, and it may result from problems with spindle formation, improper chromosome segregation, or a mitotic "catastrophe" after failure of cell cycle arrest.

Radiation Response and Sensitivity

Different tumors exhibit a wide range of sensitivities and responsiveness to radiotherapy. The cells that are most sensitive to radiation are likely to be those that undergo an interphase death, with lymphocytes being the prime example. Seminomas are also extremely radiosensitive, presumably because germs cells are also more prone to apoptosis, which perhaps makes sense on a genome-protection, teleological level. Except for cases in which interphase death is a major contributor to the overall rate of radiation-induced killing, the clinical responsiveness of a tumor depends largely on the underlying rate of turnover since radiation-induced death does not occur until cells try to divide. As a result, cancers that grow more slowly, such as prostate cancer, are likely to take longer to respond to radiation and may also be less sensitive, that is, require higher doses to be eradicated.

The radiosensitivity of cells is also modulated by oxygenation and cell-cycle phase. It has been shown that hypoxic cells are relatively resistant to radiation (2). Specifically, two to three times more radiation may be required to produce the same effect for cells in a hypoxic environment compared to those in an aerobic environment. The relevant range of oxygen tensions in these experiments was between 0 and 10 mm Hg. It is believed that oxygen is important in *fixing* or making permanent the chemical changes induced by free-radical generation during radiation exposure. Similarly, the effectiveness of radiation can vary dramatically depending on the cell-cycle phase during which radiation occurs. Exposure during G2/M phase produces much greater cell-kill than does exposure during late S phase, which is the phase most resistant to radiation-induced cell death. The relative sensitivity is also roughly two- to threefold.

Dose and Fractionation

The 4 R's of Radiotherapy

Radiotherapy is most often delivered in multiple *fractions*, or treatments, over the course of several weeks. A typical regimen for prostate cancer is to give a total of 70 Gy in daily 2 Gy fractions, 5 days per week, so that treatment takes 7 weeks.

The advantage of fractionating radiotherapy over delivering a single high-dose treatment is that the therapeutic index (i.e., the effect of radiation on tumor relative to normal tissue) is generally increased with fractionation for several reasons. First, tumors that have hypoxic cores may shrink over the course of therapy, so *reoxygenation* of hypoxic areas may occur, enhancing the effect of later fractions. Second, with each fraction, cells in the most sensitive portion of the cell cycle will be selectively killed by the radiation, and between fractions, cells in less sensitive phases may move into a more sensitive phase for the next fraction. This process, commonly referred to as *reassortment*, may occur in both tumor and normal tissue but is likely to play a greater role in rapidly cycling cell populations. Finally, by giving multiple small fractions, some degree of *repair* is permitted between treatments. This opportunity for repair generally favors normal tissue over cancer cells, whose repair mechanisms are more likely to be defective. These three R's—reoxygenation, reassortment, and repair—generally increase the effectiveness of radiation with fractionation. In considering the impact of the fractionation schedule on outcome, however, there is generally a fourth R—*repopulation*—that must be included since repopulation of tumor cells over time precludes the use of an excessively protracted course of radiotherapy.

Linear-Quadratic Model

A simple mathematical model, known as the linear-quadratic model, has been developed to predict the effects of different fractionation schedules (3). This model is based on experimental measurements of cell-killing as a function of radiation dose. These measurements show that the relationship between the surviving fraction of cells and dose delivered is not linear. For example, if a treatment of 2 Gy resulted in a 50% reduction in cell survival, a simple linear model would predict that treating with 4 Gy would result in a surviving fraction of 25% (the result of giving 2 Gy twice). In fact, however, the surviving fraction after a single dose of 4 Gy is observed to be substantially smaller than that. The difference between the observed effect and the effect that would be predicted based on a linear model alone can be estimated by a quadratic function; that is, it varies as the square of dose. Thus, the linear-quadratic model includes two parameters, α and β, that quantify the linear and quadratic contributions to cell-killing.

Note that the quadratic component is the one that yields different effects depending on fractionation. Therefore, the ratio of α to β, which may be different from one tissue (or effect) to another, provides a measure of sensitivity to fractionation, with smaller α/β ratios reflecting relatively greater sensitivity.

Early and Late Effects

Clinically, the effects of radiation are generally divided into early and late effects. Early effects occur during the course of treatment or within the weeks immediately following radiotherapy, while late effects tend to occur 6 months or even years after radiotherapy has been completed. In prostate cancer treatment, early effects include skin reaction, cystitis, and diarrhea; late effects include fibrosis, erectile dysfunction, and rectal bleeding. Estimates of the α/β ratio for early effects are relatively high (~10) and for late effects are generally lower (~3). Furthermore, most tumors are thought to have α/β similar to that of early responding tissues (~10). These estimates corroborate the empirical observation that schedules employing larger fraction sizes tend to increase late effects, assuming a fixed rate of tumor control. Early effects, on the other hand, are unlikely to be substantially affected by changes in fractionation.

Altered Fractionation

Experience has shown that 1.8- to 2-Gy fractions seem to provide a good therapeutic ratio in most cases being treated with definitive radiotherapy. However, there are situations in which it may be beneficial to use different fraction sizes, and the linear-quadratic formula is helpful for determining the appropriate total dose when using either smaller or larger fractions. Given the fraction size (d), total dose (D), and α/β, one can compute the *biologically equivalent dose* (BED), which is given by the following linear quadratic formula:

$$BED = D(1 + d/(\alpha/\beta))$$

The BED normally carries a subscript corresponding to the assumed α/β since it is clearly different for large and small α/β. Thus, for any given fractionation schedule, one must determine BED for both early (including tumor) and late effects.

Two alternatives to a standard (1.8 to 2 Gy) fractionation schedule are known as *hyperfractionation* and *hypofractionation*. In a hyperfractionated schedule, smaller than standard fraction sizes are used, usually to a higher total dose, so that a higher rate of tumor control might be achieved for a fixed rate of late complications. In contrast, with hypofractionation, relatively large fractions are used to a lower total dose. The main benefit of such a schedule is a shorter overall course of treatment, but the risk of long-term complications may be relatively higher. In palliative cases, it often makes sense to expedite treatment, and late effects may be less important in patients with a limited prognosis.

Interestingly, there is also some evidence that a hypofractionated schedule may also be beneficial in the definitive treatment of prostate cancer. This speculation arises from studies of dose and tumor control following treatment of prostate cancer with either external radiation or brachytherapy. Because different brachytherapy sources emit radiation at different rates, it is possible to get rough estimates of the α/β for prostate cancer; and some studies suggest that prostate cancer may have, among common human neoplasms, a uniquely low α/β of ~1.5. If these estimates are accurate, then the therapeutic ratio for prostate cancer relative to late effects may, in fact, be optimized by using larger than standard fractions. Trials of hypofractionation are in progress, but until they are complete, the standard of care is still to use the standard fractions (1.8 to 2 Gy) (4).

New Technologies and Equipment

Three-Dimensional Conformal Radiotherapy and Intensity-Modulated Radiotherapy

Along with innovations in computing and imaging, radiotherapy techniques have improved. Powerful workstations facilitate the examination of multiple treatment strategies and allow radiation oncologists to optimize the ratio of dose delivered to the tumor target and minimize the dose absorbed by uninvolved normal structures (5).

Three-dimensional conformal radiotherapy (3DCRT) is defined as treatment using a volumetric imaging data set, such as computed tomography (CT) or magnetic resonance imaging (MRI), and segmentation of that data set into relevant structures, usually tumor targets (e.g., prostate and seminal vesicles) and normal structures (e.g., rectum and bladder). Multiple beams are selected by the oncologist based on separation of tumor from normal, and the beams are each sharply collimated with movable lead leaves (multileaf collimation). The multiple beams (commonly four to six for prostate cancer) intersect at the target resulting in a high dose and uniform dose delivery. For 3DCRT, each beam is relatively "flat," that is, the dose is uniform as one traverses the beam aperture. The dose received by normal tissues is also calculated and can be displayed volumetrically using a dose-volume histogram, which shows the percent of the structure that receives above a certain dose. The dose-volume histogram can be analyzed to predict the risk of toxicity, since toxicity is related to the dose received by a certain volume of an organ. For example, many prostate cancer treatments are designed to treat the prostate fully to up to 78 Gy, but to limit the rectum such that no more than 25% of the rectum receives more than 70 Gy.

Intensity-modulated radiotherapy (IMRT) is a more recent extension of the 3DCRT principles. However, as implied by the name, the intensity of each beam is nonuniform across the aperture. This allows even more conformal dose distributions and greatly increases the therapeutic ratio of external beam radiotherapy. Figure 10.1 illustrates schematically the variation in intensity across an IMRT aperture and illustrates the improvement in conformality that can be achieved with IMRT versus 3DCRT for prostate cancer.

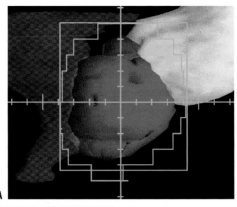

A

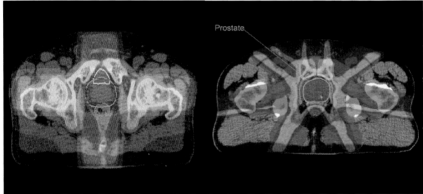

B

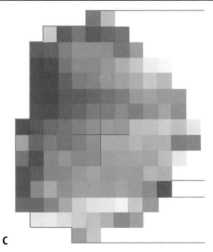

C

FIGURE 10.1. (A) Beam's-eye view display showing prostate (red) surrounded by custom aperture (green), which avoids rectum (blue) and bladder (yellow). (B) Three-dimensional conformal radiotherapy (3DCRT) dose distribution (left) and intensity-modulated radiotherapy (IMRT) dose distribution (right). The prostate target is outlined in pink and the high-dose region is in red. Note the uniform intensity across the beam in the 3DCRT plan versus the modulated intensity across the beams in the IMRT plan. (C) Grayscale view of the intensity map of a single prostate IMRT beam showing the variation in intensity that, when combined with multiple similarly modulated beams, results in the highly conformal treatment seen in B.

As mentioned above, ionizing radiotherapy can be delivered with particles as well as with photons or x-rays. Electrons are commonly employed to treat superficial targets, as these light particles have little ability to penetrate deeply into tissue. High-energy protons, which weigh 2000 times more than an electron, are capable of penetrating deeply into tissue. Because protons are charged particles, they deposit their energy via electromagnetic interaction with the charged particles in tissue (electrons and nuclei). Interestingly, as the proton begins to give up its energy and slow down, this increases its energy deposition, which makes it slow down even more quickly, increasing further the energy deposition, and so it stops quite abruptly.

This leads to a relatively large amount of ionization and subsequent DNA strand breaks near the end of the protons range, and this is called the Bragg peak. This peak in ionization is favorable for radiation planning and dose delivery and has led to the proliferation of somewhat expensive proton treatment facilities at selected locations worldwide. Clinical trials are required to determine whether proton beam treatment is more favorable than the widely available IMRT techniques.

Daily Localization

As radiotherapy techniques (IMRT in particular) result in more focused radiation doses, there is more concern about accuracy in targeting. After all, the careful planning that goes into an IMRT treatment plan is only put to good use if patients are treated in the same position as they were in during the imaging data set used in the planning process. Traditionally this was done by obtaining bone images during treatment. However, if the target is movable with respect to the skeleton (as the prostate can be, depending on bladder and rectal filling), bone imaging may be inadequate. One strategy for daily location verification is to implant fiducial markers into the target organ, imaging these radiopaque markers prior to therapy, and then correcting the patient's position, if necessary (6) (Fig. 10.2). Other strategies use daily pretreatment ultrasound (7) or, for pelvic tumors, inflated rectal balloons (8).

Brachytherapy

Prostate tumors are often treated by implanting the prostate with radioactivity. There are two main approaches: low-dose rate radiotherapy, which commonly uses permanently implanted iodine-125 seeds that have a half-life of approximately 60 days and thus deliver a continuous and ultimately high cumulative dose of radiation over several months, and high-dose rate radiotherapy, that employs a highly radioactive wire that moves quickly—total treatment length is typically less than an hour—under computer guidance through temporarily placed catheters inserted through the perineum. These two approaches are widely used and, because the sources are inserted directly into the prostate gland, allow for a relatively conformal dose distribution by taking advantage of rapid dose absorption and the effect of the inverse square law.

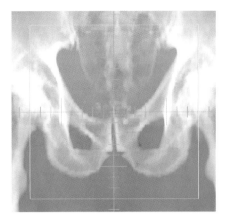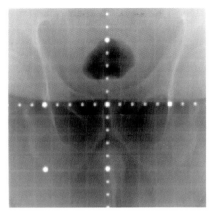

FIGURE 10.2. Left: Digitally reconstructed radiograph (DRR), obtained from treatment planning CT with gold fiducial markers noted in the prostate by colored x's. Right: An anterior image taken of the patient before treatment. Note that the gold markers are about 1 cm inferior compared with the DRR but that the center of the beam has been adjusted to account for the shift in prostate position.

For prostate cancer, compared to external beam IMRT, however, these two approaches may be accompanied by more acute and chronic urinary toxicity (9). Both of the brachytherapy techniques—because of the nature of the rapid dose fall off—are often combined with 5 weeks of external beam radiotherapy that is used to broaden the treatment area to encompass microscopic extension that may be outside of the high-dose brachytherapy volume and to homogenize the overall dose distribution by additional dosage to the prostate gland itself to fill in any inadvertent low-dose regions. Generally the lowest risk prostate cancer patients are treated with monotherapy techniques and intermediate- and high-risk patients undergo the combined approach, which may add toxicity and decreases the convenience associated with the brachytherapy monotherapy strategy.

Systemic Radiotherapy

For prostate cancer, bone seeking radioactively labeled molecules have been used for diagnostic purposes extensively—that is, bone scans. More recently, therapeutic amounts of radiation have been delivered to take advantage of the propensity that metastatic prostate cancer has for the skeleton. Strontium-89 is a β-emitting isotope with a physical half-life of approximately 50 days and a shorter biological half-life secondary to excretion, although it may be retained in metastatic bone longer than in normal bone, providing a therapeutic advantage (10). This agent has a role in the palliation of metastatic skeletal disease, especially when there is widespread involvement not easily encompassed by a focal external beam field, which can conveniently deliver adequate palliation using a single 8-Gy fraction (11). Interestingly, this agent is being tested along with chemotherapy as a possible life-prolonging strategy. Another agent used in this situation is samarium-159. Samarium was superior to placebo in providing pain relief in randomized studies (12). While systemic therapy is generally well tolerated, there can be hematologic toxicity, especially thrombocytopenia, because of radiation effects on bone marrow. Although not formally tested, toxicity may be less for samarium than for strontium, and multiple courses of samarium have been safely given. Because these agents can lead to prolonged bone marrow depression, and especially thrombocytopenia, these agents are sometimes withheld when active chemotherapy is still under consideration.

References

1. Fei P, El-Deiry WS. P53 and radiation responses. Oncogene 2003;22(37):5774–5783.
2. Corry J, Rischin D. Strategies to overcome accelerated repopulation and hypoxia— what have we learned from clinical trials? Semin Oncol 2004;31(6):802–808.
3. Fowler JF. The radiobiology of prostate cancer including new aspects of fractionated radiotherapy. Acta Oncol 2005;44(3):265–276.
4. Fowler JF, Ritter MA, Chappell RJ, Brenner DJ. What hypofractionated protocols should be tested for prostate cancer? Int J Radiat Oncol Biol Phys 2003;56(4): 1093–1104.
5. Lichter AS, Lawrence TS. Recent advances in radiation oncology. N Engl J Med 1995;332(6):371–379.
6. Litzenberg D, Dawson LA, Sandler H, et al. Daily prostate targeting using implanted radiopaque markers. Int J Radiat Oncol Biol Phys 2002;52(3):699–703.
7. McGahan JP, Ryu J, Fogata M. Ultrasound probe pressure as a source of error in prostate localization for external beam radiotherapy. Int J Radiat Oncol Biol Phys 2004;60(3):788–793.
8. Bastasch MD, Teh BS, Mai WY, et al. Tolerance of endorectal balloon in 396 patients treated with intensity-modulated radiation therapy (IMRT) for prostate cancer. Am J Clin Oncol 2006;29(1):8–11.
9. Wei JT, Dunn RL, Sandler HM, et al. Comprehensive comparison of health-related quality of life after contemporary therapies for localized prostate cancer. J Clin Oncol 2002;20(2):557–566.
10. Crawford ED, Kozlowski JM, Debruyne FM, et al. The use of strontium 89 for palliation of pain from bone metastases associated with hormone-refractory prostate cancer. Urology 1994;44(4):481–485.
11. Hartsell WF, Scott CB, Bruner DW, et al. Randomized trial of short- versus long-course radiotherapy for palliation of painful bone metastases. J Natl Cancer Inst 2005;97(11):798–804.
12. Sartor O, Reid RH, Hoskin PJ, et al. Samarium-153–Lexidronam complex for treatment of painful bone metastases in hormone-refractory prostate cancer. Urology 2004;63(5):940–945.

11
Clinical Emergencies in Genitourinary Cancers

Lewis W. Chan and Andrew J. Richards

Profuse Hematuria

Painful or painless hematuria is an important symptom in genitourinary malignancy and warrants thorough evaluation. It is unusual for gross hematuria to present as an acute emergency unless it is associated with other symptoms such as loin pain or urinary retention.

Causes

Upper Urinary Tract

- Transitional cell carcinoma (renal pelvis, ureter)
- Renal cell carcinoma
- Metastatic tumors in the kidney
- Retroperitoneal tumors (testis, lymphoma, sarcoma)
- Iatrogenic: percutaneous surgery/nephrostomy

Lower Urinary Tract

- Transitional cell carcinoma of bladder
- Pelvic cancer: cervix, rectum (with fistula to bladder), and prostate
- Iatrogenic [radiation cystitis, cyclophosphamide cystitis, postoperative, e.g., transurethral resection of prostate (TURP) or bladder tumor (TURBT)]

Clinical Presentation

Patients who present with hematuria may have associated lower urinary tract symptoms (frequency, urgency, dysuria) or clot retention.

In upper tract bleeding patients may present with ureteric colic/loin pain due to blood clots in the ureter. Unusually a patient may present with shock secondary to excessive loss of blood or associated sepsis.

Investigations

These have been described in detail in Chapter 3. Baseline investigations include full blood count, coagulation screen, electrolytes, urea, and creatinine. A midstream urine (MSU) sample is sent to the laboratory to rule out infection. When the diagnosis is not known, urine cytology is an useful investigation. Imaging should include ultrasound or computed tomography (CT) scan of the upper urinary tract, and rigid cystoscopy to evaluate the bladder and urethra.

Management

Fluid Resuscitation

Accurate assessment of hemodynamic status is the key to management of patients with profuse hematuria. Intravenous fluids and blood transfusion should take into account the age of the patient, site of bleeding, degree of anemia, hemodynamic stability, and presence of coexisting cardiac, pulmonary, or vascular conditions.

Transfusing one unit of red cells increases the hemoglobin by approximately 1 g/dL and the hematocrit by 2% to 3% in the average 70 kg adult. Adequate oxygen-carrying capacity can be met by a hemoglobin of 7 g/dL (a hematocrit value of approximately 21%) or even less when the intravascular volume is adequate for perfusion.

Catheter Irrigation

A three-way irrigation catheter [size 22 French (F)] is placed and continuous bladder irrigation is set up if the patient is in clot retention.

Rigid cystoscopy and bladder lavage to evacuate clots may be necessary after the patient's condition is stabilized. This will also help in the diagnosis of the cause of the bleeding.

Hemorrhagic Cystitis

This condition is seen in patients who had pelvic irradiation or systemic treatment with oxazaphorine alkylating agents (cyclophosphamide) and warrants special mention. In a series of 1784 patients treated with radiotherapy for carcinoma of the cervix, the incidence of hemorrhagic cystitis was 6.5% and the median interval before bleeding occurred was 35.5 months (1). Management is based on the severity of hematuria, the treatment facilities available, the risks and severity of complications, as well as the prognosis of the patient.

Placement of a large catheter (usually 20–22F three-way irrigation catheter) to allow bladder irrigation is the basic management in all patients. Periodic evacuation of clots is necessary in most cases. Coagulation defects if present should be corrected.

Cystoscopic assessment under anesthesia allows diathermy of bleeding areas, resection of tumor, and washout of clots. Intravesical irrigation with 1% alum (50 g alum in 5 L sterile water), via a three-way catheter at 250 to 300 mL/h is generally a safe, effective, and well-tolerated method of treatment. It is important to make sure that the renal function is not compromised, as alum-induced encephalopathy can occur in these patients (2).

Intravesical irrigation of alum has also been used for intractable hemorrhage from carcinoma of prostate after radiotherapy (3). Oral sodium pentosanpolysulfate (100 mg tds) has been used successfully in bleeding secondary to pelvic radiation. The dosage is gradually reduced to a maintenance dose of 100 mg until the cessation of bleeding (4).

Hyperbaric oxygen treatment is effective in 80% to 90% of cases but is not widely available. Intravesical formalin and silver nitrate have an efficacy of 70% in intractable hematuria, but there is risk of serious complications (5).

Embolization of internal iliac artery (unilaterally or bilaterally) under local anesthesia may help to control bleeding. Complications of embolization include gluteal pain and dislodgment of atherosclerotic plaques with distal embolization.

Surgical Measures

In refractory cases when conservative measures fail, surgical procedures such as urinary diversion and cystectomy may be necessary.

Urinary Retention

Urinary retention may occur due to bladder outlet obstruction or detrusor failure. This may be acute, chronic, or acute-on-chronic retention.

Causes

1. Obstruction: locally advanced prostate cancer, coexistent benign prostatic hypertrophy (BPH), or urethral stricture. Clot retention may occur due to bleeding from a tumor or hemorrhagic cystitis related to radiation or cyclophosphamide. Other less common causes include urethral cancer, advanced penile or vaginal cancer, or a tumor at the base of the bladder causing outlet obstruction.

2. Detrusor failure: Urinary retention is also caused by the inability of the detrusor muscle to contract (underactive or acontractile bladder) resulting from previous pelvic surgery/radiation, spinal or meningeal metastases, or neuropathy from chemotherapy. *BEWARE: Urinary retention may be the first sign of spinal cord compression particularly in prostate cancer.*

3. Other causes include drugs (e.g., antidepressants, opiates, analgesics, and antipsychotics), constipation, poor mobility, and urinary infection.

4. Iatrogenic: postbrachytherapy for prostate cancer.

Clinical Presentation

Acute painful retention is of short duration and is usually due to bladder outlet obstruction.

Chronic retention may present with symptoms of overflow incontinence, nocturnal enuresis, worsening lower urinary tract symptoms (LUTS), urinary tract infection, or uremia. Physical examination may reveal a palpable bladder or localized pelvic/suprapubic discomfort.

Investigations

- Serum electrolytes, urea, creatinine, calcium, prostate-specific antigen (PSA), MSU, urine cytology
- Renal ultrasound (to check for hydronephrosis/obstructive uropathy)

Other investigations may include CT scan, transrectal ultrasound (TRUS), and biopsy of prostate (if prostate cancer is suspected) and MRI of spine (if there is a concern about spinal cord compression).

Management of Acute Retention

The discomfort and pain of acute urinary retention is relieved by placement of urethral or suprapubic catheter (SPC). However, an SPC should be avoided in cancer of the bladder.

In patients with large-volume retention there may be hematuria following bladder decompression. Using a large-caliber (e.g., 18 or 20F) catheter reduces the problem of intermittent catheter blockage by clots. There is no evidence to suggest that clamping the catheter is useful in reducing the risk of bleeding.

If there is evidence of neurological signs indicating spinal cord compression, urgent MRI of the spine and neurological assessment are necessary (see below).

A trial without a catheter can be arranged once all the predisposing factors including mobility and constipation are optimized. It is usually necessary to wait at least 2 to 3 days after acute retention before attempting a trial without a catheter. Patients with chronic retention may need to wait 4 weeks or longer. A short course of α-blockers (tamsulosin or alfuzosin) may increase the chance of a successful trial of void if retention is thought to be uncomplicated and due to BPH.

Management of Chronic Retention

Postobstructive diuresis may occur following bladder decompression by catheter if there is renal failure. This is due to loss of concentrating ability of the kidneys and is managed as follows:

- Closely monitor intake/output and clinical state of hydration.
- Replace urinary volume losses with normal saline/Hartman's solution intravenously.

- Check electrolytes regularly: watch serum levels of Na, K, and Mg particularly, as patients can become hypokalemic rapidly and require K replacement.
- Admit patient to a high-dependency (critical care) ward if there are significant difficulties with fluid or electrolyte balance and involve a renal physician early.
- In patients who are fit enough to take oral fluids, IV fluid replacement can be slowed early.
- Avoid "pushing" the diuresis by giving too much IV fluids, especially when the creatinine has normalized.
- Once the general condition is stabilized, surgical intervention (e.g., TURP) may be necessary to relieve the obstruction. Patients with detrusor failure who are unable to void may be managed by long-term catheter or clean intermittent self-catheterization.

Anuria Due to Malignant Obstruction

Causes

Ureteric obstruction can result from the following:

- Muscle-invasive TCC at the base of bladder involving the trigone
- Locally advanced prostate cancer
- Bilateral ureteric TCC
- Other pelvic malignancies (colorectal, gynecological)
- Retroperitoneal lymphadenopathy (e.g., hematological malignancy— lymphoma, testicular cancer)
- Clot obstruction in a single kidney
- Rarely benign ureteric stricture after radiotherapy for pelvic tumors
- Iatrogenic: surgical damage to the ureters

Investigations

The following laboratory investigations and scans should be done:

Electrolytes, urea and creatinine, MSU, arterial blood gases
Ultrasound or noncontrast CT scan of urinary tract

Principles of Management

- Placement of urethral catheter will differentiate urinary retention/bladder outlet obstruction from ureteric obstruction. Most patients have some dehydration and will need fluid resuscitation/rehydration.
- Imaging of upper urinary tract (ultrasound or noncontrast CT scan). The findings of hydronephrosis with an empty bladder would indicate supravesical obstruction, whereas a distended bladder with bilateral hydronephrosis implies bladder outlet obstruction.

- Percutaneous nephrostomy followed by antegrade insertion of ureteric stent (cystoscopy and retrograde ureteric stenting is usually difficult if not impossible, especially in cases of locally advanced prostate cancer or a TCC bladder). Usually the kidney that has better function is drained first.

Watch for postobstructive diuresis once drainage is secured especially in cases of bilateral ureteric obstruction.

In some cases dialysis may be necessary if there is significant fluid retention and metabolic acidosis. This is discussed in Chapter 12. Close monitoring of fluid and electrolyte balance with correction of abnormalities and associated acidosis is necessary if the patient is in renal failure.

Spinal Cord Compression

Spinal cord compression should be recognized and treated promptly as it can lead to significant morbidity. Compression of the spinal cord (and its blood supply causing ischemia) is caused by metastases in the epidural space or the vertebral bodies. This affects 5% to 10% of patients with metastatic prostate cancer in the vertebral column.

Other genitourinary cancers including TCC, renal carcinoma, and testicular tumors can also cause cord compression.

Presentation

Although back pain may precede compression symptoms by months, the progression to neurological dysfunction is generally of short duration.

Localizing back pain and tenderness may be absent especially in chronic spinal cord compression. Urinary retention and constipation may be the first signs of cord compression. Neurological signs depend on the level of lesion(s).

Clinical assessment should include vital signs, full neurological assessment, palpation of back for tenderness, abdominal examination for distended bladder, and rectal examination for constipation (from associated neurogenic bowel dysfunction).

Diagnosis

Sudden development of lower motor neuron type symptoms raises the possibility of cord compression. The presentation of cauda equina lesions is gradual, with affected ankle and knee jerks, saddle anesthesia, urinary and fecal retention, or overflow incontinence. Higher level spinal cord lesions may manifest with earlier motor and sensory signs.

Investigations and Management

It is important to ascertain the diagnosis of the primary tumor, as the treatment differs according to the pathological origin of the cancer. If suspected, the management of spinal cord compression is multidisciplinary involving oncologists, neurologists, and radiotherapists (6). Urgent MRI (if available) or CT myelogram will help to assess the nature of the compression.

Intravenous dexamethasone (4 to 24 mg every 6 hours) is started immediately once cord compression is suspected. Constipation is treated with laxatives or enemas, and urinary bladder is decompressed with a catheter if the patient is in retention. Other measures include analgesics and careful nursing of the pressure areas of the back and limbs.

Spinal cord compression may be relieved by neurosurgical decompression or by radiotherapy. Surgery (laminectomy) is indicated for younger patients with a relatively good prognosis, early presentation, and a single level of compression. It is also indicated if radiation fails or if the spine is unstable. It has been shown that surgery followed by radiation is more effective than radiation alone in treating certain patients suffering from spinal cord compression caused by metastatic cancer. The outcome is related to the degree of neurological impairment at presentation. Most patients who are ambulant at presentation remain ambulant, while <40% who are not ambulant regain mobility.

Patients with spinal cord compression from metastatic prostate cancer have a poor outlook. Patients with spinal metastasis need close observation to prevent development of cord compression. In patients with hormone-resistant metastatic prostate cancer, persistent back pain can be a sign of impending compression, and imaging studies (bone scan, spine CT scan or MRI) may help to confirm the diagnosis. In such cases prophylactic local radiotherapy to the spine in the areas of bony metastases is justifiable (7).

Acute Symptoms of Testicular Cancer

Testicular cancer may present as an acute scrotal pathology or with symptoms of systemic metastases. Hemorrhage into testicular cancer may present as acute scrotal pain or swelling. There may be a history of associated minor trauma. Metastatic disease may manifest as dyspnea (extensive chest metastases), lower extremity swelling [retroperitoneal lymphadenopathy/inferior vena cava (IVC) obstruction], and renal and gastrointestinal disturbances. In rare instances spinal cord compression due to spinal metastases may occur. There may be a history of cryptorchidism/surgery for undescended testis, infertility, or testicular swelling.

Ultrasound of the scrotum and abdomen may show hemorrhage in a testicular lesion with retroperitoneal node enlargement. A CT scan of the abdomen and chest is helpful in staging. Testicular tumor markers including α-fetoprotein (AFP) and β-human chorionic gonadotropin (β-HCG) should be performed.

Management

Once the initial assessment is made and if the tumor is localized radical inguinal orchidectomy is the initial step in the management. This is followed by a CT scan of the chest and abdomen to stage the extent of the disease. In the presence of extensive metastases, chemotherapy may need to precede inguinal orchidectomy. Neurological symptoms arising due to spinal cord compression are treated by chemotherapy. The management of advanced testicular cancer is discussed in detail in Chapter 17.

Malignant Priapism

Priapism is a persistent erection not accompanied by sexual desire or stimulation lasting for more than 6 hours and typically involving only the corpus cavernosa (8). For clinical management purposes, priapism is classified as low- flow and high-flow types.

Low-flow priapism is more common and is due to occlusion of venous outflow from the corpus cavernosa. This causes pain and ischemia of the corporal smooth muscle. High-flow priapism is rare and is usually due to continuous arterial blood flow into the sinusoidal spaces of the corpora. It may occur with vascular injury following pelvic trauma.

Priapism may also be caused by vasoactive drugs (such as intracavernosal prostaglandin injections) used for treatment of impotence, hematological causes associated with hyperviscosity (e.g., sickle cell disease), trauma, and neurological conditions.

The pelvic malignancies (bladder, prostate cancer) can rarely cause priapism due to direct invasion of the base of penis. Although the exact mechanism is not known, one possible explanation is venous occlusion and stasis with resultant low-flow priapism. Other cancers (renal, colonic, melanoma, and leukemia) can also cause priapism. In a patient presenting with priapism of unknown cause, it is important to rule out malignancy.

Treatment

If the patient has a known preexisting malignancy contributing to priapism, the treatment is supportive and conservative whenever possible. In addition to treating the priapism, effort is made to treat the causative factor without any delay. Cavernosal blood sample for blood gases helps in differentiating high- and low-flow priapism. In low-flow priapism, the blood gases have values similar to those of venous blood. Cavernosal aspiration of sludged blood followed by intracavernosal phenylephrine (200 μg), an α-adrenoreceptor agonist, is the first-line treatment in low-flow priapism. This may result in some detumescence, and the same dosage (200 μg) can be repeated. The patient should have blood pressure and electrocardiogram monitoring Methylene blue injection has been advocated (9). This is supposed to inhibit cyclic guanosine monophosphate (cGMP), preventing smooth muscle relaxation. If these simple measures fail, then surgical shunting is necessary, although this may not be effective in malignant priapism. The commonest procedure is the Winter shunt, which utilizes a Tru-cut biopsy needle to create a communication between the glans and corpus cavernosa (10).

Perioperative Hypotension in Adrenal Neoplasms

Causes

1. Hypotension may be due to common postoperative causes such as blood loss, hypovolemia, cardiogenic shock, or sepsis.
2. The remaining adrenal tissue may not be able to respond to the stress of surgery (especially in the presence of preoperative adrenal suppression). This often becomes apparent after perioperative hydrocortisone has worn off.
3. In the setting of pheochromocytomas, hypotension can be related to decreased intravascular volume or catecholamine withdrawal after removal of tumor and can be prevented by volume expansion prior to surgery.

Diagnosis

Knowing the pathology of the adrenal lesion, perioperative medication (especially steroids, antihypertensives, and antibiotics) helps in assessment of the cause of hypotension. Clinical signs of bleeding or hypovolemia, cardiogenic shock, sepsis, or anaphylaxis will help to differentiate among other causes of hypotension.

Management

Management should be according to the underlying cause (transfuse and volume replacement if hypovolemic, inotropes if cardiogenic shock, etc.). If thought to be addisonian, give 100 mg IV hydrocortisone. There is usually a component of hypovolemia and fluid replacement with close monitoring of hemodynamic status and urine output is necessary in most cases.

Prevention

Consultation with an anesthetist and endocrinologist regarding preoperative admission, antihypertensives (alpha- or beta-blockade), cortisone replacement, and fluid replacement is vital prior to surgery for adrenal tumors, especially pheochromocytoma. These patients require close intra- and postoperative monitoring.

Malignancy Associated Hypercalcemia

Hypercalcemia is commonly due to hyperparathyroidism or malignancy. The basic mechanism for malignancy-associated hypercalcemia is increased bone reabsorption (osteolytic) leading to calcium mobilization. In addition, there is inadequate calcium clearance in the kidneys. Malignant cells may secrete para-thyroid hormone (PTH)-like protein (PTHrP) (11), which increases serum calcium levels in the absence of demonstrable bony lesions.

Hypercalcemia usually occurs in the setting of advanced disease [renal cancer, TCC bladder, carcinoma of the penis, and uncommonly in prostate cancer]. This may also be a paraneoplastic syndrome associated with renal cancer.

Clinical Presentation

Patients may present with vague abdominal pain, anorexia, diarrhea, thirst, polyuria, or nocturia. Other manifestations include bony pain, psychological disturbance, nephrocalcinosis, and urinary calculi if chronic hypercalcemia. If very severe, hypercalcemia may lead to obtundation or death.

Diagnosis

Normal calcium levels vary between 2.25 and 2.57 mmol/L for men and 2.22 and 2.54 mmol/L for women. It is important to note that serum protein concentrations affect serum calcium levels but not unbound fraction of calcium. So it is necessary to correct the total plasma calcium concentration for the percent calcium level measured at normal albumin levels:

$$\text{Total Serum Calcium (Corrected for Albumin Level)} =$$
$$(\text{Normal Albumin} - \text{Patient's Albumin}) \times 0.8 +$$
$$\text{Patient's Measured Total Calcium}$$

Other laboratory investigations include renal function studies (creatinine, urea, and electrolytes including magnesium and phosphate), PTH, serum 1,25-dihydroxyvitamin D, and immunoreactive PTH (iPTH).

Management

Hydration with intravenous normal saline is the mainstay of treatment together with frusemide (not thiazides). Intravenous bisphosphonates (pamidronate) is indicated if there is a lack of response to hydration, very high calcium levels, obtundation, or severe symptoms. Patients with renal failure may need dialysis.

Calcitonin is a very expensive option; it works very quickly but exhibits tachyphylaxis.

Treatment of underlying disease would depend on the stage of the tumor, patient comorbidities, and prognosis (e.g., localized renal carcinoma vs. end-stage metastatic bladder TCC). Ongoing control may involve oral bisphosphonates or periodic IV treatments (12,13).

References

1. Levenback C, Eifen PJ, Burke TW, Morris M, Gershenson DM. Hemorrhagic cystitis following radiotherapy for stage 1b cancer of the cervix. Gynecologic Oncol 1994; 55:206–210.
2. Phelps KR, Naylor K, Brien TP, Wilbur H, Haggie SS. Encephalopathy after bladder irrigation with alum: case report and literature review. Am J Med Sci 1999;318: 181–185.
3. Thompson IM, Teague JL, Mueller EJ, Rodriguez FR. Intravesical alum irrigation for intractable bleeding secondary to adenocarcinoma of the prostate. J Urol 1987;137: 525–526.
4. Sandhu SS, Goldstraw M, Woodhouse CR. The management of haemorrhagic cystitis with sodium pentosan polysulphate. BJU Int 2004;94(6):845–847.
5. Rigaud J, Hetet JF, Bouchot O. Management of radiation cystitis. Prog Urol 2004;14: 568–572.
6. Kovner F, Spigel S, Rider I, et al. Radiation therapy of metastatic spinal cord compression: multidisciplinary team diagnosis and treatment. J Neuro-Oncol 1999;42: 85–92.
7. Tazi H, Manunta A, Rodriguez A, et al. Spinal cord compression in metastatic prostate cancer. Eur Urol 2003;44(5):527–532.
8. Keoghane SR, Sullivan ME, Miller MAW. The aetiology, pathogenesis and management of priapism. BJU Int 2002;90(2):149–154.
9. Martinez Portillo FJ, Hoang-Boehm J, Weiss J, Alken P, Junneman KP. Methylene blue as a successful treatment alternative for pharmacologically induced priapism. Eur Urol 2001;39:20–23.
10. Winter CC, McDowell G. Experience with 105 patients with priapism. J Urol 1988; 140:980–983.
11. Potts JT. Diseases of the parathyroid gland and other hyper and hypocalcaemic disorders. In: Fauci AS, et al., eds. Harrison's Principles of Internal Medicine, 4th ed. New York: McGraw-Hill, 1998:2227–2240.
12. Bilezikian JP. Management of acute hypercalcemia. N Engl J Med 1992;326(18): 1196–1203.
13. Novick A, Howards S. The adrenals. In: Gillenwater J, et al., eds. Adult and Pediatric Urology, 4th ed. Philadelphia: Lippincott Williams & Wilkins, 2002:546–549.

12
Renal Failure, Dialysis, and Transplantation: Management of Tumors in Solitary Kidney and Bilateral Renal Tumors

Raj C. Thuraisingham

This chapter discusses the renal problems encountered in the management of adult genitourinary cancers. Maintenance of renal function is crucial in the management of most malignancies including genitourinary cancer, as optimal renal function is necessary for multimodal cancer therapy. There are a number of scenarios in which renal function is likely to be compromised as a result of either the cancer itself or the treatment:

1. Obstructive uropathy, which can be bilateral or unilateral, supravesical (above the vesicoureteric junction) or infravesical (below the vesicoureteric junction) (Table 12.1)
2. Renal cell carcinoma in solitary kidney
3. Preexisting renal disease in a patient with cancer
4. Nephrotoxicity induced by high-dose chemotherapy
5. Malignancies in renal transplant patients
6. Effects of previous cancer treatment: radiotherapy, chemotherapy
7. Renal damage as a result of nephrotoxicity due to analgesics and antibiotics
8. Paraneoplastic syndromes

Patient Assessment

When assessing these patients, a few key questions are essential in the overall decision-making process:

TABLE 12.1. Cancers that cause unilateral or bilateral obstruction

Infravesical: transitional cell carcinoma (TCC) bladder, prostate cancer, urethral carcinoma, carcinoma cervix/ uterus or rectum
Supravesical: TCC ureter and renal pelvis, bladder, primary or secondary retroperitoneal lymph node involvement, malignant retroperitoneal fibrosis

1. What is the likely course and prognosis of the disease process? This is the most crucial question in planning treatment:
2. What are the comorbid conditions, some of which may be more serious than the cancer process itself?
3. What is the overall level of renal function? What is the differential renal function? This basic information is required and forms the basis for the rest of the assessment.
4. Has the patient got a solitary kidney? How much function is likely to be lost (partial or total) following surgery?
5. Is the potential loss of function likely to render the patient dialysis-dependent? If so, is it short-term or long-term?
6. What would the prognosis of the patient be without treatment compared to dialysis?
7. Is further treatment (e.g., chemotherapy) likely to make the renal function deteriorate?

Blood Tests

Blood tests are the simplest way of measuring the serum concentrations of urea and creatinine. Blood urea is not generally thought to be a marker of renal function, as urea clearance is 50% to 60% of the glomerular filtration rate (GFR) (1). Urea levels are influenced by the patient's age, dietary protein intake, and protein metabolism. Blood urea nitrogen (BUN), a product urea, is affected similarly.

Serum creatinine (SCr) levels are more reliable than urea however they reflect not only renal excretion, but also the generation, intake, and metabolism of creatine and phosphocreatine (2). Other factors also influence SCr, such as the patient's age, weight, nutritional status, gender, and ethnicity. Serum creatinine levels may not rise above the normal range until the kidney function has become significantly impaired (3). For example, an elderly malnourished patient may have an SCr within the normal range but may well have a markedly impaired GFR. Conversely, a young muscular man may have an SCr that is above the normal range but have a normal GFR. In most instances, therefore, the SCr is insufficient to assess renal function, but it is important to remember that serum creatinine levels are also influenced by nonrenal factors.

Creatinine Clearance

As creatinine is not metabolized in the kidney and freely filtered by the glomeruli, it is a simple way of measuring GFR. The urinary creatinine *(U)* excretion over 24 hours when divided by the SCr *(P)* provides a measure of creatinine clearance: $(U \times \text{Urine Volume})/P$. However, as creatinine is also secreted by the proximal tubule, the creatinine clearance usually exceeds the GFR (4). This test is used frequently in clinical practice but is subject to error in that it is highly dependent on an accurate 24-hour urine collection.

Glomerular Filtration Rate

The GFR gives a fairly accurate assessment of functioning nephrons, but it is not frequently measured directly in clinical practice (5). It can be estimated using several validated formulas. The Cockcroft-Gault formula (6) uses the patient's weight, age, and serum creatinine (μmol/L). There are likely to be errors in measurements and it is difficult to ensure the quality of the variables (5). The Cockcroft-Gault formula is as follows:

$$\text{GFR} = K^* \times \text{Weight} \times (140 - \text{Age})/\text{SCr}$$

where $K^* = 1.23$ for males and 1.03 for females.

In contrast the Modification of Diet in Renal Disease in the United States (MDRD) study equation does not require the weight, not does it use the body surface area (7). Although it has been validated in many clinical situations, the adjustment for ethnicity is limited to African Americans, which may affect the result in other ethnic groups. However, increasingly the MDRD formula is being used as the preferred method of estimating the GFR (eGFR):

$$\text{GFR} = 186 \times (\text{SCr} - 1.154) \times (\text{Age} - 0.203) \times 0.742 \text{ (for females)} \times 1.212$$
$$\text{(for blacks)}$$

These GFR formulas have their strengths and weaknesses. Neither formula has been validated in the context of acute renal failure, which again limits their use. Their main strength is that finally we can estimate the GFR with some degree of accuracy without having to resort to expensive and time-consuming tests. However in the context of cancer these equations also have their problems. In a study of 122 cancer patients, GFR estimated by these equations was compared with technetium 99 m (^{99m}Tc) diethylenetriamine pentaacetic acid (DTPA) clearance. There were significant limitations, and the results were a biased and imprecise estimate of GFR (8).

Radioisotopes/Radiocontrast Studies

These techniques are the most accurate methods of measuring the GFR in clinical practice (8). The success of these methods relies on the use of radiopharmaceuticals that are freely filtered by the glomerulus and are neither reabsorbed nor secreted by the tubules. The principles of isotope renography are discussed in Chapter 5. These methods, however, are invasive and expensive, and may not be available in all clinical settings.

How Much Function Is Likely to Be Lost Following Surgery/Treatment?

To estimate the potential loss of function postoperatively, it is clearly important to know the contribution each kidney makes to the total GFR. As mentioned earlier, this can be assessed using isotope renography. These techniques employ radiopharmaceutical agents that are either glomerular filtration agents (DTPA) or tubular secretion agents [mercaptoacetyltriglycine (MAG3), or dimercapto-succinic acid (DMSA)]. Following intravenous administration, it is possible to measure renal blood flow and renal cortical function by the isotope activity, which is then computed using scintigraphic techniques (9).

By using this information combined with the assessment of the overall GFR, the single kidney GFR can be determined. As an example, if a nephrectomy is being planned and the contribution of the problem kidney is 10% for someone with an overall GFR of 80 mL/min (problem kidney has a GFR of 8 mL/min), then there should be more than sufficient residual renal function postoperatively. If, however, the affected kidney contributes 50% or more to overall function in someone with a total GFR of 20 mL/min, the planned nephrectomy may render the patient dialysis dependent. The impact on renal function following nephron-sparing surgery is more difficult to predict, but at least patients can be counseled regarding the worst-case scenario.

The information regarding the degree of residual renal function postsurgery is extremely important as it enables clinicians to advise the patients on the potential need for dialysis postoperatively on either a temporary or permanent basis. This is discussed in more detail below.

Is the Potential Loss of Function Likely to Render the Patient Dialysis Dependent?

The threshold GFR at which renal support is required varies according to the individual patient and to the standard practice in the specific renal unit. Most clinicians would agree that a GFR of 10 mL/min/1.73 m^2 or less is an indication for dialysis [National Kidney Foundation Kidney Disease Outcomes Quality Initiative (NKF-DOQI) clinical practice guideline] (10). Based on the measurements discussed above, one may be able to predict, with some degree of certainty, the likely need for dialysis support postoperatively. This information should be relayed to patients, as it may inform their choice of treatment options. As mentioned above, in the case of nephron-sparing surgery (or partial nephrectomy), it is more difficult to predict the impact of surgery on renal function.

There are several postoperative scenarios for renal support in genitourinary cancer patients with compromised renal function:

1. Patients with sufficient residual function who do not require postoperative dialysis: Their remaining nephron mass is sufficient for them not to need renal replacement therapy.

2. Patients who need dialysis in the short term but then become dialysis independent: In this scenario the patient is left with sufficient nephron mass not to require long-term dialysis but the operative procedure has caused acute tubular necrosis and temporary renal shut down. This usually recovers but may take up to 6 weeks.

3. Patient regains independent renal function postoperatively but over subsequent months/years develops remnant nephropathy and end-stage renal failure: Once a critical nephron mass is lost, a maladaptive response known as hyperfiltration ensues irrespective of original pathology (11,12). In simple terms the remaining glomeruli of the kidney(s) hypertrophy. In the short term this serves to maintain the GFR but in the long term it leads to focal glomerulosclerosis and remnant nephropathy and ultimately to end-stage renal failure.

4. Patient will need dialysis henceforth: Sufficient renal mass has been removed such that the patient does not have independent kidney function and will thus require long-term/permanent dialysis.

Based on the results garnered from the investigations outlined above (overall renal function and split renal function) it is possible, with a modest degree of certainty, to predict which of these scenarios is likely. This information should be passed on to the patient. It is also extremely important for the physicians and surgeons to be aware of this as it may influence the decisions regarding surgery. This is especially true if the likely prognosis on dialysis is poor, in which case surgery may not be in the patient's best interest.

Prognosis of Tumor Versus Dialysis

When deciding treatment options, it is important to bear in mind the prognosis of the individual patient on long-term dialysis if that is a likely scenario. The prognosis of a young dialysis patient with no comorbidity is very different from an elderly patient with serious comorbidities such as heart disease and diabetes on dialysis in relation to survival. These points need to be borne in mind because the prognosis of the underlying tumor may be significantly better with conservative management in certain individuals.

It is worth remembering that for a debilitated dialysis-dependent patient, quality of life may be very poor, often with multiple admissions to the hospital

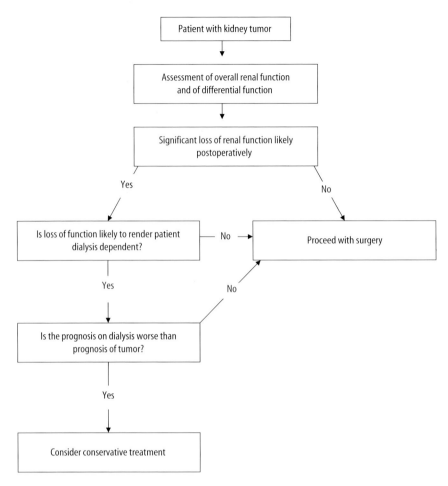

FIGURE 12.1. Treatment decision flowchart.

for initiation and maintenance of dialysis. These facts may also influence treatment decisions (Fig. 12.1).

Perioperative Management

The preoperative management of patient undergoing radical nephrectomy with a normally functioning contralateral kidney does not need any specific measures. Special precautions, however, are necessary in patients undergoing nephron-saving surgery. Fluid balance is the mainstay of maintaining renal function over the perioperative period.

Preoperative Management

Patients should be volume replete at the time of surgery, which often means they will require a continuous intravenous infusion during the nil-by-mouth period. Although there are little data on preoperative fluid regimens, studies examining hydration prior to contrast examinations have shown crystalloid infusions (at 1 mL/kg/h for 12 hours) to be very effective in preventing subsequent renal dysfunction (13). This regimen, however, must not be applied to patients who are anuric (e.g., on dialysis) as they run the danger of becoming volume overloaded.

During nephron-saving surgery temporary occlusion of the renal artery is required to achieve a bloodless field. To prevent ischemic injury to the kidney, the patient should be hydrated, and intravenous mannitol is given 5 to 10 minutes prior to renal artery occlusion to prevent intracellular edema (14). Mannitol could be repeated after removal of the vascular clamp to induce diuresis. Cooling the kidney with ice slush to decrease the core temperature to 15° to 20°C allows the surgeon 2 to 3 hours of safe ischemia (15).

Postoperative Fluid Management

The principles of postoperative fluid management very much depend on the patients' urine output and other fluid losses such as that from drains and nasogastric drainage. Other important parameters include daily weights, blood pressure, pulse rate, central venous pressure (CVP), and daily blood chemistry. Central venous pressure measurements should not replace the simple clinical parameters listed above.

The Patient with Good Urine Output

Patients need to remain on intravenous fluids until they are able to eat and drink without restriction. As a rough guide, if there is renal impairment, then the patient requires only 1 to 1.5 L per day of crystalloid adjusted according to input-output charts, serum biochemistry, and daily weights.

The Patient with Poor Urine Output/Anuria

Intravenous fluid should not be prescribed unless required as judged by the parameters outlined above. If the oliguria is felt to be secondary to volume depletion, then diuretics should be avoided but fluid prescribed instead. The signs of volume depletion include tachycardia, hypotension (especially postural hypotension), a fall in weight, nonvisible jugular venous pulse, and a low CVP. Signs such as dry mucous membranes and poor skin turgor are unreliable and should not be used. Urea and electrolytes will need to be checked immediately postoperatively and daily thereafter. Dialysis is required if there is hyperkalemia, profound acidosis, or fluid overload.

The Dialysis Patient

Managing a dialysis patient postoperatively requires special attention. Fluids should be administered using the guidelines above for the anuria/oliguric patient. In addition, daily assessments of the chemistry should be carried out and dialysis recommenced when required. If the peritoneum in patients on peritoneal dialysis (PD) has been breached, they will require temporary hemodialysis for a period prior to recommencing PD. For hemodialysis patients dialysis should be carried out with as little anticoagulation as possible.

The Transplant Patient

The fluid management of transplant patients postoperatively is dependent on their urine output as discussed above, but the key issues revolve around their medication. Where possible they should continue with their oral immunosuppressive medication; however, most would need an increase in their steroid dose (if on steroids) during the immediate postoperative period, as these patients may have adrenal suppression. If the patient is unable to tolerate steroids orally then administration by intravenous route is necessary (e.g., hydrocortisone can be used instead of prednisolone). Cyclosporin and tacrolimus (immunosuppressants) doses need adjusting if IV administration is needed, whereas the dose of intravenous azathioprine and mycophenolate mofetil is the same as for the oral route. Rapamycin is not available for intravenous use.

Dialysis Modality

In the acute postoperative period most clinicians advocate the use of hemodialysis as opposed to peritoneal dialysis for patients who were not previously on dialysis. If the patient is stable, intermittent hemodialysis via a central venous catheter would be the method of choice. The timing of initiation depends on the patients' blood chemistry, pH, and fluid status.

Because of the need for anticoagulation during the dialysis procedure, it may be preferable to delay the treatment until absolutely necessary in order to minimize the risk of bleeding, although dialysis can often be carried out with little or no anticoagulation. In the case of the hypotensive or hemodynamically unstable patient, continuous venovenous hemodialysis or diafiltration is usually employed, but in these situations the patient is usually on intensive care. The danger of these modalities is bleeding, as patients need to be continuously anticoagulated. In patients who need long-term renal replacement therapy, peritoneal dialysis can be successful especially if their renal surgery has been carried out via the retroperitoneal approach. For others, hemodialysis can be carried out.

Transplantation

Patients rendered dialysis dependent postsurgery could potentially be listed for transplantation following a detailed assessment. Most of the best practice guide lines suggest an observation period to ensure no recurrence. Although the current policy for patients with end-stage renal disease and localized prostate cancer is to wait 5 years after primary therapy, it is reasonable to assess these patients for transplantation on an individualized risk assessment (16). For most patients with renal tumors, a delay of about 2 years is probably sufficient (17). But a waiting period of 5 years for patients with urothelial tumors is prudent, as a late recurrence may occur (17).

Genitourinary Cancers in Patients with Renal Failure

The incidence of genitourinary (GU) tumors is increased in patients on dialysis (18,19). For kidney cancers the risk is increased roughly threefold compared to the normal population and more so in the younger age group (19). The main reason for this is the increased incidence of acquired cystic disease of the kidney, which occurs in between 40% and 80% of patients on dialysis.

Multicystic disease puts patients at increased risk of developing renal parenchymal cancers, which appear to be largely independent of the primary renal diagnosis. In conditions such as analgesic nephropathy, however, the kidney cancers are more often of urothelial origin. The risk of bladder cancer is also increased (50% increase) in patients on dialysis but to a lesser extent compared to the normal population. The incidence of bladder cancer decreases with time on dialysis, whereas that of kidney cancers increases with time on dialysis (19).

Renal transplant recipients are also at increased risk of developing renal and urinary tract cancers. Kidney tumors may appear in donor kidney or in the native kidneys. Renal carcinomas develop in 0.5% to 3.9% of transplant recipients, which is a roughly 10 to 100 times higher than in the general population (20). Those most at risk are patients with acquired cystic disease of the kidney (50-fold increase) (21) and those with a history of analgesic nephropathy or renal tract tumors (22). Rarely renal tumors may occur in the transplant kidney. In this case the management is to stop the immunosuppression and remove the kidney.

Diagnosis of Genitourinary Tumors in End-Stage Renal Failure

One cannot rely on urine screening to pick up GU tumors in anuric patients, but they may occasionally present with the passage of blood per urethra. Polycythemia is associated with renal tumors, but in patients with end-stage renal failure this may present as a steady unexplained decline in the need for erythropoietin. Conversely patients with any form of cancer often suffer from relative erythropoietin resistance and hence unexplained anemia in the context of erythropoietin therapy. All the other symptoms and signs are the same as in patients with normal renal function.

The diagnosis of prostatic cancer is also difficult in the anuric patient as the symptoms of prostatism cannot be relied upon. Total prostate-specific antigen (PSA) measurements are as valid in these patients as they are in the general population, though, and hence may be of some help.

Treatment of Genitourinary Cancers in Dialysis Patients

The treatment principles are the same as in a nondialysis patient; however, assessment of split function and overall renal function, as discussed above, becomes irrelevant. The surgical technique, however, does matter as any transperitoneal approach in a patient on continuous ambulatory peritoneal dialysis (CAPD) is likely to require a permanent transfer to hemodialysis thereafter; hence a retroperitoneal approach is preferred to transperitoneal approach.

Tumors in Solitary Kidney and Bilateral Renal Tumors

In a rare patient with solitary kidney and severe comorbid conditions, the best option could be masterly inactivity. Various surgical options include radical surgery (radical nephrectomy or nephroureterectomy) followed by dialysis, enucleation of the tumor, partial nephrectomy, and rarely bench surgery with autotransplantation (see Chapters 7 and 15). It is also possible to treat small tumors with cryosurgery, high-intensity focused ultrasound (HIFU), or radiofrequency ablation (23). As patients undergoing nephron-saving surgery may end up having total removal of kidney depending on technical problems and findings at the time of surgery, it is important to get a preoperative nephrological assessment. As mentioned earlier, postoperative dialysis support may be required for a limited period in patients who had nephron-saving surgery.

Acute Renal Failure

In acute renal failure (ARF), there is rapid deterioration of renal function leading to a progressive rise in serum creatinine levels. This is further characterized by failure to excrete nitrogenous products from the blood and ensuing metabolic acidosis. Acute renal failure could be the first manifestation of GU cancers, and can also occur later during the course of treatment or progression of the malignancy. Acute renal failure causes substantial morbidity and

TABLE 12.2. Possible causes of acute renal failure in genitourinary (GU) cancer patients

Prerenal	Hemorrhage and shock
	Sepsis
	Dehydration
	Drugs: NSAIDs, ACE inhibitors
	Acute tumor lysis syndrome
Renal	Renal ischemia: shock, sepsis
	Chemotherapeutic agents: ifosfamide, methotrexate, carboplatin, and cisplatin
	Antimicrobial agents: aminoglycosides, amphotericin, rifampicin, quinolones
	Pyelonephritis
	NSAIDs
Postrenal	GU malignancies: bilateral ureteric TCC, prostate cancer, TCC bladder, urethral carcinoma, retroperitoneal fibrosis, pelvic malignancies (uterine, ovarian, cervical, colorectal cancers)
	Benign conditions: BPH, uterine prolapse

ACE, angiotensin-converting enzyme; BPH, benign prostatic hypertrophy; NSAID, nonsteroidal antiinflammatory drug.

mortality in cancer patients (24). The causes of ARF are prerenal, renal and postrenal (Table 12.2).

Prerenal

Renal failure associated with renal hypoperfusion responds well to appropriate fluid replacement. Hypoperfusion leads to reduced GFR and drastic reduction in volume of urine.

Drug Toxicity

There are two broad mechanisms of renal drug toxicity: biochemical (direct and indirect) and immunological. The kidney is susceptible to drug toxicity due to its high blood flow, capacity to concentrate drugs, and its ability to metabolize the drugs. It is important to note that nonsteroidal antiinflammatory drugs (NSAIDs) increase the risk of ARF through products of prostaglandin metabolism (25), and this is dose dependent. Concurrent medication with other nephrotoxic agents could enhance worsening of the renal function (26).

Acute Tumor Lysis Syndrome

Acute tumor lysis syndrome is a life-threatening complication of cancer chemotherapy in chemosensitive tumors due to the rapid release of intracellular contents into the extracellular space. This is generally seen in hematological cancers, although it has been reported in germ cell tumors (27).

Renal

The majority of hospital-acquired acute renal failure cases are due to acute tubular necrosis (ATN) (28), which is multifactorial in origin and usually due to renal hypoperfusion, use of nephrotoxic drugs, and sepsis. Prolonged episodes of renal hypoperfusion lead to cortical necrosis. Patients who are likely to be vulnerable to ATN include the elderly, diabetics, patients with pre-existing renal disease or congestive cardiac failure, and those who have volume depletion.

Chemotherapy Agents

The two main drugs used in urological cancers are cisplatin and methotrexate.

Cisplatin-Induced Renal Toxicity

Most cisplatin is cleared through the kidneys. It has a direct effect on the proximal tubule, and its nephrotoxic effect is exacerbated in a low-chloride environment (29). Doses of cisplatin greater than $50\,mg/m^2$ have the potential to cause renal insufficiency, and doses in excess of $100\,mg/m^2$ can cause irreversible renal damage (30). Hydration and avoidance of concomitant nephrotoxic agents (e.g., aminoglycosides) is essential to prevent cisplatin toxicity. Amifostine (inorganic thiophosphates) has been shown to prevent renal failure (24). Cisplatin also causes nausea and vomiting, which may exacerbate dehydration and electrolyte disturbances. Monitoring renal function, therefore, is of the utmost importance in cisplatin therapy.

Methotrexate

Methotrexate is excreted primarily by the kidney. High doses of methotrexate are associated with renal failure due to precipitation of methotrexate or its metabolites in the tubular lumen (31). Monitoring methotrexate levels is necessary to prevent nephrotoxicity. Intravenous fluids are given during methotrexate administration to maintain high urine output. Alkalization of urine to pH 7.5 is recommended (24). Fortunately, methotrexate is removed by hemodialysis (24).

Antimicrobial Agents

Other drugs commonly used are antimicrobial agents. Amphotericin is an effective antifungal agent that can cause acute renal failure by its toxic effects on renal tubular cells, resulting in acute tubular necrosis (32).

Aminoglycosides such as gentamicin are commonly used in urological practice in the treatment of gram-negative bacterial infection. They are not metabolized in the body and are freely filtered through the glomeruli. A sizable amount accumulates in the renal cortex leading to cellular damage (33,34).

Obstructive Uropathy

The total renal mass needs to be completely obstructed in order for the renal function to deteriorate; hence a unilateral transitional cell carcinoma of the ureter will cause acute renal failure only if the contralateral kidney is diseased or absent.

The mainstay of management is to effectively diagnose outflow obstruction. A history of anuria is suggestive, but imaging is required. An ultrasound scan is probably the initial investigation of choice as it avoids the use of potentially nephrotoxic contrast agents. It is important to note, however, that obstruction cannot necessarily be ruled out on the basis of a nondilated renal pelvis nor can the diagnosis be made with complete certainty in cases with hydronephrotic kidneys. Improvement in renal function following drainage is occasionally the only way of being certain if obstruction was present. In acute cases of bilateral obstruction, drainage (nephrostomy or J-stenting) followed by resuscitation by correcting fluid balance and metabolic acidosis is necessary prior to staging and planning definitive management. Once the obstruction is relieved, there is a phase of diuresis leading to fluid loss, decreased urine concentrating ability, and electrolyte imbalance. This condition requires careful correction in high-risk patients.

References

1. Bankir L, Trinh-Trang-Tan M-M. Urea and the kidney. In: Breener BM, ed. Brenner and Rector's Kidney, 6th ed. Philadelphia: WB Saunders, 2000:637–679.
2. Levey AS, Perrone RD, Madias NE. Serum creatinine and renal function. Annu Rev Med 1988;39:465–490.
3. Doolan PD, Alpen EL, Theil GB. A clinical appraisal of the plasma concentration and endogenous clearance of creatinine. Am J Med 1962;32:65–79.
4. Levy AS, Madaio MP, Perrone RD. Laboratory assessment of renal disease: clearance, analysis and biopsy. In: Brenner BM, Rector FC, eds. The Kidney, 4th ed. Philadelphia: WB Saunders, 1991:919–968.
5. Position statement: chronic kidney disease and automatic reporting of estimated glomerular filtration rate. Med J Aust 2005;183:138–141.
6. Cockcroft DW, Gault MH. Prediction of creatinine clearance from serum creatinine. Nephron 1976;16:31–31.
7. Levey AS, Bosch JP, Lewis JB, et al. A more accurate method to estimate glomerular filtration rate from serum creatinine: a new prediction equation. Modification of Diet in Renal Disease Study Group. Ann Intern Med 1999;130:461–470.
8. Poole SG, Dooley MJ, Rischin D. A comparison of bedside renal function estimates and measured glomerular filtration rate (Tc^{99m} DTPA clearance) in cancer patients. Ann Oncol 2002;13:949–955.
9. Peters AM. Quantification of renal haemodynamics with radionuclides. Eur J Nucl Med 1991;18(4):274–286.
10. NKF-DOQI clinical practice guidelines for hemodialysis adequacy. National Kidney Foundation. Am J Kidney Dis 1997;30(3 suppl 2):S15–66.

11. Stahl RAK, Löw I, Schoeppe W. Progressive renal failure in a patient after one and two-thirds nephrectomy. J Mol Med 1988;66:508–510.

12. Abdi R, Dong VM, Rubel JR, et al. Correlation between glomerular size and long-term renal function in patients with substantial loss of renal mass. J Urol 2003;170(1): 42–44.

13. Solomon R, Werner C, Mann D, D'Elia J, Silva P. Effects of saline, mannitol, and frusemide to prevent acute decreases in renal function induced by radiocontrast agents. N Engl J Med 1994;331:1416–1420.

14. Novick AC, Derweesh I. Open partial nephrectomy for renal tumours: current status. BJU Int 2005;95(Suppl 2):35–40.

15. Novick AC. Renal hypothermia: in vivo and ex vivo. Urol Clin North Am 1983;10: 637–644.

16. Secin FP, Carver B, Kattan M, Eastham JA. Current recommendations for delaying renal transplantation after localized prostate cancer treatment: are they still appropriate? Transplantation 2004;78:710–712.

17. Kasiske BL, Cangro CB, Hariharan S, et al. The evaluation of renal transplantation candidates: clinical practice guidelines. Am J Transplant 2001;1(suppl 2):3–95.

18. Maisonneuve P, Agodoa L, Gellert R, et al. Cancer in patients on dialysis for end-stage renal disease: an international collaborative study—group of 3. Lancet 1999;354: 93–99.

19. Stewart JH, Buccianti G, Agodoa L, et al. Cancers of the kidney and urinary tract in patients on dialysis for end-stage renal disease: analysis of data from the United states, Europe, and Australia and New Zealand. J Am Soc Nephrol 2003;14: 197–207.

20. Doublet JD, Peraldi MN, Gattegno B, Thibault P, Sraer JD. Renal cell carcinoma of native kidneys: prospective study of 129 renal transplant patients. J Urol 1997; 158(1):42–44.

21. Truong LD, Krishnan B, Cao JT, Barrios R, Suki WN. Renal neoplasm in acquired cystic disease. Am J Kidney Dis 1995;26:1–12.

22. Bokemeyer C, Thon WF, Brunkhorst T, et al. High frequency of urothelial cancers in patients with kidney transplantations for end-stage analgesic nephropathy. Eur J Cancer 1996;32A(1):175–176.

23. Weld JK, Landman J. Comparison of cryoablation, radiofrequency ablation, land HIFU for treating small renal tumours. BJU Int 2005;96:1224–1229.

24. Darmon M, Ciroldi M, Thiery G, et al. Clinical review: specific aspects of acute renal failure in cancer patients. Crit Care 2006;10:211.

25. Murray MD, Brater DC. Renal toxicity of the nonsteroidal anti-inflammatory drugs. Annu Rev Pharmacol Toxicol 1993;32:4350–4365.

26. Gutthann SP, Rodriguez LAG, Raiford DS, Oliart AD, Romeu JR. Non-steroidal anti-inflammatory drugs and the risk of hospitalization for acute renal failure. Arch Intern Med 1996;156:2433–2439.

27. Pentheroudakis G, O'Neill VJ, Vasey P, Kaye SB. Spontaneous acute tumour lysis syndrome in patients with metastatic germ cell tumours. Report of two cases. Support Care Cancer 2001;9(7):554–557.

28. Myers BD, Moran SM. Hemodynamically mediated acute renal failure. N Engl J Med 1986;314:97–105.

29. Arany I, Safirstein RL. Cisplatin nephrotoxicity. Semin Nephrol 2003;23:460–464.

30. Ries F, Klastersky J. Nephrotoxicity induced by cancer chemotherapy with special emphasis on cisplatin toxicity. Am J Kidney Dis 1986;8:368–379.

31. Condit PT, Chanes RE, Joel W. Renal toxicity of methotrexate. Cancer 1969;23: 126–131.

32. Wall et al. Effective clearance of methotrexate using high-flux hemodialysis membranes. Am J Kidney Dis 1996;28:86–54.

33. Walker RJ, Duggin GG. Drug nephrotoxicity. Annu Rev Pharmacol Toxicol 1988; 28:331–345.

34. Nagai J, Takano M. Review: molecular aspects of renal handling of aminoglycosides and strategies for preventing the nephrotoxicity. Drug Metab Pharmacokinet 2004; 19:159–170.

13
Diet and Genitourinary Cancer

Sona Kapoor and Jeetesh Bhardwa

The Role of Diet in Cancer

There has long been debate over a link between diet and cancer. From the initial observations that esophageal cancers were more common in people with a high consumption of smoked fish and the link between smoking and lung cancer, it has been obvious to some that there exists a link between what we eat and the development of certain types of cancers. Similarly there has been much written in the popular press about complementary and alternative medicine (CAM) for cancers, including the role of trace elements and antioxidants, which may actually prevent the development of certain types of cancers. The reasons as to why this may be the case are the subjects of ongoing research, and in this chapter we explore the pro- and anticarcinogenic effects of certain foodstuffs on urological cancer. These effects may have additional implications, as patients also want to avoid any factors that may cause their cancer to have a poorer prognosis and are increasingly open to modulating their diet and embracing alternative/complementary health regimes.

An important question is whether isolated vitamin, mineral, and antioxidant supplements are as effective as those naturally present in fruits and vegetables. There are increasing reports that the interaction of the natural vitamins and antioxidants make them more effective than the isolated compounds. Thus there has been an increased awareness of the benefits of eating fruits and vegetables to prevent or hinder cancer progression rather than just ingesting proprietary makes of multivitamins and other trace elements.

Based on statistical and epidemiological data, Doll and Peto (1) reported that 10% to 70% (average 35%) of human cancer mortality was attributable to diet. There is compelling evidence of a wide range of dietary factors stimulating the development, growth, and spread of tumors in experimental animals. There is also a marked difference in the total cancer burden between developed and developing countries. The main reason for this variation is probably related to environmental and lifestyle factors rather than genetic factors (2). Dietary habits coupled with a sedentary lifestyle influence the proportion of body fat present in an individual, and excessive fat leads to obesity. It should not be forgotten that there are confounding variables, such as the link between obesity and cancer, which may influence the interpretation of certain dietary associations. Obesity's relationship with cancer is being currently investigated in several studies. Renal carcinoma seems to be associated with excess weight (see below) (3).

Prostate Cancer

Prostate cancer is the most commonly diagnosed malignancy in men in industrialized countries and the second leading cause of male cancer-related death. It is thus of great importance that any factor that may lead us to decrease the risk of developing or progressing of prostate cancer be explored.

Fat Intake

A close correlation exists between average per capita fat intake and prostate cancer mortality in numerous countries around the world. Japanese and Chinese men who migrate to the United States experience dramatic increases in prostate cancer risk within one generation compared with their Caucasian neighbors and with Japanese and Chinese men who have remained on a traditional diet in their homeland (4). It is also noteworthy that there has been an increase in prostate cancer among Asians in Singapore and Hong Kong who have adopted a Western lifestyle, including diet. The Physician's Health Study by Gann et al. (5) found an association between red meat consumption and prostate cancer risk, but this association was not statistically significant. Linoleic acid, which is the major polyunsaturated fat in most diets, has been associated with an increased risk of prostate carcinoma in some studies. There was no obvious association between prostate cancer and alcohol consumption (6).

Calorie Intake

In a study investigating the relationship between prostate cancer and calorie intake in rats, reduction in tumor growth was observed in rats that were fed an energy-restricted diet, regardless of whether they had a high-fat or a high-carbohydrate intake. Thus reduction in energy intake, not just fat, is needed to reduce prostate cancer growth in an experimental model (7).

Agents that May Protect Against Prostate Cancer

A large amount of epidemiological and some molecular data support the use of selenium, vitamin E, vitamin D, lycopene, and green tea as potential preventatives possibly by reducing the oxidative damage in prostatic tissue (8,9). Long-term supplementation with α-tocopherol, a form of vitamin E, significantly reduced prostate cancer incidence and mortality in smokers (10). Some of these agents are being tested in new large-scale phase III clinical trials.

A long-term randomised study, known as SELECT (Selenium and Vitamin E Cancer Prevention Trial) is currently evaluating vitamin E and selenium, although, as yet, no results are available (11). Common usage has identified the dose for selenium as 200 µg/day. Similarly common usage for vitamin E has just been reduced to 150 IU/day because of possible cardiovascular effects of higher doses. Omega-3 fatty acids, obtained mainly from fatty fish, have been shown to inhibit prostate cancer cell lines in laboratory experiments. The Netherlands Cohort Study found a potential protective effect of omega-3 fatty acids, but this was not statistically significant (12,13).

Soy products may reduce the level of androgenic steroids, the driving factor for prostate cancer. This has been attributed to isoflavonoids, plant pigments found in soybean. A large-scale cross-national study in 59 countries showed that soy products were significantly protective ($p < .001$), with an effect size per kilocalorie at least four times as large as that of any other dietary factor (14).

Bladder Cancer

Procarcinogenic Factors in Diet

The evidence linking diet and the development of bladder cancer is not strong. Environmental toxins (such as used in dye, rubber, and textile manufacturing) seem to predominate as the major factors affecting the incidence of bladder cancers and have been estimated to be responsible for up to 20% of bladder cancer cases. Aromatic amines from occupational exposures are activated and detoxified through the same reactions that aromatic amines in cigarette smoke are activated and detoxified.

It also means that exposures to occupational agents and cigarette smoke may be additive. In clinical oncology practice, more than 80% of patients with bladder cancer have a significant smoking history.

Some studies have indicated an increased risk of bladder cancers and coffee drinking (15–17), although this association remains controversial. The role of alcohol in increasing the risk of prostate, renal, and bladder cancer is still uncertain, because of the confounding variables of smoking and dietary fat. The exact role of fat intake in bladder cancer is unclear (18).

The high levels of arachidonic acid and its derivatives in meat products are postulated to have a promoting effect on prostate cancer in animals and the same may be true in bladder cancer (19,20). Several studies have reported correlation between total fluid intake and the risk of developing bladder cancer. Greater fluid intake of water could reduce the risk of bladder cancer by 50% (21).

Anticarcinogenic Factors in Diet

A reduction in risk of bladder cancer was observed in nonsmokers with a high intake of cruciferous vegetables (cabbage, Brussels sprouts, broccoli, and cauliflower) (18). Protective effects of cruciferous vegetables were thought to be due to their high concentration of the carotenoids lutein and zeaxanthin. In vitro studies have shown isoflavonoids, found in soy, to inhibit bladder cancer cells (18).

Renal Cancer

Investigators have shown an increase in renal cell carcinoma (RCC) among men consuming high-fat diets (22). There seems to be an increased risk of RCC with high energy intake, especially from increased consumption of fried meats (22,23). Chow et al. (24) reported that high protein consumption was associated with other chronic renal diseases that may predispose to RCC, while others did not. Increased consumption of chlorination by-products also appears to increase the risk (25,26). Recurrent urinary tract infections, increased intake of protein and fried foods, as well as female sex appear to increase the risk of renal cancer. Thus, dietary modification and other public health measures directed at environmental carcinogens have the potential to reduce the incidence of urological malignancies (27).

Nutritional Effects of Anticancer Treatments

Radiotherapy

Most of the side effects of radiotherapy are felt around the second or third week of the treatment and subside 3 to 4 weeks after finishing radiotherapy. Chronic side effects appear after a period of long duration, that is, after many years (28).

Nearly 70% of patients receiving radiotherapy to the pelvis experience acute gastrointestinal symptoms, as healthy bowel is inevitably included in the radiation field and 50% of these patients go on to develop chronic bowel symptoms, which affect their quality of life (29). There is no evidence base for the use of nutritional interventions to prevent or manage bowel symptoms attributable to radiotherapy. Diarrhea is treated by high liquid intake and reduced fiber content of the diet. It is also important to prescribe a high potassium diet. Low-fat diets, probiotic supplementation, and elemental diet merit further investigation. One year after pelvic radiotherapy, dietary manipulation was found to be generally unhelpful for gastrointestinal symptoms, although the role of eliminating raw vegetables may benefit from further evaluation.

Chemotherapy

Systemic chemotherapy leads to more severe side effects than radiation or surgical treatment. Most side effects are of short duration and subside once the treatment has been discontinued. The main areas that are affected by chemotherapy are those where cell division and growth is rapid, such as oral mucosa, the gastrointestinal tract, skin, hair, and bone marrow. Anorexia, altered taste sensation, nausea, vomiting, stomatitis, mucositis/esophagitis, diarrhea, and constipation are some well known side effects.

Nutritional Needs of Patients Undergoing Radiotherapy or Chemotherapy

It has been suggested that cancer patients need up to 20% more calories and 50% more protein than they needed before having cancer. People have a much easier time tolerating their treatments for cancer when they are well nourished. They usually have fewer side effects, better wound healing, and fewer infections, and are able to be more active. To prevent malnutrition from the cancer itself and chemotherapy, it is essential that patients are educated about nutritional needs.

Malnutrition and weight loss lead to poor immunity and weakness, which subsequently affect a patient's ability to regain health and acceptable blood counts between chemotherapy cycles. This can affect treatment regimes and the ability of the patient to stay on treatment schedules, which is important in achieving a successful outcome.

Patients need to be educated about neutropenic diets that are supposed to give their immune systems a boost by including lots of yogurt that contains live active cultures of *Lactobacillus bulgaricus* and *Streptococcus thermophilus*. Some other specific foods to include are garlic, and foods high in zinc such as oysters, pot roast, dark meat turkey, pumpkin, squash seeds, and shiitake mushrooms. A neutropenic diet includes all well-cooked foods and excludes foods that may contain potential disease-causing microorganisms. However, this needs further elucidation by more specific studies.

Maintaining nutrition is an integral part of patient care, and when it is possible enteral nutrition is regarded as superior to parenteral nutrition. However, when it is not possible to eat or ingest high-calorie drinks, then enteral nutrition via nasogastric route is preferable. Postpyloric feeding may enable enteral feeding to be maintained in patients who cannot tolerate nasogastric feeding. Postpyloric feeding can be successfully used to maintain enteral nutrition in patients who would otherwise require parenteral nutrition.

Parenteral nutrition is the last step, and it is reserved for patients whom it is not possible to feed enterally, especially as there may be some worry about the tumor-boosting activity of parenteral feeding and the invasiveness of this approach along with risk of infection and the morbidity associated with inserting a line.

Anorexia is present in 15% to 25% of cancer patients and is nearly as present in patients with metastasis (30). It is further aggravated by depression, loss of personal interests, loss of hope, and anxiety, resulting in protein-calorie malnutrition (31).

Immunotherapy

This modality of treatment is now increasingly used for bladder and renal tumors. Monoclonal antibodies are used to block cancer-cell receptors for growth-stimulating factors, which also cause the side effect from this form of treatment. Interferon (nonspecific immunotherapy agent) and other immune therapy agents affect the nutritional status of the patients. They cause fever, nausea, vomiting, diarrhea, and fatigue. These side effects are also experienced by patients receiving interleukin-2 for metastatic renal cell cancer, though some patients have reported weight gain (32).

Granulocyte-macrophage colony-stimulating factor (GM-CSF), a very commonly used treatment to increase the production of white blood cells, may also cause fever, nausea, vomiting, and diarrhea. These symptoms can lead to gradual or drastic weight loss causing malnutrition and complicate the expected healing and recovery process. These can be avoided by screening and assessing the patient. This should be done before starting the anticancer treatment and should continue during and after treatment. Screening is useful in identifying patients at risk of developing malnutrition during the course of illness and treatment.

Surgery

Radical or salvage surgery is another option for cancer treatment. Poorly nourished patients are at increased risk of postoperative morbidity and mortality. Every attempt should be made to correct nutritional deficiencies prior to surgery (33). Preoperative assessment and correction of the nutritional deficiencies with oral supplements, enteral or parental nutrition, or the use of pharmacological therapies to suppress nausea should be actively practiced.

Surgery, depending on the procedure (ileal conduit, transperitoneal nephrectomy, retropubic prostatectomy, retroperitoneal lymph node dissection) may cause mechanical or physiological obstruction to adequate nutrition (33). Surgery causes an immediate metabolic demand that increases nutritional requirements essential for wound healing and recovery. Many patients are unable to eat a normal diet and experience loss of appetite, fatigue, and pain as a result of surgery. Malnutrition leads to prolonged recovery time and wound healing complications.

Aims of Nutritional Therapy in Cancer Patients

Nutritional management of genitourinary cancer patient is a team effort and should include a physician/surgeon, specialist nurse, and registered dietitian. The goals of the nutrition therapy for cancer patients in active treatment and recovery are aimed at restoring healthy nutrition, correcting malnutrition, and preventing muscle wasting and immunodeficiency.

In the management of cancer patients, nutritional optimization is an important goal. The goals of the nutrition therapy for cancer are aimed at correcting malnutrition, and preventing muscle wasting and a catabolic state.

The benefit of optimal caloric and nutritional intake is well documented in patients undergoing treatment or recovering and also in patients remission and aiming to avoid cancers (34–36).

In individuals with advanced cancer, the goal of nutrition therapy should not be weight gain or reversal of malnutrition, but rather comfort and symptom relief. Nutrition continues to play an integral role for individuals whose cancer has been cured or who are in remission (37). Many patients undergoing cancer treatment use dietary supplements, particularly antioxidants, in the hope of reducing the toxicity of chemotherapy and radiotherapy. Preclinical data are inconclusive and it is advisable to not to use any agent that is not beneficial (38). Following a healthful nutrition program might help prevent another malignancy from developing.

References

1. Doll R, Peto R. The causes of cancer: quantitative estimates of avoidable risks of cancer in the United States today. J Natl Cancer Inst 1981;66:1191–1308.
2. Bingham S, Riboli E. Diet and Cancer—The European Prospective Investigation into Cancer and Nutrition. Nature Rev Can 2003;4:206–215.
3. Benichou J, Chow WH, McLoughlin JK, et al. Population attributable risk of renal cell cancer in Minnesota. Am J Epidemiol 1998;148:424–430.
4. Muir CS, Nectoux J, Staszewski J. The epidemiology of prostatic cancer: geographical distribution and time trends. Acta Oncol 1991;30:133–140.
5. Gann PH, Hennekens CH, Sacks FM, et al. Prospective study of plasma fatty acids and risk of prostate cancer. J Natl Cancer Inst 1994;89:281–286.
6. Dennis LK. Meta-analysis for combining relative risks of alcohol consumption and prostate cancer. Prostate 2000;42:56–66.
7. Mukherjee P, Sotnikov AV, Mangian HJ, et al. Energy intake and prostate tumour growth, angiogenesis, and vascular endothelial growth factor expression. J Nat Cancer Inst 1999;91:512–523.
8. Giovannucci E. Tomatoes, tomato-based products, lycopene, and cancer: review of the epidemiologic literature. J Natl Cancer Inst 1999;91:317–331.
9. Levy J, Bosin E, Feldman B, et al. Lycopene is a more potent inhibitor of human cancer cell proliferation than either α-carotene or β-carotene. Nutr Cancer 1995;24:257–266.
10. Heinonen OP, Albanes D, Virtamo J, et al. Prostate cancer and supplementation with α-tocopherol and β-carotene: incidence and mortality in a controlled trial. J Natl Cancer Inst 1998;90:440–446.
11. Klein, Eric A, Thompson, Ian M. Update on chemoprevention of prostate cancer. Curr Opin Urol 2004;14(3):143–149.
12. Mazhar D, Waxman J. Diet and prostate cancer. BJU Int 2004;93(7):919–922.
13. Schuurman AG, van den Brandt PA, Dorant E, et al. Association of energy and fat intake with prostate carcinoma risk: results from the Netherlands Cohort Study. Cancer 1999;86:1019–1027.

14. Herbert JR, Hurley TG, Olendzki BC, et al. Nutritional and socioeconomic factors in relation to prostate cancer mortality: a cross-national study. J Natl Cancer Inst 1998;90:1637–1647.

15. Donato F, Boffetta P, Fazioli R, et al. Bladder cancer, tobacco, coffee and alcohol drinking in Brescia, northern Italy. Eur J Epidemiol 1997;13:795–800.

16. Rebelakos A, Trichopoulos D, Tzonou A, et al. Tobacco smoking, coffee drinking, and occupation as risk factors for bladder cancer in Greece. J Natl Cancer Inst 1985; 75:455–461.

17. Vena JE, Freudenheim J, Graham S, et al. Coffee, cigarette smoking, and bladder cancer in western New York. Ann Epidemiol 1993;3:586–591.

18. Moyad MA. Bladder cancer prevention. Part I: what do I tell my patients about lifestyle changes and dietary requirements? Curr Opin Urol 2003;13:363–378.

19. Ghosh J, Myers C Jr. Arachidonic acid metabolism and cancer of the prostate. Nutrition 1998;14:48–57.

20. Fraser GE. Associations between diet and cancer, ischemic heart disease, and all-cause mortality in non-Hispanic white California Seventh–day Adventists. Am J Clin Nutr 1999;70(suppl 3):532–538.

21. Michaud DS, SPiegelman D, Clinton SK, et al. Fluid intake and the risk of bladder cancer in men. N Engl J Med 1999;340:1390–1397.

22. Wolk A, Gridley G, Niwa S, et al. International renal cell cancer study: the role of diet. Int J Cancer 1996;65:67–73.

23. Lindblad P, Wolk A, Bergstrom R, et al. The role of obesity and weight fluctuations in the aetiology of renal cell cancer: a population-based case-control study. Can Epidemiol Biomark Prev 1994;3:631–639.

24. Chow WH, Gridley G, McLaughlin JK, et al. Protein intake and risk of renal cell cancer. J Natl Cancer Inst 1994;86:1131–1139.

25. Bruemmer B, White E, Vaughan TL, Cheney CL. Nutrient intake in relation to bladder cancer among middle-aged men and women. Am J Epidemiol 1996;144: 485–495.

26. Shirai T, Fradet Y, Huland H, et al. The etiology of bladder cancer-are there any new clues or predictors of behavior? Int J Urol 1995;2:64–76.

27. Mydlo JH, Kanter JL, Kral JG, et al. The role of obesity and diet in urological carcinogenesis. BJU Int 1999;84:225–234.

28. Donaldson SS. Nutritional consequences of radiotherapy. Cancer Res 1977:37 (7 Pt 2):2407–2413.

29. McGough C, Baldwin C, Frost G, Andreyev HJ. Role of nutritional intervention in patients treated with radiotherapy for pelvic malignancy. Br J Cancer 2004;14;90: 2278–2287.

30. Langstein HN, Norton JA. Mechanisms of cancer cachexia. Hematol Oncol Clin North Am 1991;5:103–123.

31. Breura E. ABC of palliative care. Anorexia, cachexia and nutrition. BMJ 1997;315: 1219–1222.

32. Samlowski WE, Wiebke G, McMurry M, et al. Effects of total parental nutrition (TPN) during high-dose interleukin-2 treatment for metastatic cancer. J Immunother 1998; 21:65–74.

33. McGuire M. Nutritional care of surgical oncology patients. Semin Oncol Nurs 2000; 16:128–134.

34. McCallum PD, Polisena CG, eds. The Clinical Guide to Oncology Nutrition. Chicago: American Dietetic Association, 2000.

35. Blosch AS. Nutrition Management of the Cancer Patient. Rockville, MD: Aspen, 1990.
36. Rivlin RS, Shils ME, Sherlock P. Nutrition and cancer. Am J Med 1983;75:843–854.
37. Brown J, Byers T, Thompson K, et al. Nutrition during and after cancer treatment: a guide for informed choices by cancer survivors. CA Cancer J Clin 2001;51:153–87; quiz 189–192.
38. D'Andrea GM. Review: use of antioxidants during chemotherapy and radiotherapy should be avoided. CA Cancer J Clin 2005;55(5):319–321.

Part III
Systemic Genitourinary Oncology

14
Renal Cell Carcinoma

14.1
Renal Cell Carcinoma: Overview

Ziya Kirkali and Cag Cal

Epidemiology

Renal cell carcinoma (RCC) accounts for 3% of all adult cancers. The incidence rates for kidney cancer are highest in European and Scandinavian countries and North America (1). It is estimated that 36,160 new cases of kidney and renal pelvis cancer were diagnosed in 2005, with an estimated 12,660 resulting deaths in the United States (2). There has been a 30% increase in incidence in the last 20 years. Although this increased incidence is partly a result of more widespread and aggressive imaging, current reports show a real increase in incidence. Renal cell carcinoma is a tumor of adults occurring primarily after the 5th decade of life. It occurs one-and-a-half times as often in men as in women (3:2) (3). Childhood RCC is uncommon, representing only 2% to 6% of all renal tumors in children. Bilateral tumors are identified in 2% to 5% of the patients.

Etiology

The exact cause of RCC is not known. However, there are many risk factors that have been identified for RCC.

Tobacco Smoking

The only accepted risk factor for RCC is tobacco use. The relative associated risks have been modest and the effect is not as strong as for lung and bladder cancers. Relative risk is directly related to duration of smoking, cumulative dose, or pack-years.

Hereditary Factors

Approximately 4% of RCCs are familial, and this is likely to rise with better understanding of genomics and advances in imaging techniques (4). Hereditary RCCs are different from sporadic renal cancers; they are often multiple and occur much earlier in life. Patients need lifelong monitoring, and relatives might require screening. The hereditary tumors are described below (see Natural History and Pathology).

Obesity

A meta-analysis by Bergstrom et al. (5) found an equal association of risk among men and women and estimated the kidney cancer risk to be 36% higher for an overweight person and 84% higher for an obese person compared to those with a normal weight. The exact mechanism by which obesity increases RCC risk is not well understood. An increased exposure to insulin-like growth factor and the sex steroids estrogen and androgen is a possible mechanism. There are other risk factors, such as atherosclerosis, and hypertension caused by obesity may also contribute to the susceptibility to RCC. Reversal of obesity following bariatric surgery does not eliminate the risk for RCC (6).

Chronic Renal Failure, Dialysis, and Renal Transplantation

The risk of developing RCC increases in patients with polycystic kidney disease or chronic renal failure, and in patients who are undergoing hemodialysis and have acquired cystic disease. Renal transplantation does not reduce the malignant potential of acquired cystic disease in the native kidneys.

Diet

The difference in incidence of RCC between industrialized Western countries and Asian countries suggests that dietary factors may have some role in the development of RCC. A typical Western diet, with increased calorie intake, containing high fat, protein, and dairy products and low intake of fruits and vegetables, has a higher propensity for causing RCC.

Occupational and Environmental Effects

There is a slightly increased risk of RCC in workers exposed to asbestos, cadmium, steel, petroleum, trichloroethylene, and perchloroethylene.

Drugs

Certain drugs such as diuretics and antihypertensive medications have been shown to be associated with RCC; again relative risks are low. However, it is not clear whether the risk is associated with hypertension itself or the antihypertensive medication used to treat the condition.

Miscellaneous

There is an association of RCC with hypertension and amphetamine diet pills (6). In comparison with the general population, patients with diabetes mellitus have an increased risk of renal cell cancer (7).

Preventative Measures

The risk of RCC may be decreased with regular recreational physical activity and keeping a normal body mass index (BMI) of 18.5 to $25\,kg/m^2$. Cessation of smoking and consumption of a diet with increased fruits and vegetables also play a preventive role for RCC. There is, at present, insufficient evidence for specific dietary recommendations.

Screening

The general consensus in the literature is that the yield of screening the general population for RCC is low and not cost-effective; screening is limited to target population (Table 14.1.1) (8).

Natural History and Pathology

Renal cell carcinoma originates from mature tubular renal structures with the exception of pediatric tumors (9). It remains asymptomatic until locally advanced or there is metastatic disease. More than 50% of the renal cancers are detected incidentally in asymptomatic patients *(incidentalomas)*, whereas in the past most RCC cases were diagnosed because of investigations for classical symptoms of loin pain, hematuria, or mass. There is a corresponding decrease in the mean size of the tumor at presentation (10). These asymptomatic small tumors tend to be in an early stage and grade compared to symptomatic large tumors. The 5-year survival rate for incidentalomas of less than 4 cm with nephron-sparing or radical surgery is in the region of 95% to 100% (10).

TABLE 14.1.1. Indications for screening in target population

1. Patients with end-stage renal failure (on hemodialysis and long life expectancy)
2. Patients with von Hippel–Lindau (VHL) syndrome
3. Relatives of VHL patients who have gene defects
4. Familial forms of RCC
5. Patients with tuberous sclerosis

Bosniak et al. (11) reviewed 40 incidental tumors of less than 3.5 cm over a period of 3 years, and the growth rate of neoplasms was 0 to 1.1 cm/year (mean of 0 to 0.36 cm/year). Even though nine patients had multiple neoplasms, no patient developed metastatic disease. Similar studies of active surveillance have been reported, albeit with a short follow-up period and a small number of patients. All these studies indicate a slow growth rate and generally that there is no tendency for metastasis.

Pathology

As mentioned earlier, RCCs originate from mature tubular structures, mostly from the proximal tubule, although collecting duct carcinoma and chromophobe RCCs are supposed to originate from the lower part of the nephron, namely the collecting duct. The pathological classification of adult renal tumors is shown in Table 14.1.2. Nearly 5% of tumors do not belong to any of these categories (RCC unclassified).

TABLE 14.1.2. Pathological classification of the adult renal tumors (9)

Epithelial tumors
Benign: Cortical papillary adenoma
Renal oncocytoma
Juxtaglomerular cell tumour
Metanephric adenoma
Malignant: Renal cell carcinoma
Clear/or granular cell carcinoma (conventional)
Chromophobe type
Papillary type
Collecting duct carcinoma with medullary carcinoma
Unclassified
Mesenchymal tumors
Benign: Angiomyolipoma
Medullary fibroma
Leiomyoma
Lipoma
Hemangioma
Lymphangioma
Malignant: Sarcoma (leiomyosarcoma, liposarcoma, malignant fibrous histioma)
Lymphoma
Blastemal tumors: metastatic nephroma, adult Wilms' tumour, clear cell carcinoma
Neuroendocrine: Carcinoid, neuroectodermal tumour
Metastatic: Lung, thyroid

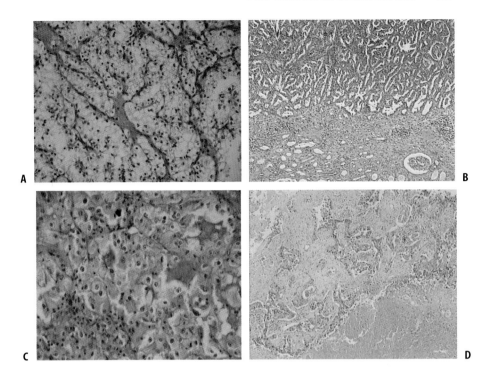

FIGURE **14.1.1.** Major histological types of renal cell carcinoma. (A) Clear cell (×100). (B) Papillary (×100). (C) Chromophobe (large cells with granular cytoplasm and perinuclear halo; × 100). (D) Collecting duct carcinoma (×100).

Conventional Renal Cell Carcinoma (Clear or Granular Cell Carcinoma)

This is the most common variety and accounts for 70% to 80% of all RCCs (Fig. 14.1.1A). These RCCs are often large and peripherally located, with a pseudo-capsule. The cut surface has areas of necrosis, hemorrhage, and calcification. Although most of these tumors are isolated, 4% of the tumors could be multifocal in one kidney and bilateral in 0.5% to 3% of cases. The clear cell RCC presents with tumors of higher stage and grade compared with patients with papillary and chromophobe RCC. It also has a worse prognosis compared with other types. The tumor may invade the renal vein or vena cava. The cells are rich in cholesterol and glycogen, showing a clear cytoplasm and cell wall. These cells are mixed with eosinophilic cells.

Papillary (Chromophilic) Renal Cell Carcinoma

This is the second most frequent tumor, accounting for 10% to 15% of cases (Fig. 14.1.1B). It is often multifocal (39%), and bilateral tumors are seen in 4%

of the patients. Papillary RCCs have predominantly papillary or tubular architecture without any clear cell. There are two main types of papillary carcinoma: type 1, small cells with pale cytoplasm and small nuclei; and type 2, large eosinophilic cells with large nuclei, often pseudostratified, and prominent nucleoli, giving a higher Fuhrman grading.

Chromophobe Renal Cell Carcinoma

This type accounts for 5% of cases (Fig. 14.1.1C). It originates from intercalated cells of collecting duct. Macroscopically it is well circumscribed without hemorrhage or necrosis. Chromophobe RCC is composed of broad sheets of a mixture of cells with eosinophilic and clear cytoplasm arranged along thin vascular septa. The cells have irregular nuclei, and perinuclear halos are a characteristic feature. This variant of RCC needs to be differentiated from oncocytoma, which shares a common cellular origin (12). The cells vary in size, with pale abundant cytoplasm and a well-defined cell membrane.

Collecting Duct Carcinoma (Bellini's Duct Carcinoma)

This is a rare tumor (<1%) (Fig. 14.1.1D). It is composed of variable-sized tubules and papillae with a single layer of cuboidal cells like a hobnail arrangement. Deletions on chromosome 1q and monosomy of chromosomes 6, 14, 15, and 22 have been reported. It is usually located in the renal medulla. Most collecting duct RCCs are high grade and at advanced stage at diagnosis, and do not respond to conventional therapies.

Sarcomatoid changes occur in nearly all types of RCC and are considered as a manifestation of aggressive behavior of the tumor. Microscopically the cells are atypical and spindle-shaped, resembling sarcomatous cells.

Fuhrman grading is the most commonly used system in RCCs and correlates well with survival (13). The nuclear features such as size, shape, chromasia, and nucleolar prominence are used in this system on a scale of 1 through 4, with grade 1 being more like normal kidney cells. Nuclear grade means that the system is based on just the appearance of the nuclei of the cancer cells, rather than on the appearance or structure of the cells as a whole. Nuclear characteristics used in the Fuhrman grade particularly indicate how actively the cells are making protein. Fuhrman grading is appropriate for most common variants of RCC. Its prognostic significance is described later.

Hereditary Renal Tumors

Like many other malignant tumors, renal cancer occurs in hereditary and non-hereditary forms. There are four well-described forms of inherited kidney tumors:

1. Von Hippel–Lindau (VHL): inherited clear-cell RCC
2. Hereditary papillary renal cell carcinoma (HPRC): Type I papillary RCC

3. Hereditary leiomyoma RCC (HLRCC): Type II papillary RCC
4. Birt-Hogg-Dubé syndrome (BHD): risk of developing several types of renal tumors, including chromophobe RCC and oncocytoma

Von Hippel–Lindau disease is a relatively rare autosomal-dominant disorder. The *VHL* gene, which is located on the short arm of chromosome 3p25.5, has now been completely sequenced, and its role as a tumor suppressor gene for both the sporadic and the familial forms of clear cell RCC has been confirmed (14). The *VHL* gene is also mutated or displays a loss of heterozygosity in a high percentage of nonhereditary renal carcinomas. Clinical features include clear cell RCC, cysts of the kidney, and adrenal tumors (pheochromocytoma). There is also predisposition to multiple tumors of the eyes (retina), central nervous system hemangioblastoma, endolymphatic sac, and epididymis. Renal cell carcinoma develops in approximately 40% of patients with VHL disease and is a major cause of death among these patients. The renal cancers could be bilateral, multifocal, and appear at an early age. Mutations of the *VHL* gene are found in patients with clear-cell RCC. Patients with papillary, chromophobe RCC and oncocytoma do not have *VHL* gene mutations (15).

Hereditary papillary renal carcinoma (HPRC) is an autosomal dominant inherited disorder. These patients have bilateral, multifocal type I papillary renal carcinoma. The gene for HPRC is the *Met* proto-oncogene located at 7q31.

Birt-Hogg-Dubé (BHD) syndrome is an autosomal dominant disease with benign cutaneous tumors (hair follicle or fibrofolliculomas), pulmonary cysts, and renal neoplasms. The tumor types in BHD syndrome can be chromophobe, oncocytoma, or clear-cell RCC. The *BHD* gene is mapped to chromosome 17p11.2. Since patients with BHD are at risk for multiple renal tumors that are often malignant and can metastasize, they should be radiographically screened at periodic intervals. The best treatment modality is nephron sparing surgical approaches (16).

Management

The standard approach is to carry out nephron-sparing surgery (NSS) by removing the tumor(s) when it reaches a size of 3 cm. Observation and surveillance is required for tumors less than 3 cm. The investigational treatments like radiofrequency ablation are being investigated.

Hereditary Leiomyomatosis Renal Cell Carcinoma

Hereditary leiomyomatosis RCC (HLRCC) is a syndrome in which patients develop painful cutaneous leiomyomata, uterine fibroids, and type 2 papillary RCC. These tumors are often solitary but grow rapidly and early metastases are common.

The disease is inherited typically as autosomal dominant, and there is a germline defect of the loss or mutation of one copy of fumarate hydratase on chromosome 1q.

Clinical Features Including Paraneoplastic Syndromes and Metastasis

At initial presentation, approximately 30% of patients with RCC have metastatic disease, and 20% have locally advanced disease, with the remainder having localized tumors.

Symptoms and Signs

Most renal tumors are asymptomatic and nonpalpable until advanced disease develops. Today, tumors are mostly identified incidentally during a radiological examination obtained for other reasons. Local symptoms arise only after the tumor reaches a considerable size to displace or invade other organs. Frequently, the first symptoms are from metastatic lesions or paraneoplastic syndromes described below.

The classic symptoms of pain, macroscopic hematuria, and palpable mass are seen in less than 10% of the patients. Patients may also have nonspecific signs and symptoms such as weight loss, fever, malaise, and anemia. A minority of patients present with symptoms due to metastatic disease, such as bone pain or persistent cough (due to phrenic nerve stimulation). The other indicators of advanced disease include palpable cervical lymphadenopathy or varicocele, or lower extremity edema, which suggests venous involvement.

Paraneoplastic syndromes are found in 10% to 40% of patients with RCC. Nonmetastatic hepatic dysfunction (Stauffer's syndrome) is characterized by elevated serum hepatic enzymes values, prolonged prothrombin time, fever, weight loss, and fatigue. Hepatic function normalizes after nephrectomy in 60% to 70% of cases. Persistence or recurrence of hepatic dysfunction is almost always indicative of the presence of viable tumor and thus represents a poor prognosis. Hypertension, polycythemia, and hypercalcemia are other important paraneoplastic syndromes in patients with RCC.

Among patients who present with metastatic disease, 75% have lung metastases. Other sites of metastases are soft tissues, bone, liver, skin, and nervous system.

Due to its retroperitoneal location, only patients with advanced disease may have clinical findings. A palpable flank mass or lymphadenopathy and a rapidly developing varicocele may be some of the findings.

Investigations

Laboratory Tests

Full blood count may show anemia or polycythemia. Urea and electrolytes are generally normal. Urine cytology may be useful in differentiating RCC from transitional cell carcinoma (TCC) of the renal pelvis. Liver function tests may show elevated serum alkaline phosphatase. There are no specific tumor markers for RCC.

Initial Imaging Investigations (Intravenous Urogram and Ultrasound)

Most of the renal tumors are initially detected by abdominal ultrasound (US) for some other indications. The detection of kidney tumors mainly depends on the size, location, and echogenicity of the lesion. The main limitation of US is with small isoechoic intraparenchymal tumors. It can detect masses less than 3 cm with 80% sensitivity. Renal cell carcinoma can be isoechoic, hypoechoic, hyperechoic, or complex. Color Doppler ultrasonography can be very useful in the differential diagnosis. Ultrasound also helps in differentiating solid from cystic masses. Intravenous urography when used alone is not helpful and does not distinguish between cystic and solid masses.

Staging Investigations

Computed tomography (CT) scanning is more useful in detecting, and characterizing kidney masses and staging of RCC than is US, with an accuracy of 50% to 80%. A typical finding of renal cancer on a CT scan is a renal mass that enhances with intravenous contrast medium. In early acquisition after injection of contrast agent, most clear-cell RCCs are hypervascular, while papillary carcinomas appear almost isodense or poorly enhanced and homogeneous. Recent evidence shows that at least 15% of the CT-detected lesions are benign. The suspected lesion could be isodense, hypodense, or hyperdense on unenhanced images.

Thin slice scans before and after contrast medium injection are essential. Enhancement up to 20 Hounsfield units (HU) is a criterion for diagnosis of a mass (17).

Patients with an enlarged adrenal gland on CT, upper pole tumor location, or extensive malignant replacement of the kidney are at risk for ipsilateral adrenal involvement. The detection of lymph node involvement is based on a size limit of 1 cm. Enlarged hilar or retroperitoneal lymph nodes greater than 2 cm diameter are likely to harbor malignancy. Many smaller nodes are inflammatory rather than neoplastic. The assessment of the renal vein and inferior vena cava is essential.

Magnetic resonance imaging (MRI) produces high-resolution multiplanar images and is very helpful for differential diagnosis. It has a unique role in patients who cannot be assessed by CT because of allergy to iodinated contrast media and patients with renal insufficiency. Magnetic resonance imaging is highly efficient for the evaluation and staging of tumor in the inferior vena cava. Another advantage is the avoidance of radiation exposure.

The staging of renal masses must include a *routine chest radiograph*. A chest CT can be saved for patients with pulmonary symptomatology or an abnormal chest radiograph. The bone scan has to be performed in patients with elevated serum alkaline phosphatase or bone pain.

The indications for *percutaneous biopsy* or *fine-needle aspiration cytology* in the evaluation of renal masses are limited, owing to the improved diagnostic accuracy of cross-sectional imaging techniques (CT and MRI). More importantly, the accuracy of biopsy or aspiration is low because of sampling error or difficult interpretation. There are also potential complications such as bleeding, infection, arteriovenous fistula, needle tract seeding, and pneumothorax. Biopsy is mainly used to differentiate RCC from conditions such as abscess, lymphoma, and metastatic disease. The indications for biopsy will probably increase with the developments of new forms of minimally invasive treatments for RCC.

Differential Diagnosis of Renal Mass Lesion

The differential diagnosis is broad, and some features could be defined by imaging (US, CT, and MRI) and clinical history. Benign conditions such as cysts, pseudotumors, columns of Bertin, hypertrophied parenchyma, inflammatory lesions, abscess, hematoma, infarction, vascular malformations, angiomyolipoma, and neoplasia may mimic RCC. The urothelial carcinoma of the renal pelvis should be considered in tumors located centrally in the kidney. Metastatic tumors to the kidney are frequently multifocal and hypovascular. Lung and breast cancer, melanoma, gastrointestinal tract, or ovarian cancers may spread to the kidney. Lymphoma may present in various clinical forms. The majority of patients have bilateral renal involvement.

Tumor Staging

The tumor, node, metastasis (TNM) classification system (Table 14.1.3) assesses the anatomical extension and spread of the disease. Although RCC TNM staging has undergone revision in 1997, the criteria are still the subject of controversy (18). There are number of staging models for RCC, of which the Kattan et al. (19) nomogram predicts recurrence in patients undergoing radical nephrectomy. Kattan et al. included various prognostic indicators, such as symptoms, histology, tumor size, and TNM staging to predict the chances of recurrence.

Prognostic Factors

Prognostic factors can be arbitrarily classified as tumor-, patient-, and treatment-related factors. The key factors include performance status, tumor stage, histological type, and grade (20).

Tumor Related

Stage of the Tumor

Stage is one of the principal prognostic factors. The 5-year survival rates vary between 57% and 92% for T2 tumors and 35% and 77% for T3 tumors.

TABLE 14.1.3. Tumor, node, metastasis classification in kidney tumors

T: Primary tumor
Tx: Primary tumor cannot be assessed
T0: No evidence of primary tumor
T1: Tumor ≤7 cm in greatest dimension, limited to the kidney
T1a: Tumor ≤4 cm in greatest dimension, limited to the kidney
T1b: Tumor size is 4–7 cm in greatest dimension, limited to the kidney
T2: Tumor >7 cm in greatest dimension, limited to the kidney
T3: Tumor extends into major veins or invades adrenal gland or perinephric tissues but not beyond Gerota's fascia
T3a: Tumor invades adrenal gland or perinephric tissues but not beyond Gerota's fascia
T3b: Tumor grossly extends into renal vein(s) or vena cava below diaphragm
T3c: Tumor grossly extends into vena cava above diaphragm
T4: Tumor invades beyond Gerota's fascia
N: Regional lymph nodes (hilar, abdominal paraaortic, paracaval nodes)
Nx: Regional lymph nodes cannot be assessed
N0: No regional lymph node metastasis
N1: Metastasis in a single regional lymph node
N2: Metastasis in more than one regional lymph node
M: Distant metastasis
Mx: Distant metastasis cannot be assessed
M_0: No distant metastasis
M_1: Distant metastasis

The 5-year survival rates for organ-confined disease are reduced by 15% to 20% with invasion of the perinephric fat. Lymphatic spread indicates a poor prognosis.

However, most patients with tumor thrombi can be saved with an aggressive surgical approach. The number of metastatic sites provides more prognostic value than the location of metastases.

Fuhrman Grade

The commonly used tumor grading system for RCC is the Fuhrman nuclear grading system. According to the Fuhrman system, the 5-year survival rates of grade I, II, III, and IV tumors are 65% to 70%, 30% to 70%, 20% to 50% and 10% to 35%, respectively. Aneuploid tumors have an adverse prognosis compared with diploid tumors.

Histological Type

Patients with clear-cell RCC have a poorer prognosis compared with patients having papillary and chromophobe RCC. Cancer-specific survival rates at 5 years for patients with clear cell, papillary, and chromophobe RCC are 69%, 87%, and 88%, respectively. The presence of sarcomatoid differentiation, collecting duct, or medullary cell histological subtypes denotes a poor prognosis.

Tumor Size

Although tumor size is covered by pathological stage, it has recently been shown to be an independent prognostic factor. The 5-year survival rates of patients with tumor diameter less than 5 cm is 84%, for tumors between 5 and 10 cm it is 50%, and for tumors more than 10 cm in diameter it is 0%.

Microvascular Invasion

Microvascular invasion has an adverse relationship to metastasis and survival. The tumor could spread inside the lumen and under the endothelium (20).

Biomolecular Markers

Although a number of markers including nuclear DNA, p53, Bcl-2, growth factors, carbonic anhydrase, and adhesion molecules have been extensively studied, they do not have any role in management decisions.

Patient Related

Clinical Presentation

Patients presenting with symptoms related to the tumor usually do worse than the incidentally detected RCC. The median survival for incidental, classic triad (hematuria, pain, and mass), and generalized symptoms (weight loss, paraneo-plastic syndrome, etc.) was 117, 56, and 29 months, respectively (21).

C-Reactive Protein and Erythrocyte Sedimentation Rate

A raised C-reactive protein and erythrocyte sedimentation rate indicate a less favorable prognosis, as does a low hemoglobin.

Disease-Free Interval

Since the most efficient treatment for RCC is surgery, the prognosis may be negatively affected by insufficient or nonsurgical treatments. Aggressive surgery in patients with locally advanced disease seems to be the best treatment modality.

Additionally, metastasectomy or radical nephrectomy in metastatic RCC patients produces a better survival than nonsurgical treatments. The prognosis is better if the interval between the initial tumor and the occurrence of metastases or recurrence is longer.

Management

Surgery still remains the only curative treatment for localized RCC. Aggressive surgery can even cure some patients with locally advanced or metastatic RCC.

Localized Disease (T1–2, N0, M0)

Nephron-Sparing Surgery

Elective partial nephrectomy is an accepted line of management for RCCs of ≤4.0 cm in size in the presence of normal contralateral kidney (22). In selected patients localized tumors of larger size (4 to 7 cm) could be treated by nephron-sparing surgery (NSS) (23). Patients with bilateral tumors, tumor in a solitary kidney, or decreased renal function are candidates for partial nephrectomy to preserve the renal function. Nephron-sparing surgery is also the treatment of choice in patients with hereditary forms of RCC who may have multiple tumors. Another group of patients for NSS is those with a unilateral tumor and functioning contralateral kidney affected by renal artery stenosis, hydronephrosis, chronic pyelonephritis, reflux, calculous disease, or systemic conditions such as hypertension or diabetes (24).

Lately, NSS has been widely used in patients with sporadic RCC with normal contralateral kidney. Peripherally located, easily resectable tumors less than 4 cm in young healthy individuals can be treated by NSS. In more experienced centers centrally located or tumors even larger (less than 7 cm) can be treated by NSS. Similar results have been achieved with laparoscopic techniques.

Surgical Principles

Surgical procedures include wedge resection, polar (lower or upper), segmental nephrectomy, and heminephrectomy. Cooling and temporary clamping of renal hilum are not necessary for all patients. Leaving perinephric fat overlaying the tumor is important to establish correct tumor staging.

A rim of only a few millimeters of normal renal parenchyma around the tumor is sufficient for cancer control. It is useful to get a frozen section histological examination of the wound margin of the remaining kidney so that further resection is done if there is a positive histology.

Complications

Complications include hemorrhage, urinary fistula, injury to surrounding organs (spleen), infection, reexploration, and renal insufficiency (see Chapter 12).

The local recurrence after NSS is seen in 1.4% to 10% of patients. Such patients with no signs of metastasis should be considered for secondary surgical treatment, that is, radical nephrectomy, unless a second NSS is unavoidable.

Radical Nephrectomy

Radical nephrectomy is the gold-standard treatment for localized RCC. It is also treatment of choice for locally invasive tumors and tumors invading the lymphatics and veins.

Surgical Principles

Surgery entails early ligation of the renal artery and vein and removal of the kidney with Gerota's fascia, ipsilateral adrenal gland, and regional lymph nodes. However, adrenalectomy can be avoided if it appears normal on imaging and at the time of surgery, and the tumor is at low risk for adrenal involvement (i.e., small and not involving the upper pole). Resection of enlarged regional lymph nodes enables accurate staging, but may be of limited benefit in terms of survival because of the relatively rare occasion of node positivity in the absence of distant metastasis. There is a growing trend in clinical practice toward laparoscopic nephrectomy as an effective minimally invasive treatment of RCC.

Complications

Intraoperative hemorrhage can occur from injuries to the renal vein, inferior vena cava (IVC), and their tributaries. Other intraoperative complications to be avoided include gastrointestinal, pleural, or splenic injuries. Postoperative ileus, deep vein thrombosis, and chest complications are other preventable complications.

Extracorporeal Renal Surgery and Autotransplantation (Bench Surgery)

The kidney is removed and extracorporeal dissection is carried out. The kidney is then transplanted back into the patient. This technique has been used in the past (25). It may be feasible in rare cases where the tumor is large and has a complicated anatomy.

Minimally Invasive Treatments

Radiofrequency Ablation

Radiofrequency ablation (RFA) provides heat-based tissue destruction with a high-frequency electrical current (400 to 500 kHz), creating molecular friction, denaturation of cellular proteins, and cell membrane disintegration. In patients with contraindications to nephrectomy, in von Hippel–Lindau (VHL) disease, and in unfit elderly patients, RFA is an alternative treatment.

Radiofrequency ablation seems to be promising, but patient selection criteria are still evolving. In a series of 277 cases with a mean follow-up of 10 months, the recurrence rate was 7.9%, with a complication rate of 13.9% (26).

Cryoablation

The tumor is rapidly frozen and gradually thawed, and the freeze-thaw cycles are repeated. Renal cryoablation is a rising nephron-sparing treatment alternative in patients with RCC. The current indication for renal cryoablation is a small (<3 cm) solitary renal tumor located away from the collecting system in an elderly patient.

High-Intensity Focused Ultrasound

High-intensity focused ultrasound (HIFU) employs beams of ablative ultrasound frequency generated by a cylindrical piezoelectric element focused by a paraboloid reflector. Thermal destruction results in localized hemorrhage, coagulative necrosis, and chronic inflammatory infiltration. High-intensity focused ultrasound may become an effective technique once the technical problems of visualizing the target lesions, protecting against skin burns, and precisely controlling the lesion size have been solved.

Locally Advanced Disease (T3a–c, T4, N0–2, M0)

Vena Cava Involvement

Inferior vena caval involvement has been reported in 4% to 23% of RCC patients. Venous extension is frequently associated with adverse prognostic factors such as lymph node involvement and metastases. Although local tumor stage and grade are better predictors of prognosis than extent of venous involvement for patients with pT3b disease, patients with IVC involvement above the diaphragm (T3c) have a significantly worse survival rate. Tumor extension into IVC or even into the right atrium, can be removed, with cardiopulmonary bypass if necessary. Resection of the vena cava may be necessary when the tumor extends directly into the wall of the vena cava. This is a major undertaking with high rates of morbidity and mortality and has to be performed in specialist centres.

Locally Invasive Renal Cell Carcinoma

Renal cell carcinoma can invade any structure in the area such as the liver, pancreas, colon, duodenum, spleen, psoas muscle, and diaphragm. Although long-term survival in these patients is low, palliation and local control are reasonable. Additional resection of nonvital, invaded structures during nephrectomy may be necessary. Radiation therapy in the treatment of locally extensive RCC has no place and does not improve overall survival.

Local Recurrence After Surgery

Local recurrence following radical nephrectomy can be observed in 5% to 27% of the patients. Advanced T stage and positive lymph nodes increase the risk of renal fossa recurrence. Local disease recurrence in the renal bed usually heralds the presence of metastatic disease. Long-term survival can be achieved by resecting the solitary metastatic deposit and by giving systemic therapy. Radiation therapy may be of value for palliation of symptomatic local recurrences in patients who are not operative candidates.

Surgical Management of Advanced Disease (Any T, Any N, M1)

Nephrectomy in metastatic RCC improves survival in patients with good performance status. It also improves the quality of life of the patient by relieving symptoms such as hematuria, pain, or paraneoplastic symptoms. As surgical resection of metastatic disease does produce long-term survivors occasionally, it is a reasonable option in selected patients. In general, better prognosis is observed when the solitary resected metastatic lesion involves the lung, adrenal gland, or brain. A single organ of first recurrence, curative resection of first metastasis, a long disease-free interval (longer than 12 months) after nephrectomy, a solitary site of first metastasis, and metachronous presentation with recurrence are favorable predictors of survival in these cases (27).

Other Tumors of the Kidney

Oncocytoma

Oncocytoma represents 3% to 7% of all solid renal masses arising from intercalating cells of the cortical collecting ducts. Grossly, these tumors are light brown or tan colored, homogeneous, and well circumscribed. A central scar is commonly found, but prominent necrosis or hypervascularity is lacking. Microscopically, uniform round or polygonal eosinophilic cells predominate, most commonly arranged in an organoid, tubulocystic, solid, or mixed growth pattern. Common cytogenetic findings for oncocytomas include loss of the first and Y chromosomes, loss of heterozygosity on chromosome 14q, and rearrangements at 11q13 (28).

Angiomyolipoma

A benign tumor, angiomyolipoma (AML) can cause life-threatening conditions. It consists of varying amounts of mature adipose tissue, smooth muscle, and thick-walled vessels. The incidence is 0.3% of all autopsies and 0.13% in the population when screened by US. It is most likely derived from the perivascular epithelioid cells, and its growth may be hormone dependent, as suggested by its female predominance and its rarity before puberty.

Angiomyolipoma often express receptors for both estrogen and progesterone. Angiomyolipoma can be associated with tuberous sclerosis syndrome or lymphangioleiomyomatosis. It can be detected in 10% to 20% of patients with tuberous sclerosis and is more likely to be bilateral and multicentric.

Angiomyolipoma can occur as a spontaneous massive retroperitoneal hemorrhage in 25% to 30% of cases (Wunderlich syndrome). Although AML is diagnosed incidentally in more than half of the patients, anemia and hypertension are common clinical findings. It may lead to renal failure, which is the most common cause of death in patient with tuberous sclerosis syndrome. Angiomyolipoma is also associated with lymphangioleiomyomatosis (LAM) characterized by smooth muscle infiltration into the wall of alveoli and small airways especially in young females. This can lead to cystic degeneration of lung tissue, impaired gas exchange, respiratory failure, and death. Recent evidence show that LAM may be caused by metastases of angiomyolipoma cells to the lung. There are two different forms of AML: the classical form, which contains vascular structures, smooth muscle, and adipose tissue; and the epithelioid variant.

The presence of even a small amount of fat within a renal lesion on CT scan (confirmed by HU ≤ 10) virtually excludes the diagnosis of RCC and is considered diagnostic of AML. The typical, but not diagnostic, finding of AML on

US is a well-circumscribed, highly echogenic lesion, often associated with shadowing.

Asymptomatic, small AMLs (less than 4 cm) can be followed expectantly, with repeat evaluation and imaging at 12-month intervals to define the growth rate and clinical significance. Intervention, usually NSS, should be considered for larger tumors, particularly if the patient is symptomatic, taking into account the patient's age, comorbidities, and other related factors.

Adenoma

Renal adenoma of the kidney is a benign, small, and solid lesion. Although the incidence of adenoma increases with age, it is most commonly seen in patients with VHL disease and acquired renal cystic disease. The histology of adenoma is a small, well-circumscribed lesion characterized by uniform basophilic or eosinophilic cells with monotonous nuclear and cellular feature, often arranged in a papillary growth pattern. However, there is no exact histopathologic, ultra-structural, or immunohistochemical parameter to distinguish benign from malignant renal epithelial neoplasms. Larger tumors or any tumor with clear cell histology or any degree of cytological atypia should not be classified as renal cortical adenoma. Renal papillary adenoma is considered a precursor of papillary carcinoma.

References

1. Parkin DM, Muir CS, Whelan S, et al. Cancer Incidence in Five Continents, vol VI. IARC Scientific Publication No. 120. Lyon, France: World Health Organization, International Agency for Research on Cancer, 1992.
2. Jemal A, Murray T, Ward E, et al. Cancer statistics 2005. CA Cancer J Clin 2005; 55:10–30.
3. Landis SH, Murray T, Bolden S, Wingo PA. Cancer statistics 1999. CA Cancer J Clin 1999;49:8–31.
4. Choyke PL, Glenn GM, Walther MM, et al. State of the art: hereditary renal cancers. Radiology 2002;226:33–46.
5. Bergstrom A, Hsieh CC, Lindblad P, et al. Obesity and renal cell cancer—a quantitative review. Br J Cancer 2001;85:984–990.
6. Srikanth MS, Fox SR, Oh KH, et al. Renal cell carcinoma following bariatric surgery. Obes Surg 2005;15(8):1165–1170.
7. Lindblad P, Chow WH, Chan J, et al. The role of diabetes mellitus in the etiology of renal cell cancer. Diabetologia 1999;42(1):107–121.
8. Kirkali Z, Obek C. Clinical aspects of renal cell carcinoma. EAU Update Ser 2003;1: 189–198.
9. Lindner V, Lang H, Jacqmin D. Pathology and genetics in renal cell cancer. Eur Urol 2003;suppl 1:197–208.
10. Lee CT, Katz J, Shi W, et al. Surgical management of renal tumors 4 cm or less in a contemporary cohort. J Urol 2000;163:730–736.
11. Bosniak MA, Birnbaum BA, Krinsky GA, et al. Small renal parenchymal neoplasms: further observations on growth. Radiology 1995;197:589–597.

12. Wu SL, Kothari P, Wheeler TM, Reese T, et al. Cytokeartins 7 and 20 immunoreactivity in chromophobe renal cell carcinomas and renal oncocytomas. Mod Pathol 2002; 15:712–717.
13. Fuhrman SA, Lasky LC, Limas C. Prognostic significance of morphologic parameters in renal cell carcinoma. Am J Surg Pathol 1982;6:655–663.
14. Linehan WM, Lerman MI, Zbar B. Identification of the von Hippel-Lindau (VHL) gene. Its role in renal cancer. JAMA 1995;273:564–570.
15. Linehan WM, Grubb RL, Coleman JA, et al. The genetic basis of kidney cancer: implications for gene specific clinical management. BJU Int 2005;95(suppl 2):2–7.
16. Pavlovich CP, Grubb RL 3rd, Hurley K, et al. Evaluation and management of renal tumors in the Birt-Hogg-Dubé syndrome. J Urol 2005;173:1482–1486.
17. Isreal GM, Bosniak MA. Renal imaging for diagnosis and staging of renal cell carcinoma. Urol Clin North Am 2003;30:499–514.
18. Shvarts O, Lam JS, Kim L, Belldegrun AS. Staging of renal cell carcinoma: current concepts. BJU Int 2005;95(suppl 2):8–13.
19. Kattan MW, Reuter V, Motzer RJ, Katz J, Russo P. A postoperative prognostic nomogram for renal cell carcinoma. J Urol 2001;166:63–67.
20. Lang H, Jacqmin D. Prognostic factors in renal cell carcinoma. Eur Urol Update Ser 2003;1(4):215–219.
21. Pantuck AJ, Zisman A, Rauch MK, Belldegrun AS. Incidental renal tumors. Urology 2000;56:190–196.
22. Campbell S, Novick A. Expanding the indications for elective nephrectomy: Is this advisable? Eur Urol 2006;49:952–954.
23. Becker F, Siemer S, Hack M, et al. Excellent long-term cancer control with elective nephron saving surgery for selected renal cell carcinomas measuring more than 4 cm. Eur Urol 2006;49:1058–1064.
24. Uzo RG, Novick AC. Nephron-saving surgery for renal tumors: indications, techniques and outcomes. J Urol 2001;166:6–18.
25. Wickham JE. Conservative renal surgery for adenocarcinoma. The place of bench surgery. Br J Urol 1975;47:25–36.
26. Weld JK, Landman J. Comparison of cryoablation, radiofrequency ablation, land HIFU for treating small renal tumors. BJU Int 2005;96:1224–1229.
27. Hofmann HS, Neef H, Krohe K, et al. Prognostic factors and survival after pulmonary resection of metastatic renal cell carcinoma. Eur Urol 2005;48:77–81.
28. Romis L, Cindolo L, Patard JJ, et al. Frequency, clinical presentation and evolution of renal oncocytomas: multicentric experience from a European database. Eur Urol 2004;45:53–57.

14.2
Nonsurgical Management of Metastatic Renal Cell Carcinoma

Brian I. Rini and Ronald M. Bukowski

The management of advanced renal cell carcinoma (RCC) has evolved greatly in recent years. The role and benefit of debulking nephrectomy has been more clearly defined. Long-considered an immunoresponsive tumor, cytokines such as interferon-α (IFN-α) and interleukin-2 (IL-2) evolved into the standard initial treatment for advanced RCC through clinical trials in the 1980s and 1990s. More recently, a growing understanding of the biology underlying some RCC tumors has led to the clinical testing of therapeutics that target vascular endothelial growth factor (VEGF). These recent trials have produced robust clinical results that have evolved the standard of care and introduced new treatment options in this historically treatment-refractory disease. This chapter focuses on standard cytokine therapy for advanced RCC as well as VEGF-targeted approaches. In addition, certain aspects of supportive care, including treatment of central nervous system (CNS) metastases and use of bisphosphonates for bone metastases, are discussed.

Debulking Nephrectomy

Debulking nephrectomy has become a standard of care in selected metastatic RCC patients on the basis of two identically designed, prospective randomized trials (1). Eligibility for both trials, based on the tumor, node, metastasis (TNM) grade, included biopsy-proven T_{any}, N_{any}, M1 RCCs with a primary tumor amenable to resection as determined by the operating surgeon. Additional eligibility included Eastern Cooperative Oncology Group (ECOG) performance status 0 or 1, no prior radiotherapy or systemic treatment of any kind, and adequate end-organ function. Eligible patients were randomized to radical nephrectomy (with or without lymphadenectomy), followed within 1 month after surgery by interferon-α (5 million units subcutaneously 3 × /week) or to immediate interferon without preceding nephrectomy. Both trials were powered to detect an overall survival improvement, with analysis based on intent-to-treat criteria using Kaplan-Meier technique for survival duration. A combined analysis of 341 total randomized patients demonstrated an overall survival advantage for the nephrectomized group of 13.6 months versus 7.8 months ($p = .002$). Not surprisingly, the benefit was most pronounced in performance status 0 patients, but was not dependent on the site of metastasis or disease measurability. The combined response rate in 253 patients with measurable disease revealed a 6.9% response rate in the nephrectomy arm vs. a 5.7% response rate in the interferon only arm ($p = .60$). Surgical morbidity and mortality were acceptable and did not prevent subsequent administration of interferon in 95% of nephrectomized patients a median of 19 days after surgery.

These trials provide convincing evidence of an overall survival benefit in appropriately selected patients. These data have been translated into the clinical practice of initial debulking nephrectomy followed by systemic therapy. Importantly, proper patient selection can maximize the benefit of this approach. Patients with good performance status, a resectable primary tumor representing the majority of tumor burden, and without rapidly progressing extrarenal disease or medical comorbidities should be considered for initial nephrectomy.

Cytokine Therapy in Advanced Renal Cell Carcinoma

Although a mainstay of cancer therapeutics for decades, the exact mechanism of IL-2 in RCC is largely unknown. Interleukin-2 is a cytokine that stimulates activated T cells and natural killer (NK) cells, inducing an antitumor immune response (2). Interferon-α is a naturally occurring glycoprotein produced in response to viral infections and foreign antigens. It has been investigated as an antitumor agent in a variety of diseases including RCC with postulated mechanisms of action including immunomodulation (3,4), antiproliferative activity (5), and inhibition of angiogenesis (6). In metastatic RCC, varying doses, schedules, and combinations of these cytokines have been investigated.

High-Dose Interleukin-2

Two large randomized trials have examined the benefit of high-dose (HD) IL-2 in comparison to low-dose cytokine regimens. The Cytokine Working Group randomized 193 cytokine-naive metastatic RCC patients to HD IL-2 (600,000 units/kg IV q8h × 14 doses; maximum three cycles) or low-dose subcutaneous (sc) IL-2 [5 million units (MU)/m^2 5 days/week + IFN 5 MU/m^2 3 days/week] (7). The primary end point was progression-free survival at 3 years. The overall response rate was 23% for HD IL-2 vs. 10% for low-dose cytokines ($p = .018$), and the median response duration for HD IL-2 was 24 months, compared with 15 months for IL-2 and IFN ($p = .18$). However, no significant difference in 3-year progression-free survival (10% vs. 3%; $p = .082$) or overall survival (17 months vs. 13 months; $p = .21$) was observed. There were a substantially increased number of grade 3/4 toxicities in HD IL-2 arm.

The second trial conducted by the National Cancer Institute randomized 283 mostly untreated metastatic RCC patients to one of three treatment regimens: HD IL-2 (720,000 units/kg IV q8h) or low-dose IV bolus IL-2 (72,000 units/kg IV q8h) or low-dose subcutaneous IL-2 (125,000 units/kg sc 5 days/week × 6-week cycles) (8). Overall response rate was 21% for HD IL-2 vs. 10% for low-dose sc IL-2 ($p = .033$), but there was no significant difference in overall survival ($p = .34$). There was a substantial increase in grade 3/4 toxicities in the HD IL-2 arm. The percentage of durable complete responders to HD IL-2 appears to be on the order of 5% based on these and other series (9,10). Taken together, these data suggest that HD IL-2 has a higher overall and complete response rate compared with low-dose therapy, with the major benefit realized in patients who achieve a durable complete response. There is no proven benefit, however, in disease-free or overall survival with HD IL-2 for the entire cohort, likely due to the low overall response rates. Toxicity is substantial with HD IL-2 and highlights the need for stringent patient selection.

Low-Dose Cytokine Therapy

Interferon-α

Both IFN-α and IL-2 have been investigated in low-dose regimens for the treatment of advanced RCC. IFN-α therapy has employed both recombinant interferon-α2a (Roferon, Hoffmann-La Roche, Basel, Switzerland) and interferon-α2b (Intron A, Schering Plough International, Kenilworth, NJ). No difference in the clinical effect between these two agents has been demonstrated in RCC. Overall response rates between approximately 15% have been repeatedly demonstrated in large series (11). To investigate a possible survival benefit to interferon-α in RCC, several randomized trials have been performed. Investigators have used "placebo-equivalent" control arms with agents such as medroxyprogesterone (MPA) or vinblastine to address possible low compliance with placebo-controlled trials (Table 14.2.1).

Three-hundred fifty patients with metastatic RCC were randomized to receive interferon-α2b 10 million units (MU) three times a week (TIW) × 12 weeks or MPA 300 mg QD × 12 weeks (12). The primary end point of this trial was overall survival (OS), designed to detect a 12% difference in 2-year OS. This trial was closed at an interim analysis when the stopping boundary for a survival advantage of interferon had been reached. At that time, 236 patients had died, 90% from metastatic RCC. Intent-to-treat analysis demonstrated a significant overall survival advantage for patients randomized to interferon, with a hazard ratio of 0.72 [95% confidence interval (CI) 0.55–0.94; $p = .017$). The median overall survival was 8.5 months in the interferon arm and 6.0 months in the MPA arm, an improvement of 2.5 months (95% CI 0.5–5.0 months). The 1-year survival rates were 43% for interferon and 31% for MPA, an improvement of 12% (95% CI 3–22%).

TABLE 14.2.1. Selected randomized trials evaluating cytokine therapy in patients with metastatic renal cell carcinoma

Reference	Treatment	Overall response (%)	Complete response (CR) (%)	Durable CR[a] (%)	Overall survival (months)
McDermott (7)	HD IL-2	23	8.4	7.4	17
	Low-dose IL-2/IFN-α	10	3.3	0	13
Yang (8)	HD IL-2	21	6	5	NS
	Low-dose IL-2	10	2	1	NS
MRC (12)	IFN-α	14	2	2	8.5
	Medroxyprogesterone	7	0	0	6.0
Pyrhonen (13)	Interferon-α2a plus vinblastine	16.5	8.9	0	15.8
	Vinblastine	2.4	1.2	1.2	8.8

[a]Defined as CR beyond 3 years in McDermott et al. study; durable CR rate for Yang et al. study in HD IL-2 arm derived from eight durable CRs of 11 total CRs in 155 patients two-arm study; defined as CR beyond 6 months in MRC study; defined as CR at time of publication for Pyrhonen et al. MRC, medical research council. NS, not stated.

Another study randomized 160 patients with advanced, progressive RCC to receive interferon-α2a 18 MU TIW plus vinblastine 0.1 mg/kg IV q 3 weeks or the same dose and schedule of vinblastine alone (13). The primary end point of this trial was overall survival, with 80% power to detect a difference in median overall survival of 12 versus 8 months. A significant overall survival advantage was demonstrated with a median OS of 15.8 months for the interferon-α2a arm versus 8.8 months for the vinblastine arm ($p = .0049$).

Survival rates favored the interferon arm at 1 year (55.7% vs. 38.3%). Significant differences in overall response rates (16.5% vs. 2.4%; $p = .0025$), complete response rates (8.9% vs. 1.2%), and median time to disease progression (3 months vs. 2 months; $p = .0001$) were also observed, all favoring the interferon-α2a arm and implicating the response to interferon in the survival advantage. Thus, the available data demonstrate a modest but clinically significant overall survival advantage.

Low-Dose Interleukin-2

Low dose IL-2 comprises a spectrum of doses from intravenous dosing of approximately 10% of high-dose levels or subcutaneous dosing. Various dosing regimens have consistently produced response rates in the 15% range, with a limited number of durable and complete responses (14,15). Although randomized trials have not been reported for low-dose IL-2 compared to inactive therapy as have been performed for IFN-α, it is likely that there is a comparable modest survival advantage for these regimens.

Cytokine Combination Therapy

Given the modest benefits of cytokine monotherapy, investigators have attempted to augment the benefit of cytokine therapy in a myriad of ways: combination therapy with IL-2 and IFN-α (16,17), hormone therapy (18,19), other immunologically active cells such as lymphokine-activated killer (LAK) cells (20,21) or tumor-infiltrating lymphocytes (TILs) (22), cis-retinoic acid (23), or chemotherapy (24). Although some of these approaches have produced high response rates in single-arm studies, none has demonstrated significant clinical benefit when compared to a standard cytokine control arm in a randomized trial.

Thus, good performance status patients with access to experienced centers may appropriately receive HD IL-2 after consideration of the relative risks and benefits. Alternatively, low-dose, single-agent cytokine regimens are acceptable and confer a modest survival benefit. There is no proven advantage to combination therapy with cytokines, and thus cytokine monotherapy remains the standard of care against which new agents should be compared. It is obvious that only a small minority of patients derive ultimate benefit from cytokine therapy, and thus molecularly targeted therapy based on the underlying biology of RCC has been recently pursued.

Vascular Endothelial Growth Factor–Targeted Therapy in Renal Cell Carcinoma

Von Hippel–Lindau Pathway Biology in Renal Cell Carcinoma

The von Hippel–Lindau (*VHL*) gene encodes a 213 amino acid protein (pVHL), which plays an integral role in regulating the normal cellular response to oxygen deprivation. In conditions of physiologic oxygen availability and normal *VHL* gene function, pVHL is the substrate recognition component of an ubiquitin ligase complex that targets a family of protein transcription factors, the hypoxia-inducible factors (HIF-1α and HIF-2α) for proteolysis (25–27). In conditions of hypoxia, the pVHL-HIF interaction is disrupted and stabilization of the HIF transcription factors occurs (Fig. 14.2.1). Activated HIF translocates into the nucleus and leads to transcription of a large repertoire of hypoxia-inducible genes (28). Several of the hypoxia-inducible genes induced by this process have been identified as critical mediators of the tumorigenesis process, including VEGF (28), platelet-derived growth factor (PDGF) (29,30), and TGF-α (31–33).

The *VHL* gene has been mapped to chromosome 3p25-26 (34). In sporadic (noninherited) RCC, *VHL* gene allele deletion (loss of heterozygosity) has been demonstrated in 84% to 98% of sporadic renal tumors, and mutation in the remaining *VHL* allele has been observed in 34% to 57% of clear-cell RCC tumors

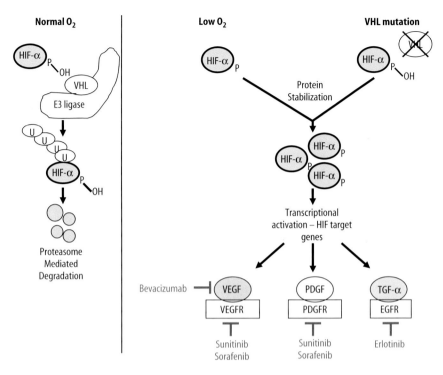

FIGURE 14.2.1. Von Hippel–Lindau biology in renal carcinoma and resulting therapeutic targets. In conditions of normoxia and normal *VHL* gene function, von Hippel–Lindau protein (pVHL) binds a hydroxylated proline residue of hypoxia-inducible factor-α (HIF-α), leading to ubiquitin attachment and degradation in the proteasome. In hypoxia or with defective pVHL function, binding between pVHL and HIF-α does not occur, HIF-α is constitutively expressed and leads to transcription of hypoxia-inducible genes, including vascular endothelial growth factor (VEGF), platelet-derived growth factor (PDGF), and transforming growth factor-α (TGF-α). Bevacizumab binds VEGF protein, preventing ligand interaction with receptor. sunitinib, AG013736 and sorafenib inhibit phosphorylation of the VEGF receptor. Sorafenib additionally inhibits Raf kinase enzyme involved in one of the intracellular pathways activated after VEGF binding. Erlotinib inhibits epidermal growth factor receptor (EGFR). (Adapted from Rathmell WK. *Expert Review of Anticancer Therapy*, Future Drugs Ltd., London, with permission.)

(35–39). *VHL* gene inactivation in RCC may also occur through gene silencing by methylation as observed in an additional 10% of RCC tumors (37,39–41). Non–clear-cell tumors do not demonstrate significant VHL gene inactivation (42). Taken together, the above data provide compelling evidence for *VHL* gene inactivation in the majority of clear-cell RCC tumors leading to overexpression of VEGF and other factors as a driving force in renal tumor angiogenesis. In fact, RCC almost universally develops highly vascular features in both the primary and metastatic sites of disease, an observation that led to the initial suggestion that liberation of an angiogenic factor may be uniquely correlated with this disease (43). Thus, with the development of effective agents targeting the angiogenesis signaling pathway, inhibition of VEGF has been aggressively pursued as a therapeutic target in RCC.

Vascular Endothelial Growth Factor

Vascular endothelial growth factor is a dimeric glycoprotein and a member of the PDGF superfamily of growth factors and composes a family of closely related isoforms.

There are six described members of the VEGF family, but VEGF-A (referred to as vascular permeability factor or VEGF) appears to exert the primary influence on angiogenesis in the setting of carcinogenesis. Vascular endothelial growth factor is the primary mediator of both normal and tumor-associated angiogenesis through increased microvascular permeability (44), induction of endothelial cell division and migration (45,46), promotion of endothelial cell survival through protection from apoptosis (47,48), and reversal of endothelial cell senescence (49). Vascular endothelial growth factor exerts its biologic effect through interaction with receptors (VEGF receptors 1, 2, and 3) present on the cell surface (44). These receptors provide unique regulation and tissue specificity to the angiogenic process (Fig. 14.2.2). VEGFR-1 is a receptor for both VEGF and VEGF-B and functions in physiological and developmental angiogenesis. VEGFR-2 mediates the majority of VEGF effects in angiogenesis including

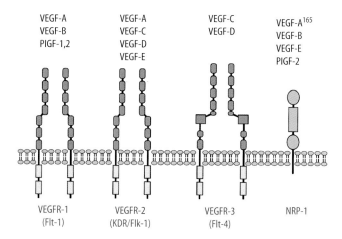

FIGURE 14.2.2. Interaction of VEGF ligands with VEGF receptors. VEGF is a dimeric glycoprotein and a member of the platelet-derived growth factor (PDGF) superfamily of growth factors that includes VEGF-B, VEGF-C, VEGF-D, VEGF-E, and placenta growth factor (PIGF). These protein ligands bind to and activate different receptors present on the endothelial cell surface. NRP-1, neuropilin receptor-1. (From Dvorak HF. Vascular permeability factor/vascular endothelial growth factor: a critical cytokine in tumor angiogenesis and a potential target for diagnosis and therapy. J Clin Oncol. 2002;20(21):4368–4380, with permission from the American Society of Clinical Oncology.)

endothelial cell proliferation, invasion, migration, and survival. VEGFR-3 is activated by VEGF-C and VEGF-D, and exclusively mediates embryonic angiogenesis and in the adult expression is limited to lymphatic endothelial cells. Upon binding of VEGF to the extracellular domain of its receptor, dimerization and autophosphorylation of the intracellular receptor tyrosine kinases occurs and cascade of downstream proteins are activated.

Vascular Endothelial Growth Factor–Targeted Therapy

Strategies to inhibit VEGF activity in renal cell carcinoma, including binding of the VEGF protein and blockade of the VEGF receptor, have recently been developed and have undergone clinical testing in the setting of metastatic RCC (see Fig. 14.1.1 in Chapter 14.1).

Anti-Vascular Endothelial Growth Factor Antibody (Bevacizumab)

A recombinant human monoclonal antibody against VEGF [rhuMAb VEGF (bevacizumab), Avastin®; Genentech, South San Francisco, CA] binds and neutralizes all biologically active isoforms of VEGF (50). In vitro studies have demonstrated that bevacizumab causes decreased survival of human vascular endothelial cells (HUVEC) and decreases VEGF-induced HUVEC permeability (51). This humanized antibody inhibits bovine capillary endothelial cell proliferation in response to VEGF and initially showed antitumor effects in sarcoma and breast cancer cell lines (50).

The clinical utility of bevacizumab in metastatic RCC has been investigated in a randomized phase II trial in which 116 patients with treatment-refractory, metastatic clear-cell RCC were randomized to receive placebo, low-dose (3 mg/kg) bevacizumab, or high-dose (10 mg/kg) bevacizumab given intravenously every 2 weeks (52). There were four partial responses, all in the high-dose bevacizumab arm (10% objective response rate). An intent-to-treat analysis demonstrated a significant prolongation of time to progression in the high-dose bevacizumab arm compared to placebo (4.8 vs. 2.5 months; $p < .001$ by log rank test). The primary toxicities observed in this study were hypertension and asymptomatic proteinuria. Follow-up has demonstrated no further toxic side effects, including four patients who have continued on therapy without progression for 3 to 5 years (53).

Based on these data, an Intergroup phase III trial investigating the addition of bevacizumab to initial systemic therapy in RCC has been undertaken (54). Patients with metastatic clear-cell RCC without prior systemic therapy were randomized to either low-dose interferon-α2b (Intron A, Schering-Plough, Kenilworth, NJ), 9 MU subcutaneously three times weekly or the same dose and schedule of interferon-α2b in combination with bevacizumab, 10 mg/kg IV every 2 weeks. The primary end point of the trial is overall survival, designed to detect an improvement in median survival from 13 months for interferon-α alone to 17 months for the combination. A similarly designed phase III trial has also been undertaken in Europe using interferon-α2a (Roferon; Hoffmann-LaRoche, Grenzach-Wyhlen, Germany) instead of interferon-α2b. These trials will evaluate the effect of adding bevacizumab to front-line therapy in RCC to possibly establish a new standard of care.

Clinical trials of HD IL-2, in combination with bevacizumab, are also underway. The rationale for this combination includes the suggestion that bevacizumab may prevent much of the tumor-induced immunosuppression attributed to VEGF and thereby enrich the immune-enhancing effects of IL-2 (55,56). In addition, IL-2 toxicity may be reduced by the vascular effects of bevacizumab. Bevacizumab may decrease the significant vascular leak syndrome associated with IL-2 and allow more IL-2 doses to be administered with less toxicity. Bevacizumab in combination with low-dose IL-2 is also planned for investigation in a separate trial.

Combination therapy of bevacizumab and other targeted agents has also been investigated in metastatic RCC. Transforming growth factor-α (TGF-α) is VHL-regulated growth factor for RCC, with biologic effect through interaction with the epidermal growth factor receptor (EGFR) (31–33). Although single-agent studies with anti-EGFR compounds have demonstrated limited antitumor effects (57–59), the combination of bevacizumab and erlotinib may have additive or synergistic effects in RCC. Sixty-three patients with metastatic RCC (68% with no prior treatment) received bevacizumab 10 mg/kg intravenously every 2 weeks and erlotinib 150 mg orally daily in a single-arm phase II trial. Fifteen patients (25%) had objective responses. Thirty-six (61%) patients had stable disease (SD), and 13 of the SD patients (22%) had tumor shrinkage. Grade 3 toxicities associated with this regimen included rash (13%), diarrhea (13%), nausea/vomiting (10%), hypertension (8%), proteinuria (6%), and bleeding (5%). These results provide early evidence that targeting both VEGF and EGFR pathways may be an effective strategy in RCC. The additive or synergistic potential of this regimen was further evaluated in a randomized phase II trial of bevacizumab plus placebo versus bevacizumab plus erlotinib. Preliminary results failed to demonstrate an advantage to the combination arm and thus further development is uncertain.

Small Molecule Vascular Endothelial Growth Factor Receptor Inhibitors

An alternative approach to VEGF inhibition involves targeting the signaling cascade initiated by cell surface receptor activation using small molecule tyrosine kinase inhibitors. These agents inhibit not only VEGFR-2, the major pro-angiogenic receptor for VEGF, but also other receptors in the split kinase domain superfamily of receptor tyrosine kinases, including the platelet-derived growth factor receptor (PDGFR). The ligand for this receptor, PDGF, is also regulated by the HIF factors, and is thus expressed at high levels in VHL mutation-driven RCC. PDGFR is expressed in pericytes, which serve as structural supporting cells for endothelial cells, and thus PDGFR inhibition may have therapeutic relevance.

Sunitinib

Sunitinib (Sutent®, Pfizer Inc. La Jolla, CA) is an orally bioavailable oxindol small molecule tyrosine kinase inhibitor of VEGFR-2 and PDGFR-B. This compound was initially selected from a screen of substituted indolin-2-one analogues for potent and selective inhibitors of VEGFR-2, PDGFR-B, and fibroblast growth factor receptor-1 (60).

In vitro assays with sunitinib have demonstrated inhibition of ligand-dependent VEGFR-2 and PDGFR-B phosphorylation as well as inhibition of VEGF-induced proliferation of endothelial cells and PDGF-induced proliferation of mouse fibroblast cells (61). Investigation in mouse xenograft models demonstrated growth inhibition of various implanted solid tumors and eradication of larger, established tumors (62).

Two phase II trials of sunitinib in cytokine-refractory, metastatic RCC have been conducted (62). Both trials enrolled cytokine-refractory metastatic RCC patients with measurable disease. Sunitinib was administered as 50 mg daily for the first 4 weeks of repeated 6-week cycles. The first trial included all histological subtypes and demonstrated an objective partial response in 25 of 63 total patients (objective response rate 40%). The second trial restricted eligibility to clear-cell RCC and required both prior nephrectomy and response evaluation criteria in solid tumors (REGIST)-defined progression after prior cytokine therapy. This trial of 106 patients reported one complete and 40 partial responses (objective response rate 39%). Toxicity in these trials, most commonly grade 1 or 2, included fatigue/asthenia, nausea, diarrhea, stomatitis, and cytopenias. sunitinib has also been investigated in untreated, metastatic RCC patients in a phase III trial versus interferon-α, demonstrating a superior progression-free survival for sunitinib (11 versus 5 months), establishing a new front-line standard therapy.

Sorafenib

Activating mutations of the *ras* family of oncogenes have been demonstrated in solid tumors. The resulting Ras protein activity contributes to pathways involved in a myriad of cellular functions including cell survival and motility, which have been comprehensively reviewed elsewhere (63,64). Among other effects, activated Ras initiates the Raf/MEK/ERK pathway by binding to and activating Raf kinase. Sorafenib (Nexarn; Bayer Pharmaceuticals, West Haven, CT, and Onyx Pharmaceuticals, Richmond, CA) is an orally bioavailable bi-aryl urea Raf kinase inhibitor, with demonstrated inhibition of Ras-dependent human tumor xenograft models (65). Sorafenib has also demonstrated direct inhibition of VEGFR-2, VEGFR-3, and PDGFR-B (66). Xenograft models treated with daily sorafenib demonstrated significant inhibition of tumor growth and tumor microvessel density, as measured by anti-CD31 immunostaining (66).

A phase II randomized discontinuation study with sorafenib has been reported in 202 patients with metastatic RCC. Tumor shrinkage was observed in 144 patients (71%) at 12 weeks and a progression-free survival advantage of

24 versus 6 weeks ($p = .0087$) was demonstrated in the randomized cohort of 55 patients (67). These data prompted a subsequent 905 patient, placebo-controlled, randomized trial of sorafenib in cytokine refractory RCC. This trial reported a progression-free survival (PFS) advantage in the treatment arm of 24 versus 12 weeks ($p < .000001$) (68). This PFS advantage was demonstrated in the sorafenib arm despite a 2% RECIST-defined objective response rate. However, a substantial proportion of patients in the sorafenib arm (74% of that cohort) were recorded as stable disease yet experienced tumor shrinkage, likely accounting for the PFS benefit.

Supportive Care

Central Nervous System Metastases

The presence of CNS metastases is a poor prognostic sign in RCC patients, associated with a median survival of 7 to 9 months, compared with 12 to 14 months in patients without CNS metastases (69,70). Surgical resection of isolated CNS metastases can provide reasonable disease-free survival, similar to metastasectomy in other organs. However, multiplicity of tumors, anatomic location, or other systemic disease preclude the majority of RCC patients from surgical resection. There is a growing clinical experience with stereotactic radiosurgery (SRS) for RCC metastatic to the CNS (71–73). This technique involves administration of focused radiation to tumors, allowing for much higher radiation doses to be delivered to the tumor than conventional whole-brain radiotherapy (WBRT). Table 14.2.2 summarizes the contemporary series of these patients with regard to outcome. Although small patient numbers preclude reaching conclusions with statistical confidence, SRS appears to offer excellent local control of CNS metastases from RCC. Given that the addition of WBRT was not standardized within or across series, the true benefit of WBRT addition awaits the results of randomized trials. A retrospective examination of predictors of outcome after stereotactic radiosurgery was undertaken in 69 metastatic RCC patients in a separate series (74).

In a multivariate analysis, factors significantly affecting the rate of survival included the following: (1) younger patient age ($p = .0076$); (2) preoperative Karnofsky Performance Scale score ($p = .0012$); (3) time from initial cancer

TABLE **14.2.2.** Select series evaluating stereotactic radiosurgery (SRS) in metastatic renal cell carcinoma

First author	No. of patients	Radiotherapy dose (range)	Median overall survival (months)	Local control rate (%)
Schoggl (73)	14	18 Gy at tumor margin (10–22 Gy)	11	96
Goyal (71)	29	18 Gy to 60% isodose line (7–24 Gy)	6.7	91
Hernandez (72)	29	16.8 Gy at 50% isodose line (13–30 Gy)	7	NR

Gy, gray; NR, not reported.

diagnosis to brain metastasis diagnosis ($p = .0017$); (4) treatment dose to the tumor margin ($p = .0252$); (5) maximal treatment dose ($p = .0127$); and (6) treatment isodose ($p = .0354$). Prior tumor resection, chemotherapy, immunotherapy, or WBRT did not correlate with extended survival. Stereotactic radiosurgery thus represents a viable option for a select group of metastatic RCC patients and should be considered in the context of the overall treatment plan.

Bisphosphonates

Bisphosphonates are osteoclast-inhibiting agents that have been utilized in the treatment of bone metastases for many solid tumors. In metastatic RCC, a study examined patients with solid tumors other than prostate or breast cancer and at least 1 bone metastasis (75). Patients were randomized to receive either 4 mg of zoledronate, 8 mg of zoledronate, or placebo given IV every 3 weeks for 9 months, in addition to standard anticancer therapy administered at the treating physician's discretion. The primary end point of the study was incidence of skeletal related events (SRE) defined as pathologic bone fracture, requirement for radiotherapy, spinal cord compression, or bone surgery (but not including hypercalcemia of malignancy). Patients in the zoledronate 8-mg arm were subsequently dose-reduced to 4 mg based on unacceptable renal toxicity, and the results for this group are not presented here.

In a subset of 74 patients with RCC, zoledronic acid (4 mg) was found to significantly reduce the proportion of patients with an SRE (37% vs. 74% for placebo; $p = .015$) and extended the time to the first skeletal event (median not reached vs. 72 days for placebo; $p = .006$). The median time to progression of bone lesions was significantly longer for patients who were treated with zoledronic acid ($p = .014$ vs. placebo). This hypothesis-generating subgroup analysis suggests that zoledronate may prevent or delay skeletal events in metastatic renal carcinoma patients with bone metastases. Given Food and Drug Administration (FDA) approval of this agent for patients with solid tumors metastatic to bone, it is unlikely that randomized, prospective trials will be performed in RCC to further evaluate the utility of zoledronic acid or any bisphosphonate in RCC. As such, it is reasonable to utilize these agents in RCC with bone metastases mindful of complications including renal failure and rare but serious osteonecrosis of the jaw (ONJ).

Conclusion

Cytokine therapy has an established role in the treatment of metastatic RCC. Good performance status patients may appropriately receive HD IL-2 after consideration of the relative risks and benefits. Alternatively, low-dose, single-agent cytokine regimens are acceptable and confer a modest survival benefit. There is no proven advantage to combination therapy with cytokines and thus cytokine monotherapy remains a standard of care against which new agents should be compared. Vascular endothelial growth factor is a powerful proangiogenic factor impacting tumor angiogenesis. Clear-cell RCC is characterized by *VHL* gene inactivation and subsequent VEGF overexpression, identifying RCC as particularly susceptible to VEGF blockade. Therapeutic inhibition of VEGF with a neutralizing antibody or VEGF receptor inhibition results in antitumor activity in RCC patients. The clinical response data with VEGF inhibition in RCC has provided an opportunity for treatment advances in this historically resistant malignancy and will establish a new treatment paradigm. Supportive care including aggressive treatment of CNS and bone metastases remains an important part of the management of metastatic RCC patients.

References

1. Flanigan RC, Mickisch G, Sylvester R, et al. Cytoreductive nephrectomy in patients with metastatic renal cancer: a combined analysis. J Urol 2004;171:1071–1076.
2. Smith KA. Lowest dose interleukin-2 immunotherapy. Blood 1993;81(6):1414–1423.
3. Luft T, Pang KC, Thomas E, et al. Type I IFNs enhance the terminal differentiation of dendritic cells. J Immunol 1998;161(4):1947–1953.
4. Tompkins WA. Immunomodulation and therapeutic effects of the oral use of interferon-alpha: mechanism of action. J Interferon Cytokine Res 1999;19(8):817–828.
5. Nanus DM, Pfeffer LM, Bander NH, et al. Antiproliferative and antitumor effects of alpha-interferon in renal cell carcinomas: correlation with the expression of a kidney-associated differentiation glycoprotein. Cancer Res 1990;50(14):4190–4194.
6. Lindner DJ. Interferons as antiangiogenic agents. Curr Oncol Rep 2002;4(6):510–514.
7. McDermott DF, Regan MM, Clark JI, et al. Randomized phase III trial of high-dose interleukin-2 versus subcutaneous interleukin-2 and interferon in patients with metastatic renal cell carcinoma. J Clin Oncol 2005;23(1):133–141.
8. Yang JC, Sherry RM, Steinberg SM, et al. Randomized study of high-dose and low-dose interleukin-2 in patients with metastatic renal cancer. J Clin Oncol 2003;21(16):3127–3132.
9. Fyfe G, Fisher RI, Rosenberg SA, et al. Results of treatment of 255 patients with metastatic renal cell carcinoma who received high-dose recombinant interleukin-2 therapy. J Clin Oncol 1995;13(3):688–696.
10. Fyfe GA, Fisher RI, Rosenberg SA, et al. Long-term response data for 255 patients with metastatic renal cell carcinoma treated with high-dose recombinant interleukin-2 therapy. J Clin Oncol 1996;14(8):2410–2411.
11. Bukowski RM. Cytokine therapy for metastatic renal cell carcinoma. Semin Urol Oncol 2001;19(2):148–154.
12. Interferon-alpha and survival in metastatic renal carcinoma: early results of a randomised controlled trial. Medical Research Council Renal Cancer Collaborators. Lancet 1999;353(9146):14–17.
13. Pyrhonen S, Salminen E, Ruutu M, et al. Prospective randomized trial of interferon alfa-2a plus vinblastine versus vinblastine alone in patients with advanced renal cell cancer. J Clin Oncol 1999;17(9):2859–2867.

14. Sleijfer DT, Janssen RA, Buter J, et al. Phase II study of subcutaneous interleukin-2 in unselected patients with advanced renal cell cancer on an outpatient basis. J Clin Oncol 1992;10(7):1119–1123.

15. Stadler WM, Vogelzang NJ. Low-dose interleukin-2 in the treatment of metastatic renal-cell carcinoma. Semin Oncol 1995;22(1):67–73.

16. Atkins MB, Sparano J, Fisher RI, et al. Randomized phase II trial of high-dose interleukin-2 either alone or in combination with interferon alfa-2b in advanced renal cell carcinoma. J Clin Oncol 1993;11(4):661–670.

17. Negrier S, Escudier B, Lasset C, et al. Recombinant human interleukin-2, recombinant human interferon alfa-2a, or both in metastatic renal-cell carcinoma. Groupe Francais d'Immunotherapie. N Engl J Med 1998;338(18):1272–1278.

18. Lissoni P, Barni S, Tancini G, et al. Immunoendocrine therapy with interleukin-2 (IL-2) and medroxyprogesterone acetate (MPA): a randomized study with or without MPA in metastatic renal cancer patients during IL-2 maintenance treatment after response or stable disease to IL-2 subcutaneous therapy. Tumori 1993;79(4): 246–249.

19. Porzsolt F, Messerer D, Hautmann R, et al. Treatment of advanced renal cell cancer with recombinant interferon alpha as a single agent and in combination with medroxyprogesterone acetate. A randomized multicenter trial. J Cancer Res Clin Oncol 1988;114(1):95–100.

20. Rosenberg SA, Lotze MT, Yang JC, et al. Prospective randomized trial of high-dose interleukin-2 alone or in conjunction with lymphokine-activated killer cells for the treatment of patients with advanced cancer. J Natl Cancer Inst 1993;85(8):622–632.

21. Law TM, Motzer RJ, Mazumdar M, et al. Phase III randomized trial of interleukin-2 with or without lymphokine-activated killer cells in the treatment of patients with advanced renal cell carcinoma. Cancer 1995;76(5):824–832.

22. Figlin RA, Thompson JA, Bukowski RM, et al. Multicenter, randomized, phase III trial of CD8(+) tumor-infiltrating lymphocytes in combination with recombinant interleukin-2 in metastatic renal cell carcinoma. J Clin Oncol 1999;17(8):2521–2529.

23. Motzer RJ, Murphy BA, Bacik J, et al. Phase III trial of interferon alfa-2a with or without 13–cis-retinoic acid for patients with advanced renal cell carcinoma. J Clin Oncol 2000;18(16):2972–2980.

24. Atzpodien J, Kirchner H, Hanninen EL, et al. Interleukin-2 in combination with interferon-alpha and 5–fluorouracil for metastatic renal cell cancer. Eur J Cancer 1993;29A(suppl 5):S6–8.

25. Kibel A, Iliopoulos O, DeCaprio JA, Kaelin WG, Jr. Binding of the von Hippel-Lindau tumor suppressor protein to Elongin B and C. Science 1995;269(5229):1444–1446.

26. Maxwell PH, Wiesener MS, Chang GW, et al. The tumour suppressor protein VHL targets hypoxia-inducible factors for oxygen-dependent proteolysis. Nature 1999; 399(6733):271–275.

27. Cockman ME, Masson N, Mole DR, et al. Hypoxia inducible factor-alpha binding and ubiquitylation by the von Hippel-Lindau tumor suppressor protein. J Biol Chem 2000;275(33):25733–25741.

28. Iliopoulos O, Levy AP, Jiang C, et al. Negative regulation of hypoxia-inducible genes by the von Hippel-Lindau protein. Proc Natl Acad Sci USA 1996;93(20):10595–10599.

29. Kourembanas S, Morita T, Liu Y, Christou H. Mechanisms by which oxygen regulates gene expression and cell-cell interaction in the vasculature. Kidney Int 1997; 51(2):438–443.

30. Wiesener MS, Munchenhagen PM, Berger I, et al. Constitutive activation of hypoxia-inducible genes related to overexpression of hypoxia-inducible factor-1alpha in clear cell renal carcinomas. Cancer Res 2001;61(13):5215–5222.
31. Knebelmann B, Ananth S, Cohen HT, Sukhatme VP. Transforming growth factor alpha is a target for the von Hippel-Lindau tumor suppressor. Cancer Res 1998;58(2): 226–231.
32. Gunaratnam L, Morley M, Franovic A, et al. Hypoxia inducible factor activates the transforming growth factor-alpha/epidermal growth factor receptor growth stimulatory pathway in VHL(-/-) renal cell carcinoma cells. J Biol Chem 2003; 278(45):44966–44974.
33. de Paulsen N, Brychzy A, Fournier MC, et al. Role of transforming growth factor-alpha in von Hippel–Lindau (VHL)(-/-) clear cell renal carcinoma cell proliferation: a possible mechanism coupling VHL tumor suppressor inactivation and tumorigenesis. Proc Natl Acad Sci USA 2001;98(4):1387–1392.
34. Latif F, Tory K, Gnarra J, et al. Identification of the von Hippel-Lindau disease tumor suppressor gene. Science 1993;260(5112):1317–1320.
35. Gnarra JR, Tory K, Weng Y, et al. Mutations of the VHL tumour suppressor gene in renal carcinoma. Nat Genet 1994;7(1):85–90.
36. Shuin T, Kondo K, Torigoe S, et al. Frequent somatic mutations and loss of heterozygosity of the von Hippel-Lindau tumor suppressor gene in primary human renal cell carcinomas. Cancer Res 1994;54(11):2852–2855.
37. Herman JG, Latif F, Weng Y, et al. Silencing of the VHL tumor-suppressor gene by DNA methylation in renal carcinoma. Proc Natl Acad Sci USA 1994;91(21): 9700–9704.
38. Gnarra JR, Lerman MI, Zbar B, Linehan WM. Genetics of renal-cell carcinoma and evidence for a critical role for von Hippel-Lindau in renal tumorigenesis. Semin Oncol 1995;22(1):3–8.
39. Kondo K, Yao M, Yoshida M, et al. Comprehensive mutational analysis of the VHL gene in sporadic renal cell carcinoma: relationship to clinicopathological parameters. Genes Chromosomes Cancer 2002;34(1):58–68.
40. Brauch H, Hoeppner W, Jahnig H, et al. Sporadic pheochromocytomas are rarely associated with germline mutations in the VHL tumor suppressor gene or the ret protooncogene. J Clin Endocrinol Metab 1997;82(12):4101–4104.
41. Clifford SC, Prowse AH, Affara NA, et al. Inactivation of the von Hippel-Lindau (VHL) tumour suppressor gene and allelic losses at chromosome arm 3p in primary renal cell carcinoma: evidence for a VHL-independent pathway in clear cell renal tumourigenesis. Genes Chromosomes Cancer 1998;22(3):200–209.
42. Kenck C, Wilhelm M, Bugert P, et al. Mutation of the VHL gene is associated exclusively with the development of non-papillary renal cell carcinomas. J Pathol 1996;179(2):157–161.
43. Bard RH, Mydlo JH, Freed SZ. Detection of tumor angiogenesis factor in adenocarcinoma of kidney. Urology 1986;27(5):447–450.
44. Hicklin DJ, Ellis LM. Role of the vascular endothelial growth factor pathway in tumor growth and angiogenesis. J Clin Oncol 2005;23(5):1011–1027.
45. Dvorak HF, Brown LF, Detmar M, Dvorak AM. Vascular permeability factor/vascular endothelial growth factor, microvascular hyperpermeability, and angiogenesis. Am J Pathol 1995;146(5):1029–1039.
46. Ferrara N, Davis-Smyth T. The biology of vascular endothelial growth factor. Endocr Rev 1997;18(1):4–25.

47. Benjamin LE, Golijanin D, Itin A, et al. Selective ablation of immature blood vessels in established human tumors follows vascular endothelial growth factor withdrawal. J Clin Invest 1999;103(2):159–165.

48. Jain RK, Safabakhsh N, Sckell A, et al. Endothelial cell death, angiogenesis, and microvascular function after castration in an androgen-dependent tumor: role of vascular endothelial growth factor. Proc Natl Acad Sci USA 1998;95(18):10820–10825.

49. Watanabe Y, Lee SW, Detmar M, et al. Vascular permeability factor/vascular endothelial growth factor (VPF/VEGF) delays and induces escape from senescence in human dermal microvascular endothelial cells. Oncogene 1997;14(17):2025–2032.

50. Presta LG, Chen H, O'Connor SJ, et al. Humanization of an anti-vascular endothelial growth factor monoclonal antibody for the therapy of solid tumors and other disorders. Cancer Res 1997;57(20):4593–4599.

51. Wang Y, Fei D, Vanderlaan M, Song A. Biological activity of bevacizumab, a humanized anti-VEGF antibody in vitro. Angiogenesis 2004;7(4):335–345.

52. Yang JC, Haworth L, Sherry RM, et al. A randomized trial of bevacizumab, an anti-vascular endothelial growth factor antibody, for metastatic renal cancer. N Engl J Med 2003;349(5):427–434.

53. Yang JC. Bevacizumab for patients with metastatic renal cancer: an update. Clin Cancer Res 2004;10(18 pt 2):6367S–6370S.

54. Rini BI, Halabi S, Taylor J, et al. Cancer and Leukemia Group B 90206:A randomized phase III trial of interferon-alpha or interferon-alpha plus anti-vascular endothelial growth factor antibody (bevacizumab) in metastatic renal cell carcinoma. Clin Cancer Res 2004;10(8):2584–2586.

55. Gabrilovich DI, Chen HL, Girgis KR, et al. Production of vascular endothelial growth factor by human tumors inhibits the functional maturation of dendritic cells. Nat Med 996;2:1096–1103.

56. Gabrilovich DI, Ishida T, Nadaf S, et al. Antibodies to vascular endothelial growth factor enhance the efficacy of cancer immunotherapy by improving endogenous dendritic cell function. Clin Cancer Res 1999;5(10):2963–2970.

57. Motzer RJ, Amato R, Todd M, et al. Phase II trial of antiepidermal growth factor receptor antibody C225 in patients with advanced renal cell carcinoma. Invest New Drugs 2003;21(1):99–101.

58. Drucker B, Bacik J, Ginsberg M, et al. Phase II trial of ZD1839 (IRESSA) in patients with advanced renal cell carcinoma. Invest New Drugs 2003;21(3):341–345.

59. Dawson NA, Guo C, Zak R, et al. A phase II trial of gefitinib (Iressa, ZD1839) in stage IV and recurrent renal cell carcinoma. Clin Cancer Res 2004;10(23):7812–7819.

60. Sun L, Liang C, Shirazian S, et al. Discovery of 5-(5-fluoro-2-oxo-1,2-dihydroindol-(3Z)-ylidenemethyl)-2,4-dimethyl-1H-pyrrole-3-carboxylic acid (2-diethylamino-ethyl) amide, a novel tyrosine kinase inhibitor targeting vascular endothelial and platelet-derived growth factor receptor tyrosine kinase. J Med Chem 2003;46(7):1116–1119.

61. Mendel DB, Laird AD, Xin X, et al. In vivo antitumor activity of SU11248, a novel tyrosine kinase inhibitor targeting vascular endothelial growth factor and platelet-derived growth factor receptors: determination of a pharmacokinetic/pharmacodynamic relationship. Clin Cancer Res 2003;9(1):327–337.

62. Motzer RJ, Rini BI, Michaelson MD, et al. Phase 2 trials of SU11248 show antitumor activity in second-line therapy for patients with metastatic renal cell carcinoma (RCC). Proc Am Soc Clin Oncol 2005;23(16S):4508.

63. Joneson T, Bar-Sagi D. Ras effectors and their role in mitogenesis and oncogenesis. J Mol Med 1997;75(8):587–593.

64. Bar-Sagi D. A Ras by any other name. Mol Cell Biol 2001;21(5):1441–1443.

65. Lyons JF, Wilhelm S, Hibner B, Bollag G. Discovery of a novel Raf kinase inhibitor. Endocr Relat Cancer 2001;8(3):219–225.

66. Wilhelm SM, Carter C, Tang L, et al. Sorafenib exhibits broad spectrum oral antitumor activity and targets the RAF/MEK/ERK pathway and receptor tyrosine kinases involved in tumor progression and angiogenesis. Cancer Res 2004;64(19):7099–7109.

67. Ratain MJ, Eisen T, Stadler WM, et al. Final findings from a Phase II, placebo-controlled, randomized discontinuation trial (RDT) of sorafenib (BAY 43-9006) in patients with advanced renal cell carcinoma (RCC). Proc Am Soc Clin Oncol 2005; 23(16S):4544.

68. Escudier B, Szczylik C, Eisen T, et al. Randomized Phase III trial of the Raf kinase and VEGFR inhibitor sorafenib (BAY 43-9006) in patients with advanced renal cell carcinoma (RCC). Proc Am Soc Clin Oncol 2005;23(16S):4510.

69. Culine S, Bekradda M, Kramar A, et al. Prognostic factors for survival in patients with brain metastases from renal cell carcinoma. Cancer 1998;83(12):2548–2553.

70. Decker DA, Decker VL, Herskovic A, Cummings GD. Brain metastases in patients with renal cell carcinoma: prognosis and treatment. J Clin Oncol 1984;2(3):169–173.

71. Goyal LK, Suh JH, Reddy CA, Barnett GH. The role of whole brain radiotherapy and stereotactic radiosurgery on brain metastases from renal cell carcinoma. Int J Radiat Oncol Biol Phys 2000;47(4):1007–1012.

72. Hernandez L, Zamorano L, Sloan A, et al. Gamma knife radiosurgery for renal cell carcinoma brain metastases. J Neurosurg 2002;97(5 suppl):489–493.

73. Schoggl A, Kitz K, Ertl A, et al. Gamma-knife radiosurgery for brain metastases of renal cell carcinoma: results in 23 patients. Acta Neurochir (Wien) 1998;140(6): 549–555.

74. Sheehan JP, Sun MH, Kondziolka D, et al. Radiosurgery in patients with renal cell carcinoma metastasis to the brain: long-term outcomes and prognostic factors influencing survival and local tumor control. J Neurosurg 2003;98(2):342–349.

75. Lipton A, Zheng M, Seaman J. Zoledronic acid delays the onset of skeletal-related events and progression of skeletal disease in patients with advanced renal cell carcinoma. Cancer 2003;98(5):962–969.

15
Tumors of the Adrenal Gland

Veronica Moyes and Shern L. Chew

It is often possible to reach the correct diagnosis of an adrenal tumor preoperatively, based on clinical assessment and noninvasive radiological and endocrinological investigations. This important feature facilitates safe and well-planned treatment strategies, with avoidance of unpleasant surprises. An expert radiologist is vital in sorting out renal from adrenal lesions and whether adrenal lesions are invading the adjacent kidney.

A major problem in adrenal disease is that the glands frequently become nodular with age, presumably as part of a degenerative process, followed by a regenerative cycle. This tendency to nodularity is seen commonly in other endocrine glands, classically the thyroid. One task is to separate such natural nodularity from the diseases that require treatment. Another difficulty in adrenal pathology is distinguishing benign from malignant adrenal tumors by histological analysis. This lack of histological certainty means that careful clinical follow-up is often required.

Adrenal Incidentalomas

With the widespread availability of imagery including ultrasound and computed tomography (CT) scan, more incidental adrenal masses are being detected for unrelated reasons. Autopsy rates indicate a prevalence of incidental adrenal masses of 2% to 9% (1,2). Computed tomography scan studies have demonstrated 0.5% to 4.4% detection rates of adrenal masses (3–5). The majority are benign and nonfunctioning, and show no progression in size (6), but up to 20% are functioning or malignant, and are therefore of great clinical significance.

The prevalence of incidentalomas peaks between the ages of 50 and 60 years, with a slight female preponderance (7). The prevalence increases with patient age, with 0.2% in young patients and 6.9% in patients older than 70 years of age (4). Incidentalomas are particularly common in patients with features of the metabolic syndrome (insulin resistance, dyslipidemia, obesity, and hypertension).

TABLE 15.1. Differential diagnosis of incidentalomas (6,8)

Benign adrenal (cortical and medullary)
Adrenal cortical tumors
Adrenal adenoma (nonfunctioning)
Adrenal adenoma functioning (cortisol-secreting)
Adrenal adenoma functioning (androgen-secreting)
Adrenal nodular hyperplasia
Pheochromocytoma
Ganglioneuroma
Neuroblastoma
Ganglioneuroblastoma

Miscellaneous benign lesions
Cysts and pseudocysts
Myelolipoma
Schwannoma
Hemorrhage
Hemangioma
Granulomatosis and infections
Pseudoadrenal masses (stomach, kidney, pancreas, liver, lymph nodes)

Malignant
Carcinoma
Pheochromocytoma
Neuroblastoma
Metastatic tumors (breast, kidney, lung, ovarian, melanoma, leukemia)

Causes of Incidentalomas

Evaluation and management of adrenal incidentalomas requires an understanding of differential diagnoses of adrenal masses (Table 15.1), their biochemical profile, and the risk factors for malignancy.

Assessment of Malignant Potential

A definitive preoperative diagnosis of primary malignancy is difficult because the tumors are generally symptomless and hormonally inert. The risk of malignancy, however, increases with the size of the incidentaloma. Adrenal adenomas are rarely larger than 6 cm, and hypersecreting adenomas are often small (9). Metastatic disease must be suspected in any patient with a history of cancer; up to three quarters of incidental adrenal masses prove to be metastatic in patients with such a history (10,11). This higher incidence is due to the fact that most of the times patients with known malignancies are included as incidentalomas, although by definition these are not incidentalomas. In patients with no prior history of cancer, more than two thirds of incidentally found adrenal lesions are reported to be benign (6).

Imaging Investigations

Ultrasonography

Ultrasonography is not a reliable investigation to differentiate between benign and malignant adrenal lesions (12). (This is discussed in detail in Chapter 3.) Recently endoscopic ultrasound-guided fine-needle aspiration has been used for assessing adrenal masses (13).

Computed Tomography

Computed tomography (CT) scanning is effective in distinguishing benign adrenal disease from malignancy. The main indicator of malignancy is size. For example, adrenocortical carcinoma was detected in 2% of masses <4 cm in diameter, 6% of masses 4.1 to 6.0 cm, and 25% of masses >25 cm (14). Assessment of CT radiographic absorption (expressed as Hounsfield units, HU) of adrenal masses suggests that a value of >10 HU is an indicator of malignant potential, with specificity of 96% to 100% and sensitivity of 68% to 79% (15,16). Other radiographical features such as heterogeneous appearance of the gland, irregular border of the mass, and involvement of surrounding structures are sinister.

Magnetic Resonance Imaging

The finding of intracellular lipid in a solid adrenal lesion by magnetic resonance imaging (MRI) is suggestive of an adrenocortical adenoma. Pheochromocytomas are characterized by hypointensity on T1-weighted MRI and hyperintensity on T2-weighted MRI. The presence of fat in the lesion may suggest a myelolipoma, which are benign nonfunctioning neoplasms consisting of mature adipose cells and hemopoietic tissue (15).

Positron Emission Tomography

Positron emission tomography (PET) scanning has sensitivities of over 90% in identifying malignant adrenal masses, particularly metastases (17,18), and in distinguishing them from benign adrenocortical adenomas. However, a number of cases of false-positive PET studies are reported in nonmalignant adrenal pathologies (19–22). Most studies have evaluated fluorodeoxyglucose as a tracer, with metomidate also showing potential (23). Thus, PET scanning has a role in the assessment of an adrenal mass, but CT and MRI are close to PET in their clinical usefulness.

Assessment of Functional Status

The main concern is whether an adrenal incidentaloma is secreting cortisol, as adrenalectomy may be more hazardous. In these cases, first, the contralateral adrenal may be suppressed, with a hypoadrenal crisis and hypotension when the adenoma is removed as the circulating cortisol falls to low levels. Second, postoperative complications of infection, poor wound healing, and hemorrhage are more likely if high preoperative cortisol levels are not detected and treated prior to surgery. An elevated serum cortisol level and suppressed serum adrenocorticotropin (ACTH) or dehydroepiandrosterone sulfate (DHEAS) are very suggestive of autonomous adrenal cortisol production. However, patients with mild oversecretion may have serum cortisol levels within the normal range and a low-dose dexamethasone suppression test is often useful. This test entails administering dexamethasone 0.5 mg every 6 hours for 48 hours with measurement of urine free cortisol and/or 17-hydroxycorticosteroids (17-OH-corticosteroids). Serum cortisol is measured at 0 and 48 hours. There is complete suppression in normal individuals (<50 nmol/L).

Conn's syndrome should be suspected in any patient with hypertension with or without hypokalemia. As a screening measure, patients should have an assessment of their electrolytes including bicarbonate and measurement of plasma aldosterone concentration and plasma renin activity with assessment of the ratio.

Other biochemical tests include assessment of androgens, looking for evidence of virilization. It may also be helpful to assess serum DHEAS as levels may be increased in adrenocortical carcinoma. For completion 17-hydroxyprogesterone should be assessed in view of the possibility of congenital adrenal hyperplasia.

Clinically silent pheochromocytomas account for 0.04% to 11% of incidentalomas (4,6,7,24). These frequently present with no specific symptoms and should be excluded in any patient with an incidentaloma. Twenty-four-hour urinary catecholamines provide a useful screening tool with 96% sensitivity and are widely available.

Management

Adrenalectomy is recommended for masses greater than 6 cm in diameter. Homogeneous lesions less than 4 cm in diameter are considered low risk and may be followed by scanning. Masses that measure 4 to 6 cm, or that have heterogeneity, may be followed up or excised, although if features of rapid growth or decreased lipid content are present, surgery would be advisable. Over a 10-year follow-up, less than 30% of the masses increase in size and less than 20% develop biochemical abnormalities (14).

Tumors of the Adrenal Cortex

Benign (Adenomas)

Functioning Adrenocortical Adenomas

Adrenal Cushing's syndrome accounts for approximately 10% all cases of Cushing's syndrome. The most common cause is a unilateral benign adenoma.

In severe, untreated cases it is associated with 50% mortality at 5 years (25), while less clinically obvious cases have a significantly increased morbidity and mortality due to hypertension and secondary diabetes mellitus. Clinical manifestations vary according to the degree of levels of cortisol.

In adrenal Cushing's, the serum cortisol usually remains high throughout the day and night, or pulses up and down with no relation to time of day. The midnight cortisol in adrenal Cushing's syndrome is usually very similar to the morning cortisol. A low-dose dexamethasone suppression test in adrenal Cushing's syndrome usually shows no suppression of the serum cortisol. The high circulating cortisol levels suppress the hypothalamopituitary axis, resulting in undetectable serum ACTH levels and often mild reductions in luteinizing hormone (LH) and thyroid-stimulating hormone (TSH) levels.

The mainstay of treatment for adrenal Cushing's syndrome is ipsilateral adrenalectomy. Serum cortisol levels can be lowered with metyrapone for at least 6 weeks before surgery. Ketoconazole may also be used for this purpose but has a slower time of onset and offset. The anesthetic agent etomidate provides an effective short-term method of controlling very severe hypercortisolemia (26). Hydrocortisone cover should be administered with the induction of anesthesia and continued during the peri- and postoperative period due to hypothalamo-adrenal axis suppression. One regimen is a hydrocortisone infusion of 2 mg per hour, or 100 mg intramuscularly every 6 hours until the patient is able to swallow tablets again (usually within 8 hours). The oral hydrocortisone is rapidly tapered to a physiological replacement dose of 10 mg on waking, 5 mg at lunch, and 5 mg at 5 p.m.

The patient is readmitted about 3 months after surgery to withdraw hydrocortisone and to check the recovery of the hypothalamopituitary axis and endogenous cortisol from the contralateral adrenal gland. If the patient is still dependent on hydrocortisone, reassessments are done every 6 months. Most patients recover the function of the contralateral adrenal by about 18 months after surgery, but a small number continue to need hydrocortisone replacement for the long-term. Adrenal adenomas treated successfully by surgery have a good prognosis with a low risk of recurrence.

Conn's Syndrome (Primary Hyperaldosteronism)

Aldosterone is the main mineralocorticoid produced by the zona glomerulosa, the outer portion of the adrenal cortex. Hyperaldosteronism most commonly occurs as a result of a unilateral adenoma or idiopathic hyperaldosteronism (also known as bilateral adrenal hyperplasia). Rarer causes include glucocorticoid-suppressible hyperaldosteronism and aldosterone-producing adrenocortical carcinoma.

Many antihypertensive drugs interfere with the assessment of hyperaldosteronism, but patients may be controlled on calcium antagonists or α-adrenoreceptor blockers during investigation. Diuretics, β-adrenoceptor antagonists, angiotensin-converting enzyme inhibitors, and angiotensin-2 receptor antagonists should be withdrawn for at least 2 weeks prior to investigations. Initial simple investigations include measurement of serum potassium and bicarbonate and urinary potassium; the presence of a hypokalemic alkalosis and raised urinary potassium of >30 mmol/24 hours is highly suggestive of hyperaldosteronism.

The aldosterone/renin ratio (ARR) has been used as the initial test for Conn's syndrome. An aldosterone/renin ratio is suggestive of Conn's syndrome at >800 (when expressed in SI units; aldosterone in pmol/L and renin activity in pmol/L/h) or >67 (when expressed in conventional units: aldosterone ng/dL; renin activity ng/mL/h). Conn's syndrome is unlikely when the ratio is <300 (in SI units) or <24 (in conventional units). More complex dynamic tests may be used, including the response of aldosterone to posture and circadian rhythm.

Computed tomography or MRI of the adrenal is done to identify whether a single adenoma or bilateral adrenal hyperplasia is present. Further information may be provided by adrenal vein sampling in specialist centers.

Where there is a unilateral adenoma, surgery is the treatment of choice leading to a cure of hypertension in 70% of cases. Surgery is not advised in cases of idiopathic hyperaldosteronism due to the inability to cure the condition, even with bilateral adrenalectomy. Medical treatments include the mineralocorticoid receptor antagonists. Spironolactone is used in doses of 200 to 400 mg/day, but the main limitation to use is gynecomastia and impotence in men. Eplerenone is a newer specific mineralocorticoid receptor antagonist, and can be started at doses of about 50 mg per day with some patients requiring more than 200 mg per day

Nonfunctioning Adrenocortical Adenomas

This is a common lesion and usually does not need active treatment. Multiple adrenocortical adenomas are seen in multiple endocrine neoplasia type I (MEN-I). MEN-I is an autosomal dominant genetic tumor syndrome with high penetrance and with equal sex distribution, causing parathyroid adenomas, pituitary adenomas, and pancreatic islet cell tumors. The disease is caused by mutations in the *MENIN* gene on chromosome 11q13 (27). There are over 20 different combinations of endocrine and nonendocrine tumors causing MEN-I, and no simple definition could cover all index cases or all families (27). The investigations, management, and follow-up were discussed above (see Adrenal Incidentalomas).

Adrenocortical Carcinoma

Epidemiology

Malignant adrenal tumors may be primary adrenocortical carcinoma or secondary metastases to the adrenal from other cancers. Adrenocortical carcinomas are rare tumors accounting for only 0.05% to 2% of all cancers. The reported incidence is 2 per million of population per year, and there is a female preponderance. Any age may be affected from infants to the elderly, although the peak age of presentation is 30 to 50 years. Approximately 2% to 10% are bilateral. It has a poor prognosis, with an overall 5-year mortality rate of 75% to 90% (28,29).

Clinical Presentation

Patients present as a result of the mass itself or as hormone secreting tumors in approximately 50% of cases. When presenting with a nonsecreting tumor, the symptoms are often vague, such as abdominal pain or anorexia, or the result of metastatic disease. When functional, patients may present with a range of endocrine conditions: Cushing's syndrome, virilization or feminization, or Conn's syndrome. Sudden and late-onset virilization and an increase in libido in females may indicate very high circulating testosterone levels from a virilizing carcinoma. Tumors may secrete multiple hormones, a characteristic feature of adrenocortical carcinomas.

Functional Assessment

Functional assessment involves measurement at 9 a.m. of serum cortisol, ACTH, aldosterone, plasma renin activity, and the androgens]androstenedione, DHEAS, testosterone/sex hormone–binding globulin (SHBG), estradiol, and 17-hydroxyprogesterone]. A low-dose dexamethasone suppression test is often needed where there is clinical or biochemical evidence of hormonal excess.

Staging Investigations

A CT scan of the abdomen, chest, and pelvis should be performed for metastases, and invasion of local structures such as the kidney and the inferior vena cava. Involvement of the inferior vena cava may also be via tumor thrombus via the adrenal vein. An MRI scan may also demonstrate the presence of thrombus in the inferior vena cava. Both CT and MRI have been shown to significantly underestimate adrenal size by about 20% (30). If there is significant distortion of the kidney by the tumor, an isotope renogram [mercaptoacetyltriglycine (MAG3) renogram] may help define differential function of the kidney in case of nephrectomy. An isotope bone scan and plain chest radiograph are also needed.

Prognosis

Staging the tumor is done by imaging to assess tumor size, local invasion, and lymph node involvement (Table 15.2).

Treatment

Surgery is the only realistic hope of cure. Radical excision with en bloc resection of any local invasion has proven to be the most effective method.

TABLE 15.2. Staging and prognosis of adrenocortical carcinoma (31)

Stage	Size	Lymph nodes	Local invasion	METs	5-year survival (%)
I	<5 cm	–	–	–	60
II	>5 cm	–	–	–	58
III	Any	+	+	–	24
IV	Any	+	+	+	0

METs, metabolic equivalents.

Cytotoxic Chemotherapy

A range of palliative chemotherapeutic agents have been tested, often in a small number of patients, and are largely ineffective, except when used in combination with mitotane. Several phase II studies have been performed using cisplatin and etoposide with response rates (partial and complete response) of 11% to 46% (32), and a trial of the combination of etoposide, doxorubicin, cisplatin, and mitotane with a response rate of 49% (33). Of these, only 6% to 7% demonstrate a complete response (32,33).

Drugs that Affect Steroid Synthesis

These drugs are mainly used as palliative treatment or in addition to surgical treatment. Mitotane is an adrenolytic agent (3 to 12 g daily) that inhibits 11β-hydroxylase, causing a reduction in cortisol levels. It has adrenolytic activity in high doses, causing a reduction in all steroid hormones, and it also alters the extraadrenal metabolism of cortisol and androgens. It results in an improvement of hypercortisolism in 60% of patients (34) and has a tumor response (complete and partial) in 13% to 33% of cases. At present it is the only effective palliative medical therapy. Mitotane is associated with gastrointestinal side effects and lethargy, dizziness, neurotoxicity, and rashes.

Other Drugs

Metyrapone blocks cortisol synthesis by inhibiting 11β-hydroxylase in adrenocortical cells. Aminoglutathamide is an aromatase inhibitor by its actions on cytochrome P-450 reduction. Newer investigational drugs including suramin, 5-fluorouracil, and gossypol have been tried but rarely employed (35).

Adrenocortical Oncocytomas and Cysts

Adrenocortical oncocytomas are rare tumors composed of oncocytes, large polygonal or round cells with abundant granular and eosinophilic cytoplasm that are packed with mitochondria. Patients of any age may be affected, with a slight preponderance of women. Presentation is often vague; abdominal pain and hematuria may occur. Up to a third are detected incidentally and are usually nonfunctioning. Size may vary from 2 to 20 cm, and while they are usually non-malignant, there have been cases of local invasion (36,37).

Adrenal cysts are most frequently benign, but may have features of malignancy, and a careful assessment, therefore, should be done. A review of 613 cases of adrenal cysts determined that 7% are malignant or potentially malignant and there was one reported case of malignancy in a cyst originally thought to be benign (38). If the suspicion of malignancy is low, and the lesion is nonfunctioning, the adrenal cyst may be managed by observation alone. The cyst may be drained percutaneously if it expands. Surgical excision is indicated if the cyst develops solid elements.

Tumors of the Adrenal Medulla

Pheochromocytomas

Pheochromocytomas are catecholamine-secreting tumors that arise from the adrenal medulla in 90% of cases; the remaining 10% arise from extraadrenal tissue and are termed paragangliomas. They occur in about 0.05% of hypertensive patients. The Mayo Clinic autopsy study indicated an incidence of 1300 cases per million. Of these 61% were reported retrospectively to have been hypertensive and 91% had nonspecific symptoms that may have been attributable to pheochromocytomas (Fig. 15.1) (39).

Pathogenesis and Physiology

Pheochromocytomas occur more frequently on the right than on the left. They are bilateral in 10% of adults and in 35% of children, usually in association with a genetic disorder. Paragangliomas arise from extraadrenal chromaffin tissue adjacent to sympathetic ganglia. Eighty-five percent are located intraabdominally; other locations include the bladder and the mediastinum. Extraadrenal

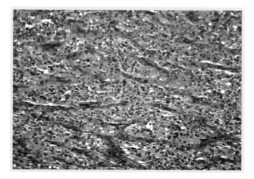

FIGURE 15.1. Pheochromocytoma of adrenal medulla. Hematoxylin and eosin stain, × 40. (Courtesy of Dr. Sohail Baithun, Royal London Hospital, London.)

paragangliomas rarely secrete adrenaline; cortisol is required for the induction of the enzyme responsible for the conversion of noradrenaline to adrenaline, and the lack of proximity to the adrenal gland precludes this. Catecholamine secretion may be increased by hemorrhage within the tumor or pressure on the tumor. Surgical manipulation of the tumor may cause a hypertensive crisis if appropriate measures are not taken preoperatively. The rate of malignancy is associated with an increased size (>6 cm).

Genetics

Approximately 10% of pheochromocytomas are associated with autosomal dominant genetic tumor syndromes: multiple endocrine neoplasia type IIA, von Hippel–Lindau disease, and familial paraganglioma syndromes. Pheochromocytomas are seen less frequently in neurofibromatosis type 1, tuberose sclerosis, and Sturge-Weber syndrome. Such patients tend to be younger and more often have bilateral or multicentric tumors and may be normotensive. Genetic testing is advisable for any patient with a family history of pheochromocytomas or paragangliomas, for patients with bilateral pheochromocytomas or features of any of the associated genetic syndromes, and in patients under the age of 50 years. Such patients should also have the following investigations: clinical thyroid examination, serum calcium, plasma calcitonin, and ophthalmoscopy.

Multiple endocrine neoplasia type IIA includes medullary thyroid carcinoma and hyperparathyroidism, and pheochromocytomas are found in 50% of patients. Extraadrenal tumors are rare. Point mutations in the *ret* oncogene cause the disease, and mutations of the tyrosine at codon 634 is most commonly associated with pheochromocytomas (40,41).

Von Hippel–Lindau (VHL) syndrome is described in Chapter 14.1. It is an autosomal dominant disease with high penetrance caused by germline mutations of the *VHL* gene (short arm of chromosome 3, 3p25.5) (42), and characterized by hemangioblastomas in the retina, cerebellum, and spinal cord, and renal cell cysts and carcinomas. Ten percent to 20% of patients develop pheochromocytoma; these mutations tend to be missense mutations in the *VHL* tumor suppressor gene rather than deletion or frameshift mutation. They can occur as early as 8 years of age. The pheochromocytomas are often bilateral and extraadrenal or malignant (43). These cases are managed by laparoscopic surgery often with partial adrenalectomy, the aim being to preserve the function of native adrenal gland (43).

Familial paraganglioma syndromes are caused by mutations in the succinate dehydrogenase B or D subunit genes. Multiple paragangliomas may be found in the sympathetic chain from the skull base to the floor of the pelvis.

Clinical Features

The characteristic feature is hypertension, with additional commonly reported symptoms including palpitations, sweating, and headaches. Other symptoms include anxiety, tremor, visual disturbance, gastrointestinal symptoms, fever, and chest pain. Paroxysms may be induced by any action that causes pressure on the tumor, such as bending over or micturition in bladder paragangliomas. Procedures such as bladder catheterization, anesthesia, and surgery may also precipitate hypertensive crises. A number of drugs may also cause an increase in catecholamine secretion, in particular unopposed beta-blockade, meto-clopramide, tricyclic antidepressants, and opiates. Other clinical findings, including evidence of cardiomegaly due to left ventricular hypertrophy, cardiac arrhythmias, and pallor, may present as a result of vasoconstriction. The tumor itself may be detected on palpation of the abdomen in the form of a mass, or a subsequent rise in blood pressure. Approximately 15% of pheochromocytomas are malignant, and evidence of metastases should be sought in the regional lymph nodes, liver, chest, and skeleton.

Biochemical Investigations

The initial screening test for pheochromocytoma is a 24-hour urine collection for free catecholamines: noradrenaline, adrenaline, and dopamine.

Levels may vary according to the intermittent secretion of catecholamines; at least two collections, therefore, must be assessed. Plasma or urinary free meta-nephrines, a metabolite of catecholamines may be more sensitive. A number of medications influence the secretion of catecholamines and must therefore be discontinued while investigations are taking place. These are listed in Table 15.3.

Plasma catecholamines may also prove to be of some benefit in the diagnosis, although levels are only increased periodically in association with paroxysms of symptoms. A normal level does not therefore exclude the possibility of a

TABLE 15.3. Medications that influence the secretion of catecholamines

	Increased	Decreased	Variable
Antihypertensives	Alpha-blockers Beta-blockers Hydralazine Sodium nitroprusside	Clonidine Adrenergic neuron blockers	Angiotensin-converting enzyme inhibitors Calcium channel blockers
Neuropsychiatric drugs	Levodopa Domperidone Metoclopramide	Monoamine oxidase inhibitor	Levodopa Tricyclics Phenothiazines Bromocriptine
Others	Containing catecholamines Decongestants—ephedrine Caffeine Amphetamine Nicotine Glyceryl trinitrate (GTN)		

pheochromocytoma. Chromogranin A may also prove to be useful as a tumor marker, but false positives may occur in renal failure.

Imaging

Pheochromocytomas have a characteristic high intense image on T2-weighted MRI scans. If an adrenal tumor is not found, further imaging of the whole body should then take place. Radionuclide scanning using iodine-131 metaiodobenzylguanidine is done to confirm the nature of a tumor as it is taken up by uptake channels on chromaffin cells. This scan may also detect any metastases. Positron emission tomography scanning with fluorodopamine may be superior to iodine-131 metaiodobenzylguanidine for detection of metastatic disease (44). High-dose iodine-131 metaiodobenzylguanidine therapy may be used as an adjunct to surgery. If imaging proves to be unhelpful in localizing the tumor, venous sampling may localize the lesion (45).

Management

Surgery leads to normotension in 75% of patients. The rate of postoperative complications correlated with the preoperative hypertension. Once the diagnosis of a pheochromocytoma is made, α-adrenoreceptor blockade should be commenced followed by β-adrenoreceptor blockade 24 hours later. Unopposed β-adrenoreceptor blockade may precipitate a hypertensive crisis and so should not be commenced until adequate α-adrenoreceptor blockade has been administered. Oral phenoxybenzamine (20 mg qds) followed by oral propranolol (80 mg tds) is commenced with monitoring of blood pressure. To ensure complete α-adrenoreceptor blockade preoperatively, intravenous phenoxybenzamine (0.5 mg/kg in 250 mL saline over 2 hours) is administered daily on the 3 days prior to the day of surgery. Reversal of α-adrenoreceptor–mediated vasoconstriction may lead to hemodilution; hemoglobin should be monitored pre- and postoperatively. Careful perioperative anesthetic management is vital as multiple complications may arise. Handling of the tumor may cause dramatic changes in blood pressure and arrhythmias. Tumor devascularization typically causes hypotension requiring volume replacement.

Laparoscopic adrenalectomy may be preferable when the tumor is less than 6 cm and noninvasive. Advantages of laparoscopic adrenalectomy include reduced postoperative pain, shorter hospital stays, and less severe and less frequent hypotensive episodes (46). A lateral or posterior approach may be used, and the pheochromocytoma should be bagged to avoid fragmentation and spread of tumor cells.

Adrenal cortex–sparing surgery may be done in patients undergoing bilateral adrenalectomies to avoid the need for lifelong glucocorticoid and mineralocorticoid replacement. There is no anatomical plane between the cortex and medulla, so this approach leaves some medulla behind and has been associated with tumor recurrence in genetic syndromes.

Treatment of malignant pheochromocytomas involves resection of large metastases, chemotherapy, and external beam radiotherapy to bony or nervous system metastases. If metastases are iodine-131 metaiodobenzylguanidine avid on the initial scan, high doses may be administered. In most patients this provides partial remission and symptomatic relief. More rarely, complete remission may occur; this tends to occur in patients with less tumor burden (47). Thalidomide and temozolomide achieve a partial radiological response in 33% of malignant pheochromocytomas (48), and the most commonly tested regimen has been cyclophosphamide, vincristine, and dacarbazine with partial responses of up to 40% and complete tumor responses in under 10% (49,50).

Prognosis

Benign pheochromocytomas have a 96% 5-year survival rate, but this drops to 44% in malignant pheochromocytomas. Rates of malignancy are reported to be 10% for adrenal pheochromocytomas and 30% to 50% for paragangliomas. Neither histological examination nor preoperative investigations can reliably confirm the presence of malignancy. Features of malignant potential include tumor diameter >6 cm, tumor necrosis, vascular invasion, and extensive local invasion. Repeat 24-hour urine catecholamines should be checked 2 weeks postsurgery; in the case of a benign tumor, levels should drop into the normal range. Patients should be followed up for life as metastases may develop up to 20 years after initial presentation.

Follow-up of patients with pheochromocytoma should involve urinary catecholamines and CT of the adrenal bed in the first year for a baseline, and in suspicious cases, annually for 5 years.

References

1. Kokko JP, Brown TC, Berman MM. Adrenal adenoma and hypertension. Lancet 1967; 7488:468–470.
2. Hedeland H, Ostberg G, Hokfelt B. On the prevalence of adrenocortical adenomas in an autopsy material in relation to hypertension and diabetes. Acta Med Scand 1968;184:211–214.
3. Peppercorn PD, Grossman AB, Reznek RH. Imaging of incidentally discovered adrenal masses. Clin Endocrinol (Oxf) 1998;48(4):379–388.
4. Kloos RT, Gross MD, Francis IR, Korobkin M, Shapiro B. Incidentally discovered adrenal masses. Endocr Rev 1995;16(4):460–484.
5. Bovio S, Cataldi A, Reimondo G, et al. Prevalence of adrenal incidentalomas in a contemporary computerized tomography series. J Endocrinol Invest 2006;29(4): 298–302.
6. Bülow B, Jansson S, Juhlin C, et al. Adrenal incidentaloma—follow-up results from a Swedish prospective study. Eur J Endocrinol 2006;154(3):419–423.
7. Mantero F, Terzolo M, Arnaldi G, et al. A survey on adrenal incidentaloma in Italy. Study Group on Adrenal Tumors of the Italian Society of Endocrinology. J Clin Endocrinol Metab 2000;85(2):637–644.

8. Barzon L, Sonino N, Fallo F, Palù G, Boscaro M. Prevalence and natural history of adrenal incidentalomas. Eur J Endocrinol 2003;149:273–285.

9. Copeland PM. The incidentally discovered adrenal mass. Ann Intern Med 1983;98:940–945.

10. Frilling A, Tecklenborg K, Weber F, et al. Importance of adrenal incidentaloma in patients with a history of malignancy. Surgery 2004;136(6):1289–1296.

11. Kumar R, Xiu Y, Yu JQ, Takalkar A, et al. 18F-FDG PET in evaluation of adrenal lesions in patients with lung cancer. J Nucl Med 2004;45(12):2058–2062.

12. Paivansalo M, Merikanto J, Kallioinen M, McAnsh G. Ultrasound in the detection of adrenal tumours. Eur J Radiol 1988;8(3):183–187.

13. Stelow EB, Debol SM, Stanley MW, et al. Sampling of the adrenal glands by endoscopic ultrasound-guided fine-needle aspiration. Diagn Cytopathol 2005;33:26–30.

14. Grumbach MM, Biller BM, Braunstein GD, et al. Management of the clinically inapparent adrenal mass ("incidentaloma"). Ann Intern Med 2003;138(5):424–429.

15. Sahdev A, Reznek RH. Imaging evaluation of the non-functioning indeterminate adrenal mass. Trends Endocrinol Metab 2004;15(6):271–276.

16. Moreira SG Jr, Pow-Sang JM. Evaluation and management of adrenal masses. Cancer Control 2002;9(4):326–334.

17. Metser U, Miller E, Lerman H, Lievshitz G, Avital S, Even-Sapir E. 18F-FDG PET/CT in the evaluation of adrenal masses. J Nucl Med 2006;47(1):32–37.

18. Jana S, Zhang T, Milstein DM, Isasi CR, Blaufox MD. FDG-PET and CT characterization of adrenal lesions in cancer patients. Eur J Nucl Med Mol Imaging 2006;33(1):29–35.

19. Shimizu A, Oriuchi N, Tsushima Y, et al. High (18F) 2-fluoro-2-deoxy-D-glucose (FDG) uptake of adrenocortical adenoma showing subclinical Cushing's syndrome. Ann Nucl Med 2003;17(5):403–406.

20. Rao SK, Caride VJ, Ponn R, Giakovis E, Lee SH. F-18 fluorodeoxyglucose positron emission tomography-positive benign adrenal cortical adenoma: imaging features and pathologic correlation. Clin Nucl Med 2004;29(5):300–302.

21. Basu S, Nair N. 18F-FDG uptake in bilateral adrenal hyperplasia causing Cushing's syndrome. Eur J Nucl Med Mol Imaging 2005;32(3):384.

22. Umeoka S, Koyama T, Saga T, et al. High 18F-fluorodeoxyglucose uptake in adrenal histoplasmosis: a case report. Eur Radiol 2005;15(12):2483–2486.

23. Minn H, Salonen A, Friberg J, et al. Imaging of adrenal incidentalomas with PET using (11)C-metomidate and (18)F-FDG. J Nucl Med 2004;45(6):972–979.

24. Kasperlik-Zeluska AA, Roslonowska E, Slowinska-Srzednicka J, et al. Incidentally discovered adrenal mass (incidentaloma): investigation and management of 208 patients. Clin Endocrinol (Oxf) 1997;46(1):29–37.

25. Plotz CM, Knowlton AI, Ragan C. The natural history of Cushing's syndrome. Am J Med 1952;13:597–614.

26. Drake WM, Perry LA, Hinds CJ, et al. Emergency and prolonged use of intravenous etomidate to control hypercortisolemia in a patient with Cushing's syndrome and peritonitis. J Clin Endocrinol Metab 1998;83:3542–3544.

27. Brandi ML, Gagel RF, Angeli A, et al. Guidelines for diagnosis and therapy of MEN type 1 and type 2. J Clin Endocrinol Metab 2001;86(12):5658–5671.

28. Wooten MD, King DK. Adrenal cortical carcinoma. Epidemiology and treatment with mitotane and a review of the literature. Cancer 1993;72:3145–3155.

29. Derneure MJ, Somberg LB. Functioning and non-functioning adrenocortical carcinoma: clinical presentation and therapeutic strategies. Surg Oncol Clin North Am 1998;7:791–805.

30. Kouriefs C, Mokbel K, Choy C. Is MRI more accurate than CT in estimating the real size of adrenal tumours? Eur J Surg Oncol 2001;27(5):487–490.

31. Icard P, Goudet P, Charpenay C, et al. Adrenocortical carcinomas: surgical trends and results of a 253–patient series from the French Association of Endocrine Surgeons study group. World J Surg 2001;25(7):891–897.

32. Allolio B, Hahner S, Weismann D, Fassnacht M. Management of adrenocortical carcinoma. Clin Endocrinol (Oxf) 2004;60(3):273–287.

33. Berruti A, Terzolo M, Sperone P, et al. Etoposide, doxorubicin and cisplatin plus mitotane in the treatment of advanced adrenocortical carcinoma: a large prospective phase II trial. Endocr Rel Cancer 2005;12:657–666.

34. Luton JP, Cerdas S, Billaud L, et al. Clinical features of adrenocortical carcinoma, prognostic factors, and the effect of mitotane therapy. N Engl J Med 1990;322:1195–1201.

35. Horstmann M, Merseburger AS, Stenzl A, Kuczyk M. Systemic therapy of malignant adrenal tumors. Urologe A 2006;45:605–608.

36. Erlandson RA, Reuter VE. Oncocytic adrenal cortical adenoma. Ultrastruct Pathol 1991;15(4–5):539–547.

37. Sasano H, Suzuki T, Sano T, et al. Adrenocortical oncocytoma. A true nonfunctioning adrenocortical tumor. Am J Surg Pathol 1991;15(10):949–956.

38. Neri LM, Nance FC. Management of adrenal cysts. Am Surg 1999;65(2):151–163.

39. Beard CM, Carney JA, Sheps SG, Lie JT, Kurland LT. Incidence of phaeochromocytoma. J Hum Hypertens 1989;3(6):481.

40. Donis-Keller H, Dou S, Chi D, et al. Mutations in the ret proto-oncogene are associated with MEN 2A and FMTC. Human Molecular Genetics 1993;2:851–856.

41. Eng C, Clayton D, Schuffenecker I, et al. The relationship between specific RET proto-oncogene mutations and disease phenotype in multiple endocrine neoplasia type 2. International RET mutation consortium analysis. JAMA 1996;276(19):1575–1579.

42. Latif F, Tory K, Guarra J, et al. Identification of the von Hippel-Lindau disease tumor suppressor gene. Science 1993;260:1317–1320.

43. Linehan WM, Walther Mc M, Zbar B. The genetic basis of cancer of the kidney. J Urol 2003;170:2163–2172.

44. Ilias I, Yu J, Carrasquillo JA, Chen CC, et al. Superiority of 6–(18F)-fluorodopamine positron emission tomography versus (131I)-metaiodobenzylguanidine scintigraphy in the localization of metastatic pheochromocytoma. J Clin Endocrinol Metab 2003;88(9):4083–4087.

45. Allison DJ, Brown MJ, Jones DH, Timmis JB. Role of venous sampling in locating a phaeochromocytoma. Br Med J 1983;286:1122–1124.

46. Vargas HI, Kavoussi LR, Bartlett DL, et al. Laparoscopic adrenalectomy: a new standard of care. Urology 1997;49(5):673–678.

47. Loh KC, Fitzgerald PA, Matthay KK, Yeo PP, Price DC. The treatment of malignant pheochromocytoma with iodine-131 metaiodobenzylguanidine (131I-MIBG): a comprehensive review of 116 reported patients. J Endocrinol Invest 1997;20(11):648–658.

48. Kulke MH, Stuart K, Enzinger PC, et al. Phase II study of temozolomide and thalidomide in patients with metastatic neuroendocrine tumors. J Clin Oncol 2006;24(3):401–406.

49. Averbuch SD, Steakley CS, Young RC, et al. Malignant pheochromocytoma: effective treatment with a combination of cyclophosphamide, vincristine and dacarbazine. Ann Intern Med 1988;109(4):267–273.

50. Edstrom EE, Hjelm Skog AL, Hoog A, Hamberger B. The management of benign and malignant pheochromocytoma and abdominal paraganglioma. Eur J Surg Oncol 2003;29(3):278–283.

16
Urothelial Tumors

16.1
Superficial Bladder Cancer

T.R. Leyshon Griffiths and J. Kilian Mellon

Epidemiology

Approximatley 357,000 new cases of bladder cancer were diagnosed worldwide in 2002, making this overall the ninth most common cancer (1). It is the fifth most common cancer in men and the eighth in women, and is three times as common in men as in women. The median age of presentation of bladder cancer is 70 years. In Europe and the United States, the incidence is typically higher in urban than in rural areas.

Risk Factors

The etiology of transitional cell carcinoma (TCC) of the bladder is dependent on chemical exposure from smoking and sometimes on occupation. Genetic polymorphisms for certain enzymes affect susceptibility. Other risk factors include pelvic radiotherapy for cervical cancer (two- to fourfold increased risk) (2,3), and cyclophosphamide treatment (ninefold increased risk) (4). Abuse of the analgesic phenacetin has also been linked with bladder cancer. A risk factor for squamous cell carcinoma of the bladder is keratinizing squamous metaplasia induced by stones, strictures, and infection by *Schistosoma haematobium*.

Smoking

Approximately two thirds of all bladder cancers may be related to tobacco smoking. The link between tobacco smoking and bladder cancer has been evident for more than four decades. In a meta-analysis of data from 43 studies, it was shown that current smokers face a threefold increased risk of developing urinary tract cancer compared with nonsmokers (5). The risk correlates with the number of cigarettes smoked, the duration of smoking, and the degree of inhalation of smoke. Within 4 years of ceasing, the risk of developing bladder cancer decreases by 30% to 60% (6). Tobacco smoke contains at

TABLE 16.1.1. Occupations associated with bladder cancer

Dye, cable textile, tire rubber, and leather workers
Painters/printers
Petroleum industry workers
Shoe manufacturers and cleaners
Hairdressers
Truck drivers
Drill-press operators
Rodent exterminators
Sewage workers

least 40 candidate carcinogens including nitrosamines, β-naphthylamine, and 4-aminobiphenyl.

Occupation

Approximately a fifth of bladder cancers may be attributable to occupational exposure to chemicals. Occupations associated with bladder cancer are outlined in Table 16.1.1.

In 1938, Heuper et al. (7) demonstrated that the aromatic amine β-naphthylamine could induce bladder cancer in dogs. Later, an epidemiological survey conducted by Case and Hosker (8) showed that exposure to α-naphthylamine, β-naphthylamine, and benzidine were the main factors associated with the development of bladder tumors. Some polycyclic aromatic hydrocarbons can also act as urinary tract hydrocarbons (9). Most carcinogens have an associated latent period of up to 20 years between exposure and the development of cancer.

Genetic Polymorphisms

Drug and carcinogen-metabolising enzymes are in part controlled by genetic polymorphism. Slow acetylation of N-acetyltransferase-2 (NAT2) (10,11), rapid CYP1A2 activity (12), and glutathione S-transferase (GST) M1 null genotype (11) are associated with an increased risk of TCC. Approximately 50% of Caucasians and 25% of Asians are slow acetylators of NAT2. Compared with NAT2 rapid or intermediate acetylators, NAT2 slow acetylators have a 40% increased risk of bladder cancer (10,11), which is stronger for cigarette smokers than for lifelong nonsmokers (11). The overall association of GSTM1 polymorphism and bladder cancer is not modified by smoking status (11).

Natural History

There are three different pathways in the history of bladder cancer following the initial treatment: patients may have no further recurrences; they may develop local recurrences; or they may progress to a local stage or develop distant metastases, which ultimatly leads to death. Local recurrence can occur on a single occasion or on multiple occasions.

The recurrences may be solitary or multifocal, but are usually of the same stage and grade as the primary tumor.

Of patients presenting with TCC, 70% have superficial tumors (50% Ta and 20% T1) not invading detrusor muscle, 5% have carcinoma in situ (Tis), and 25% have muscle-invasive tumors. Of newly diagnosed superficial bladder tumors, approximately 30% are multifocal at presentation, 60% to 70% will recur, and 10% to 20% will undergo stage progression to muscle-invasive or metastatic disease (13). Of newly diagnosed muscle-invasive tumors, 50% have occult nodal or systemic metastases that manifest within 12 months.

Pathogenesis

Molecular and Genetic Basis

Genetic alterations on chromosome 9 are an early event in bladder tumorogenesis. Chromosome 9 loss of heterozygosity (LOH) is found in more than 50% of all bladder tumors, regardless of stage and grade (14,15). Loss of function of tumor suppressor genes on both chromosome arms has been shown to contribute to tumor development.

There is now a well-defined model for the molecular pathogenesis of TCC that is consistent with clinical observations (16,17) (Fig. 16.1.1). Almost certainly, this is too simplistic, but it does provide a useful basis for further genetic studies. Mutations of the fibroblast growth factor receptor gene *(FGFR3)* on chromosome 4p and the *TP53* gene on chromosome 17p are almost mutually exclusive, each confined to one of the two major groups of TCC; low-grade superficial papillary (Ta) tumors usually harbor *FGFR3* but not *TP53* mutations, whereas carcinoma in situ (Tis) and invasive carcinomas (>T2) harbor *TP53* but not *FGFR3* mutations (16,17). However, there are several gaps in our current understanding and, for example, no significant differences have yet been found among Tis, muscle-invasive TCC, and the metastases that develop from them. Also, we are unsure if T1 tumors represent a distinct group, or are merely caught in their journey to muscle invasion.

Two theories have arisen from the observation that patients with bladder cancer often present with metachronous tumors that develop at different times and sites within the bladder: the field change (oligoclonal) and monoclonal theories (18). The field change theory attributes multifocality to individual transformation of epithelial cells at a number of sites where there is dysplasia or Tis.

In contrast, at least in some cases, molecular biological studies support a common clonal origin for concomitant urothelial tumors. This was first demonstrated in methylation studies of the X chromosome (19). For each of four female patients with multiple tumors, it was found that all the tumors from a given individual had inactivation of the same X chromosome. Lateral intra-

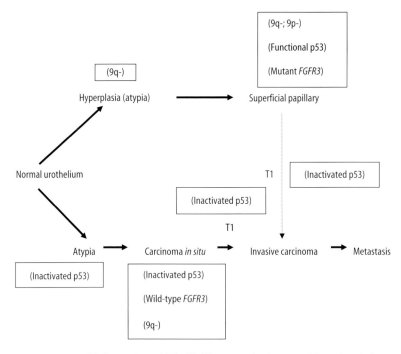

FIGURE 16.1.1. A simplified genetic model for bladder tumor development. Minus signs indicate copy number losses or loss of heterozygosity.

epithelial spread and dispersal of transformed cells are possible mechanisms underlying the monoclonal theory. Current evidence suggests that oligoclonal tumors might be more common in precursor lesions and early tumor stages. The frequent monoclonality found in patients with advanced tumors could be due to outgrowth of one tumor clone with specific genetic alterations (18).

Pathology

In Europe and the United States, almost all bladder cancers are TCC. Transitional cell epithelium lines the cavity of the renal pelvis, ureter, urinary bladder, and the proximal urethra. Transitional cell tumors of the bladder are approximately 50 times as common as those of the ureter or renal pelvis. Urothelial cancer sometimes contains squamous or glandular components. Pure squamous cell carcinoma is found in approximately 1% to 3% of cases, and pure adenocarcinomas are typically found in <1% of cases. Rarely, adenocarcinoma may arise in a urachal remnant. Small cell carcinoma comprises 0.5% to 1% of bladder tumors, and demonstrates an aggressive natural history. Other rare

FIGURE **16.1.2.** Carcinoma in situ of the
bladder. Hematoxylin and eosin Stain, ×25.
Cells show hyperchromatic nuclei with
varying size.

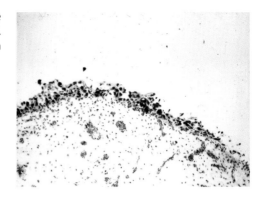

bladder cancers include sarcomas and malignant melanomas. Adenocarcinomas of the rectum, uterus, breast, ovary, and prostate may also metastasize to the bladder.

Carcinoma in situ (Cis, Tis) (Fig. 16.1.2) is charcaterized by flat and velvety erythematous patch with anaplastic urothelium. It may occur as a primary lesion or in association with superficial and muscle invasive tumors. Diagnosis is made by cytology and bladder biopsy. Its natural history is variable and it has the propensity to develop into invasive disease. Patients with Cis present with irritative bladder symptoms. Figure 16.1.2 shows variable thickness of the urothelium with cellular atypia. There is also loss of cellular denudation.

Preneoplastic Lesions

Keratinizing squamous metaplasia, detected in exstrophy, chronic bladder inflammation, and schistosomiasis is premalignant. Investigators supporting dysplasia as a premalignant condition cite the frequent coexistence of dysplastic and neoplastic lesions and the frequency of tumor recurrence and tumor progression among bladder cancer patients with dysplasia (20). One difficulty in interpreting the data is that dysplasia is often described interchangeably with Tis. Moreover, it is unclear whether dysplasia develops before or concomitantly with clinically manifest TCC.

Stage and Grade

Tumor Stage

The 2002 tumor, node, metastasis (TNM) classification of malignant tumors is currently recommended for the staging of bladder cancer (21) (Table 16.1.2; Fig. 16.1.3). Histological categories Ta, T1, and Tis are described as superficial bladder cancers.

TABLE 16.1.2. Tumor, mode, metastasis (TNM) classification of bladder cancer (2002)

T	*Primary tumor*
TX	Primary tumor cannot be assessed
T0	No evidence of primary tumor
Ta	Noninvasive papillary carcinoma
Tis	Carcinoma in situ
T1	Tumor invades subepithelial conective tissue
T2	Tumor invades muscle
T2a	Tumor invades superficial muscle (inner half)
T2b	Tumor invades deep muscle (outer half)
T3	Tumor invades perivesical tissue
T3a	Microscopically
T3b	Macroscopically (extravesical mass)
T4	Tumor invades any of the following: prostate, uterus, vagina, pelvic wall, abdominal wall
N	*Regional lymph nodes*
NX	Regional lymph nodes cannot be assessed
N0	No regional lymph node metastasis
N1	Metastasis in single lymph node ≤ 2 cm in diameter
N2	Metastasis in a single lymph node >2 cm to ≤ 5 cm in diameter/or multiple lymph nodes, none >5 cm in diameter
N3	Metastasis in a lymph node >5 cm in diameter
M	*Distant metastasis*
MX	Distant metastasis cannot be assessed
M0	No distant metastasis
M1	Distant metastases

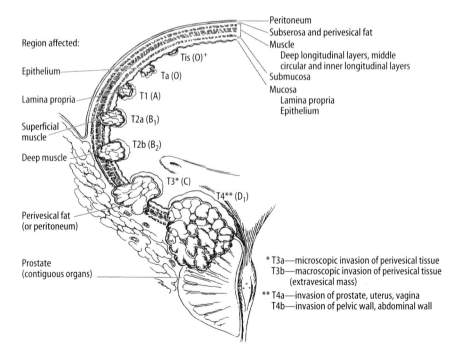

FIGURE 16.1.3. T staging of bladder cancer. (Adapted from Grossfield GD, Carroll PR. Urothelial carcinoma: cancers of the bladder, ureter, and renal pelvis. In: Tanagho EA, McAninch JW, eds. Smith's General Urology, 16th ed. New York: McGraw-Hill, 2004:324–345, with permission of McGraw-Hill.)

Subcategorization of T1 tumors based on depth of penetration relative to the muscularis mucosa has been proposed, but variability in interpretation among experienced uropathologists is a concern. Moreover, the muscularis mucosa is only apparent in 70% of cases anyway. Clinical staging is based on careful bimanual examination under anesthesia after resection. If the tumor is muscle-invasive, but there is no mass after resection, the clinical stage is T2. If despite apparent complete resection of the tumor there is a persistent mobile mass, the clinical stage is T3. If the mass is fixed or infiltrating the pelvic organs, the clinical stage is T4.

Histological Grade

Despite several more recent classifications, the favored histological grading system is still the 1973 World Health Organisation (WHO) classification (22). Tumor grade is the second important prognostic factor for TCC bladder. Tumors are classified into grades 1, 2, or 3 (G1, G2, and G3) based on the degree of nuclear anaplasia. G2 tumors are the heterogeneous group of tumors that include invasive and noninvasive lesions. Grade 3 tumors have a high risk of progression to muscle invasion particularly in association with Tis. Classifications that have not been widely adopted in the United Kingdom include a European classification (23), the 1998 WHO/International Society of Urological Pathology (ISUP) Consensus classification (24), and the 1999 WHO classification (25) (Fig. 16.1.4).

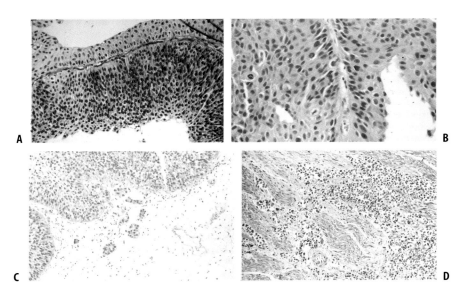

FIGURE 16.1.4. (A–C) Different grades of transitional cell carcinoma of the bladder. (D) Muscle infiltrating tumor. (A) Well differentiated TCC bladder × 25 grade 1. (B) TCC bladder × 25 G2pTa. (C) TCC bladder × 25 G3pT1 showing invasion of lamina propria. (D) TCC bladder × 25 G3pT2a showing tumor cells dispersed in the muscle layer. (Courtesy of Dr. Sohail Baithun, Royal London Hospital, London, UK.)

Clinical Features

The most common presenting symptom of bladder cancer is painless macroscopic hematuria, which is often intermittent. Approximately a quarter of adult patients with macroscopic hematuria are found to harbor bladder cancer. On the other hand, bladder cancer is detected in only 2% to 4% of adult patients with microscopic hematuria. The second most common symptom complex associated with bladder cancer is the overactive bladder syndrome, which manifests with irritative bladder symptoms. Around 5% of these patients are found to have bladder cancer, usually Tis or muscle-invasive types.

Investigations

Flexible/Rigid Cystoscopy

Cystoscopy remains the gold standard method for diagnosing new and recurrent bladder cancer.

Urine Cytology

Urine cytology was first described by Papanicolaou and Marshall (26) in 1945. The overall specificity is greater than 95% when obvious cancer cells are identified. However, the overall sensitivity of cytology in most series is only 30% to 50%. The main limitation is that low-grade tumors often shed cytologically normal-appearing cells. Urine cytology is more sensitive in patients with high-grade tumors and Tis.

New Urinary Tumor Markers

During the last decade, many new urine tumor markers have become available to aid the diagnosis of bladder cancer, but none has sufficient sensitivity to replace the need to perform a cystoscopy (27). In some centers, these tests are used to aid the decision making with regard to the frequency of surveillance cystoscopies. Point of care tests capable of being performed in the office include the the bladder tumor antigen (BTA) test and the BTA stat test. Quantitative immunoassays performed in the laboratory include the nuclear matrix protein-22 (NMP-22) immunoassay, the minichromosome maintenance protein-5 (Mcm-5) immunoassay, and the BTA-TRAK assay. A fluorescence-based cellular assay performed in the laboratory is the ImmunoCyt test.

Other investigational tests include the telomerase assay, hyaluronic acid and hyaluronidase tests, and microsatellite analysis of exfoliated urinary cells.

Intravenous Urography

This is particularly useful in examining the upper urinary tract for associated urothelial tumors or the identification of obstruction of the ureter. Approximately

5% of patients with a diagnosis of bladder cancer harbor synchronous or meta-chronous upper tract TCC. In contrast, 40% to 70% of patients diagnosed with uppper tract TCC will develop bladder TCC (see Fig. 3.1 in Chapter 3).

Cross-Sectional Imaging

Improvements in computed tomography (CT) technology, such as the develop-ment of multidetector row helical CT, have improved the resolution of CT with regard to local staging (28). Several trials have compared CT with magnetic resonance imaging (MRI) in the evaluation of bladder cancer. Although it is unclear which modality is superior, it is generally accepted that MRI produces higher resolution images of soft tissue, and potentially offers improved visual-ization of perivesical fat invasion (29). Neither MRI nor CT, however, is success-ful at distinguishing bladder cancer from inflammation following transurethral resection (TUR) of bladder tumor (28). With this caveat in mind, many centers now perform MRI before TUR if the tumor appears solid at the time of flexible cystoscopy. For the assessment of nodal and visceral metastases, CT of the abdomen and chest is preferred (see Figs. 3.12 and 3.16 in Chapter 3).

Progostic Factors

Clinical Prognostic Markers

Recurrence

In a multivariate analysis, Parmar et al. (30), on behalf of the Medical Research Council in the U.K., concluded that patients with superficial bladder cancer could be categorized into three groups according to the likelihood of recurrence after the first-check cystoscopy (30). Group 1 patients (about 60% of all new cases) present with a solitary tumor that does not recur at 3 months.

They have a low risk of recurrrence at 1 year (20%). Group 2 patients (about 30% of cases) present with a solitary tumor that recurs at 3 months, or present with multiple tumors withour recurrence at 3 months. Their risk of recurrence at 1 and 2 years is 40% and 60%, respectively. Group 3 patients (about 10% of cases) present with multiple tumors that recur at 3 months. They have a high likelihood of recurrence at 1 to 2 years (90%).

Progression

Superficial tumors show significant differences in their potential to progress. Patients with so-called high-risk superficial TCC are defined as those who harbor T1G3 TCC, TaG3 TCC, multifocal T1G2 TCC, and Tis (31); they are more likely to progress than those with other superficial tumors. Frequent disease recurrence is also associated with progression (32). Many series have shown the importance of histological grade in predicting rates of progression. The National

Bladder Cancer Collaborative Group (NBCCG) trial reported progression rates for grades 1, 2, and 3 of 2%, 11%, and 45%, respectively (33). The NBCCG also reported progression in only 3% of Ta tumors compared with 30% of T1 tumors. The likelihood of concomitant Tis is highest in those with high-grade tumors. Progression rates of approximately 77% have been reported when Tis and papillary tumors are noted together (34,35). Progression rates for untreated diffuse Tis and focal Tis are 58% and 8%, respectively (36). Tumor size >3 cm has also been correlated with poorer outcome (33).

In the European Organization for Research and Treatment of Cancer (EORTC) genitourinary analyses, the relative risk of disease progression has been assessed (32). In this multivariate analysis, the highest risk was in those with frequent disease recurrence followed by histological grade and size. T stage did not add independent prognostic value.

Multiplicity and Size of the Tumor

Multiple tumors and tumors greater than 3 cm have been shown to be risk factors of recurrence and progression (37).

Molecular Markers

A wide range of molecular alterations have been assessed, but, to date, none has sufficient power for routine use in the clinic (38).

Recurrence

An altered cytokeratin 20 staining pattern, markers associated with cell proliferation such as Ki67 labeling, four regions of LOH on chromosome 9, monosomy 9, wild-type *FGFR3*, low matrix metalloproteinase-9 (MMP-9)/tissue inhibitor of metalloproteinase-1 (TIMP-1) ratio, *CDKN2A*/p14 promoter methylation, *DAPK* (death-associated protein kinase) promoter methylation, reduced expression of E-cadherin, expression of the imprinted *H19* gene, and expression of survivin (an antiapoptotic protein) are associated with increased risk of recurrence. Perhaps the most promising marker to date is *FGFR3* mutation (39). The recurrence rate for tumors with *FGFR3* mutation appears lower than for tumors without mutation. In a recent study, combining *FGFR3* mutatation status and MIB-1 labeling was found to be superior to pathological grading for prediction of recurrence and progression (40).

Progression

Although many molecular alterations are associated with high tumor grade and advanced stage, they do not necessarily represent risk factors for progression from Ta TCC (38). For example, p53, Rb, EGFR, E-cadherin, and S100A4 are frequently dysregulated in bladder cancer and are independently associated with poor clinical outcome. However, most studies that have assessed these markers have grouped Ta and T1 tumors together, because few low-grade Ta tumors progress to muscle invasion. It is likely that in most cases, it is the T1 tumors that show molecular alterations.

Management of Superficial Bladder Cancer

Cystoscopic Surveillance

Based on Parmar's predictive model of tumor recurrence, a cystoscopic follow-up protocol was devised, which has been widely adopted (41). Patients at low risk of recurrence (group 1) can be followed safely by flexible cystoscopy at annual intervals.

For patients at intermediate risk of recurrence (group 2), flexible cystoscopic follow-up every 3 months is appropriate for the first year, and a course of adjuvant intravesical treatment may be considered. Patients in group 3 warrant rigid cystoscopy every 3 months in the first year with adjuvant courses of intravesical chemotherapy or immunotherapy.

In terms of longevity of follow-up, patients in group 1 who remain recurrence-free can be discharged after 5 years. Patients in groups 2 and 3 are usually discharged after 10 recurrence-free years.

Patients with Ta/T1G3 TCC, multifocal T1G2 TCC, or Tis have a high risk of not only recurrence but also progression to muscle-invasive TCC. They should be considered for intravesical maintenance bacille Calmette-Guérin (BCG) therapy and rigid cystoscopic follow-up every 3 months in the first year. In patients with T1G3 TCC, a re-resection at 6 weeks is recommended prior to commencing BCG. In one report, of 35 T1 cases with muscle present in the specimen, five (14%) were found to harbor muscle-invasive TCC at re-resection 2 to 6 weeks after the initial TUR (42). Moreover, these patients should also have deep TUR biopsies of their prostate as part of their initial staging. In a series of 489 men who had a radical cystoprostatectomy for TCC, 57 were staged T1 or less in the pathological specimen (P1); in this subset, the overall 5-year survival for those with prostatic stromal TCC was 64% compared with 79% for those with no prostatic TCC. The survival of patients with P1 TCC and prostatic stromal invasion was similar to that in those with muscle-invasive TCC with no stromal invasion (63%) (43).

Principles of Cystoscopy

The examination starts with bimanual vaginal or rectal examination of the bladder (and prostate in men) to note the mobility of the bladder and presence of any palpable mass or thickening. The urethra is then visualized with a 0-, 12-, or 30-degree telescope for abnormal areas, tumors, and stricture. Once the urinary bladder is entered, irrigation is stopped and the whole of the bladder is visualized without overdistending the bladder with the 70-degree telescope. The size and positions of the tumors are noted; flat, sessile, or ulcerated lesions are likely to be of higher grade and stage. Transurethral resection is carried out in two stages: whole of the tumor and base of the tumor. The two specimens are sent separately for laboratory analysis to facilitate correct pathological staging.

Bladder Mapping

Guidelines from the European Association of Urology state that random biopsies of normal mucosa are indicated in the presence of positive cytology, or if a tumor is solid in appearance (44). However, this recommendation is not without controversy. In patients with solitary papillary tumors, the rate of detection of abnormalities is approximately 4%; only 1% show Tis (45). There is a consensus that in these patients random biopsies of normal mucosa is not indicated. Indeed, there is a theoretical risk of reimplantation if they are performed.

There is agreement on the rate of abnormalities detected in random biopsies in patients with multifocal tumors, but there is disagreement on whether information arising from these biopsies would have changed management. In both the EORTC 30911 (45) and American (46) studies, the normal mucosa of patients with superficial bladder tumors at intermediate or high risk of recurrence (multifocal or recurrent tumors) was abnormal in 12%.

There were differences, though, in the detection of Tis (3% in the EORTC study versus 7% in the American study). However, it is questionable in European practice if management would have been changed in most cases, because many of these patients would be treated with adjuvant intravesical immunotherapy anyway.

This controversy using white light cystoscopy is currently being superseded by technology utilizing fluorescence cystosocopy; the latter has better sensitivity and specificity for Tis, and enables a more complete TUR. A randomized prospective trial compared TUR with fluorescence cystoscopy to white light cystoscopy (47). The intravesical agent used to label bladder tumors was 5-aminolevulinic acid (5-ALA). Recurrence-free intervals after 12 and 24 months were 90% and 90%, respectively, in the fluorescence cystoscopy group, compared with 74% and 66% in the white light cystoscopy group ($p = .004$). The superiority proved to be independent of risk groups for recurrence. Fluorescence cystoscopy was used for initial diagnosis but not for any of the follow-up visits.

A variety of intravesical fluorophores have been tested. Indeed, hexylester has been compared with 5-ALA and found to have superior fluorescence at 2 hours after instillation (48).

Intravesical Chemotherapy

The aim of the intravesical treatment is to prevent or delay the recurrence or progression. There is no evidence to suggest the superiority of one drug over other agents. Thio-TEPA (N,N',N''-triethylenethiophosphoramide), an alkylating agent, was the first cytotoxic agent used for intravesical therapy. The major systemic side effect was myelosuppression. Subsequently doxorubicin, an anthracycline and its derivative epirubicin (4′-epidoxorubicin) were used intravesically for 4 to 8 weeks. Now a single instillation of epirubicin (50 mg/50 mL) (49) or mitomycin C (40 mg/40 mL) (50) given within 24 hours of TUR of newly diagnosed bladder tumors has been shown to reduce tumor recurrence equally effectively. Four further instillations of mitomycin C administered after each check cystoscopy were not significantly better than a single instillation (50). In patients at low risk of tumor recurrence, intravesical mitomycin C and BCG are equivalent (51,52). However, mitomycin C is the preferred agent because of its lower toxicity. In a meta-analysis of phase III European trials, intravesical chemotherapy did not prevent progression (53). Phase II studies of intravesical gemcitabine, an antimetabolite have shown complete response rates comparable to, if not better than, those reported in previous similar studies on BCG and other chemotherapeutic agents (54). Moreover, its tolerability profile is excellent. However, its role in the management of superficial bladder cancer depends on its long-term durability data and cost-related issues.

Intravesical Immunotherapy

Bacille Calmette-Guérin

Mechanism of Antitumor Effect

To date, the precise mechanism of action of intravesical BCG remains unknown. Regardless of its target, it is certain that BCG exerts its antitumor effects through immune mechanisms since an immunocompetent host is required for such effects (55).

Significantly, both T-cell–deficient and natural killer (NK)-cell–deficient mice respond poorly to BCG therapy (56). Bacille Calmette-Guérin behaves as a nonspecific immune stimulant and activates a variety of cell types including dendritic cells, macrophages, T lymphocytes, B lymphocytes, and NK cells. The differentiation of naive CD4-positive T cells into the T-helper type-1 (Th1) subset is indispensable for successful treatment of superficial bladder cancer with BCG (57).

The mycobacteria are thought to bind to the bladder wall via the interaction between the bacterial antigen 85 complex and fibronectin (58). In one model, fibronectins bound to BCG bind $\alpha_5\beta_1$ integrins present on bladder cancer cells (Fig. 16.1.5).

Cross-linking of $\alpha_5\beta_1$ receptors initiates signal transduction within bladder cancer cells (59). A likely scenario is that exposure to BCG acts as a danger signal enhancing antigen presentation by means of local dendritic cell activation (60). The activated dendritic cells may then migrate to local lymph nodes where peptides of BCG and TCC origin are presented to T lymphocytes. Activated T lymphocytes then migrate to the urothelium and lyse TCC cells, either

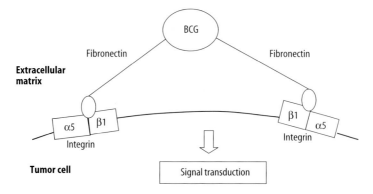

FIGURE 16.1.5. Bacille Calmette-Guérin (BCG) cross-links $\alpha_5\beta_1$ integrin on bladder tumor cells.

directly through the CD8-positive population or indirectly by activating NK cells.

Indications

Intravesical BCG should be administered to patients with so-called high-risk superficial TCC, which is defined as those with Ta/T1G3 TCC, Tis, and recurrent multifocal Ta/T1 TCC.

For these patients, the potential toxicity associated with BCG is outweighed by the potential benefits of preventing tumor recurrence (61,62) and progression (63,64). In those with Tis, a meta-analysis showed that the complete response to BCG was superior to that of mitomycin C (70% versus 40%) (64,65).

In a recent meta-analysis of nine randomized trials including 700 patients with Tis, the risk of progression was reduced by 26% in those on maintenance BCG (66).

Local Side Effects

The commonest side effects are low-grade fever (<38.5°C) and cystitis, which usually subside within 48 hours.

Complications

Allergic reactions to BCG are uncommon (<1% of cases); they include arthritis, conjunctivitis, and skin rashes. Allergic reactions can usually be treated with nonsteroidal antiinflammatory drugs (NSAIDs). In cases refractory to NSAIDs, oral steroids should be considered.

Systemic Complications. Generalized "BCG-itis" is the most serious systemic complication arising from hematogenous spread of BCG. It requires urgent treatment with four-agent antituberculous therapy. These patients usually have a high fever (>38.5°C) with impaired hemodynamic status. Systemic complications are rare provided that certain precautions are followed. Intravesical BCG should not be given within 14 days of TUR, or if there is an active urinary tract infection, frank hematuria, traumatic catheterization, or immunodeficiency. Coadministration of prophylactic isoniazid does not reduce toxicity (67).

The optimal dose remains unknown. A number of trials have compared the efficacy and toxicity of reduced doses of BCG with full doses. In a study of one-third versus full-dose BCG (68), the reduced-dose schedule did not compromise efficacy and fewer patients reported toxicity. However, the incidence of severe systemic toxicity was not reduced.

Optimal Strain

There is currently no evidence to suggest that BCG strains differ in clinical efficacy. In a meta-analysis, five different strains of BCG were included: Tice, Connaught, Pasteur, RIVM, and A. Frappier (63). Their ability to prevent progression was similar.

Maintenance Therapy

Many urologists are reluctant to use maintenance schedules of intravesical BCG for patients with superficial bladder cancer. Skeptics cite poor compliance rates of only 16% (69), and a perception that adverse events increase with further instillations.

However, a pivotal meta-analysis of 24 randomized trials carried out by the EORTC has shown that maintenance BCG but not a single induction course of BCG instillations prevents or delays progression (63). A 37% reduction in the odds of progression was observed for the 20 trials in which a maintenance BCG regimen was given. In another meta-analysis comparing the therapeutic efficacies of BCG and mitomycin C, only maintenance BCG prevented progression (64). The majority of local and systemic side effects are seen during the induction and first half-year of maintenance (70).

Clearly, a maintenance schedule of BCG is needed for optimal efficacy, but the precise regimen to achieve this remains unknown. Many different schedules have been employed, ranging from a total of 10 installations given over 18 weeks to 27 installations given over 3 years. Both the EORTC Genitourinary Group and the South West Oncology Group (SWOG) have given 27 installations over 3 years in their trials. Current evidence suggests that BCG schedules lasting at least 1 year are needed to prevent progression (63).

Intravesical Combined Chemoimmunotherapy

Several investigators have tested the hypothesis that combined chemoimmuno-therapy is more effective and less toxic than conventional chemotherapy or BCG alone.

To date, chemoimmunotherapy schedules have not been shown to improve effectiveness, but may be better tolerated. A phase III trial compared the efficacy of a sequential mitomycin C and BCG protocol with mitomycin C alone in patients with intermediate and high-risk superficial papillary bladder cancer. The sequential schedule was comparable with mitomycin C alone in terms of efficacy and toxicity (71). A subsequent study compared sequential epirubicin and BCG with BCG alone in patients with Ta/T1 TCC. The sequential protocol was comparable with BCG alone in efficacy and superior in terms of toxicity (72). More recently, a Nordic study has compared alternating mitomycin C and BCG instillations with BCG alone in the treatment of Tis. Alternating therapy was shown to be less effective but better tolerated than BCG monotherapy (73).

Transitional Cell Carcinoma Refractory to Bacille Calmette-Guérin

Interferon-α_{2b}

At present, intravesical BCG with interferon (IFN) appears to be the most effective salvage therapy for patients whose disease is refractory to BCG (74). Interferons are host-produced glycoproteins that are classified into three broad types: IFN-α, IFN-γ, and IFN-β. Interferon-α_{2b} is the most extensively studied IFN, and is most active intravesically at doses of 50 to 100 million units. Interferons stimulate NK cells, induce expression of class I major histocompatibility complex antigen, and increase antibody responsiveness. They exhibit immunomodulatory, antitumor, antiangiogenic, and antiproliferative properties. Although IFN as a single agent is not beneficial in bladder cancer, combinations of BCG and IFN-α_{2b} have demonstrated synergism (74–76). Moreover, the favorable toxicity profile of IFN-α_{2b} has allowed a reduction in the BCG dose with subsequent reduction in BCG-related toxicity.

Interim results from a multicenter phase II trial of combination BCG plus IFN-α_{2b} administered as a maintenance regimen to BCG-failure ($n = 231$) and BCG-naive ($n = 259$) patients have been published (74). After an induction course of six installations once a week, patients underwent maintenance cycles consisting of three installations once a week at 3, 9, and 15 months. Disease-free rates at 24 months were 42% for BCG-failure patients and 57% for BCG-naive patients. Patients in the BCG-failure group were treated with reduced-BCG dose plus 50 million units of IFN-α_{2b} throughout.

The dose reduction was either one-third dose BCG or one-tenth dose BCG depending on tolerance to BCG. Other investigators have reported similar encouraging results utilizing BCG/IFN protocols for patients with BCG failure. In a study of 12 BCG-failure patients, the tumor-free rate at 1 year was 50% (74); in another study of 22 BCG-failure patients, 60% were tumor-free after a median follow-up of 22 months (76).

A large phase III trial is underway comparing the efficacy of BCG to BCG plus IFN-α_{2b} as first-line therapy.

Bropiramine

In the 1990s, bropirimine emerged as a promising oral nonspecific immune response modulator in the treatment of superficial bladder cancer. This arylpyrimidinone could be absorbed orally and excreted in the urine. It induced IFNs, interleukin-1 (IL-1), and tumor necrosis factor, as well as stimulating B-cell proliferation, macrophage activity, NK cells, and lymphokine-activated killer cells. In one study, a complete response to bropirimine was observed in approximately 32% of patients with BCG-refractory or BCG–intolerant Tis (77). In a subsequent phase III trial conducted to compare oral bropirimine with intravesical BCG in patients with BCG-naive Tis, 92% of patients in the bropirimine arm were tumor-free after a mean follow-up of 12.6 months; this was similar to results in the BCG arm (78). However, subsequent monitoring revealed that bropirimine was associated with significant cardiotoxicity. Consequently, it is no longer available for general use or clinical trials.

Keyhole-Limpet Hemocyanin

The first clinical use of keyhole-limpet hemocyanin (KLH) in the immuno-therapy of superficial bladder cancer was described by Olsson et al. (79) in 1974. They observed a decreased rate of recurrence after treatment with KLH. Keyhole-limpet hemocyanin, a nonspecific immune response modifier, is a highly anti-genic extracellullar copper-containing respiratory protein. It is extracted and purified from the hemolymph of *Megathura crenulata*, a sea mollusk collected off the southern California coast. Subsequent studies have shown that although the toxicity of KLH is minimal, intravesical KLH is less effective than BCG. In a prospective randomized trial of 42 patients, recurrence rates were 41% for KLH compared with 14% for BCG after a follow-up of 20 months (80). In patients with residual papillary TCC after BCG, the overall complete response to KLH was only 26% (81). However, response rates to KLH for Tis refractory to BCG were higher. Of 18 patients with Tis without associated Ta or T1 TCC, nine (50%) had a complete response (81). The role of KLH in combination with BCG has not been investigated.

Other Conservative Treatments for Transitional Cell Carcinoma Refractory to Bacille Calmette-Guérin

In the largest series of BCG-refractory patients with Tis, complete response rates of 19 of 90 (21%) on valrubicin (82), and 21 of 36 (58%) and 13 of 27 (48%) on photodynamic therapy (83,84) have been reported. A phase I study of intravesical gemcitabine included 18 BCG-refractory patients, 14 of whom had Tis (85). Seven of the 18 (39%) had a complete response.

Role of Cystectomy for Superficial Bladder Cancer

Younger patients with multifocal T1 TCC and concomitant Tis should be given the option of primary cystectomy. For those who adopt a bladder-preserving strategy, response to intravesical BCG is best assessed at 6 months. In these patients, the purpose of the 3-month check cystoscopy is to exclude early progression to muscle-invasive TCC.

Further support for this concept can be found in the SWOG maintenance trial. After six instillations of BCG for Tis, 70% of patients were tumor free. Following three further instillations, the complete response rate increased to 82% (69). Patients with persistent high-grade TCC, Tis, or multifocal TCC after nine instillations of BCG are considered to be BCG-refractory, and should be offered radical cystectomy.

References

1. Parkin DM, Bray F, Ferlay J, Pisani P. Global cancer statistics 2002. CA Cancer J Clin 2005;55:74–108.
2. Duncan RE, Bennett DW, Evans AT, et al. Radiation-induced bladder tumours. J Urol 1977;118:43–45.
3. Sella A, Dexeus FH, Chong C, et al. Radiation therapy-associated invasive bladder tumours. Urology 1989;33:185–188.
4. Fairchild WV, Spence CR, Solomon HD, et al. The incidence of bladder cancer after cyclophosphamide therapy. J Urol 1979;122:163–164.
5. Zeegers MP, Tan FE, Dorant E, et al. The impact of characteristics of cigarette smoking on urinary tract cancer risk: a meta-analysis of epidemiologic studies. Cancer 2000; 89:630–639.
6. Hartge P, Siverman D, Hoover R, et al. Changing cigarette habits and bladder cancer risk:a case-control study. J Natl Cancer Inst 1987;78:1119–1125.
7. Heuper WC, Wiley FH, Wolfe HD. Experimental production of bladder tumours in dogs by administration of beta-naphthylamine. J Ind Hyg Toxicol 1938;20:46–84.
8. Case RAM, Hosker ME. Tumour of the urinary tract as an occupational disease in the rubber industry in England and Wales. Br J Prev Soc Med 1954;8:39–50.
9. BAUS Subcommittee on Industrial Bladder Cancer. Occupational bladder cancer: a guide for physicians. Br J Urol 1988;61:183–191.
10. Marcus PM, Vineis P, Rothman N. NAT2 slow acetylationand bladder cancer risk: a meta-analysis of 22 case-control studies conducted in the general population. Pharmacogenetics 2000;10:115–122.
11. Garcia-Closas M, Malats N, Silverman D, et al. NAT2 slow acetylation, GSTM1 null genotype, and risk of bladder cancer: results from the Spanish Bladder Cancer Study and meta-analyses. Lancet 2005;366:649–659.
12. Lee SW, Jang IJ, Shin SG, et al. CYP1A2 activity as a risk factor for bladder cancer. J Korean Med Sci 1994;9:482–489.
13. Lutzeyer W, Rubben H, Dahm H. Prognostic parameters in superficial bladder cancer: an analysis of 315 cases. J Urol 1982;127:250–252.
14. Tsai YC, Nichols PW, Hiti AL, et al. Allelic losses of chromosomes 9, 11 and 17 in human bladder cancer. Cancer Res 1990;50:44–47.
15. Cairns P, Shaw ME, Knowles MA. Initiation of bladder cancer may involve deletion of a tumour-suppressor gene on chromosome 9. Oncogene 1993;8:1083–1085.
16. Bakkar AA, Wallerand H, Radvanyi F, et al. FGFR3 and TP53 gene mutations define two distinct pathways in urothelial cell carcinoma of the bladder. Cancer Res 2003; 63:8108–8112.
17. van Rhijn BW, van der Kwast TH, Vis AN, et al. FGFR3 and P53 characterise alternative genetic pathways in the pathogenesis of urothelial cell carcinoma. Cancer Res 2004;64:1911–1914.

18. Hafner C, Knuechel R, et al. Clonality of multifocal urothelial carcinomas: 10 years of molecular genetic studies. Int J Cancer 2002;101:1–6.

19. Sidransky D, Von Eshenbach A, Oyau R, et al. Clonal origin bladder cancer. N Engl J Med 1992;326:737–740.

20. Cheng L, Cheville JC, Neumann RM, et al. Natural history of urothelial dysplasia of the bladder. Am J Surg Pathol 1999;23:443–447.

21. Sobin LH, Wittekind C, eds. Union Internationale Contre le Cancer. TNM Classification of Malignant Tumours, 6th ed. New York: Wiley-Liss, 2002.

22. Mostofi F. International histologic classification of tumours. A report by the Executive Committee of the International Council of Societies of Pathology. Cancer 1973; 33:1480–1484.

23. Pauwels RP, Smeetes AW, Schapers RF, et al. Grading in superficial bladder cancer. Morphological criteria. Br J Urol 1988;61:135–139.

24. Epstein JI, Amin MB, Reuter VR, et al. World Health Orgainisation/International Society of Urological Pathology Consensus Classification of Urothelial (Transitional Cell) Neoplasms of the Urinary Bladder. Am J Surg Pathol 1998;22:1435–1448.

25. Mostofi FK, Davis CJ, Sesterhenn IA, et al., eds. Histological Typing of Urinary Bladder Tumours. World Health Organisation International Histological Classification of tumours, 2nd ed. New York: Springer, 1999.

26. Papanicolaou GN, Marshall VF. Urine sediment smears as a diagnostic procedure in cancers of the urinary tract. Science 1945;101:519.

27. Quek ML, Sanderson K, Daneshmand S, et al. New molecular markers for bladder cancer detection. Curr Opin Urol 2004;14:259–264.

28. Kim JK, Park SY, Ahn HJ, et al. Bladder cancer:analysis of multi-detector row helical CT enhancement pattern and accuracy in tumour detection and perivesical staging. Radiology 2004;231:725–731.

29. Mallampati GK, Siegelman ES. MR imaging of the bladder. Magn Reson Imaging Clin North Am 2004;12:545–555.

30. Parmar MK, Freedman LS, Hargreave TB, Tolley DA. Prognostic factors for recurrence and follow-up policies in the treatment of superficial bladder cancer: report from the British Medical Research Council Subgroup on Superficial bladder Cancer (Urological Cancer Working Party). J Urol 1989;142:284–288.

31. Millan-Rodriguez F, Chechile-Toniolo G, Salvador-Bayarri, et al. Primary superficial bladder cancer risk groups according to progression, mortality and recurrence. J Urol 2000;164:690–691.

32. Kurth KH, Denis L, et al. Factors affecting recurrence and progression in superficial bladder tumours. Eur J Cancer 1995;31A:1840–1846.

33. Heney NM, Ahmed S, Flanagan MJ, et al. Superficial bladder cancer: progression and recurrence. J Urol 1983;130:1083–1086.

34. Althausen AF, Prout GR Jr, Daly JJ. Non-invasive papillary carcinoma of the bladder associated with carcinoma in siu. J Urol 1976;116:575–580.

35. Herr HW, Wartinger DD, Fair WR, et al. Bacillus Calmette-Guerin therapy for superficial bladder cancer: a 10-year followup. J Urol 1992;147:1020–1023.

36. Riddle PR, Chisholm GD, Trott PA, et al. Flat carcinoma in situ of bladder. Br J Urol 1975;47:829–833.

37. Millán-Rodriguez F, Chechile-Toniolo G, Bayyari-Salvador J, et al. Multivariate analysis of the prognostic factors of primary superficial bladder cancer. J Urol 2000; 163:73–78.

38. Knowles MA. Molecular biology of bladder cancer. In: Waxman J, ed. Urological Cancers. London: Springer-Verlag, 2005:115–130.

39. van Rhijn BW, Lurkin I, Radvanyi F, et al. The fibroblast growth factor receptor 3 (FGFR3) mutation is a strong indicator of superficial bladder cancer with low recurrence rate. Cancer Res 2001;61:1265–1268.
40. van Rhijn BW, Vis AN, van der Kwast TH, et al. Molecular grading of urothelial cell carcinoma with fibroblast growth factor receptor 3 and MIB-1 is superior to pathologic grade fro the prediction of clinical outcome. J Clin Oncol 2003;21: 1912–1921.
41. Hall R, Parmar M, Richards A, et al. Proposal for changes in cystoscopic follow up of patients with bladder cancer and adjuvant intravesical chemotherapy. BMJ 1994; 308:257–260.
42. Herr H. The value of second transurethral resection in evaluating patients with bladder tumours. J Urol 1999;162:74–76.
43. Esrig D, Freeman J, Elmanjian D, et al. Transitional cell carcinoma involving the prostate with a proposed staging classification for stromal invasion. J Urol 1996;156: 1071–1076.
44. Oosterlinck W, Lobel B, Jakse G, et al. Guidelines on bladder cancer. Eur Urol 2002; 41:105–112.
45. van der Meijden A, Oosterlinck W, Brausi M, et al. Members of the EORTC GU Group Superficial Bladder Committee. Significance of bladder biopsies in Ta, T1 bladder tumours: a report from the EORTC Genito-Urinary Tract Cancer Cooperative Group. Eur Urol 1999;35:267–271.
46. May F, Treiber U, Hartung R, et al. Significance of random bladder biopsies in superficial bladder cancer. Eur Urol 2003;44:47–50.
47. Filbeck T, Pichlmeier U, Knuechel R, et al. Clinically relevant improvement of recurrence-free survival with 5-aminolevulinic acid induced fluorescence diagnosis in patients with superficial bladder tumours. J Urol 2002;168:67–71.
48. Marti A, Jichlinski P, Lange N, et al. Comparison of aminolevulinic acid and hexylester aminolevulinate induced proto-porphyrin IX distribution in human bladder cancer. J Urol 2003;170:428–432.
49. Oosterlinck W, Kurth K, Schroder F, et al. A prospective European Organisation for Research and treatment of Cancer Genitourinary Group randomized trial comparing transurethral resection followed by a single intravesical instillation of epirubicin or water in single stage Ta, T1 papillary carcinoma of the bladder. J Urol 1993;149: 749–752.
50. Tolley D, Parmar M, Grigor K, et al. The effect of intravesical mitomycin C on recurrence of newly diagnosed superficial bladder cancer: a further report with 7 years of followup. J Urol 1996;155:1233–1238.
51. Vegt P, Witjes J, Witjes W, et al. A randomized study of intravesical mitomycin C, bacillus Calmette-Guerin Tice and bacillus Calmette-Guerin RIVM treatment in pTa-pT1 papillary carcinoma and carcinoma in situ of the bladder. J Urol 1995;153: 929–933.
52. Krege S, Giani G, Meyer R, et al. A randomized multicentre trial of adjuvant therapy in superficial bladder cancer: transurethral resection only versus transurethral resection plus mitomycin C versus transurethral resection plus bacillus Calmette-Guerin. Participating Clinics. J Urol 1996;156:962–966.
53. Pawinski A, Sylvester R, Kurth K, et al. A combined analysis of European Organisation for Research and Treatment of Cancer, and Medical Research Council randomized controlled trials for the prophylactic treatment of stage TaT1 bladder cancer. European Organisation for Research and Treatment of Cancer Genitourinary Tract

Cancer Cooperative Group and the Medical Research Council Working Party on superficial bladder cancer. J Urol 1996;156:1934–1940.

54. Gontero P, Casetta G, Maso G, et al. Phase II study to investigate the ablative efficacy of intravesical administration of gemcitabine in intermediate-risk superficial bladder cancer (SBC). Eur Urol 2004;46:339–343.

55. Ratliff T, Gillen D, Catalona W. Requirement of a thymus dependent immune response for BCG-mediated antitumour activity. J Urol 1987;137:155–159.

56. Brandau S, Riemensberger J, Jacobsen M, et al. NK cells are essential for effective BCG immunotherapy. Int J Cancer 2001;92:697–702.

57. Saint F, Patard J, Maille P, et al. T helper 1/2 lymphocyte urinary cytokine profiles in responding and nonresponding patients after 1 and 2 courses of bacillus Calmette-Guerin for superficial bladder cancer. J Urol 2001;166:2142–2147.

58. Zlotta A, Drowart A, Van Vooren J, et al. Evolution and clinical significance of the T cell proliferative and cytokine response directed against the fibronectin binding antigen 85 complex of bacillus Calmette Guerin during intravesical treatment of superficial bladder cancer. J Urol 1997;157:492–498.

59. Chen F, Zhang G, Iwamoto Y, et al. Bacillus Calmette-Guerin initiates intracellular signalling in a transitional cell line by cross-linking alpha 5 beta 1 integrin. J Urol 2003;170:605–610.

60. Matzinger P. An innate sense of danger. Semin Immunol 1998;10:399–415.

61. Shelly M, Wilt T, Court J, et al. Intravesical bacillus Calmette-Guerin is superior to mitomycin C in reducing tumour recurrence in high-risk superficial bladder cancer: a meta-analysis of randomized trials. BJU Int 2004;93:485–490.

62. Lundholm C, Norlen B, Ekman P. A randomized prospective study comparing long-term intravesical instillations of mitomycin C and bacillus Calmette-Guerin in patients with superficial bladder carcinoma. J Urol 1996;156:372–376.

63. Sylvester R, van der Meijden A, Lamm D. Intravesical bacillus Calmette-Guerin reduces the risk of progression in patients with superficial bladder cancer: a meta-analysis of the published results of randomised clinical trials. J Urol 2002;168:1964–1970.

64. Bohle A, Bock P. Intravesical bacille Calmette-Guerin versus mitomycin C in superficial bladder cancer: formal meta-analysis of comparative studies on tumour progression. Urology 2004;63:682–686.

65. Bouffioux C. Intravesical adjuvant treatment in superficial bladder cancer. A review of the question after 15 years of experience with the EORTC GU group. Scand J Urol Nephrol Suppl 1991;138:167–177.

66. Sylvester RJ, van der Meijden AP, Witjes JA, et al. Bacillus Calmette-Guerin versus chemotherapy for the intravesical treatment of patients with carcinoma in situ of the bladder: a meta-analysis of the published results of randomized trials. J Urol 2005;174:86–91.

67. Vegt P, van der Meijden A, Sylvester R, et al. Does isoniazid reduce side effects of intravesical bacillus Calmette-Guerin therapy in superficial bladder cancer? Interim results of European Organisation for Research and Treatment of Cancer Protocol 30911. J Urol 1997;157:1246–1249.

68. Martinez Pineiro J, Flores N, et al. Long-term follow-up of a randomised prospective trial comparing a standard 81 mg dose of intravesical bacillus Calmette-Guerin with a reduced dose of 27 mg in superficial bladder cancer. BJU Int 2002;89:671–680.

69. Lamm DL, Blumenstein B, Crissman J, et al. Maintenance bacillus Calmette-Guerin immunotherapy for recurrent Ta, T1 and carcinoma in situ transitional cell carcinoma of the bladder: a randomised Southwest Oncology study. J Urol 2000;163:1124–1129.

70. van der Meijden A, Sylvester R, Oosterlinck W, et al. Maintenance bacillus Calmette-Guerin for Ta T1 bladder tumours is not associated with increased toxicity: results from a European Organisation for Research and Treatment of Cancer Genito-Urinary Group Phase III trial. Eur Urol 2003;44:429–434.

71. Witjes J, Caris C, Mungan N, et al. Results of a randomized phase III trial of sequential intravesical therapy with mitomycin C and bacillus Calmette-Guerin versus mitomycin C alone in patients with superficial bladder cancer. J Urol 1998, 160:1668–1671.

72. Ali-El-Dein B, Nabeeh A, Ismail El-H, et al. Sequential bacillus Calmette-Guerin and epirubicin versus bacillus Calmette-Guerin alone for superficial bladder tumours: a randomized prospective study. J Urol 1999, 162:339–342.

73. Kaasinen E, Wijkstrom H, Malmstrom P-U, et al. Alternating mitomycin C and BCG instillations versus BCG alone in treatment of carcinoma in situ of the urinary bladder: a Nordic study. Eur Urol 2003;43:637–645.

74. O'Donnell M, Lilli K, Leopold C. Interim results from a national multicentre phase II trial of combination BCG plus interferon-α-2b for superficial bladder cancer. J Urol 2004;172:888–893.

75. Punnen S, Chin J, Jewett M. Management of bacillus Calmette-Guerin (BCG) refractory superficial bladder cancer: results with intravesical BCG and interferon combination therapy. Can J Urol 2003;10:1790–1795.

76. Lam J, Benson M, O'Donnell M, et al. Bacillus Calmette-Guerin plus interferon-alpha-2b intravesical therapy maintains an extended treatment plan for superficial bladder cancer with minimal toxicity. Urol Oncol 2003;21:354–360.

77. Sarosdy M, Manyak M, Sagalowsky A, et al. Oral bropirimine immunotherapy of bladder carcinoma in situ after prior intravesical bacille Calmette-Guerin. Urology 1998;51:226–231.

78. Witjes W, Konig M, Boeminghaus F, et al. Results of a European comparative randomized study comparing oral bropirimine versus intravesical BCG treatment in BCG-naive patients with carcinoma in situ of the urinary bladder. European Bropirimine Study Group. Eur Urol 1999;36:576–581.

79. Olsson C, Chute R, Rao C. Immunologic reduction of bladder cancer recurrence rate. J Urol 1974;111:173–176.

80. Kable T, Mohring K, Ikinger U, et al. Intravesical prevention of recurrence of superficial urinary bladder cancer with BCG and KLH. A prospective randomised srudy. Urologe A 1991:118–121.

81. Lamm D, DeHaven J, Riggs D. Keyhole limpet hemocyanin immunotherapy of bladder cancer: laboratory and clinical studies. Eur Urol 2000;37(suppl 3):41–44.

82. Herr H, Dalbagni G. Defining bacillus Calmette-Guerin refractory superficial bladder tumours. J Urol 2003;169:1706–1708.

83. Nseyo UO, Shumaker B, Klein EA, et al. Photodynamic therapy using porfimer sodium as an alternative to cystectomy in patients with refractory transitional cell carcinoma in situ of the bladder. Bladder Photofrin Study Group. J Urol 1998;160:39–44.

84. Manyak MJ, Ogan K. Photodynamic therapy for refractory superficial bladder cancer: long-term clinical outcomes of single treatment using intravesical diffusion medium. J Endourol 2003;17:633–639.

85. Dalbagni G, Russo P, Sheinfield J, et al. Phase I trial of intravesical gemcitabine in bacillus Calmette-Guerin refractory transitional cell carcinoma of the bladder. J Clin Oncol 2002;20:3193–3198.

16.2
Upper Urinary Tract Transitional Cell Carcinoma

D. Michael A. Wallace

Epidemiology and Etiology

The upper urinary tract is lined with urothelium that is identical to the urothelium lining the bladder. Like the bladder, this is exposed to the urine-borne carcinogens responsible for the development of urothelial cancers. Upper tract tumors are less common than tumors in the bladder, and this may be due to the shorter contact time of carcinogens with the urothelium or due to different activation mechanisms in the urine. Urothelial tumors of the renal pelvis account for approximately 10% of all renal tumors and 5% of all urothelial tumors (1).

Approximately 5% of urothelial cancers occur in the upper tracts and 95% occur in the bladder. There are rare situations where this is different, such as the Balkan nephropathy cases and the cases that occurred as a result of analgesic abuse, mainly with phenacetin, which was withdrawn in 1973. In these cases the tumors mainly in the upper tract were of low grade and more often bilateral (2). Upper tract urothelial tumors occur more frequently in men than in women and also occur more frequently in white people as compared to black people, with a white-to-black ratio of 2:1 (3). A higher risk of upper urinary tract transitional cell carcinoma (TCC) must be expected in patients with multiple primary superficial bladder TCC (4).

Upper tract tumors may occur as part of the Lynch syndrome II of hereditary nonpolyposis colorectal cancers associated with extracolonic cancer sites, especially upper tract TCC and prostate cancer (5). In these cases the upper tract TCC is frequently bilateral. It is worthwhile checking the family history in cases with colon and upper tract tumors (6). Similarly to bladder TCC, there is a strong association between cigarette smoking upper tract TCC.

Pathology

The majority of upper tract (90%) tumors are TCCs and occur in the pelvis. Ureteric tumors are more often found in the lower ureter than upper ureter.

With higher grade tumors the disease is more likely to be multifocal and associated with areas of carcinoma in situ in the upper tracts, which is often discontinuous. Synchronous bilateral tumors are extremely rare, with metachronous bilateral tumors occurring in 3% (7). Patients with a bladder TCC have approximately a 2% to 4% lifetime risk of developing a tumor in the upper tracts, whereas patients presenting with an upper tract TCC have a risk of developing a bladder cancer of 25% to 75% (8,9).

Benign tumors in the upper tracts are rare, but two tumor types can cause difficulty in diagnosis: (1) Benign ureteral polyps may mimic ureteral TCC but usually occur in younger age groups (10). Often they become pedunculated and may even prolapse into the bladder. Ureteroscopic biopsy and the radiological features usually establish the diagnosis. (2) Cholesteatomas may occur in the renal pelvis and present with similar radiological appearances to an advance TCC in the pelvis (11). Most end up being treated with radical surgery. However, the key to the diagnosis is the detection of keratinizing squamous cells on urine cytology. Unlike leukoplakia of the bladder, these cases do not seem to become malignant.

Prognostic Factors

The significant prognostic factors for survival rates are T stage, grade, multiplicity, location, and surgical modality (12). Lymphovascular invasion has also been noted as an independent prognostic marker (13). Pelvic and ureteral TCC are not the same disease in terms of invasion and prognosis. Ureteral TCC is associated with a higher local or distant failure rate than renal pelvis TCC. A radical surgical approach including meticulous lymphadenectomy may be therapeutic in patients with invasive ureteral TCC. High-grade upper urinary tract transitional cell carcinoma and a history of metachronous or synchronous bladder transitional cell carcinoma were independent adverse prognostic factors (14). Patients with transitional cell carcinoma on dialysis seem to have a higher recurrence rate in the upper urinary tract than patients not on dialysis (15).

Staging

The tumor, node, metastasis (TNM) staging of renal pelvic and ureteric TCC is analogous to that of the bladder (Table 16.2.1).

TABLE 16.2.1. Tumor, mode, metastasis (TNM) classification of renal pelvic and ureteral transitional cell carcinoma

T	*Primary tumor*
Ta	Noninvasive papillary carcinoma
Tis	Carcinoma in situ
T1	Tumor invades subepithelial connective tissue
T2	(Renal pelvis) Tumor invades beyond muscularis into peripelvic fat or renal parenchyma
T3	(For ureter only) Tumor invades beyond muscularis into periureteric fat
T4	Tumor invades adjacent organs or through the kidney into perinephric fat
N	*Regional lymph nodes*
NX	Regional lymph nodes cannot be assessed
N0	No regional lymph node metastasis
N1	Metastasis in a single lymph node, 2 cm or less in greatest dimension
N2	Metastasis in a single lymph node, >2 cm and <5 cm in greatest dimension; or multiple lymph nodes, none <5 cm in greatest dimension
N3	Metastasis in a lymph node >5 cm in greatest dimension
M	*Distant metastasis*
MX	Distant metastasis cannot be assessed
M0	No distant metastasis
M1	Distant metastasis

Note: Laterality does not affect the N classification.

Clinical Features

The majority of upper tract TCCs are picked up on investigation of macroscopic or microscopic hematuria. Upper tract TCC is an infrequent diagnosis in hematuria clinics (16) and depends on the quality of upper tract imaging and degree of suspicion. In units that screen the upper tracts of hematuria patients only by ultrasound, there is a significant risk of missing upper tract TCC, as many of these cases do not have any upper tract dilatation. All patients with hematuria, therefore, need adequate imaging of the upper tracts to give detailed anatomy of the collecting system as well as to exclude renal mass lesions (see Chapter 3). Other unusual features are hydronephrosis and loin pain.

Diagnosis and Staging

The diagnosis of an upper tract tumor depends on good-quality radiology. Intravenous urography (IVU) may be adequate to demonstrate the whole anatomy of the collecting system, but where this is not adequate then computed tomography (CT) urography or magnetic resonance (MR) urography may be used, and either of these imaging modalities may be needed when cytology indicates that the lesion may be high grade. Retrograde ureteropyelography is often used in conjunction with flexible or rigid ureteroscopy and should give full demonstration of the collecting system (see Chapter 3).

Confirmation of diagnosis may be with cytology or biopsy. Cytology samples can be taken for each renal unit with the cytology brush or by washings or just by ureteric sampling of urine. If there is synchronous tumor in the bladder, great care must be taken to avoid any carryover of malignant cells. If the tumor can be reached with ureteroscopy, then a biopsy can be taken, but the size of the sample is always small and may not be sufficient to indicate any more than the histological grade of tumor.

As part of the diagnostic workup for an upper tract tumor, the bladder should be carefully assessed cystoscopically including the taking of biopsies. These patients have a high risk of subsequently developing bladder tumors, and in situ change, particularly around the ureteric orifice, should be detected and treated synchronously.

Management of Upper Tract Transitional Cell Carcinoma

There is a wide range of treatment options for upper tract tumors, and the selection of the best option for an individual patient may be very taxing for the urologist. Treatment choice may be influenced first by patient factors such as the overall renal function, the function of the affected unit, disease in the bladder, and comorbidity. Second, it is important to have an accurate assessment of the grade of the tumor and the likelihood of the tumor being invasive and multifocal. High-grade malignant cells on cytology or high grade on biopsy are relative contraindications to conservative or nephron-sparing treatments. However, this may be compromised by significant comorbidity or renal impairment. If the diagnosis of a low-grade noninvasive tumor can be made with confidence from the radiology, cytology, and biopsy, then there are a wide range of conservative and nephron-sparing treatments to select from.

Localized Transitional Cell Carcinoma of the Renal Pelvis and Ureter

Nephroureterectomy with Cuff of the Bladder

Nephroureterectomy with removal of the whole ureter including a cuff of bladder has been the standard operation for the resection of upper tract TCC. Failure to remove the whole lower ureter leaves the patient at high risk of recurrence in the ureteric stump, which is difficult to keep under surveillance. For high-grade tumors, the nephrectomy should be radical but need not include the adrenal glands but should include the regional nodes (paraaortic and common iliac). Removal of the distal ureter from the bladder cannot usually be done reliably from an extravesical approach, and therefore the bladder needs to be opened to resect adequately a cuff of bladder around the orifice. A less invasive method of doing this is to resect the intramural ureter transurethrally into perivesical fat and then leave a catheter for several days to allow the bladder to heal as when resecting a bladder tumor in this area. When this is done the first move on exploring the kidney is to ligate the ureter in continuity to prevent tumor cells being pushed down the ureter and into the perivesical space. The risk of that happening appears to be extremely low. This method should be used only for upper ureteric or renal pelvic tumors and not for the lower ureter.

Nephroureterectomy can be carried out with equivalent oncological outcome by laparoscopy as by open surgery (17). The frequency of bladder recurrences, local recurrences, and distant metastases appears to be similar with the laparoscopic approach, although the finding of port-site metastases in 1.6% of 377 cases is cause for some concern (18). However in a 7-year outcome study Bariol et al. (19) have demonstrated that the laparoscopic approach does not affect long-term oncological control, and tumor stage and grade remain important prognostic indicators in the development of metastasis. The ureterovesical resection can be carried out endoscopically or through the lower abdominal incision used to remove the kidney. For high-grade tumors that may be invasive, a meticulous node dissection is indicated, which may favor an open operation rather than laparoscopic in these cases.

Conservative Resections for Upper Tract Transitional Cell Carcinoma

Where the anatomy is favorable and the tumor of low grade, there are a number of options for surgical resection and conservation of the kidney. These treatments have to be selected carefully on an individual basis.

Segmental Resection and End-to-End Anastomosis

This option is suitable for mid-ureteric tumors that are small where enough ureter can be mobilized to allow a tension-free anastomosis.

Segmental Resection with Ureteric Reimplant

This option can be used for lower third ureteric tumors close to the bladder. In these cases the ureteric orifice is dissected out transvesically and the bladder can then be hitched to psoas or a Boari flap constructed to allow for a tension-free reimplant. Reflux prevention is not required in these cases, and indeed it may be preferable to have a refluxing ureter so that intravesical chemotherapy can be used to treat the upper tract. The reimplant should be as straight as possible to allow subsequent ureteroscopy.

Segmental Resection with Transureteroureterostomy

For lower ureteric tumors where a tension-free reimplant is not possible, this option can be considered. It should be used only when there is a strong indication for conserving the kidney and a low risk of local recurrence. Endoscopic surveillance of the upper tract subsequently is difficult, and there is a risk of compromising the contralateral side.

Segmental Resection with Ileal Interposition

Where there is an imperative indication for conserving the kidney and there is insufficient ureter to carry out a transureteroureterostomy, an isolated segment of ileum can be used to substitute the ureter. A wide anastomosis to the bladder makes subsequent endoscopic surveillance easy and topical treatment possible.

Bench (ex vivo) surgery may be given a consideration when the whole of the ureter has to be excised in a solitary kidney, which is then reimplanted into the pelvis and anastomosed directly to the bladder.

Endoscopic Treatment of Upper Tract Transitional Cell Carcinoma

It is now possible to endoscope the whole of the upper urinary tract using percutaneous access through the kidney or in a retrograde fashion via the ureter using rigid or flexible ureteroscopes (20).

Access through the kidney enables the use of a conventional resectoscope, and therefore an adequate assessment of the histology is obtained. Selection of cases for percutaneous resection depends on the tumor being in an anatomically favorable site with a high probability of being low grade and noninvasive. Laser or diathermy coagulation of the base of the tumor or small tumors in the pelvis can be used in addition to endoscopic resection. When resection has been completed, the nephrostomy tube should be left in situ to allow the pelvis to be perfused with mitomycin C in a manner analogous to the bladder instillation used after transurethral resection (21). However, the risk with percutaneous resections of upper tract tumors is the tumor implantation into the tract used for access (22). One method of treating the tract is to irradiate it with an iridium wire before removing the nephrostomy tube (23).

Ureteroscopic treatment allows for laser destruction of small tumors, which are likely to be of low grade and noninvasive. Only a small biopsy is obtained, which may result in underestimating grade and stage of the tumor. Laser ablation of ureteric tumors is relatively safe and repeatable where it is important to conserve the kidney or avoid open surgery.

Topical Therapy for Upper Tract Tumors

Intravesical chemotherapy agents and bacille Calmette-Guérin (BCG) therapy can be used in the upper tracts as either definitive therapy or adjuvant therapy after conservative surgery. For repeated instillations, a percutaneous nephrostomy tube is more practical than having to catheterize the ureter and can be left capped off between instillations. Before each instillation into the upper tracts, care must be taken that the tube is correctly sited and not obstructed, otherwise extravasation will occur.

Topical chemotherapy with mitomycin C can be instilled into the upper tracts via a nephrostomy or via a ureteric catheter (24). The same dose of 40 mg in 40 mL as used in the bladder can be infused safely into the upper tract over 1 hour. A concentration of 2 mg/mL can also be used to minimize the effects of dilution by urine, although care must be taken as mitomycin C tends to precipitate at this concentration if not kept warm (25).

Topical BCG is the treatment of choice for cases diagnosed with in situ carcinoma of the upper tracts. The BCG can be infused into the upper tract via a nephrostomy tube using a manometer in the circuit to prevent high pressure from any obstruction causing extravasation. The total dose can be three times higher than that used in the bladder, but at the same concentration and infused over 2 hours. The results of BCG therapy for upper tract carcinoma in situ and high-grade tumors seems to be comparable to the results of BCG for similar bladder tumors (26).

Systemic Chemotherapy for Upper Tract Tumors

Upper tract tumors are an uncommon and a heterogeneous group of tumors. Good-quality evidence to support the management policies for these tumors especially randomized trials is lacking. However, as the pathology and etiology and pattern of spread are so similar to that in the bladder, it is reasonable to extrapolate from the evidence for bladder TCC to upper tract TCC. Use of neoadjuvant chemotherapy is likely to be contraindicated by the reduced renal function from obstruction with high-grade tumors. Using adjuvant chemotherapy after surgery should be considered only if the function of the remaining kidney is good enough. This can also be considered in cases with good renal function but a poor prognosis due to nodal metastases or extension through the ureter (T3 cases). A combination of methotrexate, vinblastine, doxorubicin, and cisplatin (M-VAC) is often used for upper tract tumors (27).

Radiotherapy

External beam radiotherapy has very little place in the management of upper tract tumors. It is not possible to get an adequate dose of radiation to the kidney and ureter without causing unacceptable bowel toxicity. Palliative radiation can be considered to try and control local recurrence.

Surveillance After Treatment

After either radical or conservative treatment of an upper tract TCC, both the bladder and the upper tracts require surveillance. The risk of developing a bladder tumor in these cases is between 25% and 50%, and therefore all these cases should have the same cystoscopic follow-up as cases having had a bladder tumor resection.

Close surveillance of the remaining upper tract after nephroureterectomy may not be so important because of the low risk of developing a contralateral recurrence and the need for prolonged and repeated radiological surveillance. If the patient is getting recurrent bladder tumors in addition to having had a nephroureterectomy, then this would justify radiological surveillance of the remaining upper tract.

After conservative (kidney-sparing) treatment of an upper tract tumor, surveillance is mandatory because of the risk of upper tract recurrence (28) and the risk of postsurgical complications such as stricturing of the ureter.

Surveillance may be radiological (IVU or CT urogram or retrograde pyelography) or by ureteroscopy or both. The frequency and duration of upper tract tumors vary according to the perceived risks, but it is difficult to subject patients to any upper tract surveillance for long term more than once every 6 months.

Bilateral Disease

In rare cases with panurothelial disease affecting the bladder as well as the upper tracts, usually sequentially, total excision of all the urothelium may need to be considered. As well as bilateral nephroureterectomy and cystectomy, these patients must also have the urethra excised. Later transplantation into a conduit should be considered only after an interval of 5 years recurrence free.

References

1. Fraley EE. Cancer of the renal pelvis. In: Skinner DG, de Kernion JB, eds. Genitourinary Cancer. Philadelphia: WB Saunders, 1978:134.
2. Radovanovic Z, Krajinovic, Jankovic S, et al. Family history of cancer among cases of upper urothelial tumours in the Balken nephropathy area. J Cancer Res Clin Oncol 1985;110:181–183.
3. Greenlee RT, Murray T, Bolden S, Wings PA. Cancer Statistics, 2000. CA Cancer J Clin 2000;50:7–33.
4. Millan-Rodriguez F, Chechile-Toniolo G, Salvador-Bayarri J, et al. Upper urinary tract tumours after primary superficial bladder tumours: prognostic factors and risk groups. J Urol 2000;164:1183–1187.
5. Lynch HT, Watson P Lanspa SJ, et al. Natural history of colorectal cancer in hereditary non-polyposis colorectal cancer (Lynch syndromes I and II). Dis Colon Rectum 1988;31:439–444.
6. Greenland JE, Weston PMT, Wallace DMA. Familial transitional cell carcinoma and the Lynch syndrome II. Br J Urol 1993;72:177–180.
7. Holmang S, Johansson SL. Bilateral metachronous ureteral and renal pelvic carcinomas: incidence, clinical presentation, histopathology, treatment and outcome. J Urol 2006;175:69–73.
8. Huben RP, Mounzer AM, Murphy GP. Tumor grade and stage as prognostic variables in upper tract urothelial tumors. Cancer 1988;62(9):2016–2020.
9. Sagalowsky AI, Jarrett TW. Management of Urothelial tumors of the renal pelvis and ureter. In: Walsh PC, Retik AB, Vaughan ED Jr, Wein AJ, eds. Campbell's Urology, vol 4, 8th ed. Philadelphia: WB Saunders, 2002.
10. Gana BM, Evans AT, Weaver JPA. Fibroepithelial polyp of the ureter. Br J Urol 1993; 72:660–661.
11. Park WH, Kim HG, Choi YC, et al. Upper urinary tract cholesteatoma misdiagnosed as a ureteral tumour. J Urol 2000;164:120–121.
12. Matsui Y, Utsunomiyya N, Ichioka K, et al. Risk factors for subsequent development of bladder cancer after primary transitional cell carcinoma of the upper urinary tract. Urology 2005;65:279–283.

13. Kikuchi E, Horiguchi Y, Nakashima J, et al. Lymphovascular invasion independently predicts increased disease specific survival in patients with transitional cell carcinoma of the upper urinary tract. J Urol 2005;174(6):2120–2123; discussion 2124.

14. Reitelman C, Sawczuk IS, Olsson CA, et al. Prognostic variables in patients with transitional cell carcinoma of the renal pelvis and proximal ureter. J Urol 1987; 138:1144–1145.

15. Wu CF, Shee JJ, Ho DR, Chen WC, Chen CS. Different treatment strategies for end stage renal disease in patients with transitional cell carcinoma. J Urol 2004;171: 126–129.

16. Khadra MH, Pickard M, Charlton PH, et al. A prospective analysis of 1,930 patients with haematuria to evaluate current diagnostic practice. J Urol 2000;163:524–527.

17. Matin SF. Radical laparoscopic nephroureterectomy for upper urinary tract transitional cell carcinoma: current status. BJU Int 2005;95(suppl 2):68–74.

18. Rassweiler JJ, Schulze M, Marrero R, et al. Laparoscopic nephroureterectomy for upper tract transitional cell carcinoma: is it better than open surgery? Eur Urol 2004; 46:690–697.

19. Bariol SV, Stewart GD, McNeill SA, Tolley DA. Oncological control following laparoscopic nephroureterectomy: 7-year outcome. J Urol 2004;172:1805–1808.

20. Ho KL, Chow GK. Ureteroscopic resection of upper-tract transitional-cell carcinoma. J Endourol 2005;19:841–848.

21. Lam JS, Gupta M. Ureteroscopic management of upper tract transitional cell carcinoma. Urol Clin North Am 2004;31:115–128.

22. Treuthardt C, Danuser H, Studer UE. Tumour seeding following percutaneous antegrade treatment of transitional cell carcinoma in the renal pelvis. Eur Urol 2004; 46:442–443.

23. Shepherd SF, Patel A, Bidmead AM, et al. Nephrostomy track brachytherapy following percutaneous resection of transitional cell carcinoma of the renal pelvis. Clin Oncol 1995;7:385–387.

24. Patel A, Fuchs GJ. New techniques for the administration of topical adjuvant therapy after endoscopic ablation of upper tract transitional cell carcinoma. J Urol 1998;159: 71–75.

25. Weston PMT, Greenland JE, Wallace DMA. Role of topical mitomycin C in upper urinary tract transitional cell carcinoma. Br J Urol 1993;71:624–625.

26. Thalmann GN, Markwalder R, Walter B, Studer UE. Long-term experience with bacillus Calmette-Guerin therapy of upper urinary tract transitional cell carcinoma in patients not eligible for surgery. J Urol 2002;168:1381–1385.

27. Lerner SE, Blute ML, Richardson RL, Zincke H. Platinum-based chemotherapy for advanced transitional cell carcinoma of the urinary tract. Mayo Clin Proc 1996;71: 945–950.

28. Palou J, Piovesan LF, Huguet J, et al. Percutaneous nephroscopic management of upper urinary tract transitional cell carcinoma: recurrence and long term follow up. J Urol 2004;172:66–69.

16.3
Surgical Management: Cystectomy and Urinary Diversion

Murugesan Manoharan and Alan M. Nieder

The chapter discusses the principles of surgical management of invasive bladder cancer. The muscle-invasive disease is an aggressive form of bladder malignancy and has a greater propensity for metastatic disease (1). In the last two decades, advances in chemotherapy and continent urinary diversion have given a new dimension to the management of muscle-invasive bladder cancer.

Cystectomy

Simple cystectomy is unusual in the cancer setting, although it may be necessary for a severely scarred and contracted bladder or intractable symptoms (e.g., hematuria) as palliation. Radical cystectomy is usually a radical cystoprostatectomy with or without urethrectomy in men and anterior exenteration in women (see below). It is one of the major procedures in urological surgery and involves multidisciplinary risk assessment prior to consideration for surgery. Indications for radical cystectomy are outlined in (Table 16.3.1).

Preoperative Assessment

A general outline of preoperative risk assessment is described in Chapter 6. To summarize, it is important to consider the patient's age and cardiorespiratory and vascular status, as bladder cancer patients are elderly and have comorbidities. Nutritional aspects should be evaluated in preoperative assessment.

Obesity may be associated with wound infection, dehiscence, and stomal problems.

Perioperative Complications

Due to advances in anesthesia, intensive care, prevention, and effective management of cardiovascular diseases, there is decreased mortality and morbidity following radical cystectomy (2). The complication rates following cystectomy approaches 20% to 30% in most series (Table 16.3.2).

TABLE 16.3.1. Indications for radical cystectomy

Muscle-invasive (≥T2) bladder cancer
Selected patients with recurrent high-grade noninvasive lesions (T1 or CIS)
(BCG or intravesical chemotherapeutic agent failures or for patients who present with high-risk "superficial"
   disease, e.g., high-grade, multifocal, T1 lesions, with concomitant CIS)
Recurrent T1 disease

Mortality

Mortality is usually related to the patients' comorbidities, and it has decreased substantially in the last two to three decades to approximately 1% to 2% (3,4).

Radical Cystectomy

Radical cystectomy involves the removal of the entire bladder and urethra with pelvic lymph nodes bilaterally in men, and the removal of the bladder, urethra, uterus, cervix, and cuff of the vagina in women. The procedure is carried out by either a laparoscopic or an open approach. It is an effective curative treatment for muscle-invasive urothelial cancer of the bladder. Excellent local control of the disease can be achieved. It also provides amelioration of local symptoms due to bladder cancer such as hematuria, frequency, dysuria, and clot retention.

In men, radical cystectomy is typically performed as radical cystoprostatectomy with removal of the bladder, prostate, and seminal vesicles en bloc. It may be performed with or without cavernous-nerve sparing for improved erectile function postoperatively.

Prostate-sparing cystectomy has been described to improve the potency rate (5). However, the chances of incidental prostate cancer is high, around 15% to 40%. Hence this is not widely practiced.

TABLE 16.3.2. Complications of cystectomy (3,4)

Intraoperative	Rectal injury
	Bleeding: arterial and venous
Early postoperative	Ileus/small bowel obstruction
	Wound infection/abscess/sepsis
	Anastomotic breakdown, fistula
	Deep vein thrombosis, phlebitis, pulmonary embolism
	Pneumonia, coronary problems
	Lymphatic leak/lymphocele
Late	Urinary tract infections
	Stricture, ureteral obstruction
	Bowel obstruction
	Stoma: retraction, prolapse, hernia
	Incisional hernia

In women, radical cystectomy is typically performed as anterior exenteration with removal of the bladder, uterus, ovaries, fallopian tubes, and part of the anterior vaginal wall.

Bilateral pelvic lymphadenectomy involves removal of the obturator, external iliac, and internal iliac lymph nodes bilaterally up to the common iliac artery bifurcation. It is always performed in conjunction with radical cystectomy both as a therapeutic and as a staging diagnostic procedure. Occasionally these patients may have prolonged lymphatic fluid leak and occasionally lymphocele.

Recent data suggest that an extended lymph node dissection (to the bifurcation of the aorta) may also be a therapeutic procedure for patients with minimal adenopathy (6). Patients with a greater number of removed lymph nodes may have an improved disease-free survival. Most patients with positive lymph nodes require adjuvant chemotherapy. Despite this, the 5-year survival is poor at 20%.

Partial Cystectomy

Partial cystectomy involves removal of part of the bladder wall that is involved by a discrete lesion. Patients with a solitary muscle-invasive lesion, with no evidence of carcinoma in situ (CIS) or previous history of multiple superficial tumors or metastasis, without involvement of the trigone or posterior urethra, are suitable candidates. It is desirable to have a clear margin of at least 1.5 cm around the tumor. Other indications include bladder tumors in the diverticulum and urachal adenocarcinoma in the urachus (7). Partial cystectomy is often selected for elderly patients or those with multiple comorbidities who may not tolerate an extended procedure.

Before considering the bladder-preserving procedure, the following assessment should be done: (1) bladder mapping: rule out CIS and multifocal lesions by performing systematic bladder biopsies; (2) bladder capacity should be assessed preoperatively and should be adequate to avoid postoperative voiding symptoms due to low bladder capacity.

Patients who undergo partial cystectomy require surveillance with cystoscopy and urinary cytology due to an increased risk of recurrence secondary to multifocal nature of urothelial cancer. The mean 5-year survival after partial cystectomy for T2 to T3b tumors is 67% to 80% (8,9).

Salvage Cystectomy

Salvage cystectomy is indicated in intractable hematuria following chemotherapy or radiotherapy. It is also considered in patients with local recurrence or progression following primary radiotherapy. The operation is usually considered palliative; however, well-selected patients may have significant long-term survival.

Risks

Intraoperative blood loss tends to be high, as is the risk of injury to adjacent organs (e.g., rectum, iliac vessels, etc.). Anatomical planes are not well defined in postradiotherapy patients because of desmoplastic reaction. The surgeon should be prepared to perform only a urinary diversion if the bladder cannot be safely removed. Tissue planes are often distorted secondary to radiation effects. Risks of wound infection and ileus are also increased. Survival rates after salvage cystectomy are quite low (10). Complication rates are higher with orthotopic bladder reconstruction in these cases.

Urinary Diversion in Salvage Cystectomy

The ileal conduit is the preferred method of urinary diversion in salvage cystectomy. Risk of incontinence is greater if neobladder reconstruction is attempted secondary to radiation effects on the sphincter. Assessment of the ileum must be made to ensure that there are no radiation-induced injuries, and in such cases other segments of uninvolved bowel should be used.

Sexuality Preserving Cystectomy and Neobladder

Various specialist centers in Europe and the United States have described conservative procedures involving bladder removal with pelvic lymph node dissection and preservation of the vasa deferentia, prostate, and seminal vesicles in males, and all internal genitalia in females. This is followed by an ileal neobladder reconstruction and its anastomosis to the margins of the prostate in males and urethra in females. Indications for this type of surgery are bladder cancer stages T1 to T3 with no tumor in the bladder neck and prostate in males and absent tumor in the trigone in females (11).

These patients need to undergo preoperative assessment and investigations for neoplasia of the prostate [prostate-specific antigen (PSA) and transrectal ultrasound (TRUS)], uterus, and cervix (colposcopy and cytology), and erectile dysfunction in men. The results are encouraging, but long-term follow-up results are still awaited (12).

Intraoperative Care

Radical cystectomy and urinary diversion may be complicated by significant intraoperative blood loss. The operation can be lengthy (3 to 6 hours), and patients have also typically undergone complete bowel preparation for 1 or 2 days prior to the operation. Patients may also be chronically anemic secondary to gross hematuria. Therefore, intraoperative and postoperative fluid management is critical.

Intraoperative monitoring entails the following:

1. Two large-bore intravenous lines
2. Arterial-line monitoring (if indicated)

3. Central venous line monitoring (if indicated)
4. Urine output measurement, which is often unreliable intraoperatively

Postoperative Care

Postoperative care entails the following:

1. Initial intensive care unit monitoring in selected patients (not needed in all patients)
2. Strict fluid balance
3. Nasogastric tube drainage, removed once the bowel functions recover
4. Slow advancement of diet (most common perioperative complication is ileus, necessitating replacement of nasogastric tube)
5. Antibiotics: no prospective randomized studies have demonstrated improved outcomes for prolonged prophylactic antibiotics; most urologists prefer 36 hours of broad-spectrum antibiotics; prolonged use of antibiotics is not recommended due to the risk of *Clostridium difficile* infection (pseudo-membranous colitis)
6. Deep vein thrombosis prophylaxis: sequential compression devices (SCDs) are placed on patient prior to the induction of general anesthesia
7. Subcutaneous heparin (5000 mL q12h) and low molecular weight heparin prophylaxis may be utilized; early ambulation and active chest physiotherapy are warranted

Urinary Diversion: Ileal, Jejunal, and Colonic Conduits

Bowel preparation reduces the risk of infection and provides the surgeon greater visibility in performing an ureterointestinal anastomosis. Mechanical bowel preparation combined with antibiotics is the preferred option. However, there are studies that failed to show any benefit with mechanical bowel preparation.

The typical bowel preparation includes the following:

1. Mechanical bowel prep:
   a. Liquid diet on the day prior to surgery
   b. Nil per oral after the midnight prior to surgery
   c. Go-Lytely or magnesium citrate on the day prior to surgery
   d. No intravenous fluids required the day prior to surgery (i.e., patient can complete bowel prep at home)
2. Antibiotic bowel prep: neomycin and erythromycin on the day prior to surgery

Principles of Technique of Conduit Creation

Virtually every possible type of bowel segment has been utilized in the creation of both urinary conduits and urinary diversions. Ileum is currently the preferred choice of bowel for conduits due to its low risk of metabolic abnormalities, ease of use, and length of mesentery (13). Jejunum is rarely used because of its greater risk of metabolic complications. Transverse colon is typically a second choice if ileum is not available or diseased secondary to prior pelvic radiation.

The bowel must be handled gently. The "butt" end of the conduit is usually oversewn with nonabsorbable sutures if metallic staples are used to divide the bowel. The ureterointestinal anastomosis must be widely spatulated to prevent anastomotic strictures (14). Anastomosis performed over 7-French (F) stents. Mesenteric defect should be reapproximated with nonabsorbable sutures to prevent internal herniation.

Complications of Conduit Diversions (14,15)

Surgical

Stomal stenosis (5–15%) can be exacerbated by poorly fitting appliances. Ureterointestinal anastomotic stricture is seen in 5% to 15%, and when present it is important to rule out malignancy. Chronic pyelonephritis and renal failure are seen in 15% of cases on long-term follow-up. Parastomal hernia (5%) and conduit calculi (5–20%) are also seen.

Metabolic complications include the following:

1. Ileal conduit: hyperchloremic metabolic acidosis
2. Jejunal conduit: hypochloremic hyperkalemic metabolic acidosis
3. Colonic conduit: hyperchloremic hypokalemic metabolic acidosis

Bladder Substitution

Orthotopic bladder substitutions are being increasingly offered to patients undergoing cystectomy due to documented improvement in the quality of life, our increased understanding of pelvic anatomy, and advances in the surgical techniques (16).

The pelvic anatomy should be favorable and should not compromise the functional and oncological outcomes. Meticulous preservation of the external sphincter mechanism is essential. The distal urethra should be free of malignancies and strictures. Locally advanced disease is not a strict contraindication for bladder substitution, and the decision to perform bladder substitution should be individualized. Adjuvant and neoadjuvant chemotherapy are safe in these patients, and hence orthotopic bladder substitution should not be denied unfairly to patients who may require chemotherapy (17).

Detailed preoperative discussion with the patient regarding bladder substitution is essential. Patients should always be counseled for alternate urinary diversion options, such as ileal conduit preoperatively in case the neobladder formation is not feasible. Enterostomal therapists play a pivotal role in patient education both pre- and postoperatively.

Patient Selection and Principles

The long-term outcome is dependent on careful patient selection, meticulous postoperative care, and follow-up.

Renal Insufficiency

Renal insufficiency increases the chances of complications such as metabolic acidosis and electrolyte imbalances. In patients with serum creatinine levels >2.0 mg/L, bladder substitution should be avoided. However, if the renal insufficiency is due to ureteral obstruction that can be reversed by the surgery, bladder substitution should be considered.

Bowel Disease

A history of previous bowel resection, inflammatory bowel disease, and radiation therapy increases the chances of postoperative bowel dysfunction. These patients should be fully evaluated and counseled regarding the bowel dysfunction. An attempt should be made to preserve the terminal ileum and ileocecal valve to minimize bowel dysfunction and maintain vitamin B_{12} and bile salt metabolism.

Hepatic Dysfunction

Patients with liver dysfunction are at a higher risk for hyperammonemia following neobladder formation, particularly if the patient develops infection with urease-splitting organisms.

Pelvic Floor

In patients with significant sphincter deficiency and stress incontinence, neobladder reconstruction should be avoided.

State of Urethra

It is imperative that the urethral margins at the anastomotic level be negative for malignancy to avoid tumor recurrences. The presence of carcinoma in situ, multifocal diseases, and prostatic urethral involvement increases the chances of tumor recurrence, but they are not absolute contraindications for tumor recurrence.

Psychological

Patients should be compliant and motivated. They should demonstrate good manual dexterity and hand–eye coordination.

Types of Bladder Substitution

The continent bladder substitutions can be broadly classified as continent ileocecal reservoirs and orthotopic neobladder reconstruction.

Ileocecal Reservoirs

These catheterizable reconstruction techniques involve the use of the right colon as the urinary reservoir, and continence is achieved by a variety of techniques using the ileocecal valve, appendix, and terminal ileum. The commonly used techniques include the Koch pouch, the Indiana pouch, and the T pouch (18,19). Common complications associated with continent reservoirs are listed in Table 16.3.3. Studies with long-term follow-up indicate that the need for repeat surgical procedures is high.

Orthotopic Neobladders

These diversion options are becoming more popular and increasingly replacing other methods. This method involves using the ileal segment to create a low-pressure reservoir and relies on the patient's sphincter for continence. The two common techniques used were described by Hautmann et al. (21) and Studer and Zingg (22). Several techniques have been described for improvising and modifying above techniques.

A variety of early and late complications have been described. Most of the complications are transient and self-limiting without compromising the quality of life significantly (Table 16.3.4); different institutions report a variable incidence of complications, and average incidences are shown in the table.

Techniques of Anastomosis: Suturing and Stapling

Bowel Resection and Anastomosis

Bowel resection and anastomosis are commonly performed using metallic stapling devices with gastrointestinal anastomosis (GIA) and thoracoabdominal

TABLE 16.3.3. Complications of ileocecal reservoirs (19,20)

Complication	Incidence (%)
Redo operations	25–50
Stomal stenosis	10–20
Pyelonephritis	5–10
Renal impairment	3–5
Metabolic disturbances	20
Ureteral strictures	2–4
Bowel obstructions	4
Bowel dysfunction	5
Calculus	5–10
Vitamin deficiency	5–10

(TA) staplers. This decreases the operative time, fecal spillage, and anastomotic stricture rate.

Neobladder Reconstruction

Neobladder reconstruction is best performed with hand-sewn anastomosis using absorbable sutures. The absorbable staplers can be used to reduce the operative time. However, they are bulky and cause persistent rigidity and internal septations in the neobladder. This results in poor compliance and decreased functional results compared with hand-sewn anastomosis. The absorbable staplers are more favorable for ileocolic reservoirs than for the orthotopic neobladders. Use of metallic staplers in the neobladder can result in stone formation along the suture line and hence should be avoided.

Ureteral Anastomosis

Simple nonrefluxing, end-to-side ureteroileal anastomosis provides the best results in neobladder reconstruction with the least complications and lowest reoperation rates (14). It is essential to create a well-vascularized, tension-free, and watertight anastomosis to achieve the best results. The anastomosis can be performed with either interrupted or continuous absorbable sutures. Most urologists utilize the ureteral stents to protect the anastomosis, though it may not be essential.

Local Recurrences Following Neobladder Reconstruction

Urethral recurrence is seen in 2% to 4% of patients (25,26), mostly close to the bladder neck region. Urethral wash cytology or flexible cystoscopy is recommended every 6 months in the first 2 years and yearly following that. If the recurrences are small and low grade, they can be treated with fulguration. There is always a risk of developing strictures due to fulguration. When lesions are of high grade or multiple, urethrectomy and conversion to ileal conduit is recommended.

TABLE 16.3.4. Complications of neobladder reconstruction (22–24)

Early	Incidence (%)	Late	Incidence (%)
Ureteral leak	4	Ureteral stricture	2
Ureteral stenosis	2	Bladder neck stricture	5
Retained stents	1	Fistula	2
Ileus	10	Calculus	2
Acute pyelonephritis	2	Renal impairment	4
Sepsis	2	Acidosis	4
Pelvic abscess	2	Bowel dysfunction	2
Intestinal leak	1	Bowel obstruction	3
Wound infection	3	Pyelonephritis	5

TABLE 16.3.5. Recommended follow-up scheme following urinary diversion

Evaluation	3 months	6 months	12 months	18 months	Year 2	Years 3 and 4	Year 5, then Q 2 years
Physical examination	X	X	X	X	X	X	X
CT/MRI abdomen and pelvis*	X	X[a]	X	X[a]	X	X[a]	X[a]
CT/MRI urography	X		X		X	X	X
Chest x-ray/CT chest*	X	X	X	X	X	X	X
Blood workup[b]	X	X	X	X	X	X	X
Urine cytology	X	X	X	X	X	X	X
Vitamins A, D, B₁₂, and folate					X	X	X

[a]May be omitted in patients with <T2N0M0.
[b]Electrolytes, BUN, creatinine, liver profile, lipid profile, magnesium.
*Patients with bladder cancer only.

Pelvic recurrences are seen in 10% to 15% of patients following neobladder reconstruction (27). In general these pelvic recurrences are not amenable to surgical resections and are usually treated with chemotherapy.

Up to two thirds of these patients maintain good bladder function until the last follow-up or death. The type of diversion does not affect the local recurrence rates.

Follow-Up

Lifelong follow-up is essential, and the recommended follow-up schedule is given in Table 16.3.5 (28).

Quality of Life

No randomized controlled studies assessing the quality of life (QOL) in different urinary diversions is available at present. Follow-up studies have demonstrated significant improvement in patients with a neobladder, including functional, social, emotional, and cognitive aspects of life.

Rectal/Sigmoid Neobladders

This procedure utilizes the anal sphincter to provide continent urinary diversion. This may be the procedure of choice in the presence of intractable urinary incontinence or extensive small bowel disease that is not suitable for continent urinary diversion (29). These procedures are contraindicated in patients with incompetent anal sphincter and anorectal pathology.

Ureterosigmoidostomy

Currently ureterosigmoidostomy is reserved for elderly and debilitated patients. Patient selection is very important in these situations. It is imperative to ascertain that the anal sphincter is intact. The ureters are implanted to the rectosigmoid region with an antireflux mechanism.

The Mainz II pouch is a modified ureterosigmoidostomy that consists of folded rectosigmoid pouch with suitable antireflux ureterointestinal anastomosis. The procedure follows the principles of detubularization and spherical reconfiguration to create a low-pressure reservoir and stratifying ureteric implantation between submucosal and serous-lined extramural tunnel techniques. It has shown good continence rates and better long-term preservation of the upper urinary tract than with a classical ureterosigmoidostomy (30).

Complications

A variety of complications including metabolic disturbances, hepatic dysfunction, pyelonephritis, stone formation, and bone demineralization discourage urologists from performing this form of urinary diversion. The incidence of neoplasia occurring in the ureterosigmoidostomy is high, ranging from 6% to 29%. The risk increases with time. Eighty-five percent of these tumors are adenocarcinoma and 10% are transitional cell carcinoma. Various modifications to the standard ureterosigmoidostomy have been described, but they are rarely used.

References

1. Scher HI. Systemic chemotherapy in regionally advanced bladder cancer. Theoretical considerations and results. Urol Clin North Am 1992;19(4):747–759.
2. Peyromaure M, Guerin F, Debre B, Zerbib M. Surgical management of infiltrating bladder cancer in elderly patients. Eur Urol 2004;45:147–154.
3. Messing EM, Catalona W. Urothelial tumors of the urinary tract. In: Walsh PC, Retik AB, Vaughan ED Jr, Wein AJ, eds. Campbell's Urology, 7th ed. Philadelphia: WB Saunders, 1998:2327–2410.
4. Figueroa AJ, Stein JP, Dickinson M, et al. Radical cystectomy for elderly patients with bladder carcinoma. An updated experience with 404 patients. Cancer 1998;83: 141–147.
5. Nieuwenhuijzen JA, Meinhardt W, Horenblas S. Clinical outcomes after sexuality preserving cystectomy and neobladder (prostate sparing cystectomy) in 44 patients. J Urol 2005;173(4):1314–1317.
6. Stein JP, Skinner DG. The role of lymphadenectomy in high-grade invasive bladder cancer. Urol Clin North Am 2005;32(2):187–197.
7. Mariano MB, Tefilli MV. Laparoscopic partial cystectomy in bladder cancer—initial experience. Int Braz J Urol 2004;30(3):192–198.

8. Dandekar NP, Tongaokar FIB, Dalal AV, Kulkarni SN. Partial cystectomy for invasive bladder cancer. J Surg Oncol 1995;60:24–29.

9. Novick AC, Stewart BH. Partial cystectomy in the treatment of primary and secondary carcinoma of the bladder. J Urol 1976;116:570–574.

10. Nieuwenhuijzen JA, Horenblas S, Meinhardt W, et al. Salvage cystectomy after failure of interstitial radiotherapy and external beam radiotherapy for bladder cancer. BJU Int 2004;94:793–797.

11. Nieuwenhuijzen JA, Meinhardt W, Horenblas S. Clinical outcomes after sexuality preserving cystectomy and neobladder (prostate sparing cystectomy) in 44 patients. J Urol 2005;173(4):1314–1317.

12. Vallancien G, Abou El Fettouh H, et al. Cystectomy with prostate sparing for bladder cancer in 100 patients: 10-year experience. J Urol 2002;168(6):2413–2417.

13. Bricker EM. Bladder substitution after pelvic evisceration. Surg Clin North Am 1950;30:1511–1521.

14. Manoharan M, Tunuguntla HS. Standard reconstruction techniques: techniques of ureteroneocystostomy during urinary diversion. Surg Oncol Clin North Am 2005;14: 367–379.

15. Leadbetter WF, Clarke BD. Five year's experience with the uretero-enterostomy by the "combined" technique. J Urol 1954;73:67–82.

16. Montie JE, Wie JT. Formation of an orthotopic neobladder following radical cystectomy: historical perspective, patient selection, and contemporary outcomes. J Pelv Surg 2002;8:141–147.

17. Manoharan M, Reyes MA, Kava BR, et al. Is adjuvant chemotherapy for bladder cancer safer in patients with an ileal conduit than a neobladder? BJU Int 2005;96:1286–1289.

18. Kock NG, Nilson AE, Norlen LS, et al. Urinary diversion via a continent ileal reservoir: clinical results in 12 patients. J Urol 1982;128:469–475.

19. Skinner DG, Boyd SD, Lieskovsky G, et al. Lower urinary tract reconstruction following cystectomy: experience and results in 126 patients using the Kock ileal reservoir with bilateral ureteroileal urethrostomy. J Urol 1991;146:756–760.

20. Sevin G, Kosar A, Perk H, Serel TA, Gurbuz G. Bone mineral content and related biochemical variables in patients with ileal bladder substitution and colonic Indiana pouch. Eur Urol 2002;41:655–659.

21. Hautmann RE, Egghart G, Frohneberg D, Miller K. The ileal neobladder. J Urol 1988; 139:39–42.

22. Studer UE, Zingg EJ. Ileal orthotopic bladder substitutes. What we have learned from 12 years' experience with 200 patients. Urol Clin North Am 1997;24:781–793.

23. Hautmann RE, de Petriconi R, Gottfried HW, et al. The ileal neobladder: complications and functional results in 363 patients after 11 years of followup. J Urol 1999; 161:422–427.

24. Mills RD, Studer UE. Metabolic consequences of continent urinary diversion. J Urol 1999;161:1057–1066.

25. Lebret T, Herve JM, Barre P, et al. Urethral recurrence of transitional cell carcinoma of the bladder. Eur Urol 1998;33:170–174.

26. Erckert M, Stenzl A, Falk M, Bartsch G. Incidence of urethral tumor involvement in 910 men with bladder cancer. World J Urol 1996;14:3–8.

27. Tefilli MV, Gheiler EL, Tiguert R, et al. Urinary diversion-related outcome in patients with pelvic recurrence after radical cystectomy for bladder cancer. Urology 1999; 53:999–1004.

28. Varol C, Studer UE. Managing patients after an ileal orthotopic bladder substitution. BJU Int 2004;93:266–270.
29. Wear JB, Barquin OP. Ureterosigmoidostomy: long-term results. Urology 1973;1: 192–200.
30. D'elia G, Pahernik S, Fisch M, Hohenfellner R, Thuroff JW. Mainz pouch II technique: 10 years' experience. BJU Int 2004;93(7):1037–1042.

16.4
Multidisciplinary Care of Invasive Bladder Cancer: Emerging Roles of Chemotherapy

Derek Raghavan and Howard M. Sandler

Invasive bladder cancer is associated with a cure rate of only 50%, when all stages are considered. The pattern of relapse is dominated by systemic spread, with metastases occurring despite local control. In the past two decades, strategies of treatment have been predicated on the use of systemic chemotherapy before, during, or after locoregional management in an attempt to control occult systemic disease. More recently, molecular prediction has been applied to this clinical problem, with gene expression being studied as a prognostic and predictive marker. Of particular importance, *p53* mutation and expression of the epidermal growth factor receptor may predict the natural history and response to treatment.

The Biology of Locally Advanced Bladder Cancer

Invasive bladder cancer, including tumors that penetrate through the lamina propria into muscle and beyond, constitutes around 20% of incident cases of bladder cancer. This translates into an annual incidence of about five cases per 100,000 males and one case per 100,000 females. However, the issue is more significant demographically as superficial bladder cancers may evolve into invasive disease in up to about 30% of cases. As these are not "new" cases, they are not reflected in national incidence figures.

The majority of bladder cancers (90%) are transitional cell carcinomas (TCCs) (1); less common cell types include squamous cell carcinoma, adenocarcinoma, small cell carcinoma, and rarely sarcoma, lymphoma, or melanoma (2,3). The majority of invasive bladder cancers are moderately to poorly differentiated (1). Studies in our laboratory have suggested that there is a stem cell tumor of origin in bladder cancer, which enables dominant transitional cell carcinoma to coexist with (and possibly give rise to) squamous and glandular differentiation (4). We have also shown that there is dramatic clonal heterogeneity, with regard to histological and tumor marker expression and parameters of response to chemotherapy within individual tumor deposits (4). This heterogeneity creates a more complex target for therapeutic intervention, given that the

TABLE 16.4.1. Limitations of studies of novel prognostic indicators

Parameter	Limitation	Examples
Laboratory methodology	New assay system	• Standardization in progress
		• What is "normal"?
		• Optimal technology?
		• Immunohistochemistry vs. fluorescent in-situ hybridization?
	Lab test applied to clinical samples	• RNA vs. protein?
		• Interlaboratory variation
		• Differences in fixation
		• Tumor sampling error
		• Tumor heterogeneity
		• "Live" tissue vs. fixed tissue
		• Limited range of samples tested early in history of assay
Clinical analysis	Studies not designed for marker correlation	• Missing data
		• Post hoc analysis
		• Uninformative cases
		• Case/sample selection bias
		• Limited sample size
		• Inadequate follow-up
		• Not all initial analysis is blinded

patterns of response to treatment of these histological subtypes are usually quite different (5).

Of importance in the design of management protocols is the attribution of likely prognosis, thus identifying tumors that may require more aggressive management strategies. Stage (extent of invasion) and grade (degree of differentiation) are the most important conventional prognostic determinants (1,6). In some early series, investigators did not recognize that the lamina propria is invested with a muscularis of its own, the muscularis mucosae (7), and thus some superficial tumors were overstaged when they were noted to have interspersed fibers of muscularis mucosae abutting the tumor tissue. The pattern of growth (solid rather than papillary), large size, aneuploidy, presence of hydronephrosis, and lymphatic and vascular invasion have been shown to be adverse prognostic determinants in univariate analysis (1,6,8–13).

In addition to the conventional histopathological and clinical predictors of natural history and response to therapy, a series of adverse molecular prognosticators have been identified. An important caveat in any discussion of novel prognostic markers is that many new marker technologies have important limitations with respect to execution and interpretation in this context (Table 16.4.1).

Molecular Prediction of Natural History of Bladder Cancer

Our understanding of the molecular biology of bladder cancer is still in an evolutionary state (14). The simplest molecular predictors of outcome have correlated with tumor differentiation. For example, absence of expression of ABO blood group substances on the surface of superficial bladder cancer cells is associated with higher rates of relapse and progression to invasion (15). Similarly, the presence of aneuploid populations of cells is also associated with an increased prevalence of relapse and tumor progression, although most invasive bladder cancers actually are aneuploid. Superficial and invasive bladder cancers have different patterns of molecular pathogenesis. Superficial disease is characterized by a loss of heterozygosity of chromosome 9 (16). With the development of more invasive and undifferentiated disease, aberrations of chromosome 17 are detected, in association with mutations of *p53* (17). Similarly, increased expression of *ras* and its variants appears to be associated with loss of differentiation and a worse prognosis (18,19), and may correlate with p53 function (18).

The functions of *p53* and *p21* are linked, and thus accurate molecular characterization of bladder cancer requires the study of both genes. In addition, the deletion of the *Rb* gene confers an adverse prognosis, and its normal function is influenced by the action of the *p53/p21* complex (20). Immunohistochemical studies of a relatively small number of bladder cancer specimens obtained by radical cystectomy have shown that the most favorable prognosis appears to be associated with expression of wild-type *p53* and normal expression of *p21* (21). The presence of mutant *p53* with deletion of expression of *p21* predicts for a high relapse rate. Studies from the University of Southern California (USC) have shown that expression of *p53* mutation confers prognostic information additional to that afforded by stage and grade (17,21). This has become the basis of an international randomized trial (see below), which will be reassessing the true importance of *p53* mutations in a much larger sample size.

Another protein with a locus on chromosome 9 is p16^{INK4a}, which functions as a tumor suppressor. It probably inhibits cyclin D function, and is particularly associated with the evolution of squamous carcinoma and bilharzial bladder cancer (22).

The expression of the epidermal growth factor receptor (EGFR) is another potential molecular determinant of prognosis (23). This cell surface protein, with known cell growth regulatory functions, is correlated with expression of *p53*, aneuploidy, and invasive growth (24). As discussed below, it may also play a role in resistance to cytotoxic agents, such as cisplatin. The transferrin receptor (25), also located on the surface of bladder cancer cells, appears to be another independent prognostic determinant, although the nature of this function is unknown, as is its relationship to the expression of EGFR and other molecular determinants. It is possible that gallium, one of the cytotoxic agents with modest antitumor activity against bladder cancer, may interact with these tumor cells at the level of the transferrin receptor.

The genes that control vascular invasion and angiogenesis seem to have prognostic implications. It is known that microvessel density, the extent of tumor vascularity per high power field, is associated with metastasis and prognosis; the higher the microvessel density, the worse the prognosis (26). Cote and colleagues (31) have also studied the expression of thrombospondin-1 in bladder cancer. This is a glycoprotein component of the extracellular matrix, which inhibits angiogenesis (27), and its expression is directly correlated with prognosis. These studies also have suggested that *p53* mutation is associated with suppression of expression of thrombospondin-1.

Investigators at Memorial Sloan-Kettering Cancer Center (MSKCC) have used oligonucleotide arrays to analyze the transcript profiles of bladder tumors and have carried out immunohistochemical analyses on bladder cancer tissue arrays to validate the associations among marker expression, staging, and outcome. They were able to achieve a greater than 80% accuracy in prognostication (28).

Overlapping and interacting molecular functions regulate growth, differentiation, and prognosis of bladder cancer. Several of these oncogenes and suppressor genes may be suitable candidates for gene therapy, or for downstream regulation through inhibitors of transcription and translation.

Molecular Prediction of Response to Chemotherapy

Studies in the late 1980s revealed higher objective response rates from the use of combination chemotherapy regimens than were achieved with single agents, both for the treatment of metastatic bladder cancer and in the neoadjuvant setting (5,29).

For many tumor types, there is an increasing level of focus on the molecular biology of tumor response to chemotherapy. We have previously studied the expression of the intracellular scavenger glutathione, which decreases the available level of cytotoxic agents, such as cisplatin, within tumor cells (30). In a series of bladder cancer xenografts, high levels of glutathione were identified, representing higher concentrations than are found in malignant melanoma and ovarian cancer, the classical models of the role of glutathione in cytotoxic resistance. In addition, we showed that higher levels of glutathione are expressed in human tumor biopsy specimens than in biopsies from patients with a past history of bladder cancer, and, in turn, these levels were higher than those found in normal bladder tissue.

As yet, the significance of these observations has not been clarified, although there are several sets of preliminary data that implicate glutathione and glutathione-S-transferase in the biology of responses to chemotherapy.

One controversial issue is the clinical significance of mutation of the *p53* suppressor gene in the context of resistance to cytotoxic chemotherapy. Innate resistance to chemotherapy may be a function of expression of *p53*, although there are conflicting data on whether mutation of *p53* confers increased responsiveness (31) or increased resistance (31) to the impact of chemotherapy. Cote and colleagues (31) have reported a post hoc study of immunohistochemical staining of tumor biopsies from a randomized study of adjuvant platinum-based chemotherapy (32), and suggested that tumors exhibiting mutation of *p53* benefited from adjuvant chemotherapy. By contrast, those with wild-type *p53* did not exhibit any difference in survival between the control population and those receiving adjuvant chemotherapy. The major problem with this study was small sample size and its post hoc nature, and more information on this topic will be available when the results of the international *p53* trial are known.

By contrast, studies from MSKCC initially suggested that *p53* mutation was associated with resistance to neoadjuvant chemotherapy with the methotrexate, vinblastine, Adriamycin (doxorubicin), and cisplatin (MVAC) regimen (33). A detailed study of molecular prognosticators in patients treated with the MVAC or cisplatin, methotrexate, and vinblastine (CMV) regimens for advanced bladder cancer at Princess Margaret Hospital, Toronto, did not identify any prognostic impact from expression of *p53* immunohistochemically (34). It is not clear whether this reflects a true lack of prognostic relevance or is an artifact of methodology or small sample size. That said, in this small study, another marker (metallothionein expression) did have statistically significant prognostic implications.

The data regarding the prognostic role of metallothionein expression are interesting. Metallothioneins are a family of sulfhydryl-containing cysteine residues that are involved in absorption, transport, and metabolism of heavy. Previous studies have suggested that these proteins may be related to resistance to cisplatin and alkylating agents (35). Satoh et al. (36) demonstrated that an increase in the concentration of metallothionein in mice caused a reduction of nephrotoxicity, accompanied by cisplatin resistance in a mouse bladder cancer. Siu et al. (34) showed in univariate analysis that good performance status, low percentage of metallothionein staining, and high tumor grade were significant positive predictors of response to cisplatin chemotherapy, but that the latter factor was lost in multivariate analysis.

In a detailed study of cell lines, Kielb et al. (37) showed that *p53* mutation is required for paclitaxel to induce cell death in vitro in human bladder cancer cells, whereas cells with normal *p53* function were not affected by this agent. By contrast, the cytotoxic impact of gemcitabine was not influenced by *p53* mutations, suggesting a potentially different spectrum of responses to this agent in bladder cancer.

Multidrug or pleiotropic resistance, in which cell surface protein complexes function as efflux pumps or modulators of intracellular cytotoxic drug concentrations, appears to be relevant to bladder cancer. A family of multidrug resistance (MDR) proteins, including p-glycoprotein, correlates with resistance to the taxanes, vinca alkaloids, and anthracycline antibiotics. This phenomenon has been found to be particularly relevant in ovarian cancer and multiple myeloma, but studies of expression of MDR in bladder cancer have been difficult, for reasons that are not fully clear. For example, our xenograft studies identified major clonal differences in response to doxorubicin and vinblastine, but we were unable to demonstrate clear and reproducible expression of p-glycoprotein in the tumor specimens. Others have encountered similar problems. Siu et al. (34), studying patients treated with MVAC or CMV chemotherapy, did not find any prognostic significance from expression of p-glycoprotein, although any impact for response or resistance to chemotherapy might have been overcome by the presence of cisplatin in both regimens, an agent that is not influenced by MDR expression.

However, Petrylak et al. (38) were able to demonstrate clear enhancement of expression of p-glycoprotein in pre- and posttreatment biopsies of human tumors treated with the MVAC regimen. The highest proportion of tumor cells expressing p-glycoprotein was observed in metastases from patients treated with six or more cycles of chemotherapy. These workers speculated that MDR could contribute significantly to the patterns of resistance seen in the use of the MVAC regimen.

Adopting a more technically sophisticated approach, investigators at MSKCC have studied the transcript profiles of more than 100 bladder specimens, representing the spectrum from normal to relatively benign to malignant disease, in an attempt to identify useful novel prognosticators (39). In an elegant study that requires validation, they identified a hierarchy of determinants, including peptidyl propyl isomerase A, nuclear RNA export factor 1, tetratricopeptide repeat domain G, hematopoietic cell specific Lyn substrate 1, ankyrin G, baculoviral IAP repeat-containing 3, intercellular adhesion molecule 1, and TP53-activated protein 1. In each instance, Kaplan-Meier curves identified differences in survival based on expression, but further study will be required to identify the utility of such gene expression in predicting the outcome of specific chemotherapy regimens.

In this context, Takata et al. (40), studying a small number of patients treated with MVAC-style chemotherapy, identified another series of potential genetic predictors of outcome using array techniques. Again the significance of their preliminary observations will require clarification, although it was interesting to note that these array studies further implicated *p53* gene function and mutation in predicting the outcomes of chemotherapy.

At a more pragmatic level, the Radiation Therapy Oncology Group (RTOG) has carried out retrospective analyses of their series of cases treated with radiotherapy and cisplatin-based chemotherapy, and has demonstrated that expression of EGFR is associated with improved outcome, including response to chemoradiotherapy, whereas expression of the *her-2-neu* gene correlates in univariate analysis with reduced response and survival after such treatment (41).

As outlined in Table 16.4.1, validation of these applied technologies in much larger patient sets will be required before this approach becomes a standard of care in clinical practice.

Management of T1–T2 Bladder Cancer: Impact of Molecular Biology

As noted above, mutation of *p53* has been shown to have prognostic significance independent of stage and grade (17,20,21). The experience from USC has suggested that patients with superficially invasive bladder cancer (stages P1–2) have a higher relapse rate when the tumors express mutations of *p53*. As a result, a randomized trial has studied the effect of adjuvant MVAC chemotherapy after radical cystectomy for pathological stage P1–2 tumors with negative lymph nodes and expression of mutated *p53*. The Southwest Oncology Group has recently joined this trial, which will address important questions regarding the utility of adjuvant chemotherapy and the prognostic significance of mutations of *p53, p21,* and other molecular determinants. At present, the study is on hold, pending a recommendation by the Data Safety Monitoring Committee to perform an interim analysis of data.

The Role of Surgery in Invasive Bladder Cancer

The least aggressive surgical treatment of bladder cancer is transurethral resection (TUR), in which the aim is to remove the tumor completely with endoscopic resection, while attempting to spare the bladder. Depending on the care in case selection, the extent of tumor, and the population of patients being treated, TUR may lead to 5-year survival of 30% to 69%, with the majority of patients retaining an intact bladder (42,43).

Another option that has also enabled bladder preservation has been the surgical removal of the portion of the bladder that contains the tumor—partial cystectomy (44). The general consensus is that this is a technique that should be used only in highly selected cases, provided that the following criteria are met: (1) solitary primary lesion at the dome of the bladder, well removed from the bladder neck and ureters; (2) 2-cm margin of normal bladder tissue around the tumor; (3) likelihood of good bladder capacity and function after the procedure; (4) absence of carcinoma in situ from random biopsies. When present, carcinoma in situ is associated with superficial recurrence, and lymph node involvement is associated with systemic disease (44).

However, the standard of care for most patients with invasive bladder cancer is radical cystectomy (11,45,46), as discussed in detail elsewhere in this chapter. The cure rate depends on well-defined prognostic factors, including conventional indices, such as stage and grade, and the more recent correlates discussed above. In addition, it appears that delay in cystectomy may lead to impaired survival (46). As shown, at USC, we showed that cure is even possible from surgery alone in advanced stage disease, although the chance is much lower. In well-staged patients in contemporary series, the relapse rate after surgical resection of performance status (PS) T3–4 tumors still is 50% or higher, with most relapses occurring at distant sites. As a result, and in view of the modest successes of chemotherapy for metastatic and recurrent disease (see Chapter 16.5), attempts have been made to combine systemic therapy with definitive local treatment. In addition, attempts are being made to modify surgical templates, including the creation of continent pouches and artificial neobladders (11), the use of laparoscopic approaches (47), and the avoidance of prostatectomy (48) in an attempt to ameliorate toxicity for an approach with a high relapse rate.

Radiotherapy and Bladder Preservation Techniques

The use of radiotherapy as an alternative to cystectomy for invasive bladder cancer was previously favored in parts of Europe and Canada, although the pendulum has swung back somewhat toward radical cystectomy in recent years because of the perception of higher surgical cure rates. It should be noted that this perception may be influenced heavily by the fact that comparisons in the literature, between the results of surgery and radiotherapy for bladder cancer, reflect the comparison of surgical versus clinical staging. Furthermore, patients treated in radiation series are characteristically older and less robust than those subjected to cystectomy. The traditional approaches to radiotherapy included doses of external beam irradiation in the range of 50 to 70 Gy, with a higher level of local control achieved in series reporting higher dose schedules (9,10,49–52). Ideal radiotherapy candidates have had aggressive preradiotherapy TUR, absence of extralesional carcinoma in situ, and no hydronephrosis.

The techniques used to deliver curative irradiation to the bladder tumor volume, while sparing normal tissue, vary from one institution to another, depending on the availability of equipment and the quality of physics and computer support (10,49,50). Irrespective of field size and technique, it is clear that dose is critically important, with total doses less than 60 Gy being ineffective (51). Whether the newer techniques of intensity modulated radiation therapy (IMRT) and image-guided radiotherapy will truly improve local control or reduce local tissue toxicity remains to be seen (49). What is clear is that careful treatment planning is critical and requires close collaboration between radiation oncologist and urologist (52). Of particular importance is the definition of the site and size of the tumor, and treatment planning should require a localizing cystogram or planning computed tomography (CT) scan, which is preferred as extravesical disease can be discerned, in the treatment position and periodic assessment to ensure adequacy of ongoing coverage of the tumor and tumor bed within the treatment fields. It is clear that the bladder moves to some extent, despite fixity of bony landmarks, but with appropriate treatment planning, the movement of the bladder does not appear to affect treatment outcomes (53). Various approaches have been studied in an attempt to improve local control, to shorten the duration of treatment, or to ameliorate toxicity.

To date, attenuated dose schedules with hyperfractionation appear to have increased toxicity without providing any improvement in local control or survival (54).

Preservation of a well-functioning bladder is more likely if a portion of the bladder can safely be excluded from the high dose of radiation needed for the bladder cancer itself. Treatment of the entire bladder with high doses per fraction or a high total dose is more likely to result in scarring and contracture, especially for the bladder that has sustained multiple TURs. Care should be taken with respect to the known tolerance of the surrounding normal tissues. Nevertheless, it is clear that bladder preservation maintains quality of life by preserving a functional bladder and avoiding the need for a urinary diversion or "neobladder", with concomitant improvement in sexuality, lifestyle and self image.

One of the key issues of debate has been the respective merits of surgery versus radiotherapy. However, after many decades of comparison, there is still no absolute proof regarding the superiority of radical cystectomy or radical radiotherapy. A recent report from a single institution in the Netherlands suggests that, once differences in staging techniques are taken into account, there is no major difference in outcomes between these modalities of treatment (54). However, others have claimed that, notwithstanding the problems of comparison of surgical versus clinical staging, radical cystectomy ultimately offers better local control and survival, in part because surgical resection of involved pelvic nodes will allow long-term survival in 20% to 30% of cases (11). This view remains controversial and has not been proven in randomized trials.

Chemotherapy and Combined Modality Strategies

Combined modality approaches, incorporating systemic chemotherapy with definitive local modalities, have been studied extensively in the past few years in the hope of sparing the bladder or to improve overall survival (13,55,56). This has been predicated on the following concepts:

- Systemic chemotherapy may reduce the extent of local tumor.
- It facilitates clinical assessment of the chemoresponsiveness of the tumor.
- It may control occult metastases.
- If radiotherapy is planned, it may cause enhanced radiation responsiveness via synergistic effects and radiosensitization.

However, as around 40% to 60% of tumors are absolutely or relatively chemoresistant, some patients will sustain unnecessary toxicity for no benefit, and there is the risk that effective local treatment will be delayed while ineffective systemic chemotherapy is used.

In a randomized, prospective trial assessing the utility of concurrent chemoradiation, a protocol of single-agent cisplatin administered during the period of radiotherapy resulted in 67% sustained pelvic tumor control compared to 45% from radiation alone; however, overall survival was not statistically different, although there was a survival trend in favor of the combined modality therapy (57). It should be noted that this study was not powered to demonstrate a survival benefit. We know of no other randomized trials that have tested the impact of chemoradiation, compared to radiation alone, for invasive bladder cancer, although a range of phase II trials have demonstrated antitumor efficacy and toxicity. The RTOG has completed several studies that have assessed the utility of neoadjuvant or adjuvant chemotherapy in association with concurrent chemoradiation.

The role of neoadjuvant (first-line) systemic chemotherapy, followed by definitive radiotherapy or cystectomy, has been studied in detail (13,56). The early, randomized trials, predominantly using single-agent chemotherapy, failed to show a survival benefit from a combined modality treatment. However, with the introduction of cisplatin-based multidrug regimens, such as MVAC and

TABLE 16.4.2. Results of randomized clinical trials of preemptive chemotherapy for invasive bladder cancer

Series	Regimen	Median survival (months)	Actuarial long-term survival*
Shipley	CMV → C-RT	36	48% 5-year
Shipley	C-RT	36	49% 5-year
Shearer	M → RT	23	39% 3-year
Shearer	RT Only	20	37% 3-year
Wallace	C-RT	~24	39% 3-year
Wallace	RT only	~22	39% 3-year
MRC-EORTC	RT/S Only	37.5	50% 3-year
MRC-EORTC	CMV-RT/S	44	55% 3-year
Intergroup†	MVAC	72	42% 10-year
Intergroup†	Observation	45	35% 10-year

RT, radiotherapy; C, cisplatin; M, methotrexate; A, Adriamycin (doxorubicin); V, vinblastine; S, surgery (usually radical cystectomy).
*Deaths from all causes, including death from intercurrent disease in an elderly population.
†Definitive treatment was cystectomy alone.

CMV, small but significant improvements in survival have been documented in randomized trials and in a meta-analysis (Table 16.4.2) (13,58–60). The Medical Research Council (MRC)–European Organization for Research and Treatment of Cancer (EORTC) international trial of neoadjuvant CMV was designed to identify a 10% difference in long-term survival, but failed to do so (achieving a 6% to 7% difference in outcome) and was thus reported as a "negative" trial (58). The RTOG, also testing the utility of neoadjuvant CMV chemotherapy followed by chemoradiation versus chemoradiation alone, showed identical 3-year survival (61).

Although the North American Intergroup trial of neoadjuvant MVAC revealed a very dramatic difference in median survival (6 years versus 3.8 years), the absolute improvement in long-term survival and potential cure rate was only of the order of 8% (59), a figure consistent with most other published studies (60). The difference in the RTOG trial may have reflected the use of chemoradiation (with cisplatin) in both arms.

These data suggest that, in 2006, a major component of the state of the art is neoadjuvant MVAC chemotherapy followed by cystectomy for patients with invasive bladder cancer who are deemed fit for chemotherapy and surgery. However, this precept does not address the role of radical cystectomy with adjuvant systemic chemotherapy for patients chosen on the basis of histological, biochemical, or other predictive factors. As a consequence, there is still considerable controversy regarding the true standard of care; many clinicians still believe that it is appropriate to perform radical cystectomy as the first step in management of invasive bladder cancer, with subsequent management decisions regarding chemotherapy being predicated on the pathologic stage of the tumor.

Adjuvant (postoperative) chemotherapy has shown some promise in improving survival for patients with invasive bladder cancer. Randomized trials assessing the utility of combination chemotherapy (such as the combination of methotrexate, vinblastine, and cisplatin, with or without doxorubicin or epirubicin—the CMV, MVAC, or MVEC regimens), administered after radical cystectomy for patients with deeply invasive disease or involved lymph nodes, have shown improved disease-free survival (62–65). However, the published trials have been weakened by poor statistical design or execution, and these studies have not demonstrated a statistically significant improvement in overall survival. For example, in one study, there was an uneven distribution of salvage chemotherapy, making the trial a test of chemotherapy at any time after cystectomy, rather than addressing the role of early chemotherapy as classical adjuvant treatment (63). Unfortunately, the situation has been confused by a recent flawed meta-analysis (65), which ignored the various problems of individual published and unpublished trials and grouped them together into a comparison of observed versus expected outcomes. This study erroneously concluded that there is a survival benefit from adjuvant chemotherapy. While this may ultimately prove to be correct, this specific study did not prove this point.

Accordingly, the EORTC has attempted to address this issue in a well-designed, randomized trial, in which standard local therapy has been compared to standard local therapy plus the addition of adjuvant chemotherapy. Unfortunately, this important trial has not accrued as well as had been planned, presumably because of preconceptions of participating clinicians about the true role of neoadjuvant or classical adjuvant chemotherapy, but it is continuing.

Little information is available regarding the use of newer cytotoxic agents in the adjuvant context for bladder cancer. We completed a preliminary assessment of our experience with three to four cycles of adjuvant gemcitabine plus cisplatin after radical cystectomy at the University of Southern California Norris Cancer Hospital, based on the similarity of outcomes when compared to the MVAC regimen for metastatic disease (66). We treated 25 patients with high-grade, invasive bladder cancer demonstrated to be deeply invasive or with involved lymph nodes (67). We have demonstrated that the regimen is well tolerated, and our initial report suggested that this approach yields an actuarial 3-year disease-free survival of 70% (66); however, subsequent follow-up showed that the true median survival was only 3 years. This approach requires further characterization, including long-term follow-up and validation in a randomized trial setting, which is currently the focus of a trial being developed by the Southwest Oncology Group.

Conclusion

Systemic chemotherapy has been shown in randomized trials to improve outcomes of definitive local treatment when used as first-line treatment. Classical adjuvant therapy has been shown to prolong disease-free survival, and appears to produce an improved nonsignificant trend in overall survival, but an ongoing randomized trial will require completion to resolve this issue. Novel biochemical and molecular predictors of prognosis and response to treatment are being used increasingly as aids to clinical management, although definitive trials of their utility remain in progress. However, substantial changes in diagnosis and management seem likely to improve survival from invasive bladder cancer, while reducing the toxicity of treatment.

References

1. Koss LG. Tumors of the urinary bladder. In: Atlas of Tumor Pathology, 2nd series, fascicle 11. Washington, DC: Armed Forces Institute of Pathology, 1975.
2. Johansson SL, Anderstrom CR. Primary adenocarcinoma of the urinary bladder and urachus. In: Raghavan D, Brecher MI, Johnson DH, Meropol NJ, Moots PJ, Thigpen JT, eds. Textbook of Uncommon Cancer. Chichester: Wiley-Liss, 1999:29–43.
3. Sternberg CN, Swanson DA. Non-transitional cell bladder cancer. In: Raghavan D, Scher HI, Leibel S, Lange PH, eds. Principles and Practice of Genitourinary Oncology. Philadelphia: Lippincott-Raven, 1997:315–330.
4. Brown JL, Russell PJ, Philips J, Wotherspoon J, Raghavan D. Clonal analysis of a bladder cancer cell line: an experimental model of tumour heterogeneity. Br J Cancer 1990;61:369–376.
5. Loehrer PJ, Einhorn LH, Elson PJ, et al. A randomized comparison of cisplatin alone or in combination with methotrexate, vinblastine, and doxorubicin in patients with metastatic urothelial carcinoma: a cooperative group study. J Clin Oncol 1992;10: 1066–1072.
6. Bostwick DG, Montironi R, Lopez-Beltran A, Cheng L. Pathology of urothelial tumors of the bladder. In: Droller MJ, ed. American Cancer Society Atlas of Clinical Oncology—Urothelial Tumors. Hamilton, London: BC Decker, 2004:92–111.
7. Ro JY, Ayala AG, El-Naggar A. Muscularis mucosa of urinary bladder: importance for staging and treatment. Am J Surg Pathol 1987;11:668–673.
8. Slack NH, Prout GR Jr. The heterogeneity of invasive bladder carcinoma and different responses to treatment. J Urol 1980;123:644.
9. Mameghan H, Fisher RJ, Watt WH, et al. The management of invasive transitional cell carcinoma of the bladder: results of definitive and preoperative radiation therapy in 390 patients treated at the Prince of Wales Hospital, Sydney, Australia. Cancer 1992;69:2771.
10. Gospodarowicz MK, Hawkins NV, Rawlings GA, et al. Radical radiotherapy for muscle invasive transitional cell carcinoma of the bladder: failure analysis. J Urol 1989;142:1448.
11. Stein JP, Lieskovsky G, Cote R, et al. Radical cystectomy in the treatment of invasive bladder cancer: long-term results in 1054 patients. J Clin Oncol 2001;19: 666–675.
12. Gustafson H, Tribukait B, Esposti PL. DNA profile and tumour progression in patients with superficial bladder tumours. Urol Res 1982;10:13.
13. Raghavan D, Shipley WU, Garnick MB, et al. Biology and management of bladder cancer. N Engl J Med 1990;322:1129–1133.
14. Russell PJ, Brown JL, Grimmond SM, Raghavan D. Molecular biology of urological tumors. Br J Urol 1990;65:121–130.

15. Limas C, Lange PH, Fraley EE, Vessella RL. ABH antigens in transitional cell tumors of the urinary bladder: correlation with the clinical course. Cancer 1979;44: 2099–2107.

16. Spruck CH III, Ohneseit PF, Gonzalez-Zulueta M, et al. Two molecular pathways to transitional cell carcinoma of the bladder. Cancer Res 1994;54:784–788.

17. Esrig D, Elmajian D, Groshen S, et al. Accumulation of nuclear p53 and tumor progression in bladder cancer. N Engl J Med 1994;331:1259–1264.

18. Theodorescu D, Cornil I, Fernandez BJ, Kerbel RS. Overexpression of normal and mutated forms of HRAS induces orthotopic bladder invasion in a human transitional cell carcinoma. Proc Natl Acad Sci USA 1990;97:9047–9051.

19. Theodorescu D, Sapinoso LM, Conaway MR, et al. Reduced expression of metastasis suppressor RhoGDI2 is associated with decreased survival for patients with bladder cancer. Clin Cancer Res 2004;10(11):3800–3806.

20. Cote RJ, Dunn MD, Chatterjee SJ, et al. Elevated and absent pRb expression is associated with bladder cancer progression and has cooperative effects with p53. Cancer Res 1998;58:1090–1094.

21. Stein JP, Ginsberg DA, Grossfeld GD, et al. Effect of p21$^{WAF1/CIP1}$ expression on tumor progression in bladder cancer. J Natl Cancer Inst 1998;90:1072–1079.

22. Tamimi Y, Bringuier PP, Smit F, et al. Homozygous deletions of p16(INK4) occur frequently in bilharziasis-associated bladder cancer. Int J Cancer 1996;65:840–845.

23. Neal DE, Marsh C, Bennett MK, et al. Epidermal-growth-factor receptors in human bladder cancer: comparison of invasive and superficial tumours. Lancet 1985;1: 366–368.

24. Lipponen P, Eskelinen M. Expression of epidermal growth factor receptor in bladder cancer as related to established prognostic factors, oncoprotein (c-erbB-2, p53) expression and long-term prognosis. Br J Cancer 1994;69:1120–1125.

25. Seymour GJ, Walsh MD, Levin MR, Strutton G, Gardiner RA. Transferrin receptor expression by human bladder transitional cell carcinoma. Urol Res 1987;15:341–344.

26. Bochner B, Cote RJ, Weidner N, et al. Angiogenesis in bladder cancer: relationship between microvessel density and tumor prognosis. J Natl Cancer Inst 1995;87: 1603–1612.

27. Grossfeld GD, Ginsberg DA, Stein JP, et al. Thrombospondin-1 expression in bladder cancer: association with p53 alterations, tumor angiogenesis, and tumor progression. J Natl Cancer Inst 1997;89:219–227.

28. Sanchez-Carbayo M, Socci ND, et al. Defining molecular profiles of poor outcome in patients with invasive bladder cancer using oligonucleotide microarrays. J Clin Oncol 2006;24:778–789.

29. Meyers FJ, Palmer JM, Freiha FS, et al. The fate of the bladder in patients with metastatic bladder cancer treated with cisplatin, methotrexate and vinblastine: a Northern California Oncology Group study. J Urol 1985;134:1118–1121.

30. Pendyala L, Velagapudi S, Toth K, et al. Translational studies of glutathione in bladder cancer cell lines and human specimens. Clin Cancer Res 1997;3:793–798.

31. Cote RJ, Esrig D, Groshen S, et al. P53 and treatment of bladder cancer. Nature 1997;385:123–124.

32. Skinner DG, Daniels JR, Russell CA, et al. The role of adjuvant chemotherapy following cystectomy for invasive bladder cancer: a prospective comparative trial. J Urol 1991;145:459–467.

33. Sarkis A, Bajorin D, Reuter V, et al. Prognostic value of p53 nuclear overexpression in patients with invasive bladder cancer treated with neoadjuvant MVAC. J Clin Oncol 1995;13:1384–1390.

34. Siu LL, Banerjee D, Khurana RJ, et al. The prognostic role of p53, metallothionein, P-glycoprotein, and MIB-1 in muscle invasive urothelial transitional cell carcinoma. Clin Cancer Res 1998;4:559–565.

35. Kelley SL, Basu A, Teicher BA, et al. Overexpression of metallothionein confers resistance to anticancer drugs. Science 1988;241:1813–1815.

36. Satoh M, Kloth DM, Kadhim SA, et al. Modulation of both cisplatin nephrotoxicity and drug resistance in murine bladder tumor by controlling metallothionein synthesis. Cancer Res 1993;53:1829–1832.

37. Kielb SJ, Shah NL, Rubin MA, Sanda MG. Functional p53 mutation as a molecular determinant of paclitaxel and gemcitabine susceptibility in human bladder cancer. J Urol 2001;166:482–487.

38. Petrylak DP, Scher HI, Reuter V, O'Brien JP, Cordon-Cardo C. P-glycoprotein expression in primary and metastatic transitional cell carcinoma of the bladder. Ann Oncol 1994;3:835–840.

39. Sanchez-Carbayo M, Socci ND, Lozano J, et al. Defining molecular profiles of poor outcome in patients with invasive bladder cancer using oligonucleotide microarrays. J Clin Oncol 2006;24:778–789.

40. Takata R, Katagiri T, Kanehira M, et al. Predicting response to methotrexate, vinblastine, doxorubicin, and cisplatin neoadjuvant chemotherapy for bladder cancers through genome-wide gene expression profiling. Clin Cancer Res 2005;11:2625–2636.

41. Chakravarti A, Winter K, Wu CL, et al. Expression of the epidermal growth factor receptor and Her-2 are predictors of favorable outcome and reduced complete response rates, respectively, in patients with muscle-invading bladder cancers treated by concurrent radiation and cisplatin-based chemotherapy: a report from the Radiation Therapy Oncology Group. Int J Radiat Oncol Biol Phys 2005;62:309–317.

42. Barnes RW, Dick AL, Hadley HL, Johnston OL. Survival following transurethral resection of ladder carcinoma. Cancer Res 1977;37:2895–2897.

43. Herr HW. Conservative management of muscle-infiltrating bladder cancer: prospective experience. J Urol 1987;138:1162.

44. Holzbeierlein JM, Lopez-Corona E, Bochner BH, et al. Partial cystectomy: a contemporary review of the Memorial Sloan-Kettering Cancer Center experience and recommendations for patient selection. J Urol 2004;172:878–881.

45. Solsona E, Iborra I, Dumont R, et al. Risk groups in patients with bladder cancer treated with radical cystectomy: statistical and clinical model improving homogeneity. J Urol 2005;174:1226–1230.

46. Lee CT, Madii R, Daignault S, et al. Cystectomy delay more than 3 months from initial bladder cancer diagnosis results in decreased disease specific and overall survival. J. Urol 2006;175:1262–1267.

47. Rozet F, Harmon J, Arroyo C, et al. Benefits of laparoscopic prostate-sparing radical cystectomy. Expert Rev Anticancer Ther 2006;6:21–26.

48. Pinthus JH, Nam RK, Klotz LH. Prostate sparing radical cystectomy—not for all, but an option for some. Can J Urol 2006;13(suppl 1):81–87.

49. McBain CA, Logue JP. Radiation for muscle-invasive bladder cancer: treatment planning and delivery in the 21st century. Semin Radiat Oncol 2005;15:42–48.

50. Shipley WU, Prout GR Jr, Kaufman DS, Peronne TL. Invasive bladder carcinoma: the importance of initial transurethral surgery and other significant prognostic factors for improved survival with full-dose irradiation. Cancer 1987;60:514–520.

51. Parsons JT, Million RR. The role of radiation therapy alone or as an adjunct to surgery in bladder carcinoma. Semin Oncol 1990;17:566–582.

52. Michaelson MD, Shipley WU, Heney NM, Zietman AL, Kaufman DS. Selective bladder preservation for muscle invasive transitional cell carcinoma of the urinary bladder. Br J Urol 2004;90:578–581.

53. Lotz HT, Pos FJ, Hulshof MC, van Herk M, et al. Tumor motion and deformation during external radiotherapy of bladder cancer. Int J Radiat Oncol Biol Phys 2006; 64:1551–1558.

54. Horwich A, Dearnaley D, Huddart R, et al. A randomized trial of accelerated radiotherapy for localized invasive bladder cancer. Radiother Oncol 2005;75: 34–43.

55. Nieuwenhuijzen JA, Pos F, Moonen LM, Hart AA, Horenblas S. Survival after bladder-preservation with brachytherapy versus radical cystectomy; a single institution experience. Eur Urol 2005;48:239–245.

56. Vazina A, Raghavan D, Lerner SP. Neoadjuvant and adjunctive systemic chemotherapy in the treatment of invasive urothelial cancer of the bladder. In: Droller MJ, ed. American Cancer Society Atlas of Clinical Oncology—Urothelial Tumors. Hamilton, London: BC Decker, 2004:261–271.

57. Coppin CM, Gospodarowicz MK, James K, et al. Improved local control of invasive bladder cancer by concurrent cisplatin and preoperative or definitive radiation. The National Cancer Institute of Canada Clinical Trials Group. J Clin Oncol 1996;14: 2901–2907.

58. International Collaboration of Trialists on behalf of MRC Advanced Bladder Cancer Working Party, EORTC Genitourinary Group, Australian Bladder Cancer Study Group. Neoadjuvant cisplatin, methotrexate, and vinblastine chemotherapy for muscle-invasive bladder cancer: a randomized controlled trial. Lancet 1999;354: 533–540.

59. Grossman HB, Natale RB, Tangen CM, et al. Neoadjuvant chemotherapy plus cystectomy compared with cystectomy alone for locally advanced bladder cancer. N Engl J Med 2003;349:859–866.

60. Advanced Bladder Cancer Meta-Analysis Collaboration. Neoadjuvant chemotherapy in invasive bladder cancer: a systematic review and meta-analysis. Lancet 2003;361: 1927–1934.

61. Shipley WU, Winter K, Kaufman D, et al. Phase III trial of neoadjuvant chemotherapy in patients with invasive bladder cancer treated with selective bladder preservation by combined radiation therapy and chemotherapy: initial results of Radiation Therapy Oncology Group 89–03. J Clin Oncol 1998;16:3576–3583.

62. Skinner DG, Daniels JR, Russell CA, et al. The role of adjuvant chemotherapy following cystectomy for invasive bladder cancer: a prospective comparative trial. J Urol 1991;145:459–464.

63. Lehman J, Franzaring L, Thuroff J, Wellek S, Stockle M. Complete long-term survival data from a trial of adjuvant chemotherapy vs control after radical cystectomy for locally advanced bladder cancer. BJU Int 2006;97:42–47.

64. Freiha F, Reese J, Torti FM. A randomized trial of radical cystectomy plus cisplatin, vinblastine and methotrexate chemotherapy for muscle invasive bladder cancer. J Urol 1996;155:495–500.

65. Advanced Bladder Cancer (ABC) Meta-Analysis Collaboration. Adjuvant chemotherapy in invasive bladder cancer: a systematic review and meta-analysis of individual patient data. Eur Urol 2005;48:189–201.
66. von der Maase H, Sengelov L, Roberts JT, et al. Long-term survival results of a randomized trial comparing gemcitabine plus cisplatin, with methotrexate, vinblastine, doxorubicin, plus cisplatin in patients with bladder cancer. J Clin Oncol 2005;23: 4602–4608.
67. El Khoueiry A, Tagawa S, Quinn D, Skinner DG, Raghavan D. Adjuvant gemcitabine and cisplatin chemotherapy for locally advanced carcinoma of the bladder after radical cystectomy: USC experience with molecular correlates. Proc Am Soc Clin Oncol 2004;22(suppl):4639.

16.5
Management of Metastatic Bladder Cancer

Matthew D. Galsky and Dean F. Bajorin

Despite local therapy with curative intent, a substantial proportion of patients with invasive transitional cell carcinoma (TCC) of the bladder develop distant metastases during the course of their illness. Furthermore, a subset of patients presents with advanced disease at the time of initial diagnosis. Once the cancer is metastatic, the majority of patients succumb to their disease. As a result, intense efforts over the past two decades have focused on the development of active chemotherapeutic regimens for this disease.

Methotrexate, Vinblastine, Adriamycin (Doxorubicin), and Cisplatin: The (Historical) Gold Standard

Cisplatin is among the most active single agents in urothelial TCC. During the late 1970s, several trials of single-agent cisplatin in patients with advanced TCC reported overall response (OR) rates ranging from 26% to 65% (1–8). Although uncommon, complete responses were also observed (5% to 16%). The median survival of patients treated with single-agent cisplatin in these trials was 8 to 9 months (9–11). Subsequently, additional single-agents were found to have activity in urothelial TCC. The most active of these agents included methotrexate (OR 30%), doxorubicin (OR 17%), and vinblastine (OR 22%) (12–24).

Multiagent chemotherapeutic regimens were developed during the 1980s in an attempt to improve upon the results with single-agent therapy. In 1985, investigators at Memorial Sloan-Kettering Cancer Center (MSKCC) reported a landmark trial using a regimen combining the most active agents at the time: methotrexate, vinblastine, Adriamycin (doxorubicin), and cisplatin (MVAC). In a small cohort, this regimen yielded an overall response rate of 71%. Other groups subsequently published their experience with MVAC and other multia-gent regimens, leading to a series of randomized trials that established MVAC as a standard of care during the 1980s and 1990s (Table 16.5.1).

TABLE 16.5.1. Randomized trials of cisplatin-based chemotherapy in advanced urothelial carcinoma

Treatment	Reference	OR (%)	CR (%)	Survival (months)	p
MVAC	11	36	13	12.5	<.0002
Cisplatin		11	3	8.2	
MVAC	54	65	35	12.6	<.05
CISCA		46	25	10.0	
MVAC	55	59	24	12.5	.17
FAP		42	10	12.5	
MVAC	28	58	9	14.1	.122
HD-MVAC		72	21	15.5	
MVAC	29	46	12	14.8	.746
Gemcitabine + cisplatin		50	12	13.8	
MVAC	30	54	23	14.2	.025
Docetaxel + cisplatin		37	13	9.3	
[a]MVAC	31	40	13	14.2	.41
Paclitaxel + carboplatin		28	3	13.8	

MVAC, methotrexate, vinblastine, Adriamycin (doxorubicin), cisplatin; CISCA, cyclophosphamide, cisplatin, doxorubicin; FAP, 5-fluorouracil, interferon-α-2b, cisplatin; HD-MVAC, high-dose MVAC; OR, overall response rate; CR, complete response rate.
[a]Trial terminated early with only 85 patients; definitive conclusions are not possible.

Limitations

Despite the superiority of MVAC in phase III trials, the limitations of this regimen were readily apparent. Although many patients responded to treatment, median survivals were consistently less than 13 months. Furthermore, the long-term durability of complete responses was poor, with only 3.7% of patients remaining continuously free of disease in an intergroup trial reported comparing MVAC with cisplatin (25).

Perhaps the most limiting factor associated with MVAC was the toxicity; febrile neutropenia occurred in up to 25% of patients and grade 2 to 3 mucositis developed in up to 50%. Other prominent toxicities included decreased renal function, hearing loss, and peripheral neuropathy. Treatment-related deaths occurred in 2% to 4% of patients.

Attempts to Improve MVAC

In an effort to decrease the toxicity and improve the efficacy of MVAC, several investigators evaluated the use of altered doses/schedules with colony-stimulating factor support. In a study utilizing standard dose MVAC, treatment with granulocyte colony-stimulating factor (GCSF) after chemotherapy was associated with a reduction in both hematopoietic toxicity and mucositis (26).

Based on promising phase II data with dose-dense MVAC (standard dose MVAC given every 2 weeks) with GCSF support (27), the European Organization for Research and Treatment of Cancer (EORTC) conducted a randomized trial

TABLE 16.5.2. Results with newer agents in metastatic urothelial carcinoma (cumulative results, data compiled irrespective of dose and schedule)

Treatment	Chemotherapy-naive		Previously treated	
	OR (%)	95% CI (%)	OR (%)	95% CI (%)
Paclitaxel (56–58)	42	23–63	9	0–17
Docetaxel (59,60)	31	14–48	13	4–30
Ifosfamide (61–63)	33	20–46	20	10–32
Gemcitabine (64,65)	26	16–36	23	8–38

OR, overall response rate; CI, confidence interval.

comparing this regimen to MVAC administered every 4 weeks (28). While there was a significant difference in the complete response rates (21% vs. 9%, $p = .009$) and progression-free survival [$p = .037$; hazard ratio (HR) 0.75; 95% confidence interval (CI) 0.58–0.98] favoring the every 2 week schedule, there was no significant difference in median overall survival. Of note, this trial was powered to detect a 50% difference in median survival, and a smaller benefit with this dose-dense regimen may have been missed.

Newer Regimens in Transitional Cell Carcinoma: The Post-MVAC Era

Based on the MVAC experience, it became evident that improvements in efficacy or reduction of toxicity would require new agents. Over the past decade, several new agents with activity in TCC have been identified including gemcitabine, the taxanes, and ifosfamide (Table 16.5.2). Various combinations of the older and newer active drugs have been explored (Table 16.5.3). The combinations of gemcitabine plus cisplatin, docetaxel plus cisplatin, and paclitaxel plus carboplatin have been compared with MVAC in randomized phase III trials.

TABLE 16.5.3. Phase II trials of newer doublets and triplets as first-line treatment in metastatic transitional cell carcinoma (cumulative results, data compiled irrespective of dose and schedule)

Regimen	n	OR (%) (95% CI [%])	CR (%) (95% CI [%])
Paclitaxel + cisplatin (66,67)	86	45 (34–55)	16 (2–24)
Docetaxel + cisplatin (68–70)	129	43 (34–52)	23 (16–30)
Gemcitabine + cisplatin (71–73)	112	46 (37–55)	21 (13–29)
Paclitaxel + carboplatin (74–78)	153	45 (37–53)	18 (12–24)
Gemcitabine + carboplatin (34,79,80)	90	56 (46–66)	8 (2–13)
Paclitaxel + ifosfamide (81)	13	31 (6–56)	23 (0–46)
Paclitaxel + gemcitabine (82)	39	56 (40–72)	8 (0–17)
Ifosfamide + cisplatin + paclitaxel (83,84)	44	68 (52–81)	23 (13–37)
Gemcitabine + cisplatin + paclitaxel (32)	58	78 (60–98)	28 (18–40)
Gemcitabine + carboplatin + paclitaxel (85)	47	68 (56–83)	32 (20–46)

OR, overall response rate; CR, complete response rate.

Gemcitabine and Cisplatin: A New Standard

Based on encouraging initial results with the gemcitabine plus cisplatin (GC) combination, a multicenter randomized phase III trial was performed to compare GC with MVAC in patients with advanced TCC (29); 405 chemotherapy-naive patients were enrolled, with 203 randomized to GC and 202 randomized to MVAC. The response rates on both arms were similar, with 12% complete responses and 37% partial responses on the GC arm and 12% complete responses and 34% partial responses on the MVAC arm ($p = .51$). Similarly, median overall survival was similar, 13.8 months with GC and 14.8 months with MVAC (HR 1.04; 95% CI 0.82–1.32; $p = .75$). Importantly, GC was associated with a better safety profile and tolerability.

This trial was not designed or powered to establish noninferiority. However, these data can be interpreted as showing that the response rates and overall survival achieved with GC is comparable to MVAC. Given these results, and the improved tolerability, GC has become a widely used standard treatment regimen for patients with metastatic TCC.

Docetaxel and Cisplatin

A phase III randomized trial comparing docetaxel plus cisplatin (DC) with MVAC was reported by the Hellenic Cooperative Oncology Group (30). Of the 224 patients enrolled, 109 were randomized to MVAC and 111 were randomized to DC. Although DC was better tolerated, the overall response rate (54.2 vs. 37.4; $p = .017$), median time to progression (9.4 vs. 6.1 months; $p = .003$), and median survival (14.2 vs. 9.3 months; $p = .026$) favored the MVAC arm. Notably, patients were not stratified for baseline performance status, and there were a higher proportion of patients with poor performance status on the DC arm. This imbalance may have, in part, influenced the outcome of this study.

Paclitaxel and Carboplatin

An Eastern Cooperative Oncology Group phase III trial compared MVAC with paclitaxel plus carboplatin (31). After 2½ years, the study was terminated due to poor accrual. Of the planned 330 patients, only 85 were enrolled. Compared with carboplatin/paclitaxel (CP), patients treated with MVAC had more severe myelosuppression, mucositis, and renal toxicity. At a median follow-up of 32.5 months, there was no significant difference in response rate (35.9% MVAC vs. 28.2% CP, $p = p = .34$) or median survival (15.4 months MVAC vs. 13.8 months CP, $p = .41$) between the arms. Because this trial was severely underpowered, definitive conclusions are not possible.

New Triplets in Metastatic Transitional Cell Carcinoma

Several triplet regimens incorporating the newer cytotoxic agents in TCC have been explored in recent years (Table 16.5.3). Although these regimens appear to be associated with higher overall and complete response rates than the commonly utilized doublet regimens, a definitive conclusion cannot be made in the absence of randomized trials. The promising activity of the combination of gemcitabine, paclitaxel, and cisplatin has led to an international phase III trial comparing this regimen with gemcitabine plus cisplatin (32).

Prognostic Factors in Advanced Transitional Cell Carcinoma

Baseline prognostic factors are critical in both predicting outcomes of patients with advanced TCC and in interpreting the results of phase II trials. In a retrospective study, a database of 203 patients with unresectable/metastatic TCC was subjected to multivariate analysis to determine which patient characteristics predicted survival (33). Two factors had independent prognostic significance: Karnofsky performance status (KPS) $\leq$ 80% and visceral (lung, liver, or bone) metastases. The median survival for patients with none, one, or two risk factors was 33, 13.4, and 9.3 months, respectively ($p = .0001$).

By simply altering the proportion of patients from the different risk categories, the survival of a given cohort of patients with advanced TCC could vary from 9 to 26 months.

Therefore, attention to these baseline prognostic factors is critical when comparing median survivals among different phase II studies, and stratification of phase III trials should be based on these variables.

Carboplatin Versus Cisplatin

Given the renal, neurologic, and auditory toxicity associated with cisplatin, and the elderly patient population with advanced TCC, carboplatin-based regimens have been explored extensively. The relative efficacy of carboplatin, compared with cisplatin, in advanced TCC is controversial. There have been no phase III studies performed to definitively answer this question. However, several randomized phase II trials have been performed (34–36) (Table 16.5.4), which

TABLE 16.5.4. Randomized phase II trials comparing cisplatin- and carboplatin-based combinations in advanced urothelial carcinoma

Treatment	Citation	CR (%)	OR (%)	p
MVAC	36	13	52	.3
MCAVI		0	39	
MVE-cisplatin	35	25	71	.04
MVE-carboplatin		11	41	
[a]Gemcitabine + cisplatin	34	23	66	NP
Gemcitabine + carboplatin		9	59	

MVAC, methotrexate, vinblastine, Adriamycin (doxorubicin), cisplatin; MCAVI, methotrexate, carboplatin, vinblastine; MVE, methotrexate, vinblastine, epirubicin; NP, not provided; OR, overall response; CR, complete response.
[a]Preliminary results.

consistently report higher overall and complete response rates for the cisplatin-containing regimens. As a result, in patients with advanced TCC with favorable prognostic factors, and adequate renal function, cisplatin-based therapy should be considered the treatment of choice.

New Approaches to the Treatment of Transitional Cell Carcinoma

Targeting the Epidermal Growth Factor Receptor

The human epidermal growth factor receptor (EGFR) family of tyrosine kinases is an important mediator of cell growth, survival, and differentiation. Binding of ligands to EGFR (or c-ErbB1) leads to homodimerization or heterodimerization with other members of the receptor subfamily (including c-ErbB2 or Her-2). These interactions result in autophosphorylation of the intracellular domain of EGFR and subsequent signaling through the mitogen-activated protein kinase pathway. Expression of EGFR and Her-2 has been variably demonstrated in bladder cancer specimens (2% to 74%) depending on the methodology used and the criteria utilized to define expression. Epidermal growth factor receptor expression has also been implicated as a prognostic factor in TCC. As a result, this family of receptors has been a prime target for novel treatment strategies (37).

Trastuzumab is a humanized murine monoclonal antibody directed against the extracellular domain of Her-2. A multicenter phase II study has explored a regimen integrating this novel agent with the combination of gemcitabine, carboplatin, and paclitaxel (38). Patients eligible for this trial had metastatic or recurrent urothelial carcinoma and either tissue or serum available for Her-2 testing.

Patients with evidence of either Her-2 overexpression by immunohistochemistry), fluorescent in-situ hybridization, or serum testing (>16 ng/mL) were then enrolled for treatment. In a preliminary report, of the 111 patients registered, 59 patients overexpressed Her-2, and 44 patients went on to receive treatment. Treatment with this regimen was generally well tolerated, with myelosuppression as the major toxicity. The overall response rate of 70% and median survival of 15.1 months with this regimen is promising; however, the ultimate contribution of trastuzumab can only be delineated in a random assignment trial.

Targeting Angiogenesis

Several processes central to tumor progression, including tumor growth, invasion, and metastasis, are dependent on an adequate blood supply. Angiogenesis, the process by which the neovascular blood supply is recruited, is orchestrated by a balance of stimulatory and inhibitory factors released by tumor and host cells. Over 25 years ago, Chodak et al. (39) first demonstrated that the urine of patients with TCC contained proangiogenic substances. Several mediators of angiogenesis have subsequently been identified, among which the most potent is vascular endothelial growth factor (VEGF). The major angiogenic effects of VEGF are mediated through binding to VEGFR-2 (or Flk-1), a receptor tyrosine kinase expressed on endothelial cells (40). Targeting the VEGF/VEGFR-2 axis has proven beneficial in the treatment of several solid tumors (41).

Multiple lines of evidence support targeting angiogenesis in TCC:

- Microvessel density, a histological measure of angiogenesis, has been correlated with stage, recurrence, and survival, in TCC (42–44).
- Increased expression of VEGF in the tissue, serum, and urine of patients with TCC has been correlated with stage and prognosis (45–47).
- Inhibitors of angiogenesis have shown activity in preclinical models of TCC (48–50).

Bevacizumab is a recombinant humanized monoclonal antibody that binds all isoforms of human VEGF. In clinical studies, treatment with single-agent bevacizumab has proven safe and has resulted in prolonged time to disease progression when compared with placebo in patients with metastatic renal cell carcinoma (23).

However, optimization of antiangiogenic therapy in most solid tumors will likely require coadministration with cytotoxic chemotherapy. Indeed, this approach has already proven successful. The addition of bevacizumab to cytotoxic chemotherapy has significantly improved response proportions in randomized trials in non–small-cell lung cancer, breast cancer, and colon cancer (10,24,25) and has led to a significant improvement in overall survival in phase III trials in colon cancer and non–small-cell lung cancer. Trials integrating bevacizumab, and other antiangiogenic agents, in the treatment of TCC are underway.

Special Considerations in Metastatic Transitional Cell Carcinoma

Postchemotherapy Surgery

The importance of postchemotherapy surgery in the setting of minimal residual disease after achieving a "near" complete response to chemotherapy has been highlighted in several analyses (51–53). In a retrospective study of 203 patients treated with MVAC, 50 patients underwent postchemotherapy surgery for suspected or known residual disease (51). In 17 patients, no viable tumor was found at the time of surgery. Three patients had postchemotherapy surgery aborted due to unresectable disease. In the remaining 30 patients, residual disease was completely resected, resulting in a complete response to chemotherapy plus surgery. Of these 30 patients, 10 (33%) remained alive at 5 years, similar to results attained for patients achieving a complete response to chemotherapy alone (41%). Optimal candidates were those patients with disease limited to the primary site or lymph nodes prior to initiation of chemotherapy.

Second-Line Therapy

For patients with progressive TCC after first-line chemotherapy, prognosis is poor. However, several trials have shown modest activity of both single agents and combinations in patients with refractory or recurrent disease (Table 16.5.2).

In patients with a preserved functional status, treatment with one of these agents/combinations may be appropriate. Alternatively, enrollment on a clinical trial should always be considered.

Conclusion

There have been significant advances in the management of metastatic TCC in the last 20 years. This disease has proven to be chemotherapy-sensitive, and long-term survival has been achieved in a select subgroup of patients. Recently, regimens with retained activity and improved tolerability have been introduced. Novel approaches are needed to further improve the outlook for patients with this disease.

References

1. Herr HW. Cis-diamminedichloride platinum II in the treatment of advanced bladder cancer. J Urol 1980;123:853–855.
2. Yagoda A. Phase II trials with cis-dichlorodiammineplatinum(II) in the treatment of urothelial cancer. [Review]. Cancer Treat Rep 1979;63:1565–1572.
3. Peters PC, O'Neill MR. Cis-diamminedichloroplatinum as a therapeutic agent in metastatic transitional cell carcinoma. J Urol 1991;121:375–377.
4. Merrin C. Treatment of advanced bladder cancer with cis-diamminedichloroplatinum (II NSC 119875): A pilot study. J Urol 1978;119:493–495.
5. Soloway MS, Ikard M, Ford K. Cis-diamminedichloroplatinum (II) in locally advanced and metastatic urothelial cancer. Cancer 1981;47:476–480.
6. De Lena M, Lorusso V, Iacobellis U, et al. Cis-diamminedichloroplatinum activity in bidimensionally measurable metastatic lesions of the bladder. Tumori 1984;70:85–88.
7. Oliver RTD, Newlands ES, Wiltshaw E, Malpas JS. A phase 2 study of cis-platinum in patients with recurrent bladder carcinoma. The London and Oxford Co-operative Urological Cancer Group. Br J Urol 1981;55:444–457.
8. Rossof AH, Talley RW, Stephens R, et al. Phase II evaluation of cis-dichlorodiammineplatinum (II) in advanced malignancies of the genitourinary and gynecologic organs: a Southwest Oncology Group Study. Cancer Treat Rep 1979;63:1557–1564.
9. Soloway MS, Einstein A, Corder MP, et al. A comparison of cisplatin and the combination of cisplatin and cyclophosphamide in advanced urothelial cancer. A National Bladder Cancer Collaborative Group A Study. Cancer 1983;51:767–772.
10. Hillcoat BL, Raghavan D, Matthews J, et al. A randomized trial of cisplatin versus cisplatin plus methotrexate in advanced cancer of the urothelial tract. J Clin Oncol 1989;7:706–709.

11. Loehrer PJ Sr, Einhorn LH, Elson PJ, et al. A randomized comparison of cisplatin alone or in combination with methotrexate, vinblastine, and doxorubicin in patients with metastatic urothelial carcinoma: a cooperative group study. J Clin Oncol 1992; 10(7):1066–1073.

12. Oliver RT. Methotrexate as salvage or adjunctive therapy for primary invasive carcinoma of the bladder. Cancer Treat Rep 1981;65(suppl 1):179–181.

13. Oliver RT, England HR, Risdon RA, Blandy JP. Methotrexate in the treatment of metastatic and recurrent primary transitional cell carcinoma. J Urol 1984;131(3): 483–485.

14. Turner AG, Hendry WF, Williams GB, Bloom HJ. The treatment of advanced bladder cancer with methotrexate. Br J Urol 1977;49(7):673–678.

15. Turner AG. Methotrexate in advanced bladder cancer. Cancer Treat Rep 1981;65(suppl 1):183–186.

16. Natale RB, Yagoda A, Watson RC, et al. Methotrexate: an active drug in bladder cancer. Cancer 1981;47:1246–1250.

17. Gad-el-Mawla N, Hamsa R, Cairns J, Anderson T, Ziegler JL. Phase II trial of methotrexate in carcinoma of the bilharzial bladder. Cancer Treat Rep 1978;62: 1075–1076.

18. Hall RR. Methotrexate treatment for advanced bladder cancer. A review after 6 years. Br J Urol 1980;52(5):403.

19. Pavone-Macaluso M, EORTC Genito-urinary Tract Co-Operative Group A. Single-drug chemotherapy of bladder cancer with Adriamycin, VM-26 or bleomycin. Eur Urol 1976;2:138–141.

20. O'Bryan RM, Baker LH, Gottlieb JE. Dose response evaluation of Adriamycin in human neoplasia. Cancer 1977;39:1940.

21. Yagoda A, Watson RC, Whitmore WF, et al. Adriamycin in advanced urinary tract cancer. Experience in 42 patients and review of the literature. Cancer 1977;39: 279–285.

22. Knight EW, Pagand M, Hahn RG, Horton J. Comparison of 5–FU and doxorubicin in the treatment of carcinoma of the bladder. Cancer Treat Rep 1983;67:514–515.

23. Gagliano R, Levin H, El-Bolkainy MN, et al. Adriamycin versus Adriamycin plus cis-diamminedichloroplatinum (DDP) in advanced transitional cell bladder carcinoma. A Southwest Oncology Group Study. Am J Clin Oncol (CCT) 1983;6:215–218.

24. Blumenreich MS, Yagoda A, Natale RB, Watson RC. Phase II trial of vinblastine sulfate for metastatic urothelial tract tumors. Cancer 1982;50:435–438.

25. Saxman SB, Propert KJ, Einhorn LH, et al. Long-term follow-up of a phase III inter-group study of cisplatin alone or in combination with methotrexate, vinblastine, and doxorubicin in patients with metastatic urothelial carcinoma: a cooperative group study. J Clin Oncol 1997;15(7):2564–2569.

26. Gabrilove JL, Jakubowski A, Scher H, et al. Effect of granulocyte colony-stimulating factor on neutropenia and associated morbidity due to chemotherapy for transitional-cell carcinoma of the urothelium. N Engl J Med 1988;318(22):1414–1422.

27. Sternberg CN, de Mulder PH, van Oosterom AT, et al. Escalated M-VAC chemotherapy and recombinant human granulocyte-macrophage colony stimulating factor (rhGM-CSF) in patients with advanced urothelial tract tumors. Ann Oncol 1993;4(5): 403–407.

28. Sternberg CN, de Mulder PH, Schornagel JH, et al. Randomized phase III trial of high-dose-intensity methotrexate, vinblastine, doxorubicin, and cisplatin (MVAC) chemotherapy and recombinant human granulocyte colony-stimulating factor

versus classic MVAC in advanced urothelial tract tumors: European Organization for Research and Treatment of Cancer Protocol no. 30924. J Clin Oncol 2001;19: 2638–2646.

29. von der Maase H, Hansen SW, Roberts JT, et al. Gemcitabine and cisplatin versus methotrexate, vinblastine, doxorubicin, and cisplatin in advanced or metastatic bladder cancer: results of a large, randomized, multinational, multicenter, phase III study. J Clin Oncol 2000;18(17):3068–3077.

30. Bamias A, Aravantinos G, Deliveliotis C, et al. Docetaxel and cisplatin with granulo-cyte colony-stimulating factor (G-CSF) versus MVAC with G-CSF in advanced uro-thelial carcinoma: a multicenter, randomized, phase III study from the Hellenic Cooperative Oncology Group. J Clin Oncol 2004;22:220–228.

31. Dreicer R, Manola J, Roth BJ, et al. Phase III trial of methotrexate, vinblastine, doxo-rubicin, and cisplatin versus carboplatin and paclitaxel in patients with advanced carcinoma of the urothelium. Cancer 2004;100(8):1639–1645.

32. Bellmunt J, Guillem V, Paz-Ares L, et al. Phase I-II study of paclitaxel, cisplatin, and gemcitabine in advanced transitional-cell carcinoma of the urothelium. Spanish Oncology Genitourinary Group. J Clin Oncol 2000;18(18):3247–3255.

33. Bajorin DF, Dodd PM, Mazumdar M, et al. Long-term survival in metastatic transi-tional-cell carcinoma and prognostic factors predicting outcome of therapy. J Clin Oncol 1999;17(10):3173–3181.

34. Carteni G, Dogliotti L, Crucitta A, et al. Phase II randomised trial of gemcitabine plus cisplatin (GP) and gemcitabine plus carboplatin (GC) in patients (pts) with advanced or metastatic transitional cell carcinoma of the urothelium (TCCU). Proc Am Soc Clin Oncol 2003; abstract 1543.

35. Petrioli R, Frediani B, Manganelli A, et al. Comparison between a cisplatin-containing regimen and a carboplatin-containing regimen for recurrent or meta-static bladder cancer patients. A randomized phase II study. Cancer 1996;77(2): 344–351.

36. Bellmunt J, Ribas A, Eres N, et al. Carboplatin-based versus cisplatin-based chemo-therapy in the treatment of surgically incurable advanced bladder carcinoma. Cancer 1997;80(10):1966–1972.

37. Bellmunt J, Hussain M, Dinney CP. Novel approaches with targeted therapies in bladder cancer. Therapy of bladder cancer by blockade of the epidermal growth factor receptor family. Crit Rev Oncol Hematol 2003;46(suppl):85–104.

38. Hussain M, Petrylak D, Dunn R, et al. Trastuzumab (T), paclitaxel (P), carboplatin (C), and gemcitabine (G) in advanced HER2–positive urothelial carcinoma: results of a multi-center phase II NCI trial. J Clin Oncol 2005;23(16S):abstract 4507.

39. Chodak GW, Scheiner CJ, Zetter BR. Urine from patients with transitional-cell carcinoma stimulates migration of capillary endothelial cells. N Engl J Med 1981; 305(15):869–874.

40. Ferrara N, Hillan KJ, Gerber HP, Novotny W. Discovery and development of bevaci-zumab, an anti-VEGF antibody for treating cancer. Nat Rev Drug Discov 2004;3(5): 391–400.

41. Hurwitz H, Fehrenbacher L, Novotny W, et al. Bevacizumab plus irinotecan, fluoro-uracil, and leucovorin for metastatic colorectal cancer. N Engl J Med 2004;350(23): 2335–2342.

42. Dickinson AJ, Fox SB, Persad RA, et al. Quantification of angiogenesis as an indepen-dent predictor of prognosis in invasive bladder carcinomas. Br J Urol 1994;74(6): 762–766.

43. Jaeger TM, Weidner N, Chew K, et al. Tumor angiogenesis correlates with lymph node metastases in invasive bladder cancer. J Urol 1995;154(1):69–71.
44. Bochner BH, Cote RJ, Weidner N, et al. Angiogenesis in bladder cancer: relationship between microvessel density and tumor prognosis. J Natl Cancer Inst 1995;87(21): 1603–1612.
45. Brown LF, Berse B, Jackman RW, et al. Increased expression of vascular permeability factor (vascular endothelial growth factor) and its receptors in kidney and bladder carcinomas. Am J Pathol 1993;143(5):1255–1262.
46. Chopin DK, Caruelle JP, Colombel M, et al. Increased immunodetection of acidic fibroblast growth factor in bladder cancer, detectable in urine. J Urol 1993;150:1126–1130.
47. Nguyen M, Watanabe H, Budson AE, et al. Elevated levels of the angiogenic peptide basic fibroblast growth factor in urine of bladder cancer patients. J Natl Cancer Inst 1993;85(3):241–242.
48. Inoue K, Slaton JW, Davis DW, et al. Treatment of human metastatic transitional cell carcinoma of the bladder in a murine model with the anti-vascular endothelial growth factor receptor monoclonal antibody DC101 and paclitaxel. Clin Cancer Res 2000;6(7):2635–2643.
49. Inoue K, Chikazawa M, Fukata S, Yoshikawa C, Shuin T. Docetaxel enhances the therapeutic effect of the angiogenesis inhibitor TNP-470 (AGM-1470) in metastatic human transitional cell carcinoma. Clin Cancer Res 2003;9(2):886–899.
50. Inoue K, Chikazawa M, Fukata S, Yoshikawa C, Shuin T. Frequent administration of angiogenesis inhibitor TNP-470 (AGM-1470) at an optimal biological dose inhibits tumor growth and metastasis of metastatic human transitional cell carcinoma in the urinary bladder. Clin Cancer Res 2002;8(7):2389–2398.
51. Dodd PM, McCaffrey JA, Herr H, et al. Outcome of postchemotherapy surgery after treatment with methotrexate, vinblastine, doxorubicin, and cisplatin in patients with unresectable or metastatic transitional cell carcinoma. J Clin Oncol 1999;17(8): 2546–2552.
52. Donat SM, Herr HW, Bajorin DF, et al. Methotrexate, vinblastine, doxorubicin and cisplatin chemotherapy and cystectomy for unresectable bladder cancer. J Urol 1996; 156(2 pt 1):368–371.
53. Miller RS, Freiha FS, Reese JH, Ozen H, Torti FM. Cisplatin, methotrexate and vinblastine plus surgical restaging for patients with advanced transitional cell carcinoma of the urothelium. J Urol 1993;150(1):65–69.
54. Logothetis CJ, Dexeus F, Sella A, et al. A prospective randomized trial comparing CISCA to MVAC chemotherapy in advanced metastatic urothelial tumors. J Clin Oncol 1990;8:1050–1055.
55. Siefker-Radtke AO, Millikan RE, Tu SM, et al. Phase III trial of fluorouracil, interferon alpha-2b, and cisplatin versus methotrexate, vinblastine, doxorubicin, and cisplatin in metastatic or unresectable urothelial cancer. J Clin Oncol 2002;20(5):1361–1367.
56. Roth BJ, Dreicer R, Einhorn LH, et al. Significant activity of paclitaxel in advanced transitional-cell carcinoma of the urothelium: a phase II trial of the Eastern Cooperative Oncology Group. J Clin Oncol 1994;12(11):2264–2270.
57. Vaughn DJ, Broome CM, Hussain M, Gutheil JC, Markowitz AB. Phase II trial of weekly paclitaxel in patients with previously treated advanced urothelial cancer. J Clin Oncol 2002;20(4):937–940.
58. Papamichael D, Gallagher CJ, Oliver RT, Johnson PW, Waxman J. Phase II study of paclitaxel in pretreated patients with locally advanced/metastatic cancer of the bladder and ureter. Br J Cancer 1997;75(4):606–607.

59. de Wit R, Kruit WH, Stoter G, de Boer M, Kerger J, Verweij J. Docetaxel (Taxotere): an active agent in metastatic urothelial cancer; results of a phase II study in non-chemotherapy-pretreated patients. Br J Cancer 1998;78(10):1342–1345.

60. McCaffrey JA, Hilton S, Mazumdar M, et al. Phase II trial of docetaxel in patients with advanced or metastatic transitional-cell carcinoma. J Clin Oncol 1997;15(5): 1853–1857.

61. Gad el Mawla N, Hamza MR, Zikri ZK, et al. Chemotherapy in invasive carcinoma of the bladder. A review of phase II trials in Egypt. Acta Oncol 1989;28:73–76.

62. Otaguro K, Ueda K, Niijma T, et al. Clinical evaluation of Z4942 (ifosfamide) for malignant urological tumors. Acta Urol Jpn 1981;27:459–469.

63. Witte RS, Elson P, Bono B, et al. Eastern Cooperative Oncology Group phase II trial of ifosfamide in the treatment of previously treated advanced urothelial carcinoma. J Clin Oncol 1997;15(2):589–593.

64. Stadler WM, Kuzel T, Roth B, Raghavan D, Dorr FA. Phase II study of single-agent gemcitabine in previously untreated patients with metastatic urothelial cancer. J Clin Oncol 1997;15(11):3394–3398.

65. Moore MJ, Tannock IF, Ernst DS, Huan S, Murray N. Gemcitabine: a promising new agent in the treatment of advanced urothelial cancer. J Clin Oncol 1997;15(12): 3441–3445.

66. Dreicer R, Manola J, Roth BJ, Cohen MB, Hatfield AK, Wilding G. Phase II study of cisplatin and paclitaxel in advanced carcinoma of the urothelium: an Eastern Cooperative Oncology Group Study. J Clin Oncol 2000;18(5):1058–1061.

67. Burch PA, Richardson RL, Cha SS, et al. Phase II study of paclitaxel and cisplatin for advanced urothelial cancer. J Urol 2000;164(5):1538–1542.

68. Garcia del Muro X, Marcuello E, Guma J, et al. Phase II multicentre study of docetaxel plus cisplatin in patients with advanced urothelial cancer. Br J Cancer 2002;86(3): 326–330.

69. Sengelov L, Kamby C, Lund B, Engelholm SA. Docetaxel and cisplatin in metastatic urothelial cancer: a phase II study. J Clin Oncol 1998;16(10):3392–3397.

70. Dimopoulos MA, Bakoyannis C, Georgoulias V, et al. Docetaxel and cisplatin combination chemotherapy in advanced carcinoma of the urothelium: a multicenter phase II study of the Hellenic Cooperative Oncology Group. Ann Oncol 1999;10(11): 1385–1388.

71. von der Maase H, Andersen L, Crino L, Weinknecht S, Dogliotti L. Weekly gemcitabine and cisplatin combination therapy in patients with transitional cell carcinoma of the urothelium: a phase II clinical trial. Ann Oncol 1999;10(12): 1461–1465.

72. Kaufman D, Raghavan D, Carducci M, et al. Phase II trial of gemcitabine plus cisplatin in patients with metastatic urothelial cancer. J Clin Oncol 2000;18(9):1921–1927.

73. Moore MJ, Winquist EW, Murray N, et al. Gemcitabine plus cisplatin, an active regimen in advanced urothelial cancer: a phase II trial of the National Cancer Institute of Canada Clinical Trials Group. J Clin Oncol 1999;17(9):2876–2881.

74. Redman BG, Smith DC, Flaherty L, Du W, Hussain M. Phase II trial of paclitaxel and carboplatin in the treatment of advanced urothelial carcinoma. J Clin Oncol 1998; 16(5):1844–1848.

75. Zielinski CC, Schnack B, Grbovic M, et al. Paclitaxel and carboplatin in patients with metastatic urothelial cancer: results of a phase II trial. Br J Cancer 1998;78(3): 370–374.

76. Pycha A, Grbovic M, Posch B, et al. Paclitaxel and carboplatin in patients with metastatic transitional cell cancer of the urinary tract. Urology 1999;53(3):510–515.

77. Vaughn DJ, Manola J, Dreicer R, See W, Levitt R, Wilding G. Phase II study of paclitaxel plus carboplatin in patients with advanced carcinoma of the urothelium and renal dysfunction (E2896): a trial of the Eastern Cooperative Oncology Group. Cancer 2002;95(5):1022–1027.

78. Small EJ, Lew D, Redman BG, et al. Southwest Oncology Group Study of paclitaxel and carboplatin for advanced transitional-cell carcinoma: the importance of survival as a clinical trial end point. J Clin Oncol 2000;18(13):2537–2544.

79. Carles J, Nogue M. Gemcitabine/carboplatin in advanced urothelial cancer. Semin Oncol 2001;28(suppl):19–24.

80. Bellmunt J, de Wit R, Albanell J, Baselga J. A feasibility study of carboplatin with fixed dose of gemcitabine in "unfit" patients with advanced bladder cancer. Eur J Cancer 2001;37(17):2212–2215.

81. Sweeney CJ, Williams SD, Finch DE, et al. A Phase II study of paclitaxel and ifosfamide for patients with advanced refractory carcinoma of the urothelium. Cancer 1999; 86(3):514–518.

82. Meluch AA, Greco FA, Burris HA III, et al. Paclitaxel and gemcitabine chemotherapy for advanced transitional-cell carcinoma of the urothelial tract: a phase II trial of the Minnie Pearl Cancer Research Network. J Clin Oncol 2001;19(12):3018–3024.

83. Bajorin DF, McCaffrey JA, Hilton S, et al. Treatment of patients with transitional-cell carcinoma of the urothelial tract with ifosfamide, paclitaxel, and cisplatin: a phase II trial. J Clin Oncol 1998;16:2722–2727.

84. Bajorin DF, McCaffrey JA, Dodd PM, et al. Ifosfamide, paclitaxel, and cisplatin for patients with advanced transitional cell carcinoma of the urothelial tract: final report of a phase II trial evaluating two dosing schedules. Cancer 2000;88(7):1671–1678.

85. Hussain M, Vaishampayan U, Du W, Redman B, Smith DC. Combination paclitaxel, carboplatin, and gemcitabine is an active treatment for advanced urothelial cancer. J Clin Oncol 2001;19(9):2527–2533.

16.6
Urethral Cancer (Excluding Penile Cancer)

Priyadarshi Kumar and Vinod H. Nargund

Primary neoplasm of the urethra is rare, which makes its study difficult and explains the lack of studies in the literature. The studies reported are retrospective reviews of treatment. Therefore, it has not been possible to adequately define the natural history or suggest an ideal management strategy in these tumors. At presentation it has often invaded locally, contributing to its generally poor prognosis despite the treatment modality employed. This chapter discusses primary malignancy of the urethra, with specific reference to transitional cell carcinoma.

Epidemiology

Primary urethral cancer is extremely rare, accounting for less than 1% of all malignancies. Female urethral cancer is four times more common than male urethral cancer. It typically presents after the age of 60. Primary carcinoma of the urethra accounts for only 0.02% of all malignancies in females (1). The exact etiology is not known. Caucasians seem to have a higher incidence (2). There are number of differences between male and female urethral malignancy due to anatomic and histological factors.

Risk Factors

Like many other cancers, chronic inflammation seems to play a role in the pathogenesis of urethral cancer. In males, an increased incidence of primary urethral cancer has been associated with sexually transmitted diseases and urethral stricture disease (3). There is also evidence to suggest that human papilloma virus 16 (HPV-16) is associated with the development of squamous cell cancer of the urethra (4). For females these associations are not so strong, but chronic irritation and urinary tract infections have been implicated with urethral cancer. Other factors quoted include preexisting lesions such as caruncles, papillomas, adenomas, polyps, and leukoplakia of the urethra (5). Smoking is a risk factor for bladder cancer, as well as a risk factor in the development of transitional cell urethral carcinoma.

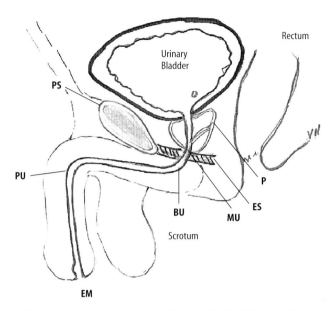

FIGURE 16.6.1. Diagrammatic representation of urethra and bladder. ES, external sphincter; BU, bulbar urethra; PU, penile urethra; P, prostate; EM, external urethral meatus; PS, pubic symphysis; MU, membranous urethra.

Anatomy

The anatomy of the urethra explains the pathological types, progression, and behavior of urethral carcinoma in both sexes.

Male Urethra

The male urethra has an approximate length of 20 cm. For descriptive purposes the male urethra is anatomically divided into penile, bulbar, membranous, and prostatic segments (Fig. 16.6.1 and Table 16.6.1).

The male urethra may be subdivided into anterior and posterior, according to the lymphatic drainage. The anterior urethra comprises the urethral meatus, fossa navicularis, and penile segment, and their lymph drainage is to the inguinal nodes. The posterior urethra comprises the bulbar, membranous, and prostatic segments, which drain to the pelvic nodes. Penile cancer is discussed in detail in Chapter 19.

TABLE 16.6.1. Urethral segments and epithelial type in the male

Urethral segment	Epithelium
Urethral meatus, fossa navicularis	Stratified squamous
Penile, bulbar	Pseudostratified and stratified columnar
Prostatic, membranous	Transitional

Female Urethra

The female urethra is shorter than its male counterpart with an approximate length of 4 cm. The distal two thirds are lined by stratified squamous epithelium, while the proximal third comprises transitional cell epithelium. The distal third or anterior urethra drains to the superficial and deep inguinal lymph nodes. The proximal two thirds or posterior urethra drains to the pelvic nodes.

Pathology

Male

Benign Tumors

Condyloma acuminatum (genital or venereal warts; human papilloma virus types 6 to 11) is slow growing, entails urethral involvement in 5% of patients, and is commonly seen on the glans, shaft, and prepuce.

Urethral polyps are fibrous (usually congenital and early presentation) or prostatic polyps (uncertain etiology and related to reactive proliferations secondary to urethral injury). The lesion could be sessile or papillary.

Premaligant

Balanitis xerotica obliterans is a genital variation of lichen sclerosis et atrophicus. Leukoplakia are whitish plaques involving the meatus and associated with in situ squamous carcinoma and verrucous cancer. Carcinoma in situ is a synonym for erythroplasia of Queyrat or Bowen's disease of the glans (6).

Malignant Tumors

Primary urethral malignancy accounts for less than 1% of genitourinary tumors in men. The common histological varieties include squamous (80%), urothelial (15%), adenocarcinoma (5%), and rarer varieties including malignant melanoma, basal cell carcinoma, and sarcomas. The commonest urethral tumor, squamous cell carcinoma, occurs in the bulbo-urethral region (60%). Ninety percent of cancers in the prostatic urethra are transitional in origin, reflecting the predominant epithelial type in this location.

Kaposi's sarcoma of the meatus has also been described, although more common areas, including the skin, oral mucosa, lymph nodes, and visceral organs, may be involved (7).

Nearly 4% to 18% of men develop urethral transitional cell carcinoma (TCC) after cystectomy (8–10).

Female

In a series of 18 female patients, Thyavihally et al. (11) found the predominant histology to be squamous cell cancer, accounting for 50% of cases. Transitional cell cancer accounted for 28% and adenocarcinoma 22%. Nearly 6% of women undergoing cystourethrectomy have urethral TCC (12).

Clinical Presentation

There is no typical clinical presentation of urethral cancer. Because of early local involvement, most of the tumors are advanced at the time of presentation. The presentation is insidious, and the symptoms are often ascribed to benign disorders. The most common presentation is with a palpable urethral lump or with lower urinary tract symptoms. Alternative presentations include urethral stricture disease, urethral fistulation, urethral diverticula, abscesses, recurrent urinary tract infections, dyspareunia, perineal pain, and lymphadenopathy. Hemospermia may be an additional symptom in men. It must be emphasized that a strong index of suspicion should be exercised with a low threshold for investigation so that any delay is avoided.

In patients who have undergone urethra-sparing cystectomy, urethral bleeding is the only sign of urethral TCC. However regular endoscopic surveillance is mandatory in these cases.

Tumor, Node, Metastasis Staging (Table 16.6.2)

Urethral cancer spreads locally to the corpora, periurethral muscle, and adjacent organs including vagina, prostate, bladder, and rectum. Palpable lymph nodes are present in 20% of patients at presentation, and most of them have tumor within these nodes. Hematogenous spread is rare and a late event.

TABLE 16.6.2. Tumor, node, metastasis (TNM) classification of urethral cancer

Primary	Tumor
Local tumor	
Tx	Primary tumor cannot be assessed
T0	No evidence of primary tumor
Ta	Noninvasive papillary, polypoid, or verrucous carcinoma
Tis	Carcinoma in situ
T1	Tumor invading subepithelial connective tissue
T2	Tumor invading any of the following: corpus spongiosum, prostate, periurethral muscle
T3	Tumor invading any of the following: corpus cavernosum, beyond prostatic capsule, anterior vagina, bladder neck
T4	Tumor invades other adjacent organs
Regional	Lymph nodes
Nx	Regional lymph nodes cannot be assessed
N0	No regional lymph node metastasis
N1	Metastasis in a single lymph node, 2 cm or less in greatest dimension
N2	Metastasis in a single lymph node, larger than 2 cm but less than 5 cm in greatest dimension; or in multiple nodes, none greater than 5 cm
N3	Metastasis in a single lymph node greater than 5 cm in greatest dimension
Distant metastasis	
Mx	Distant metastasis cannot be assessed
M0	No distant metastasis
M1	Distant metastasis

Prognostic Factors

The prognosis depends on the cancer's anatomical location and depth of invasion. Tumor stage clearly is an important prognostic indicator, with advanced tumors having poor prognosis (13). The prognosis is also poor in female urethral carcinoma involving proximal or urethral involvement (11). The clinical course of TCC of the urethra is discussed later.

Diagnostic Investigations

Apart from routine investigations like complete blood count, urea and electrolytes, liver function tests, and bone profile, urine is sent for culture and sensitivity and cytological analysis for the presence of transitional cell carcinoma cells.

Flexible cystourethroscopy facilitates inspection of the bladder and urethra and biopsies under local anesthesia. In most cases, however, general anesthesia is required to carry out rigid urethrocystoscopy and biopsy followed by examination under anesthesia (EUA). The EUA enables clinical assessment of local disease spread and provides useful staging information. If there is any suspicion of rectal invasion, then flexible sigmoidoscopy may be warranted.

Staging Investigations

Imaging

Computed tomography (CT) is used to assess the extent of local spread of urethral cancer. Magnetic resonance imaging (MRI) has also been demonstrated to be 90% accurate in evaluating local extension of urethral cancer; it also offers multiplanar imaging, which is potentially advantageous in accurately planning surgery (14). Magnetic resonance imaging is particularly useful in evaluating the female urethra and periurethral tissues (15). If the patient presents with hematuria or the histology is TCC, then evaluation of the upper tracts is required by either intravenous urography (IVU) or CT. Bone scanning and plain radiographs are required if metastasis is suspected on biochemical or clinical grounds. Barium enema may be useful in staging if rectal spread is suspected. The chest assessment is routinely done with a chest x-ray.

Treatment

It is difficult to propose the best treatment for urethral cancer in view of the small number of cases reported over a long interval. The studies in the main are comprised of retrospective reviews of treatment strategies. Traditionally surgery has been considered the mainstay in the treatment of urethral cancer.

Male

Surgery alone has not provided very good outcomes (16), and neither has the use of radiotherapy alone (17). Dalbagni et al. (3) have reported on three factors as predictive of survival: nodal status, histologic type, and site of cancer. In their study they noted that most cases at presentation were of an advanced stage (36 of 43 patients had invasive disease). Locally advanced tumors of the anterior urethra are treated by chemoradiation and penectomy (3). For advanced posterior urethral tumors, chemoradiation and cystoprostatectomy with penectomy has been suggested. There may also be a case for conservative surgical management of superficial disease by transurethral resection, fulguration, or excision, provided the cancer is of low stage and low grade (18). The treatment options are summarized in Table 16.6.3.

Nodal Management

If inguinal nodes are palpable, ipsilateral dissection is carried out after frozen section confirmation (19,20). In the absence of palpable nodes, regular clinical follow-up and assessment is needed.

Bulbomembranous Urethra

Lesions in bulbar or membranous regions are treated with cystoprostatectomy with regional (pelvic) lymphadenectomy (≥T2 lesions) (21). This may have to be supplemented with scrotectomy and resection of pubic rami depending on the depth of invasion and bulkiness of the tumor (22).

Radiation and Chemotherapy

Radiation is generally indicated for patients who refuse surgery and have early disease of the anterior urethra. The main advantage of radiotherapy is preservation of the penis, but it may result in urethral stricture, and recurrence is a possibility (23). Chemotherapy as a monotherapy needs further studies, and so far in a small number of patients the results are disappointing (24). Chemoradiation in patients with locally advanced carcinoma has been encouraging (25,26).

Gheiler et al. (27) have found the best treatment outcome with multimodality treatment of chemoradiation (Cisplatin and 5-fluorouracil plus radiation) and surgery in their series of 21 patients.

TABLE 16.6.3. Surgical management of anterior urethral carcinoma

Stage	Treatment
Ta, Tis	Transurethral resection/diathermy
T1	Transurethral resection/partial penectomy
T2–3	Partial penectomy/total penectomy

Female

Prognostic factors for female urethral cancer include stage, histology type, tumor site, and nodal status (28). Except for small tumors, the prospects of cure are limited. Again, distal tumors of low grade may be treated with conservative resection, although DiMarco et al. (28) noted a high recurrence rate with this approach and recommended radical urethrectomy. Ipsilateral lymph node dissection is carried out if the initial biopsy is positive on frozen section. For locally advanced tumors involving the posterior urethra, en-bloc resection of involved adjacent viscera is required for disease control. Tumors less than 2 cm can be treated either by radiotherapy or by surgery. For tumors 2 cm or larger, preoperative radiation followed by extirpative surgery may provide better outcome (29). There are not enough studies in the literature to comment on the usefulness of adjuvant chemoradiation as yet.

Urethral Carcinoma After the Radical Management of Transitional Cell Carcinoma Bladder

Urethral TCC occurs in association with bladder TCC as a manifestation of multicentric tumor. It is important to recognize those patients undergoing radical cystectomy who are likely candidates for urethral recurrence. Risk factors for urethral recurrence of TCC in the male patient are papillary tumors, multifocality, bladder neck involvement, associated carcinoma in situ (CIS), upper tract TCC, and prostatic and trigonal involvement with superficial TCC and invasion of the stroma (8,30).

Clinical presentation may indicate advanced disease. Clark et al. (31) noted in their review of 1054 patients who underwent radical cystectomy and urinary diversion that although most patients with urethral recurrence presented with symptoms (57%), a significant proportion (31%) were detected by screening cytology.

The median survival of patients with recurrence was only 28 months after diagnosis, with urethral stage (superficial vs. invasive) at diagnosis being the most important predictive factor (13,31). Patients undergoing continent urinary diversion seem to have a lower incidence of urethral recurrence. The exact reason for this is not known (32–34).

References

1. Dalbagni G, Zhang ZF, Lacombe L, Herr HW. Female urethral carcinoma: an analysis of treatment outcome and a plea for a standardized management strategy. Br J Urol 1998;82:835–841.
2. Ray B, Guinan PD. Primary carcinoma of the urethra. In: Javadpour N, ed. Principles and Management of Urologic Cancer. Baltimore: Williams & Wilkins 1979:445–473.
3. Dalbagni G, Zhang ZF, Lacombe L, Herr HW. Male urethral carcinoma: analysis of treatment outcome. Urology 1999;53:1126–1132.

4. Cupp MR, Reza MS, Goellner JR, et al. Detection of human papillomavirus DNA in primary squamous cell carcinoma of the male urethra. Urology 1996;48:551–555.
5. Narayan P, Konety B. Surgical treatment of female urethral carcinoma. Urol Clin North Am 1992;19(2):373–382.
6. Kim SJ, MacLennan GT. Pathology page: tumours of the male urethra. J Urol 2005; 174:312.
7. Lands RH, Ange D, Hartman DL. Radiation therapy for classic Kaposi's sarcoma presenting only on the glans penis. J Urol 1992;147(2):468–470.
8. Freeman JA, Esrig D, Stein JP, Skinner DG. Management of the patient with bladder cancer. Urethral recurrence. Urol Clin North Am 1994;21:645–651.
9. Erckert M, Stenzl A, Falk M, Bartsch G. Incidence of urethral tumour involvement in 910 men with bladder cancer. World J Urol 1996;14:3–8.
10. Schellhammer RF, Whitmore WF Jr. Transitional cell carcinoma of the urethra in men having cystectomy for bladder cancer. J Urol 1976;115:56–60.
11. Thyavihally YB, Wuntkal R, Bakshi G, Uppin S, Tongaonkar HB. Primary carcinoma of female urethra: single center experience of 18 cases. Jpn J Clin Oncol 2005;35: 84–87.
12. Coloby PJ, Kakizoe T, Tobisu K, Sakamoto M. Urethral involvement in female bladder cancer patients. Mapping of 47 consecutive cystourethrectomy specimens. J Urol 1994;152:1438–1442.
13. Eng TY, Naguib M, Galang T, Fuller CD. Retrospective study of the treatment of urethral cancer. Am J Clin Oncol 2003;26(6):558–562.
14. Hricak H, Secaf E, Buckley DW, et al. Female urethra: MR imaging. Radiology 1991; 178:527–535.
15. Israel GM, Lee VS, Resnick D, et al. Magnetic resonance evaluation of the urethra and lower genitourinary tract in symptomatic women. J Women's Imag 2002;4:165–172.
16. Dinney CP, Johnson PE, Swanson DA, et al. Therapy and prognosis for male urethral carcinoma: an update. Urology 1994;43:506–514.
17. Zeidman EJ, Desmond P, Thompson I. Surgical treatment of carcinoma of the male urethra. Urol Clin North Am 1992;19:359–372.
18. Konnak JW. Conservative management of low-grade neoplasms of the male urethra: a preliminary report. J Urol 1980;123:175–177.
19. Ray B, Canto AR, Whitmore WF Jr. Experience with primary carcinoma of male urethra. J Urol 1977;117:591–594.
20. Bracken RB, Henry R, Ordonez N. Primary carcinoma of male urethra. South Med J 1980;73:1003–1005.
21. Kaplan GW, Bulkey GJ, Greyhack JT. Carcinoma of male urethra. J Urol 1967;98: 365–371.
22. Dinney CP, Johnson DE, Swanson DA. Therapy and prognosis of male anterior urethral carcinoma: an update. Urology 1994;43:506–514.
23. Donat SM, Cozzi PJ, Herr HW. Surgery of penile and urethral carcinoma. In: Walsh PC, Retik AB, Vaughn AD, Wein AJ, eds. Campbell's Urology, 8th ed. Philadelphia: WB Saunders, 2002:2983–2991.
24. Scher HI, Yagoda A, Herr HW, et al. Neoadjuvant M-VAC (methotrexate, vinblastine, doxorubicin and cisplatin) for extravesical urinary tract tumors. J Urol 1988;139: 475–477.
25. Licht MR, Klein EA, Bukowski R, Montie JE, Saxton JP. Combination radiation and chemotherapy for the treatment of squamous cell carcinoma of the male and female urethra. J Urol 1995;153:1918–1920.

26. Oberfield RA, Zinman LN, Leibenhaut M, Girshovich L, Silverman ML. Management of invasive squamous cell carcinoma of the bulbomembranous male urethra with co-ordinated chemo-radiotherapy and genital preservation. Br J Urol 1996;78: 573–578.
27. Gheiler EL, Tefilli MV, Tiguert R, et al. Management of primary urethral cancer. Urology 1998;52:487–493.
28. DiMarco DS, DiMarco CS, Zincke H, et al. Surgical treatment for local control of female urethral carcinoma. Urol Oncol 2004;22:404–409.
29. Grigsby PW, Corn BW. Localized urethral tumors in women: indications for conservative versus exenterative therapies. J Urol 1992;147(6):1516–1520.
30. Cresswell J, Roberts JT, Neal DE. Urethral recurrence after radical radiotherapy for bladder cancer. J Urol 2001;165(4):1135–1137.
31. Clark PE, Stein JP, Groshen SG, et al. The management of urethral transitional cell carcinoma after radical cystectomy for invasive bladder cancer. J Urol 2004;172: 1342–1347.
32. Stein JP, Clark P, Miranda G, Cai J, Groshen S, Skinner DG. Urethral tumor recurrence following cystectomy and urinary diversion: clinical and pathological characteristics in 768 male patients. J Urol 2005;173:1163–1168.
33. Nieder AM, Sved PD, Gomez P, Kim SS, Manoharan M, Soloway MS. Urethral recurrence after cystoprostatectomy: implications for urinary diversion and monitoring. Urology 2004;64:950–954.
34. Hassan JM, Cookson MS, Smith JA Jr, Chang SS. Urethral recurrence in patients following orthotopic urinary diversion. J Urol 2004;172:1338–1341.

17
Testis

17.1
Germ Cell Tumors

R.T.D. Oliver, Jonathan Shamash, and Vinod H. Nargund

Germ Cell Tumors of the Testis

Testicular cancer is rare, accounting for 1% to 2% of all male malignancies. Nearly 90% to 95% of tumors arising in testis are germ cell in origin. Other sites of malignant germ cell tumors include the retroperitoneum, mediastinum, sacrococcygeal region, and pineal gland. The highest incidence is seen in Scandinavian countries, particularly Denmark (1). There has been a significant disparity in the incidence of testicular cancer among the white and black populations in the United States, with higher incidence rates in the white population. Recent studies, however, show that this is changing, with an increased incidence of testicular germ cell tumors (TGCTs) among black men (2). Though these are one of the most frequent malignancies in the 15 to 50 age group, they are still relatively rare, with the incidence in that age group being 2 to 9/100,000 per year (1).

Testicular cancer is important for several reasons:

1. The incidence of testicular cancer has been steadily rising in last 30 years in industrialized nations (3). In a study of eight northern European populations, Richiardi et al. (4) have demonstrated an increase in age-standardized annual incidence rates by 2.6% to 4.9%, with marginal differences between seminomas and nonseminomas.

2. Many risk factors—genetic and environmental—have been identified.

3. Prior to the 1950s, about 50% of patients were cured, while today in excess of 95% of all patients are rendered free of disease. Though this is mainly due to the impact of curative chemotherapy, which cures 85% to 90% of all metastatic disease, improvements in early diagnosis, radiotherapy, and retroperitoneal surgery have contributed to this success.

This chapter reviews briefly what is known about the cause of these tumors and the large rise in the incidence that has occurred during the 20th century, and then considers the contribution of improved diagnosis and the three modalities of treatment—surgery, radiotherapy, and chemotherapy—to the success of modern treatment and the challenges for the future.

TABLE 17.1.1. Summary of prenatal and postpubertal environmental
and genetic factors in germ cell cancer epidemiology

Prenatal/intrauterine factors
Estrogens/xenoestrogens
Maternal smoking (and diet)
X-linked gene (Xq27) and cryptorchidism (estrogen induced)
c-*kit* gene mutation (induced by excessive in utero estrogens)

Postpubertal factors
Increasing follicle-stimulating hormone (FSH)/cyclin D switch on
carcinoma in situ (CIS) from seminoma to nonseminoma
Decreased p53, increased bcl2, increased mdm2, increased DNA repair
activity
Trauma/surgery cryptorchidism: nonseminoma > seminoma
HIV immunosuppression: seminoma > nonseminoma
Azothiopine immunosuppression: nonseminoma > seminoma
Orchitis/atrophy secondary to viruses, e.g., mumps

Diet
High-fat diet increases xenoestrogenic chemical exposure
Low-fat diet decreases vitamin A and D, producing immunosuppression

Epidemiology and Risk Factors (Table 17.1.1)

Our understanding of testicular endocrinology, the development of testicular cancer, and the biology of germ cells and germ cell neoplasia, coupled with epidemiological studies, has helped in identifying the risk factors for testicular cancer (5).

Fertility

Men with testicular cancer most often have abnormal seminal parameters, and there is a suggestion that infertility and testicular cancer share etiological factors (6). In a large Danish study by Jacobson et al. (7) there was a strong association between subfertility and subsequent risk of malignancy (for both seminoma nad nonseminomas). This suggestion is supported by the observation that men with various types of gonadal dysfunction such as testicular dysgenesis, androgen insensitivity syndrome, and cryptorchidism have increased risk of testicular cancer. Involvement of prenatal factors is a possible explanation for this observation.

Testicular Atrophy

There is a threefold increased risk of developing testicular cancer in atrophic testis (8). Atrophy, whether induced by intrauterine exposures, such as excessive estrogens or smoking, or postpubertal events, such as trauma, infection, chemical damage, or heat, reduces feedback inhibition of the hypothalamus due to lack of inhibin production. This increases gonadotropin release, particularly the release of follicle-stimulating hormone (FSH), which accelerates cellular prolif-eration of the remaining spermatogonia. Reduced time for repair of incidental DNA damage provides the driving force for clonal evolution, with transforma-tion from the precancerous carcinoma in situ (CIS) cells into invasive germ cell cancer (9) and also possibly the progression from seminoma to nonseminoma (10).

Testicular Carcinoma in situ (Testicular Intraepithelial Neoplasia)

Almost all TGCTs originate from testicular intraepithelial neoplasia (TIN) cells, with the exception of spermatocytic seminoma, occuring in elderly men, and infantile yolk sac tumor and mature teratoma (11). Carcinoma in situ is likely to develop into invasive malignancy in 50% of patients within 10 years and 70% within 7 years (12). The cells of CIS have a number of similarities to embryonic germ cells, such as their positivity for alkaline phosphatase, increased glycogen content, and the presence of stem cell factor receptor (c-KIT). Based on immu-nohistological findings, Jørgensen et al. (13) have suggested that the cell of origin of CIS is present in the gonad around the 7th to 10th week of intrauterine life.

Moreover, 5% of cases with unilateral seminoma or nonseminoma have con-tralateral CIS, indicating major events taking place even before primordial germ cells reach the left and right gonadal blastema (14). Seminomas, nonseminomas, and CIS are consistently aneuploid, indicating that polyploidization is an early and important step in the development of these tumors. It also explains why tumors with both seminoma and nonseminoma elements behave in a manner intermediate between seminoma and nonseminoma (15).

Recent evidence from immunochemistry marker studies of CIS in normal tubules surrounding an established tumor suggest that the step from seminoma to embryonal cancer can occur within the tubule.

Berney et al. (16) found that 3% of seminomas, 25% of combined semino-mas/nonseminomas, and 65% of nonseminomas showed the nonseminoma marker CD30 (type I transmembrane glycoprotein expressed by embryonal carcinoma) expressed by scattered in situ cells. CD30 defines intratubular embryonal carcinoma, which is the intermediary step between CIS and non-seminomatous germ cell tumors (16).

Sex Hormones

The peak incidence of testicular cancer seen in younger men indicates endo-crine events during gestational development, early infancy, and puberty. Epide-miological and experimental evidence suggests a possible role of estrogens as the initial intrauterine initiating factor that is opposed by androgens, while gonadotropins, particularly FSH, act as a promoting factor driving subsequent changes (17). The role of in utero estrogen exposure has been investigated extensively in the past. One mechanism that can affect fetal cells is through catechol estrogens produced by catalyzed hydroxylation of estrogens, which are responsible for the production of reactivated oxygen species (ROS) that damage the DNA of germ cells (18).

Undescended Testis and Other Congenital Abnormalities of the Testis

There is an increased risk of testicular cancer with undescended testis (relative risk ≥3.8) (19). Orchidopexy at a younger age may not eliminate the chances of malignancy developing at a later date. There is some information suggesting that younger the age at orchidopexy, the less subsequent risk of testicular cancer.

Intersex, Gonadal Dysgenesis, and Other Rare Genetic Abnormalities

Individuals with 46,XY or 45,X/46,XY gonadal dysgenesis are at very high risk (10% to 50%) of developing germ cell tumors (20). Similarly, in the androgen insensitivity syndrome (testicular feminization syndrome) there is a high risk of gonadal germ cell cancer (21).

Familial

Various family studies show an increased risk of testicular cancer in male relatives of testicular cancer patients (22). Swerdlow et al. (23) observed a relative risk of 38 in twin brothers of men with testicular cancer (see below), though the fact that there was a higher risk in dizygous compared to monozygous twins suggests that intrauterine environmental influences are as important as genetic ones. Father–son patients who have testicular tumors are an important subset, as sons have a six- to tenfold increase in the risk of developing testicular cancer (24). Genetic anticipation may be responsible for testicular tumors in this subset of population (25). The earlier age of onset and increased severity of the disease was seen only in children whose father had seminoma (25), possibly because during the era the fathers were treated, those with nonseminomatous germ cell tumors (NSGCTs) did not survive.

Testicular Dysgenesis Syndrome

Genetic environmental factors may lead to isolated or combined genital and testicular abnormalities, including testicular cancer, hypospadias, cryptorchidism, and low sperm count. All these symptoms are grouped under testicular dysgenesis syndrome (TDS), with a common origin in intrauterine life. In the most severe cases, TDS may present with all components (26).

Atypical Nevus Syndrome

There is a significant association between multiple atypical nevi and germ cell tumors as compared with healthy individuals (27). This subgroup has a high propensity to develop melanoma (28).

Genetics of Germ Cell Tumors

Invasive germ cell tumors and their adjacent CIS are aneuploid, containing a high number of chromosomal changes—numerical and structural and generally in the triploid range. Although amplification of the short arm of chromosome 12 has already been recognized for many years as a characteristic chromosomal anomaly in TGCTs, its biological significance still remains unknown, and the clinical importance is a matter of debate (29). Nearly 80% of invasive tumors have extra copies of 12p, as shown by comparative genomic hybridization. There is also an indication that the short arm of chromosome 12 contains a gene or genes of the invasive tumor (30). Candidate overexpressed complementary DNAs mapped on 12p are shown in Figure 17.1.1. A genome-wide linkage study involving sibling-pair analyses has shown variable linkage to the regions of chromosomes 1, 4, 5, 14, and 18 (31,32).

Our understanding of the genetics of testis cancer development has come from the report by the International Consortium that has collected DNA from

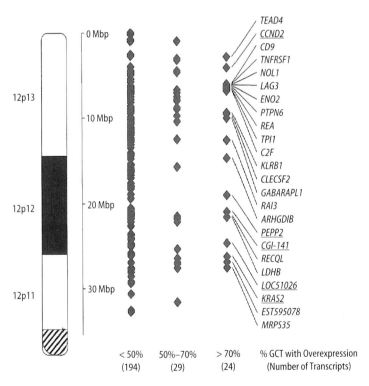

FIGURE 17.1.1. Candidate DNAs mapped on 12p. (From Houldsworth J, Bosl GJ, Chaganti RSK. Genetics and biology of adult male germ cell tumors. In: Waxman J, ed. Urological Cancers. London: Springer, 2005:223, with permission.)

a total of 134 families with 2 or more cases of TGCT, 87 of which were affected sibpairs. Brothers of men with TGCT have an eight- to tenfold risk of developing TGCT, whereas the relative risk to fathers and son is fourfold, which is much higher than that for other cancers (22,34). However, even this lower risk is much higher than that for other familial cancers. It is thought that this difference is due to environmental factors affecting the male fetus in utero based on following observations:

1. Nonidentical twins have a higher incidence than identical twins, possibly due to the fact that dizygous twins have larger placentas and the mothers have higher serum estrogen levels during pregnancy.
2. Sibling/sibling frequency of concurrent testis cancer in families is twice as frequent as father/son concurrent testis cancer in families, suggesting that there is something about the maternal environment more conducive to the early stages of testis cancer induction.
3. An environmental explanation has come from screening patients with bilateral tumors for mutations in the c-*kit* gene. This gene encodes a tyrosine kinase receptor (KIT) that is required for normal spermatogenesis.

Activation of KIT by the stem cell factor (SCF) leads to phosphorylation, including downstream pathways of regulation of cell proliferation and apoptosis (35). Kit ligand (Kitl), encoded by the Steel (Sl) locus, plays an important role in hematopoiesis, gametogenesis, and melanogenesis during both embryonic and adult life (36). Mutation of the c-*kit* gene is seen in seminomas and dysgerminomas. These mutations are much more frequent in patients with bilateral tumors but are absent from the parents. The mutation is thought to be acquired during the first trimester as those patients with bilateral tumors with a mutation have the same codon affected by a mutation in both tumors. This is likely to occur before the migration of spermatogonia from the yolk sac via the notochord into the mediastinum, and embryogenesis before separating into left and right testis.

There are also a number of other observations that indicate the involvement of genetic factors in the development of TGCTs:

1. The lower incidence of TGCTs in black men is possibly due to a higher placental testosterone concentration during pregnancy in black women compared to Caucasian women (37).
2. Familial predisposition: Nearly 2% of patients with a seminoma or nonseminoma have an affected family member (38).
3. A susceptibility gene on chromosome Xq27 has been mapped among families with two or more cases of TGCC, although the putative gene has not been identified (33).

It is possible that the failure to find a clear-cut linkage to a susceptibility gene is because there is more than one external environmental route for induction of testicular tumors. The chemical carcinogen route associated with estrogenic compounds has been clearly demonstrated to be associated with cytochrome

P-450 gene alleles involving cytochrome P-450 aromatase, which catalyzes androgens to estrogens (18). Aromatase is detected in Sertoli cells, Leydig cells, and spermatids, indicating the role of estrogens in gonadal physiology. That viruses may also play a role in initiation is more controversial, though the most clear-cut association is with postpubertal mumps viral infection.

Tumor Classification

The majority of malignant testicular tumors arise from spermatogonia and occur in teenagers and men between the ages of 15 and 50, and represent the most frequent cause of malignancy in that age group in men. Lymphomas and soft tissue sarcomas are less than 5% of all testicular malignancies.

Currently the latest World Health Organization (WHO) classification has failed to take into account the increasing evidence that tumors may progress from an intraepithelial stage via a macroscopic seminoma to a nonseminoma, and other times go to a nonseminoma directly from the intraepithelial stage (Table 17.1.2).

Much less is known about the genetic changes that determine yolk sac, choriocarcinoma, and teratocarcinomatous change, though given the considerable number of chromosomes showing loss of heterozygosity in the tumor,

TABLE 17.1.2. World Health Organization (WHO) histological classification of germ cell tumors

Germ cell tumors
Intratubular germ cell neoplasia (carcinoma in situ) unclassified
Tumors of one histological type (pure forms)
Seminoma
Seminoma with syncytiotrophoblastic cells
Spermatocytic seminoma
Spermatocytic seminoma with sarcoma
Embryonal carcinoma
Yolk sac tumor
Trophoblastic tumors
Choriocarcinoma
Trophoblastic neoplasms other than choriocarcinoma
Monophasic choriocarcinoma
Placental site trophoblastic tumor
Teratoma
Mature teratoma
Dermoid cyst
Immature teratoma
Teratoma with somatic type malignancies
Tumors of more than one histological type (mixed forms)
Mixed embryonal carcinoma and teratoma
Mixed embryonal and seminoma
Choriocarcinoma and teratoma/embryonal carcinoma
Others

more detailed microdissection genetic analysis should ultimately yield an answer.

Histological Types

Gonadal germ cell tumors have heterogeneous histological features that have important therapeutic and prognostic implications.

Carcinoma in Situ (Intratubular Germ Cell Neoplasia; Testicular Intraepithelial Neoplasia)

There is a substantial body of evidence to suggest that CIS is a precursor of testicular germ cell tumors (TGCTs) during intrauterine life, remaining dormant until the age of puberty. Thereafter, under the influence steroids and gonadotropins, CIS becomes an invasive seminomatous or nonseminomatous germ cell tumor (39). In addition, as mentioned earlier, environmental and lifestyle factors are involved.

Carcinoma in situ is randomly distributed throughout the testis, and surgical testicular biopsy measuring 3 mm × 3 mm × 3 mm (specimens sent preferably in Bouin's solution, as formalin causes shrinkage artifacts) is representative of the entire testis. The biopsy has false-negative rates of 0.5% (40). Carcinoma in situ cells are located inside the seminiferous tubules, frequently in a single row on the basement membrane, and their morphology resembles closely that of immature germ cells (gonocytes) (Fig. 17.1.2).

The cells are identified by immunohistological staining for placental alkaline phosphatase (PLAP). Leydig cell function and spermatogenesis are severely affected in the presence of testicular CIS (41). The WHO criteria for CIS are summarized in Table 17.1.3 (42).

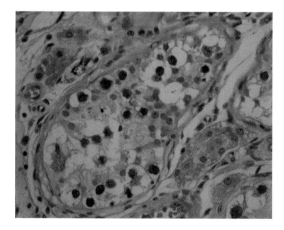

Figure 17.1.2. Carcinoma in situ. (Hematoxylin and eosin stain, ×40.) (Courtesy of Dr. Sohail Baithun, Royal London Hospital, London.)

TABLE **17.1.3.** WHO criteria for the diagnosis of carcinoma in situ of the testis (see Fig. 17.1.2)

Larger than normal spermatogonia
Clear or vacuolated cytoplasm rich in glycogen
Nuclei: large, irregular, and hyperchromatic
Nucleoli: one or more large and irregular
Abnormal mitoses
Basally located cells
Spermatogenesis commonly absent
Segmental involvement of tubules

Seminoma

Seminoma (Fig. 17.1.3) accounts for a majority of postpubertal testicular neoplasms, either in isolation or with other histological forms, with a peak incidence after the fourth decade. It resembles CIS and proliferates in a homogeneous manner. A common form of metastasis is first to lymph nodes followed by systemic spread. There are three histological subtypes of seminoma: classical (80%), spermatocytic (10–15%), and anaplastic (5–10%):

- Classical (typical) seminoma is commonly seen in the third decade. There may be an element of syncytiotrophoblast producing β-human chorionic gonadotropin (β-hCG).
- Spermatocytic seminoma accounts for less than 1% of the testicular tumors. It consists of sheets of cells of varying size with dense-staining cytoplasm and spherical nucleus. Most of these tumors occur in men over the age of 50 years. It has a favorable prognosis due to low metastatic potential, and genetic analysis suggests that it is unrelated to the commoner forms of germ cell

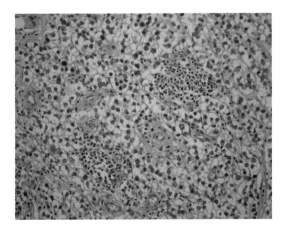

FIGURE **17.1.3.** Seminoma. (H&E stain, ×40.) (Courtesy of Dr. Sohail Baithun, Royal London Hospital, London.)

cancer. Generally it has no other germ cell elements or intratubular germ cell neoplasia, but rarely is associated with a sarcomatous component, which has an aggressive behavior and poor prognosis.

- *Anaplastic seminoma* was the term given to classical seminoma associated with high mitotic activity and nuclear pleomorphism with increased potential for local invasion and metastatic spread. Although it was thought to have higher metastatic potential and mostly presented in advanced stage, the prognosis did not differ much from classical seminoma (43). These so-called seminomas with atypia have a high proliferation activity as judged by Ki67 reactivity and expression of a marker for epithelial differentiation, Cam 5.2 (43).

Markers in Seminoma. Most seminomas produce hCG in small quantities. Elevated serum hCG level (hCG-positive seminoma) is regarded as more malignant than marker-negative seminoma, although its prognosis is still unclear (44). The tumor cells express PLAP and c-*kit*. C-*kit* (CD-117) is regularly expressed in seminoma (see below). Cytokeratin expression, on the other hand, is weak and infrequent.

Nonseminomatous Germ Cell Tumors

These tumors have embryonic elements. They differentiate along embryonic lineage (embryonal carcinoma, teratoma, teratocarcinoma) or extraembryonic tissue components (yolk sac tumor and choriocarcinoma).

Embryonal Cell Carcinoma. Histologically, embryonal cell carcinoma is extremely pleomorphic and shows a variety of patterns forming glands, tubules, papillary structures, and even primitive embryo-like structures. Many mitotic figures are present. Embryonal cell carcinoma can present as a component of mixed germ cell tumor or as a pure embryonal cell carcinoma (Fig. 17.1.4).

The other variety of yolk sac tumor (endodermal sinus tumor) is seen in infants and children but can be seen in a mixed pattern in adults. It may be

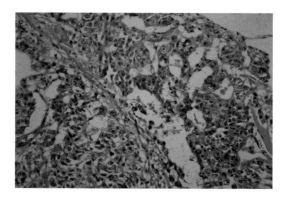

FIGURE 17.1.4. Embryonal cell carcinoma. (H&E stain, ×40.) (Courtesy of Dr. Sohail Baithun, Royal London Hospital, London.)

TABLE 17.1.4. Panel of immunostaining profile of main germ cell tumors of the testis

Immunostain marker	IGCN (CIS)	Seminoma	Spermatocytic seminoma	Embryonal cell carcinoma	Yolk sac tumor	Choriocarcinoma
AFP	−	−	−	±	+	−
C-kit	+	+	±	−	−	−
PLAP	+	+	−	±	±	−
Oct $\frac{3}{4}$	+	+	−	+	−	−
hCG	−	−	−	−	−	+
Cytokeratin	−	−	−	+	+	+
CD30	+	−	−	+	−	−

AFP, α-fetoprotein; CIS, carcinoma in situ; hCG, human chorionic gonadotropin; IGCN, intratubular germ cell neoplasia; PLAP, placental alkaline phosphatase; +, indicates positive staining; −, indicates mostly negative staining; ±, indicates variable staining.

positive for α-fetoprotein. The panel of immunostains that confirm the diagnosis include CD30 and OCT 3/4 (octamer binding transcription factor for POU5F1).

Embryonal carcinoma metastasizes early in an extensive manner by both lymphatic and hematogenous routes.

Choriocarcinoma. These tumors contains cytotrophoblast, which is the stem cell of this tumor, and syncytiotrophoblast (nonproliferating) elements (placental elements), and tend to occur in combination with other tumors. Their clinical behavior is aggressive, characterized by early hematogenous spread.

Teratoma. Teratoma denotes a neoplasm with tissues derived from three embryonic layers—ectoderm, mesoderm, and endoderm—either in isolation or in combination. They occur in both children and adults. Mature teratoma contains elements that resemble tissues derived from ectoderm, endoderm, and mesoderm. Mature teratomas are seen in partial remission following chemotherapy. In contrast, immature teratomas contain undifferentiated tissue, giving a heterogeneous appearance.

Mixed Tumors. The mixed tumors contain seminomatous and nonseminomatous elements and are treated as nonseminomas. Frequently occurring combinations are of embryonal cell carcinoma, yolk sac tumor, and teratoma (teratocarcinoma).

Gonadoblastoma. Gonadoblastoma is seen in children or adolescents who have sex chromosome abnormalities (45,XO/46,XY). The histology shows cells that resemble gonocytes or CIS with small stromal cells. The clinical course is benign but can become malignant germ cell tumor (Table 17.1.4).

Clinical Features

1. Painless testicular mass, usually noted by the patient or by his partner.
2. Testicular pain (acute or chronic orchalgia): Rarely, patients may present with a painful testicular mass, which is generally due to bleeding or infarction

within the tumor. More common is a minor testicular discomfort due to the enlargement of the testis, though it may precede the testicular enlargement.

3. Hematospermia, infertility, increase in the size of atrophic testis.

4. Systemic symptoms: Gynecomastia due to hCG-induced adrenal production of estrogen.

5. Metastatic lesions: Testicular cancer patients can present to other specialties due to metastatic lesions. These include chest or neurological symptoms. Backache, abdominal pain, erectile dysfunction (retroperitoneal masses), hemoptysis, cough, dyspnea (lung metastases), and supraclavicular mass due to enlarged lymph glands. Patients may present with atypical neurological symptoms from brain metastases or spinal cord compression.

About 25% of seminoma patients have metastases at the time of diagnosis compared to 65% nonseminoma, though the frequency of metastases is decreasing with increasing testis cancer awareness among the largest population at risk, that is, the age group of 15 to 50.

Clinical examination includes systematic palpation of the affected testis and its appendages and cord, without unduly pressing the swelling or the testis. The tumor is felt to be hard with variable consistency. The abdomen is examined for any lumps and the neck area for any lymph nodes.

Differential Diagnosis of a Testicular/Scrotal Swelling

Any acute or subacute intrascrotal swelling should be considered to be a testicular tumor unless otherwise proved. Other conditions that are likely to mislead include epididymo-orchitis, torsion, hydrocele, hematocele, spermatocele, large epididymal cysts, hernia, gumma, and trauma to the testis. Among these conditions, the two that can mimic testicular tumor are acute torsion and epididymo-orchitis. Syphilitic (gumma) and tuberculous lesions of the testis may also present with painless testicular swelling.

Spread of Malignant Testicular Tumors

The tumors have specific mode of spread, with the metastases occurring through lymphatic and vascular routes. Local spread is limited by the tunica albuginea of the testis. The lymphatic spread is a common form of metastasis, with all histological types. Hematogenous spread occurs to the lungs, liver and brain.

Anatomy of Lymphatic Drainage of the Testes (Fig. 17.1.5)

As testes develop in the retroperitoneum in the abdomen, their lymph drains to paraaortic and other lymph nodes in the infrarenal region. The lymphatics from the epididymis drain into testicular lymphatics.

The testicular lymphatics join lymphatics from the tunica albuginea in rete testis and proceed to the spermatic cord (45).

The lymphatics initially accompany testicular vessels. After crossing the ureter they spread out to join retroperitoneal lymph nodes anterior to the

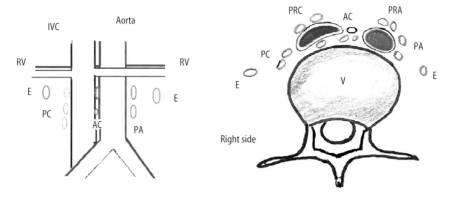

FIGURE 17.1.5. Diagrammatic representation of lymphatic drainage of testes. In addition, there are precaval nodes on the right side and preaortic nodes on the left side (not shown). IVC, inferior vena cava; Aorta, abdominal aorta; RV, renal vessels; PA, paraaortic group; PC, paracaval group; AC, aortocaval group; E, echelon nodes.

lumbar vessels (46,47). The right testicular vein drains into the anterior aspect of the inferior vena cava and the left testicular vein drains into left renal vein. Right-sided tumors metastasize to the infrarenal aortocaval, precaval, right paracaval, and retrocaval lymph nodes. Left-sided tumors spread to the left paraaortic and preaortic lymph nodes.

The echelon lymph nodes are lateral to the paracaval and paraaortic lymph nodes in the region between the first and third lumbar vertebra on the iliopsoas muscle, which can get involved particularly in cases with relapse (48). When the anatomy of the inguinoscrotal region is disturbed by surgical procedures like orchidopexy or scrotal exploration, there is likely to be a direct spread to the iliac or inguinal lymph nodes, which normally drain scrotal skin.

Diagnostic Investigations and Staging

Initial Investigations

All suspected cases should have the following investigations.

Scrotal Ultrasonography (Fig. 17.1.6)

This is a simple noninvasive investigation that gives a fair assessment of the testis and tumor and also helps to differentiate other scrotal conditions. Simultaneous abdominal scanning can be done to rule out masses and liver metastasis, but subsequent staging by computed tomography (CT) scanning is still a standard and mandatory step. Conversely, in young men presenting with retroperitoneal mass and elevated testicular tumor markers, testicular ultrasound is a crucial investigation. The ultrasonographic findings are summarized in Table 17.1.5.

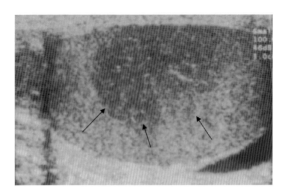

FIGURE 17.1.6. Ultrasound of testis showing seminoma. (Courtesy of Dr. Anju Sahadev, St. Bartholomew's Hospital, London.)

Chest X-Ray

Chest x-ray is done to exclude lung metastases at the initial assessment.

Tumor Markers

As germ cell tumors produce marker proteins, a blood sample is sent to the laboratory for estimation of α-fetoprotein, β-hCG (oncofetal), PLAP, and lactate dehydrogenase (LDH) (cellular enzymes).

These tumor marker assays are sensitive indicators of testicular cancer in men under 50 but are occasionally positive in undifferentiated variants of the common adult solid cancers, and thus cannot be relied on totally as specific markers of germ cell cancer.

α-Fetoprotein. α-Fetoprotein (AFP) has a half-life of 4 to 6 days. It is an oncofetal glycoprotein (molecular weight 70,000) produced by the fetal yolk sac, liver, and gastrointestinal tract, and it is present in trace amounts 1 year after birth. Elevated AFP is seen in NSGCTs including pure embryonal cell carcinoma, teratocarcinoma, yolk sac tumor, or combined tumors. Probably it reflects evolution from a seminoma to a nonseminoma (50).

β-Human Chorionic Gonadotropin. Human chorionic gonadotropin has a half-life of 24 to 48 hours. It is secreted by trophoblastic tissue (placenta) for the main-

TABLE 17.1.5. Ultrasound findings in germ cell tumors of the adult testis

Type of testicular tumor	Ultrasound findings
Seminoma	Invariably large homogeneous, mostly hypoechoic tumors with or without calcifications, rarely cystic areas showing necrosis (49)
Teratoma	Large heterogeneous (bone, cartilage), cystic areas
Choriocarcinoma	Usually small with hemorrhagic nodules, calcifications
Yolk sac	Large, heterogeneous
Embryonal cell carcinoma	Large, heterogeneous

tenance of the corpus luteum. The hCG has α and β units—the α-subunit has a glycoprotein similar to thyroid-stimulating hormone (TSH), luteinizing hormone (LH) and FSH; therefore, the β subunit is similar to luteinising hormone (LH). The β-subunit (half life 24–36 hours) is rarely produced outside pregnancy with the exception of trophoblastic tissues of germ cell tumors. Choriocarcinoma, embryonal cell carcinoma, and, as mentioned already, 5% of seminomas contain syncytiotrophoblast elements that secrete β-hCG.

Placental Alkaline Phosphatase. Placental alkaline phosphatase is a fetal isoenzyme that may be elevated in patients with advanced disease. However, it is not commonly used, as it is elevated in other conditions including smoking and several other tumors.

Lactic Dehydrogenase. Lactic dehydrogenase, a cellular enzyme, is raised with a high tumor burden. Rising LDH levels after treatment may indicate relapse.

Fertility Assessment and Semen Cryopreservation

Jacobson et al. (7) have noted the existence of common etiological factors for low semen quality and testicular cancer.

Moreover, testicular cancer patients are young at presentation and have a reasonable life expectancy after successful testicular cancer management, which raises the fertility issue as one of the future expectations for the patient. This is particularly important in patients with tumor in the solitary testis, and in these patients chemotherapy, radiotherapy, or retroperitoneal surgery is indicated. Similarly, it is also important in patients who have contralateral atrophic testis, as the sperm present may only be coming from the normal seminiferous tubules of the tumor-bearing testis.

Seminal analysis and cryopreservation should be discussed with the patient. It may be necessary to obtain a full endocrine profile including FSH, LH, and testosterone to complete the fertility assessment. There are changes in semen and the reproductive hormone profile after radical orchidectomy (51). Semen changes include a fall in sperm concentration and in some cases azoospermia. There is an increase in serum FSH in patients who have detectable pre-orchiectomy serum hCG (51). The serum levels of testosterone and serum sex binding globulin are not affected by orchiectomy.

High Inguinal Orchiectomy (Radical)

In this procedure the testis and the cord as far as the internal inguinal ring are removed through an inguinal incision. This is curative in more than two thirds of those without metastases at presentation. Radical orchidectomy should not be performed in those presenting with symptomatic metastases as the metastases can occasionally progress to become life-threatening during the postoperative phase. Once chemotherapy is instituted, complete remission of symptoms is to be expected within 24 to 48 hours. Positive tumor markers with or without fine-needle biopsy histology is usually sufficient for diagnostic purposes in these patients.

The only other indication for delaying the orchidectomy is in a patient with a small tumor where clinical examination of the non–tumor-bearing testis suggests poor function. In such patients it is preferable to arrange sperm storage first as they may be rendered azoospermic after removing the tumor-bearing testis, which begs the question of testis conserving surgery.

Testis-Preserving Surgery

The issue of orchiectomy is a difficult one for the patient when there are bilateral tumors or when the solitary testis is affected. Bilateral orchiectomy or removal of the solitary testis results in permanent sterility, with a need for lifelong replacement therapy of androgens. This imposes a psychological burden on a young patient, which raises quality of life issues. This burden may be even greater in patients who have not yet had children and are threatened with being rendered sterile by the diagnostic orchidectomy.

Heidenreich et al. (52) have described surgical enucleation of the tumor and preservation of testis.

They proposed certain prerequisites for considering this approach: (1) an organ-confined tumor with no involvement of the rete testis, (2) tumor size <20 or 25 mm, (3) normal testosterone levels, and (4) procedure performed under cold ischemia. In their 13 patients with a 6- to 30-mm tumor range, 12 patients remained recurrence free at the end of 5 years. The main advantage of testis-preserving surgery seems to be that patients do not need androgen replacement. The size criterion mentioned in this series is not applicable in all cases, particularly in patients with tumor in an atrophic testis.

It is also worrying that there is high incidence of associated carcinoma in situ in non–tumor-bearing areas of the testis. For example, in a study of 73 patients from the German Testicular Cancer Study Group, 82% of patients had associated testicular intraepithelial germ cell neoplasia, which necessitated local radiation; hypogonadism developed in 10% of patients, and there was one death due to systemic tumor progression (53). Moreover, close follow-up and patient compliance are required following this procedure. This is essentially an investigational operative technique that is highly controversial and needs a large-scale clinical trial with long-term follow-up before it can be accepted as a standard procedure. With recent advances in assisted conception techniques (in vitro fertilization, IVF) and cryopreservation of testicular tissue and semen being possible in most specialist centers, organ-preserving testicular surgery becomes obsolete except for psychological reasons or for the purpose of avoiding androgen replacement.

Staging Investigations

Imaging

A CT scan of the chest, abdomen, and pelvis is standard for routine staging postorchidectomy in those patients without obvious metastases. As mentioned already, chest x-ray and ultrasound of the testis and abdomen are basic investigations prior to orchiectomy. If either tumor marker AFP or β-hCG was positive preoperatively, it is important to arrange to take regular weekly markers, as failure to decline is an early indication of active metastasis even if the CT scan is normal. Magnetic resonance imaging (MRI) offers no advantage over CT scan except in those patients who have acute renal failure due to bilateral ureteric obstruction.

Positron Emission Tomography. This investigation involves measuring the uptake of fluorodeoxyglucose specifically to detect residual active tumor masses that have incompletely regressed after chemotherapy. This is not a routine staging investigation in patients with testicular cancer. Larger series are needed to assess its true utility over CT scan.

For all established testicular tumors, it is mandatory to assess the nodal status in the abdomen (CT), thorax (CT), and supraclavicular regions (clinical examination); visceral involvement (ultrasound and CT); and brain (CT, MRI) and skeletal involvement (bone scan). In addition, the half-life kinetics of serum tumor markers need to be assessed.

TNM Classification and Staging

The tumor, node, metastasis (TNM) classification was developed from stage groupings of the American Joint Committee on Cancer (AJCC) and International Union Against Cancer (UICC) (Table 17.1.6), and the latest version was adopted in 1997. It is based on the anatomic extent of the disease and assessment of serum tumor markers.

In stage I, the disease is confined to the testis; stage II indicates the extent of the disease in retroperitoneum; stage III indicates the extent of supradiaphragmatic disease or nodal sites or other visceral sites or markedly increased serum tumor markers. Patients with advanced disease are classified according to the International Germ Cell Cancer Collaborative Group (IGCCCG), which is defined as a prognostic-factor based staging system for metastatic testicular cancer after analyzing the data from a large pool of patients treated with platinum-based chemotherapy(54).

This scheme, though acknowledging that seminoma has a better prognosis, merged good-prognosis seminoma and nonseminoma. This is discussed later in the section on management of advanced NSGCT. As histology, site of metastasis, and serum tumor marker concentrations are independent prognostic markers indicating the outcome of the treatment, these are included in IGCCCG classification.

Surgical Staging with Retroperitoneal Lymph Node Dissection

In the United States primarily and in some centers in Europe and Australasia, staging is not complete without a template retroperitoneal lymph node dissection except in those patients who have positive chest x-ray and defined retroperitoneal masses. The reason for this is that all radiological staging procedures tend to be inaccurate to a certain degree.

It has only been through surgical staging that we are aware that CT has 25% to 35% false-negative rate, mainly due to small microscopic foci. Even

TABLE 17.1.6. Testicular cancer staging of American Joint Committee on Cancer (AJCC) and the International Union Against Cancer (UICC): tumor, node, metastasis (TNM) classification (55)

Primary tumor (pT)

pTX:	Cannot be assessed
pT0:	No evidence of primary tumor
pTis:	Intratubular germ cell neoplasia only (carcinoma in situ)
pT1:	Tumor limited to the testis and epididymis without vascular/lymphatic invasion (tumor may invade tunica albuginea but not tunica vaginalis)
pT2:	Tumor limited to the testis and epididymis with vascular/lymphatic invasion or tumor extending through tunica albuginea with involvement of tunica vaginalis
pT3:	Tumor invades spermatic cord with or without vascular/lymphatic invasion
pT4:	Tumor invades scrotum with or without vascular/lymphatic invasion

Regional lymph nodes (pN)

pNX:	Cannot be assessed
pN0:	No regional lymph node metastasis
pN1:	Metastasis with a lymph node mass less than 2 cm in greatest dimension and five or fewer positive nodes, none more than 2 cm in greatest dimension
pN2:	Metastasis with a lymph node mass greater than 2 cm but not more than 5 cm in greatest dimension, or more than five nodes positive, none greater than 5 cm; or evidence of extranodal extension of tumor
pN3:	Metastasis with a lymph node mass greater than 5 cm in greatest dimension
Specify:	Number examined: _____
	Number involved: _____

Distant metastasis (pM)

pMX:	Cannot be assessed
pM1:	Distant metastasis present
pM1a:	Nonregional lymph nodes or pulmonary metastasis
pM1b:	Distant metastasis other than to nonregional lymph nodes and lungs
Specify site(s), if known: _____	

Serum tumor markers (S)

SX:	Serum marker studies not available or performed				
S0:	Serum marker study levels within normal limits				
	LDH		HCG (mIU/mL)		AFP (ng/mL)
S1:	<1.5	and	<5000	and	<1000
S2:	1.5–10	or	5000–50,000	or	1000–10,000
S3:	>10	or	>50,000	or	>10,000

Stage grouping

Stage category	TNM
Stage 0	
Stage I: lesion confined to the testis	T1–4 N0 M0
Stage II: testicular cancer involves the testis and the retroperitoneal or paraaortic lymph nodes usually in the region of the kidney)	
Stage IIA (lymph node size <2 cm): any	T1–4 N1 M0
Stage IIB (lymph node size 2–5 cm)	T1–4 N2 M0
Stage IIC (lymph node size >5 cm)	T1–4 N3 M0
Stage III (supradiaphragmatic nodal or visceral involvement)	T1–4 N1–3 M1a
Stage IIIa	T1–4 N1–3 M1 1a
Stage IIIb	T1–4 N1–3 M1 1a 1b

Source: Used with the permission of the American Joint Committee on Cancer (AJCC), Chicago, Illinois. The original source for this material is the AJCC Cancer Staging Manual, Sixth Edition (2002) Published by Springer-New York, www.springerlink.com.

experienced radiologists can occasionally miss disease between the vena cava and aorta, which is the first site of spread for right-sided tumors. In addition, there are a further 8% to 10% of false positives in those with CT measurable (i.e., >2 cm) retroperitoneal nodes due to reactive hyperplasia either in response to the malignancy or due to postorchidectomy tissue reaction. Centers practicing primary medical management are well aware of this and do not treat patients on the basis of small retroperitoneal shadows unless the tumor markers are rising, serial CT scans show progressive enlargement, or the patient has malignant cells on fine-needle biopsy. A well-performed transabdominal retroperitoneal lymph node dissection (RPLND) is a safe staging and therapeutic procedure with minimal morbidity and negligible mortality (56), but it should always be performed with therapeutic intent. The principles of RPLND are described later in the chapter.

Laparoscopic Retroperitoneal Lymph Node Dissection. Due to advances in minimally invasive approaches in surgery, laparoscopic RPLND (LRPLND) may eventually replace open RPLND for stage I and II disease. The proponents claim less postoperative morbidity, shorter convalescence, better cosmetic results, and equal diagnostic efficacy (57). The main primary landing site in some of the laparoscopic templates is anterior to the lumbar vessels (58). It is likely that primary lymphatic metastatic spread in testicular cancer occurs anterior to the lumbar vessels, and these authors believe that removal of lymphatic tissue behind the lumbar vessels for diagnostic procedures is not necessary (58). Currently, LRPND should still be considered an investigational and diagnostic procedure to be performed by specialist surgeons with dual experience in RPLND and minimally invasive surgery because of the occasional need to convert to an open procedure. The role of LRPLND in the management of postchemotherapy masses is still not well defined.

Sentinel Lymph Node Biopsy

In many cancers including melanoma, sentinel lymph node biopsy (SLNB) has gained acceptance. Using technetium-99m–labeled phytate, Satoh and colleagues (59) have been able to map the sentinel lymph nodes in clinical stage I germ cell testicular tumors. They were able to demonstrate micrometastasis in two of their 21 patients. They also identified precaval and aortocaval groups as sentinel nodes on the right side and renal hilar lymph nodes on the left side. According to these authors, the sensitivity of the intraoperative pathological examination and technique of LRPLND are the issues to be resolved before making SLNB routine.

Treatment

Testicular Intraepithelial Neoplasia (Carcinoma in Situ)

The only way of diagnosing CIS is by biopsy. Although there is general agreement that CIS is a precursor of testicular germ cell tumor, its management is far from ideal and until recently was not dictated by the needs of the patients. *Surveillance* is not the best option, as the majority of CIS cases progress to invasive disease. In addition, patients with CIS generally have poor semen quality even before radiotherapy (see below). Fertility issues are considered first, either sperm banking or cryopreservation of testicular tissue by testicular sperm extraction (TESE) for future assisted conception where indicated. The usual clinical scenario is the case of CIS in contralateral testis after orchiectomy. If the patient insists on surveillance, it is necessary to make the patient aware of the fact that an invasive germ cell tumor may develop and metastasis could occur. As most late recurrences are stage I seminomas, orchiectomy alone may be sufficient.

Local radiotherapy, with 20 Gy in single fractions of 2 Gy, is the treatment of choice, as below that dosage recurrences have been noted. At these doses, infertility uniformly occurs, and impaired Leydig cell function requiring testosterone supplementation occurs in approximately 50% of patients (60). The same principle applies to the management of solitary testis after testis-conserving surgery.

Chemotherapy is a less reliable option for the management of CIS because as long as spermatogenesis persists, there is a risk of relapse of CIS. On the basis of the occurrence of contralateral germ cell cancer it is thought that this risk may persist for 20 years or longer. Some patients who have not yet had children may accept the short-term risk of recurrence after chemotherapy, with relapse rates at 5 and 10 years of 20% and 30%, respectively, until they have children (61).

Orchiectomy is a safe alternative but may be a difficult decision for the patient, particularly if the contralateral testis has already been removed.

Testicular Cancer

Stage I Seminoma

Radical Orchiectomy and Active Surveillance. All patients undergo radical orchiectomy as a primary procedure. The size of the primary tumor and the rete testis, and vascular invasion are important prognostic factors for relapse in patients with stage I seminoma managed with surveillance (62).

With a median follow-up of 7 years, the actuarial 5-year and 10-year relapse-free rates were 82.3% and 78.7%, respectively, in a meta-analysis undertaken from four large studies (62). The main drawback of surveillance is the need for intensive follow-up and repeated imaging for at least 5 to 10 years after radical orchidectomy. Spermatocytic seminomas are also managed by radical orchiectomy alone.

Radical Orchidectomy and Adjuvant Radiotherapy. Seminoma cells are extremely radiosensitive, and this approach has been widely used and has an excellent long-term track record. This modality is a standard management in pure seminomas. Details of radiotherapy are described separately in the radiotherapy section (see below).

Radical Orchidectomy and Adjuvant Chemotherapy. The role of adjuvant chemotherapy using one or two cycles of carboplatin has also been investigated. Based on the results of a randomized trial on 1477 patients, it has been established that there is no difference in recurrence rates between single dose of carboplatin therapy [area under the curve (AUC) ×7] and radiotherapy for a median follow-up of 4 years. The relapse rate after one cycle of adjuvant carboplatin is 3% (63), and more interesting is the observation that it reduces second contralateral primary germ cell tumor incidence by 72% at 5 years compared to radiotherapy. Some authors argue that this approach should still be regarded as investigational rather than a standard regimen as there are concerns regarding late failures and the long-term effects of chemotherapy, and there remain questions regarding the ability to use additional chemotherapy to salvage carboplatin failures. All these arguments equally apply to the newer schedules of radiotherapy, where there are reports of late relapse outside the radiation field. Thus adjuvant carboplatin therapy can be considered an alternative to radiotherapy or surveillance in stage I seminoma. Given the still unquantified late relapse risk of all these approaches, it is our policy to discuss all three options (surveillance, radiotherapy, and chemotherapy) in a multidisciplinary setting with the patient and match the selected option with the patient's circumstances at the time.

Radical Orchidectomy and Retroperitoneal Lymph Node Dissection. Retroperitoneal lymph node dissection is not recommended in stage I seminoma due to the high success rates seen with both one-dose carboplatin and radiation.

Surveillance Protocol. There is no consensus regarding the optimum follow-up for these patients (62). Patients are followed up with regular physical examination, measurement of serum tumor markers, and imaging for retroperitoneal and chest disease.

Patients are followed up at 4-month intervals for the first 3 years, 6-month intervals in years 4 to 7, and at yearly intervals in years 8 to 10.

At each visit, a CT scan is taken of the abdomen and pelvis. Chest x-rays are obtained at alternate visits. Serum tumor marker levels are estimated at each visit for the first 3 years of surveillance (62). Some clinicians feel that there are an unnecessary number of CT scans with this scheme.

Nonseminomatous Germ Cell Tumors Stage I

Though clinical stage I NSGCT on surveillance has a 30% incidence of occult retroperitoneal metastasis, it is a highly curable disease, so that the overall survival approaches 100% (64).

The main predictors of relapse in stage I NSGCT are vascular and lymphatic invasion of the primary tumor and the presence of embryonal/undifferentiated areas in the tumor and absence of yolk sac elements (65,66). The current management options for stage I NSGCT are surveillance, RPLND, or adjuvant chemotherapy. Radiation therapy has no role in the initial management of NSGCT.

Radical Orchidectomy and Adjuvant Chemotherapy. Patients with vascular invasion, embryonal carcinoma, or undifferentiated areas are recommended by some investigators to undergo two courses of bleomycin, etoposide, and Platinol (cisplatin) (BEP) chemotherapy (67). This reduces the relapse rate from 45% to 2–3% with very little toxicity, and this is even less after one course of BEP, which is increasingly recognized as producing equivalent results.

There is, however, a very small risk of slow-growing retroperitoneal teratomas after chemotherapy, which if undetected can lead to the development of chemo-resistant cancer relapse, and these patients run an uncertain risk of late effects including acute leukemia. For this reason, most investigators in the United States still prefer to use RPLND as the first-line treatment (Figure 17.1.7).

Radical Orchidectomy and Retroperitoneal Lymph Node Dissection. The risk of relapse depends on the volume of the retroperitoneal disease resected. Williams et al. (68) have shown that two courses of cisplatin-based chemotherapy given adjuvant to RPLND in node-positive disease reduces the relapse rate to less than 2%. Retroperitoneal lymph node dissection is carried out with a modified template to reduce the morbidity, mainly the incidence of retrograde ejaculation.

Radical Orchidectomy and Surveillance. With proper patient selection and management, the overall survival of patients for stage I NSGCT approaches 100%. Eighty percent of relapses occur during the first 12 months' follow-up, 12% during the second year, and 6% in the third year (69,70). It is not uncommon to see patients who have relapses but with normal serum markers.

Currently there is a need for diagnosing small-volume disease accurately prior to considering chemotherapy or RPLND. Sentinel node biopsy techniques, as already mentioned, may be the future modality for such cases.

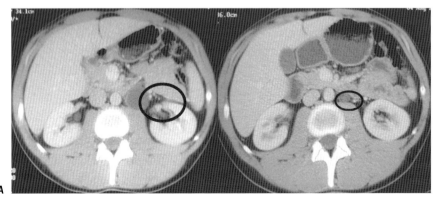

FIGURE 17.1.7. (A) Computed tomography of prechemotherapy teratoma. (B) Computed tomography postchemotherapy. (Courtesy of Dr. Anju Sahadev, St. Bartholomew's Hospital, London.)

Metastatic Germ Cell Tumors

Stage II A/B Seminoma

Radical Orchidectomy and Radiotherapy. The standard treatment for stage IIA and IIB seminoma is radiotherapy, as the majority of patients are cured with this treatment alone. Chemotherapy is the treatment of choice for stage IIC seminoma (71). The most important prognostic factor for stage II seminoma is the size of the lymph node mass in transverse diameter as seen on CT. In most centers, a size of 5 cm-subdiaphragmatic disease (IIB N1 disease) is taken as a cutoff for radiation therapy.

Chemotherapy in IIA and IIB Disease.

Single-Agent Carboplatin Therapy in Stage IIA/IIB Disease. In a pooled analysis of a study comparing single-agent carboplatin and cisplatin-based combination chemotherapy for metastatic seminoma, the progression-free survival was better for combination chemotherapy (72).

Combination Chemotherapy and Radiotherapy vs. Radiotherapy Alone. In an attempt to minimize toxicities, a combination of single-course carboplatin chemotherapy and radiotherapy has been studied in a small series of 30 patients by Patterson et al. (73). They reported a 5-year relapse-free survival (RFS) of 96.9% compared with 80.7% using single-agent carboplatin followed 4 to 6 weeks later by infradiaphragmatic radiotherapy and radiotherapy alone. In this study the radiotherapy cohort came from the patient group treated between 1970 and 1998. Confirmation of findings would require a further phase III randomized comparison.

Recurrence After Radiotherapy. Involvement of the supradiaphragmatic lymph nodes (mediastinal and supraclavicular), lung, and bone is a common form of metastasis after radiotherapy. These relapsing cases are salvaged with chemotherapy. This is discussed in detail later (see Salvage Chemotherapy).

Stage IIC Seminoma

Radiotherapy. Although local control is possible with radiotherapy, there is a 50% risk of distant metastasis, and salvage may not be possible in all cases (74). Radiotherapy, therefore, has no major role in this stage of metastatic seminoma, as BEP combination chemotherapy cures 95% of patients (75).

In addition, radiation to the involved fields after chemotherapy has been shown in a retrospective analysis to add no survival benefit (76). Today BEP chemotherapy, as with more advanced stages, remains the standard of care, though increasing attention has been given to late toxicity of the treatment, and there is increased interest in further study of a single agent (72).

Nonseminomatous Germ Cell Tumor Stage II

Nonseminomatous germ cell tumor stage II is highly curable (>95%). The general consensus in the United Kingdom and most centers in Europe is that

TABLE 17.1.7. Bleomycin, etoposide, and Platinol (cisplatin) (BEP) regimen (78,80)

Drug	BEP (5 days)	BEP (3 days)
Cisplatin	20 mg/m^2 (days 1–5)	50 mg/m^2 (days 1–2)
Etoposide	100 mg/m^2 (days 1–5)	165 mg/m^2 (days 1–3)
Bleomycin	30,000 units (days 1, 8, 15)	30,000 units (day 1, 8, 15)

all patients start with initial chemotherapy after radical orchidectomy, provided that rising tumor markers or enlarging mass on serial CT scan indicates active tumor growth. This is followed by RPLND for residual masses in the one in five patients who do not respond completely. The alternative strategy favored in the U.S. is to do an RPLND because CT scan changes in the absence of tumor markers have a high incidence of false positivity (77,78), and then to give two courses of adjuvant BEP chemotherapy if extensive malignancy is demonstrated. It should also be noted that in North America there is a greater tendency to select RPLND in patients with elements of immature teratoma in the primary tumor because of late teratomatous relapse.

Advanced Metastatic (Stage III and IV, N4, M+ Disease) Germ Cell Cancer

A risk-adapted approach based on IGCCCG criteria is recommended for advanced NSGCT. In patient with a good prognosis, the standard treatment consists of three BEP cycles, and where bleomycin is contraindicated four cycles of Platinol (cisplatin) and etoposide (PE) are recommended (79).

Currently combination chemotherapy consisting of BEP has become the standard of care for these patients, given either over 3 days, as developed in the U.K. or 5 days as used in U.S. trials (Table 17.1.7). The administration of chemotherapy in good-prognosis germ cell cancer over 3 days has no detrimental effect on the effectiveness of the BEP regimen (80). However, in a EORTC/Medical Research Council (MRC) data comparing 3- and 5-day regimens, the 3-day regimen was shown to have a marginally worse short-term toxicity including ototoxicity, peripheral neuropathy, and Raynaud's phenomenon (81), though this difference resolves on prolonged follow-up.

In intermediate and poor prognosis groups of patients, four cycles of the 5-day BEP regimen remains the standard treatment with chemotherapy given without dose reduction at 22-day intervals (82).

Trials in Intermediate and Poor Prognosis Disease

To date, despite multiple trials, there has been no combination that has improved on BEP, which remains the standard of care. Four cycles of etopside, ifosfamide, and Platinol (cisplatin) (VIP) are equally effective but are associated with myelotoxicity (82) and therefore not recommended as a standard therapy. An alternating combination chemotherapy for advanced NSGCT that has been in use since 1977 is POMB/ACE [Platinol (cisplatin), vincristine, methotrexate, bleomycin, actinomycin D, cyclophosphamide, and etoposide]. The results over 8-year follow-up show equivalent response rates and survival in men with a good prognosis and appears to achieve better survival in patients with a poor prognosis (83), and the toxicity is equivalent to that described for simpler regimens.

A more recently developed combination regimen based on a similar attempt to achieve accelerated cisplatin dosage [CBOP/BEP: carboplatin, bleomycin, vincristine, and Platinol (cisplatin), followed by bleomycin, etoposide, and cis-platin] is now undergoing testing in a randomized trial in the U.K. (84).

Retroperitoneal surgery for Surgery for Testicular Cancer

Surgical Anatomy

The original operative procedure included extensive dissection of retroperitoneal lymph nodes extending from the suprahilar region of the kidneys down to the bifuraction of the common iliac vessels with the ureters as a lateral limit. The major side effect was the loss of ejaculation secondary to the damage of lumbar sympathetic nerves. Subsequent understanding of specific sites of nodal metastasis and retroperitoneal autonomic nerve distribution has led to modified RPLND templates without compromising therapeutic benefits of RPLND. The details of lymphatic drainage have been described previously (see Fig. 17.1.5) in this chapter.

Neuroanatomy of the Lumbar Sympathetic Nervous System

One of the key structures in male ejaculation is the lumbar sympathetic system, the fibers of which are derived from the T12 to L3 thoracolumbar spinal cord. The lumbar sympathetic chain runs on either side of the vertebral column parallel to and behind the great vessels (inferior vena cava on the right side and aorta on the left side) located on the anterolateral aspect of the vertebral body at the attachment of the psoas major to the vertebral body.

The nerves from the T12 to L3 segments travel along the sympathetic chain and participate in a series of nerve plexuses (superior mesenteric, inferior mesenteric, superior hypogastric, and inferior hypogastric plexuses) (85). Ejaculation occurs as a result of combined autonomic and somatic nerve action. Sympathetic fibers are responsible for tightening the preprostatic sphincter, while somatic fibers (pudendal nerves S2–4) are responsible for rhythmic contraction of the bulbocavernosus muscles and relaxation of the external sphincter (85).

The structures to be protected from harm include the lumbar sympathetic trunks, the postganglionic fibers situated on the vertebral bodies, and the superior hypogastric plexus. The superior hypogastric plexus is situated in front of the L5 vertebral body at the level of the bifurcation of aorta. Among these three structures, the hypogastric plexus is the most important, as dissection of this plexus consistently results in loss of ejaculation. The postganglionic fibers are also important, as they contribute to the lower level plexuses. In a study by

Whitelaw and Smithwick (86), bilateral resection of up to three sympathetic ganglia between T12 and L3 did not abolish ejaculation in 46% of men. Obviously the incidence of ejaculatory problems is therefore related to the extent of the dissection.

The indications for sympathetic nerve-sparing RPLND include NSGCT stage I and early stage II tumors along with some of late stage II and postchemotherapy cases.

Retroperitoneal Lymph Node Dissection

Retroperitoneal lymph node dissection is one of the major urological procedures and takes resolution and patience to remove residual large retroperitoneal masses.

Preoperative Preparation

Patients are counseled regarding the extent of surgery and its complications, particularly retrograde ejaculation. Cryopresevation of semen should be considered wherever indicated. Bowel preparation is necessary, as bowel injury can occur during mobilization. Hydration should be adequate and may be accomplished by intravenous fluids if necessary. The operating surgeon should work out the template plan (in conjunction with radiologists) and limits of dissection before surgery. The operation is likely to be prolonged, and there may be bleeding; an adequate amount of blood must be cross-matched and postoperative care in the intensive care/high-dependency unit may be needed. Patients who had chemotherapy usually wait for 4 to 6 weeks before normalizing for surgery. Pulmonary assessment is necessary in patients who had chemotherapy.

Principles of Technique

The retropertonem is exposed either by the thoracoabdominal or abdominal approach. The main advantage of the thoracoabominal approach is that thoracic and suprahilar lesions can be dealt with simultaneously. The incision for thoracoabdominal approach starts over the eighth or ninth rib in the midaxillary line. Transabdominal RPLND is carried out through a long midline incision. The retroperitoneum is exposed by mobilization of the ascending colon and the third part of the duodenum, followed by ligation of the inferior mesenteric vein. At this stage the operating surgeon identifies the superior mesenteric artery, the renal vessels, the inferior margin of pancreas, the inferior mesenteric artery, and the ureters. The "split and roll" technique involves incising the parietal peritoneum over the inferior vena cava (IVC) and aorta vertically, and mobilizing the tissue laterally, which contains lympahtics and lymph nodes.

Stage I and II Tumors

As the primary landing site is anterior to the lumbar vessels, some authors do not advocate division of these vessels in low-volume disease (58). The boundaries for the right-side template include the right ureter to the left border of the aorta horizontally, and from the right renal vein to the right common ilica vessels vertically, excluding the inferior mesenteric artery. On the left side tissue between the left ureter and the aortocaval region horizontally, and from the left renal vein to the left common iliac vessels vertically, excluding the inferior mesenteric artery, is included. For bilateral dissections the infrahilar tissue mass between the two ureters down to bifuraction is included.

Postchemotherapy Masses

Surgery is necessary in any patient with residual disease after tumor markers have been negative for more than 6 weeks. More controversial is the question of whether surgery should be done in patients with positive tumor markers if technically feasible. With the possible exception of patients with multiple small β-hCG positive lung metastasis, it is now increasingly accepted that surgery should be done provided complete excision is possible, particularly in AFP-positive tumors, to exclude the rare mature teratoma with fetal gut-derived elements. If cystic, they can have a very slow tumor marker decline due to slow release from cyst fluid. If the excision is complete, surgery is often curative even if viable cancer is excised.

The rationale for postchemotherapy RPLND is threefold: (1) diagnostic, to help in accurate histopathological assessment; (2) therapeutic, for removal of residual disease; and (3) to prevent mechanical problems.

The surgery of postchemotherapy RPLND differs from the RPLND for stages I and II in three ways: (1) Postchemotherapy RPLND might require excision of adjacent organs (e.g., kidney). (2) These patients may have effects of chemotherapy on hematological, renal, and pulmonary functions. (3) The surgical field may have a postchemotherapy desmoplastic reaction.

Principles of Postchemotherapy Retroperitoneal Lymph Node Dissection

If the patient requires extensive surgery, he should be warned of the likelihood of retrograde ejaculation, and arrangements should be made for sperm banking if appropriate. In exceptional cases, such as patients who have evidence of post-chemotherapy mature teratoma or necrosis and who have not yet had children, deferral of surgery for 2 to 3 years (for the recovery of spermatogenesis) may be permissible. When dissection proceeds below the aortic bifurcation, loss of ejaculation is not uncommon. The aim of the operation is to remove all macroscopic tumor from around the great vessels without endangering vital organs. The histology findings of the postchemotherapy RPLND generally show necrosis in 45%, mature embryonal elements in 45%, and persistent germ cell tumor in 10% of patients (87).

Limits of the Postchemotherapy Retroperitoneal Lymph Node Dissection Dissection

The extent of surgery depends on the laterality of the mass. In patients with bilateral disease (prior to chemotherapy), a bilateral template dissection is done. Similarly in patients with large masses, bilateral dissection is carried out.

A unilateral template is indicated in patients who had prechemotherapy unilateral disease. The ureters form the lateral limit of the dissection, with the minimum vertical limits being the renal veins and bifurcation.

Although the tumor mass often appears to be firmly attached to the great vessels, a plane can be developed and the tissue separated by the split and roll technique. If there is any difficulty in mobilizing the mass, it is wise to achieve proximal control by putting a sling around the aorta or vena cava, or both, above the upper limit of the intended dissection. Retroaortic and retrocaval access is obtained by ligation and division of lumbar vessels, which also penetrate the tumor. Tumor above the renal vessels can be approached through the lesser sac, but access is poor, and it can be very difficult indeed to stop a major bleed in this region. For this reason, if there is a residual mass at the level of the diaphragmatic crura or above, a transthoracic approach may be necessary.

In clearing the lymph node mass from the paravertebral gutter, the sympathetic chain comes into view. By preserving the chain and its rami communicantes on at least one side, it may be possible to preserve ejaculatory function. Usually, however, it is the size and layout of the tumor rather than the skill of the surgeon that determine whether this can be done.

Postoperative Complications of Retroperitoneal Lymph Node Dissection

The general abdominal surgical complications such as ileus, obstruction, and sepsis can be anticipated after RPLND, although they are extremely rare. Postoperative retroperitoneal hemorrhage is not common. The overall complication rate after postchemotherapy RPLND is 20.7% (88). Chylous ascites or lymphocele formation are usually treated conservatively. Adult respiratory distress syndrome (ARDS) is seen in 1% of patients who have received bleomycin (88). Other respiratory complications include pulmonary embolism, atelectasis, and pneumonia.

Consolidation Chemotherapy After Postchemotherapy Surgical Resection

Complete resection of the residual tumor is critical in the postchemotherapy setting. If there is tumor necrosis or a mature teratoma in the excised specimen, no further treatment is necessary. The role of chemotherapy in patients with immature teratoma or active disease is equivocal.

In a retrospective study there was evidence of progression-free survival but no improvement in overall survival rates (89). This may justify a watchful monitoring policy in such patients (82). Patients with a poor prognosis with active disease or immature teratoma in the residual masses need further chemotherapy (82).

Management of Relapse or Refractory Disease

The prognostic factors for NSGCT in cases of relapse or progress after the first-line treatment include the location and histology of the primary tumor, the duration of previous remission, the level of tumor markers at the time of relapse, and the degree of response to the first-line treatment (90). These cases are best managed by combination of chemotherapy and surgery.

Salvage Chemotherapy

Combination chemotherapy (with or without surgical resection) containing cisplatin achieves a complete response in 70% to 80% of patients with advanced germ cell tumor. There is a relapse rate of 5% to 10% after first-line chemotherapy (91). Between 20% and 30% of patients with disseminated disease do not achieve a durable complete response to conventional BEP treatment. Nearly 50% of these patients achieve a complete response to second-line therapy with VEIP with 25% of these alive in the long-term (92). The treatment is supplemented with surgery where there are residual masses in NSGCT. Third-line therapy consisting of two cycles of high-dose carboplatin, etoposide with or without cyclophosphamide, or ifosfamide followed by peripheral-blood–derived stem cell (PBSC) support gives a 15% to 25% complete response rate (92). Patients with unresolved or recurrent tumors should be treated in experienced centers as there is no single salvage regimen that has unequivocal superiority.

Conventional Salvage Regimens for Nonseminomatous Germ Cell Tumors

Patients with relapsed testicular tumors are still curable and should be given further treatment with chemotherapy with this intention in mind. Recurrences can be divided into three categories:

1. Recurrence after RPLND: The majority of patients with post-RPLND recurrences have >90% complete response rates with cisplatin-based chemotherapy (82).
2. Recurrence after first-line chemotherapy with or without RPLND.
3. Multiple relapses and cisplatin refractory disease.

Recurrences after cisplatin-based chemotherapy with or without surgical resection as a first-line treatment are managed with other combination regimens including PEI [Platinol (cisplatin), etoposide, ifosfamide]/VIP (cisplatin, etoposide, ifosfamide), VeIP (vinblastine, ifosfamide, cisplatin), and TIP (paclitaxel, ifosfamide, and cisplatin).

Vinblastine or Etoposide, Ifosfamide, Cisplatin

Ifosfamide, an alkylating agent, has a significant single-agent activity in patients with germ cell tumors.

Four cycles of combination chemotherapy with ifosfamide, cisplatin, and vinblastine or etoposide has become a standard first-line salvage chemotherapy with disease-free survival rates up to 25% (95).

The results of the ifosfamide-based regimen as a first-line therapy were slightly better, but there was no statistically significant difference between the two, with BEP being less toxic. For individual patients for whom there is a

TABLE 17.1.8. Platinol (cisplatin), etoposide, ifosfamide (PEI) and vinblastine, ifosfamide, cisplatin (VeIP) regimens

Regimen	Dosage	Duration of cycle
VIP		
Cisplatin	20 mg/m^2 days 1–5 (hydration)	
Etoposide	75–100 mg/m^2 days 1–5	
Ifosfamide	1.2 g/m^2 days 1–5 (Mesna)	21 days
VeIP		
Vinblastine	0.11 mg/kg days 1 and 2	
Ifosfamide	1.2 g/m^2 days 1–5 (Mesna)	
Cisplatin	20 mg/m^2 days 1–5	

concern about bleomycin-induced pulmonary fibrosis, the VIP regimen is an attractive first-line alternative (93). The dosage of the PEI and VeIP regimens used for relapsed germ cell tumors (GCTs) (seminomas or nonseminomas) is given in Table 17.1.8 (94,95).

Paclitaxel

Unlike other cytotoxic agents, paclitaxel interferes with the normal function of microtubule growth, resulting in disruption of cytoskeleton function and ultimately causing cellular death. Paclitaxel has been used as a single agent on a small number of patients in many centers with an average response of 21% (95). This has led to further evaluation of paclitaxel in combination with ifosfamide and cisplatin (TIP). In a completed trial (phase I and II), 46 patients who had gonadal GCT with favorable prognostic factors for conventional dose chemotherapy and a prior complete response to first-line chemotherapy program were treated with four cycles of TIP adminstered 21 days apart (96). In the phase I triall, the paclitaxel dose was increased until the maximum tolerated dose (MTD) of 250 mg/m^2 was reached. After 30 patients were treated, the 6-day regimen was changed to a 5-day course for the same dosage (Table 17.1.9). The overall complete response was in the region of 70%. Myelosuppression was the

TABLE 17.1.9. Paclitaxel, ifosfamide, and cisplatin (TIP) regimen as used in the Memorial Sloan-Kettering Cancer Center TIP regimen (96)

Regimen	Dosage	Duration of cycle
Paclitaxel	250 mg/m^2	Day 1; 24-hour infusion
Dexamethasone	20 mg orally 14 and 7 hours before paclitaxel	
Diphenhydramine	50 mg IV; 1 hour before paclitaxel	
Cimetidine	300 mg IV; 1 hour before paclitaxel	
Ifosfamide	1500 mg	Days 2–5; 60-minute infusion
Mesna	500 mg/m^2	Before ifosfamide given and 4–8 hours after ifosfamide administration on days 2–5
Cisplatin	25 mg/m^2	Days 2–5; 30-minute infusion

main toxicity. Other toxicity included grade II neurotoxicity and renal toxicity. There was only one treatment-related death.

Similar results were demonstrated in the German Testicular Cancer Study Group involving 80 patients. The regimen however was different in dosage (paclitaxel 175 mg/m^2 on day 1; ifosfaamide 1200 mg/m^2 on days 1 to 5; cisplatin 20 mg/m^2 on days 1 to 5), and responders were treated with further high-dose chemotherapy consisting of carboplatin, etoposide, and thiotepa (CET regimen: carboplatin 500 mg/m^2 × 3; etoposide 600 mg/m^2 × 4; and thiotepa 150 to 250 mg/m^2 × 3). The response to TIP was 69% and to TIP and CET was 78% (97).

Gemcitabine

Gemcitabine is a deoxycytidine analogue with a lower toxicity profile. It has been used as a monotherapy in patients who had at least two previous salvage regimens tried. It has also been combined with paclitaxel. Responses with both these regimens have been between 15% and 21% (95). The main toxicity is hematological.

Other Agents

Other agents that have been used include oxaliplatin, temozolomide, and irinotecan (95).

High-Dose Chemotherapy and Stem Cell Support

Earlier trials involving high doses of etoposide, carboplatin, and ifosfamide either as a single agent or in combination showed dose-response efficacy and safety; subsequent regimens were designed by increasing the dose intensity of chemotherapy or by using other drugs with known activity in GCTs (98). However, all high-dose chemotherapy (HDCT) regimens have acute and late toxicity that are related to three main classes of drugs used in the management of GCTs: the platinum group of drugs (cisplatin and carboplatin), the epidophyllotoxins (etoposide), and the oxazaphosphorines (cyclophosphamide and ifosfamide). Initially autologous bone marrow transplantation was used in conjunction with HDCT, which was associated with significant morbidity and mortality.

In the 1990s, HDCT regimens were scheduled with peripheral blood stem cells in clinical trials for salvage therapy or first-line treatment of poor-risk disease (99). Currently the choice of regimen for HDCT and hemopoietic stem cells (HSCs) remains one of the unresolved issues in the management of advanced GCTs. The key to success depends on better patient selection and improved supportive care (Table 17.1.10).

El-Helw et al. (98) have identified three groups of patients:

Group I: Patients with high-risk diseminated disease at presentation scheduled for HDCT and HSCs as a first-line therapy after induction chemotherapy

TABLE **17.1.10.** Definitions in high-dose chemotherapy (HDCT) (98)

1. Relapse: recurrence of disease: after a complete response (CR) or partial response (PR with negative serum amrkers) ≥4 weeks
2. Relative refractory disease: postchemotherapy marker plateau but failure of markers to normalize
3. Absolute refractory disease: an increase in marker levels or clinical/radiographic detectable disease during chemotherapy or ≤4 weeks of completing the treatment with cisplatin
4. Clinical complete response (CR): total disappearance of tumors radiologically with normalization of β-hCG and AFP with chemotherapy alone for ≥1 month
5. Surgical CR: complete excision of viable malignancy or immature NSGCT with no evidence of residual disease
6. Pathological CR: complete excision of nonviable malignancy (necrosis/fibrosis) or mature NSGCT with no evidence of residual disease and clear surgical margins
7. Partial response (marker negative) PR m−: reduction in radiologically measurable disease by more than a half and normal values of β-hCG and AFP
8. Partial response (marker positive): reduction in radiologically measurable disease by more than a half and raised values of β-hCG and AFP
9. Progressive disease (PD): an icrease in radiologically measurable tumor by 25% or markers by >10%
10. Stable disease: no CR, PR m−, or PRm+, or PD
11. Progression free survival (PFS): from the first day of HDCT until the date of treatment failure as defined by progression of the disease or relapse
12. Overall survival (OS): period from the first day of HDCT until the day of death or last follow-up

Good prognosis

Nonseminoma:
Testis/retroperitoneal primary, and
No nonpulmonary visceral metastases, and
Good markers—all of:
α-fetoprotein (AFP) <1000 ng/mL, and
Human chorionic gonadotrophin (hCG) <5000 IU/mL (1000 ng/mL), and
Lactate dehydrogenase (LDH) <1.5 × upper limit of normal
(56% of nonseminomas; 5-year progression-free survival (PFS) is 89%; 5-year survival is 92%)

Seminoma:
Any primary site, and
No nonpulmonary visceral metastases, and
Normal AFP, any hCG, any LDH
(90% of seminomas; 5-year PFS is 82%; 5-year survival is 86%)

Intermediate prognosis

Nonseminoma:
Testis/retroperitoneal primary, and
No nonpulmonary visceral metastases, and
Intermediate markers–any of:
AFP ≥1000 and ≤10,000 ng/mL, or
hCG ≥5000 IU/L and ≤50,000 IU/L, or
LDH ≥1.5 × N* and ≤10 × N*
(28% of nonseminomas; 5-year PFS is 75%; 5-year survival is 80%)

Seminoma:
Any primary site, and
Nonpulmonary visceral metastases, and
Normal AFP, any hCG, any LDH
(10% of seminomas; 5-year PFS is 67%; 5-year survival is 72%)

TABLE 17.1.10. *Continued*

Poor prognosis
Nonseminoma:
Mediastinal primary, or
Nonpulmonary visceral metastases, or
For markers–any of:
AFP >10,000 ng/mL, or
hCG >50,000 IU/mL (10,000 ng/mL), or
LDH >10 × upper limit of normal
(16% of nonseminomas; 5-year PFS is 41%; 5-year survival is 48%)
• Seminoma: no patients classified as poor prognosis

*N indicates the upper limit of normal for the LDH assay.

Group II: Patients who relapsed after previous chemotherapy either after a complete response or after a partial radiological response with negative serum markers for ≥4 weeks

Group III: Relatively cisplatin-refractory patients who had a marker plateau, but never became marker negative

Hematopoetic growth factors including granulocyte and granulocyte-macrophage colony-stimulating factors (G-CSF, GM-CSF) are used to ameliorate chemotherapy-induced myelosuppression, to facilitate dose-intensity treatment, and to generate granulocytes in HDCT (100). They also stimulate in low concentration the survival and proliferation of granulocyte progenitor cells and mature neutrophils.

Salvage Therapy in Relapsed Seminomas

The relapse of seminoma following first-line radiotherapy is treated with cisplatin-based chemotherapy, and the cure rates approach 90%.

Conventional BEP therapy induces long-term remission in ≤50% of patients (101). Other regimens of choice include four cycles of PEI, VeIP, or TIP (see above). Relapsed spermatocytic seminomas usually have associated sarcomatous elements and carry a poor prognosis. These are treated with chemotherapy, but close follow-up is necessary.

Salvage Surgery

Residual masses are excised 4 to 6 weeks after normalization of markers has been reached. Surgical excision is also considered when tumor markers progress after salvage chemotherapy or there are no other treatment options left.

Late Relapse (>2 Years After the First-Line Treatment)

If feasible, patients with late relapse with negative markers should undergo radical surgery.

In patients with positive tumor markers and small tumor masses, complete resection if possible is the main goal. In unresectable tumors, biopsy is taken to assess the histology and biological behavior of the tumor, and salvage chemotherapy is considered. For postchemotherapy residual masses, surgery should be considered (82).

Practical Issues with Chemotherapy for Training Germ Cell Tumors

Acute Side Effects

Gastrointestinal

Nausea and Vomiting. Prior to the advent of modern antiemetic regimens of 5-hydroxytryptamine (5-HT$_3$) antagonists combined with dexamethasone, vomiting several times a day on cisplatin treatment was universal, and the chemotherapy-induced nausea and vomiting (CINV) was often aggravated by changes in taste and loss of appetite. Nausea and vomiting are less severe with carboplatin. In addition to standard antiemetic protocols, two recently introduced agents—palonosetron, a longer acting serotonin antagonist, and aprepitant, a neurokinin-1 antagonist—can be used in refractory CNIV (102).

Gastrointestinal Symptoms Related to Myelosuppression. Myelosuppression produces mouth ulcers, oral thrush, herpes simplex, and perianal infections. Oral thrush is treated by oral nystatin or amphotericin. Herpetic ulcers can be treated by local acyclovir application or systemically in severe infections.

Myelosuppression

Cytotoxic drugs damage the integrity of rapidly dividing bone marrow cells, which are responsible for hemopoiesis. This can lead to anemia, granulocytopenia, and thrombocytopenia. Granulocytopenic sepsis manifests as fever, chills, and rigors. Sepsis is generally caused by gram-ve bacteria, such as *Escherichia coli* and *Pseudomonas*. Skin commensals like staphylococci can infect through venepuncture sites. Platelet counts below 20×10^9/L may manifest as epistaxis, ecchymosis, or purpura. Similarly respiratory and urinary infections can overwhelm the immunosuppressed patient.

Treatment-related death is avoided by intensive treatment of neutropenic sepsis with appropriate antimicrobial agents over the neutropenic phase, avoiding aminoglycoside use; if this is the only antibiotic that can be used, extremely careful dosage control is exercised. Etoposide in particular is bone marrow suppressant leading to granulocytopenia.

Nephrotoxicity

Cisplatin is a highly nephrotoxic drug, and nephrotoxicity is its dose-limiting factor. Induction of nephrotoxicity by cisplatin is supposed to be a rapid process involving proteins in the renal tubules. Renal function is likely to get worse during repeated cycles, and a regular check on serum creatinine is advisable. A recently identified risk has been the use of intravenous contrast agents in the week after cisplatin is given.

Monitoring for cisplatin-induced magnesium leak in sick patients and adjusting the bleomycin dosage in the event of any cisplatin-induced reduction of renal function to avoid bleomycin lung are other critical aspects of management.

Aminoglycosides synergize with cisplatin leading to acute renal failure and should be avoided if possible. Carboplatin, an analogue of cisplatin, has reduced side effects, particularly cisplatin's nephrotoxic effects. Bleomycin clearance is affected in the presence of renal failure.

Neurotoxicity

Cisplatin is retained in the peripheral nervous system, particularly in the region of dorsal root ganglia (103). Central structures including brain and spinal cord are protected from cisplatin accumulation (103). Bilateral hearing deficits occur with cisplatin-based chemotherapy due to the effect on auditory nerve.

Pulmonary Toxicity

Bleomycin is commonly associated with pulmonary toxicity in 3% to 40% of patients, and fatal toxicity in 1% to 15% of cases (104). Clinically, pulmonary toxicity is characterized by cough, dyspnea, fever, tachypnea, and cyanosis due to pneumonitis or pulmonary fibrosis. Concurrent administration of G-CSF is supposed to potentiate pulmonary toxicity (105). The factors that predisposes to bleomycin-induced toxicity include increasing age, high cumulative bleomycin dose, concurrent chest radiation therapy, and oxygen administration. This problem is of particular importance if a patient is to undergo RPLND, as anesthetic problems could ensue during surgery.

Acute Vascular Toxicity

The acute and chronic vascular effects of cisplatin- and bleomycin-containing chemotherapy is well known. In vitro studies have demonstrated endothelial injury after the administration of cisplatin and bleomycin in vitro (106). Several patients have also been reported with acute myocardial infarction occurring during or shortly after the administration of cisplatin (107). In most cases, chemotherapy-induced vascular toxicity may not result in acute cardiovascular complications during treatment but manifest at a later period.

Long-Term Effects

Fertility and Leydig Cell Failure

The relationship between infertility and testicular cancer has already been discussed earlier in this chapter. Many patients have oligospermia and other sperm abnormalities. Patients with a normal sperm count also become oligospermic or azoospermic with chemotherapy, though usually it is only temporary as spermatogenesis recovers at between 18 and 36 months, depending on intensity of the treatment and whether ifosfamide has been used. Once recovered, patients are able to father children. Once cured, monitoring for relapse on follow-up ensues, and it is also important to assess testicular endocrine function and organize testosterone replacement for any patients with Leydig cell failure. This occurs in the majority of patients in the first 6 months after chemotherapy, and for some of these patients a short period of monthly intramuscular testosterone replacement can be immensely helpful. Only a small minority require continuous replacement.

Testis Conservation with Chemotherapy

This is a highly debatable issue. Until recently it was thought that the risks of second cancers from CIS precluded the use of chemotherapy for testes conservation. However, attitudes are now changing, for two reasons: first, it is now increasingly accepted that more than 70% of patients with GCTs are subfertile due to testicular atrophy; and second, there is increasing evidence that the atrophy might be contributing to the higher incidence of weight gain and noncancerous causes of death seen even in patients treated by orchiectomy alone. Because of a report that 1 in 10 patients with sperm in ejaculate preorchidectomy actually became azoospermic after orchidectomy, more attention is being paid to this issue. In one study 14 of 42 with metastases and 3 of 10 with stage I tumor were salvaged by chemotherapy, although there were two recurrences salvaged by orchidectomy. So far there have been one pregnancy, and two other patients have recovered spermatogenesis (108).

Long-Term Vascular Effects

Cardiovascular effects in the form of Raynaud's phenomenon (RP) and myocardial infarction are seen following chemotherapy in GCTs. Raynaud's phenomenon is the main late vascular toxicity, affecting one third of patients after curative chemotherapy, although major vascular events are rare. The incidence of RP following BEP (5 days) therapy, in contrast to Platinol (cisplatin), vinblastine, and bleomycin (PVB) therapy, appears to be lower (109). A trend of an increased frequency of RP is observed in patients who receive bleomycin as a bolus instead of continuous infusion (109). Hypertension is another long-term effect of platinum-based chemotherapy. In a study of long-term follow-up of 5 to 20 years after cisplatin-based chemotherapy, cured testicular cancer patients had significantly higher levels of blood pressure, a higher prevalence of hypertension, and excessive weight gain compared with patients treated with other modalities and compared with healthy controls (110).

The role of mediastinal radiotherapy in increasing the risk of myocardial infarction is described in the radiotherapy section.

Second Cancers. Second primary cancers have emerged as a leading cause of death among testicular cancer survivors (111). There is a strong age dependence of excess cancers, and statistically significantly increased risks of cancer persist for at least 35 years after a testicular cancer diagnosis. Though there is some evidence for statistically significant associations between the receipt of chemotherapy and the risk of a second cancer, more significant is the risk of radiation and even more so the risk of radiation combined with chemotherapy. There is also evidence to suggest an increased association of cancers of the pleura (mesothelioma) and esophagus in these patients (112). Patients receiving high doses of etoposide, however, are notably susceptible to chemotherapy-related leukemia, though there is possibly also a contribution of cisplatin chemotherapy to this risk.

Quality of Life. In a study of 149 testicular cancer survivors with no evidence of disease at the end of 3 years, Kaasa et al. (113) reviewed responses to questionnaires which covered well-being, working ability and use of analgesics/tranquilisers. They found no systematic differences between the treatment groups as the analyses were undertaken with all patients combined. The patients felt significantly less exhausted after a working day, were more satisfied with life and felt stronger and more fit than their age-matched controls. The patients however reported a significantly higher incidence of anxiety and depression than the normal population. The results indicate that patients treated for a malignant disease may have greater fluctuations in mood and affect than the general population. Furthermore, another study (114) has shown reduced QOL in subgroups of patients (particularly after intensive chemotherapy), such as those who are single, who have a low education, and who have sexual problems (114). In a study of 1409 patients treated between 1980 and 1994, Mykletun et al. (114) concluded the following:

1. Testicular cancer survivors, in general, do not suffer from reduced QOL, and interventions to improve long-term QOL in testicular cancer survivors should be offered only to identified subgroups with low QOL.
2. Testicular cancer treatment modality does not predict long-term QOL in testicular cancer survivors; therefore, as a general rule, QOL considerations should not have a major impact on choice of treatment in testicular cancer patients.
3. Testicular cancer survivors who report more side effects or more testicular cancer–related stress are more likely to show reduced QOL, but these associations are not attributable to testicular cancer treatment strategies.

Extragonadal Germ Cell Tumors

Extragonadal germ cell tumors are rare and account for 2% to 3% of all germ cell cancers. They can occur in the midline from the pineal gland to the coccyx, with the mediastinum being the most common site (115). It is likely that these germ cell tumors are derived from primordial germ cells misplaced during embryogenesis.

Retroperitoneal extragonadal germ cell tumors (EGGCTs) are thought to be metastasis from the testis, whereas the exact origin of mediastinal and higher lesions is unclear (116). Histologically they have the same components as their gonadal counterparts. They also share features of tumor markers with testicular germ cell tumors. Comparative genomic hybridization analysis has shown universal overrepresentation of 12p DNA in both gonadal and extragonadal germ cell tumors (117).

Clinical features depend on the site and volume of the tumor. For example, mediastinal tumors may present with respiratory symptoms, while abdominal lesions could present with pain or palpable mass. Pineal tumors may present with visual disturbances. The initial diagnosis is made on the basis of imaging (CT scan, chest x-ray, ultrasonography) and tumor markers.

The principles of management are the same as for testicular GCTs. In pooled data from the U.S. and Europe, Bokemeyer et al. (116) reported the clinical and biological features of EGGCTs and the outcome of treatment strategies. They observed that nonseminomatous histology, nonpulmonary visceral metastasis, primary mediastinal GCT location, and elevated β-hCG were independent prognostic factors. Patients with pure seminomatous EGCT had a long-term chance of survival, irrespective of the primary site, of 90%.

Non–Germ Cell Tumors

Leydig cell tumors comprise 1% to 2% of all testicular tumors, with 10% being malignant. Prepubertal tumors are usually benign and may be active, leading to precocious puberty (118). In adult patients a characteristic combination of gynecomastia, impotence, and testicular mass may be evident. Excision of the tumor invariably relieves these symptoms. Malignant Leydig cell tumors are staged by imaging.

Sertoli cell tumors are usually benign. In more than 20% of patients signs of feminization are seen (119). Management is by orchidectomy.

Gonadoblastomas are usually seen in relation to gonadal dysgenesis. Patients may present with hypospadias and cryptorchidism.

Lymphoma of the testis is usually a secondary tumor of the testis. Painless enlargement in a man over the age of 50 should raise the suspicion of lymphoma. Radical orchidectomy is necessary to make a histological diagnosis. Subsequent management and follow-up require a referral to a radiation or medical oncologist, which depends on histological type and the extent of the disease.

References

1. Parkin DM, Muir CS, Whelan SL, et al. Cancer Incidence in Five Continents, vol 6. Lyon, France: IARC Scientific Publications, 1997.
2. McGlynn KA, Devesa SS, Graubard BI, Castle PE. Increasing incidence of testicular germ cell tumors among black men in the United States. J Clin Oncol 2005; 23(24):5757–5761.
3. Huyghe E, Matsuda T, Thonneau P. Increasing incidence of testicular cancer worldwide: a review. J Urol 2003;170(1):5–11.

4. Richiardi L, Bellocco R, Adami HO, et al. Testicular cancer incidence in eight northern European countries: secular and recent trends. Cancer Epidemiol Biomarkers Prev 2004;13(12):2157–2166.

5. Moller H, Jorgensen N, Forman D. Trends in incidence of testicular cancer in boys and adolescent men. Int J Cancer 1995;61:761 764.

6. Moller H, Skakkebaek NE. Risk of testicular cancer in subfertile men: case-control study. BMJ 2005;318:559–562.

7. Jacobson R, Bostofte E, Engholm G, et al. Risk of testicular cancer in men with abnormal semen characteristics: cohort study. BMJ 2000;321:789–792.

8. Moller H, Prener A, Skakkebaek NE. Testicular cancer, cryptorchidism, inguinal hernia, testicular atrophy and genital malformations: case controlled studies in Denmark. Cancer causes and control 1996;7:264–274.

9. Nouri AME, Hussain RF, Oliver RTD, et al. Immunological paradox in testicular tumours: the presence of a large number of activated T cells despite the complete absence of MHC antigens. Eur J Cancer 1993;29A:1895–1899.

10. Skakkebaek N, Rajpert-DeMayts E, Jorgensen N, et al. Germ cell cancer and disorders of embryonal genesis: an environmental connection? APMIS 1998;106(1):3–11.

11. Skakkebaek NE. Possible carcinoma in situ of the testis. Lancet 1972;2:516–517.

12. von der Maase H, Rorth M, Walbom-Jorgensen S, et al. Carcinoma in situ of contralateral testis in patients with testicular germ cell cancer: study of 27 cases in 500 patients. BMJ 1986;293:1398–1401.

13. Jørgensen N, Rajpert-De Meyts E, Graem N, et al. Expression of immunohistochemical markers for testicular carcinoma in situ by normal fetal germ cells. Lab Invest 1995;72:223–231.

14. Dieckman KP, Skakkebaek NE. Carcinoma in situ of the testis: review of biological and clinical features. Int J Cancer 1999;83:815–822.

15. De Graafe WE, Oosterhuis JW, De Jong B, et al. Ploidy of testicular carcinoma in situ. Lab Invest 1992;66:166–168.

16. Berney DM, Lee A, Randle SJ, et al. The frequency of intratubular embryonal carcinoma: implications for the pathogenesis of germ cell tumours. Histopathology. 2004;45(2):155–161.

17. Rajpet-De Meyts E, Skakkebaek NE. The possible role of sex hormones in the development of testicular cancer. Eur Urol 1993;23:54–59.

18. Starr JR, Chen C, Doody DR, et al. Risk of testicular germ cell cancer in relation to variation in maternal and offspring cytochrome p450 genes involved in catechol estrogen metabolism. Cancer Epidemiol Biomarkers Prev 2005;14(9):2183–2190.

19. Dearnley DP, Huddart RA, Horwich A. Managing testicular cancer. BMJ 2001;322:1583–1588.

20. Verp MS, Simpson JL. Abnormal sexual differentiation and neoplasia. Cancer Genet Cytogenet 1987;25:191–218.

21. Collins GM, Kim DU, Logrono R, et al. Pure seminoma arising in androgen insensitivity syndrome (testicular feminization syndrome):a case report and review of the literature. Mod Pathol 1993;6:89–93.

22. Heimdal K, Olsson H, Tretli K, et al. Risk of cancer in relatives of testicular cancer patients Br J Cancer 1996;73:970–973.

23. Swerdlow AJ, De Stavola BL, Swanwick MA, Maconochie NES. Risks of breast and testicular cancers in young adult twins in England and Wales: evidence on prenatal and genetic aetiology. Lancet 1997;350:1723–1728.

24. Pottern LM, Brown LM, Devesa SS. Epidemiology and pathogenesis of testicular cancer. In: Ernstoff MS, Heaney JA, Peschel RE, eds. Testicular and Penile Cancer. Malden, MA; Cambridge, UK: Blackwell Science, 1998:2–10.

25. Han S, Peschel RE. Father-son testicular tumors. Evidence for genetic anticipation? A case report and review of the literature. Cancer 2000;88(10):2319–2325.

26. Skakkebaek NE, Rajpet-De Meyts E, Main KM. Testicular dysgenesis syndrome: an increasingly common developmental disorder with environmental aspects. Hum Reprod 2001;16:972–978.

27. Raghavan D, Zalcberg JR, Grygiel JJ, et al. Multiple atypical nevi: a cutaneous marker of germ cell tumors. J Clin Oncol 1994;12(11):2284–2287.

28. Avril MF, Chompret A, Verne-Fourment L, et al. Association between germ cell tumours, large numbers of naevi, atypical naevi and melanoma. Melanoma Res 2001;11(2):117–122.

29. Sandberg AA, Meloni AM, Suijkerbuijk RF. Reviews of chromosome studies in urological tumors. 3. Cytogenetics and genes in testicular tumors. J Urol 1996;155: 1531–1556.

30. van Echten-Arends J, Oosterhuis JW, Looijenga LHJ, et al. No recurrent structural abnormalities in germ cell tumours of the adult testis apart from i(12p). Genes Chromosom Cancer 1995;14:133–144.

31. Leahy MG, Tonks S, Moses JH, et al. Candidate regions for a testicular cancer susceptibility gene. Hum Mol Genet 1995;4:1551–1555.

32. Bishop DT. Candidate regions for testicular cancer susceptibility genes. APMIS 1998;106:64–72.

33. Rapley E, Crockford G, Teare D, et al. Localisation to Xq27 of a susceptibility gene for testicular germ cell tumours. Nature Genetics 2000;24:197–200.

34. Forman D, Oliver RTD, Brett AR, et al. Familial testicular cancer: a report of the UK family register, estimation of risk and an HLA Class 1 sib-pair analysis. Br J Cancer 1992;65:255–262.

35. Heinrich MC, Blanke CD, Druker BJ, Corless CL. Inhibition of KIT tyrosine kinase activity: a novel molecular approach to the treatment of KIT-positive malignancies. J Clin Oncol 2002;20:1692–1703.

36. Chandra S, Kapur R, Chuzhanova N, et al. A rare complex DNA rearrangement in the murine Steel gene results in exon duplication and a lethal phenotype. Blood 2003;102:3548–3555.

37. Moul JW, Schanne FJ, Thompson IM, et al. Testicular cancer in blacks. A multicenter experience. Cancer 1994;73(2):388–393.

38. Nicholson PW, Harland SJ. Inheritance and testicular cancer. Br J Cancer 1995;71: 421–426.

39. Giwercman A, Dezuyei N, Lundwall A, et al. Testicular cancer and molecular genetics. Andrologia 2005;37:224–225.

40. Dieckman K-P, Loy V. False negative biopsies for the diagnosis of testicular intraepithelial neoplasia (TIN): an update. Eur Urol 2003;43:516–521.

41. Petersen PM, Giwercman A, Hansen SW, et al. Impaired testicular function in patients with carcinoma in situ of the testis. J Clin Oncol 1999;17(10):173–179.

42. Elbe JN, Sauter G, Epstein JI, Sesterhenn IA. Pathology and Genetics of Tumours of the Urinary System and Male Genital Organs. Lyon, France: IARC Press, 2004.

43. Tickoo SK, Hutchinson B, Bacik J, et al. Testicular seminoma: a clinicopathological and immunohistochemical study of 105 cases with special reference to seminoma with atypical features. Int J Surg Pathol 2002;10:23–32.

44. Hori K, Uematsu K, Yasoshima H, et al. Testicular seminoma with human chorionic gonadotropin production. Pathol Int 1997;47(9):592–599.
45. Holstein AF, Orlandini GE, Moller R. Distribution and fine structure of the lymphatic system in the human testis. Cell Tissue Res 1979;200(1):15–27.
46. Husband JE, Koh D-M. Testicular germ cell tumours. In: Husband JE, Reznek RH, eds. Imaging in Oncology, 2nd ed. London: Taylor & Francis, 2004:401–427.
47. Holtl L, Pescel R, Knapp R, et al. Primary lymphatic metastatic spread in testicular cancers occurs ventral to the lumbar vessels. Urology 2002;59:114–118.
48. Williams MP, Cook JV, Duchesne GM. Psoas nodes: an overlooked site of metastasis from testicular tumours. Clin Radiol 1989;40:607–609.
49. Schwerk WB, Schwerk WN, Rodeck G. Testicular tumors: prospective analysis of real time US patterns and abdominal staging. Radiology 1987;164:369–374.
50. Oliver RTD, Leahy M, Ong J. Combined seminoma/non-seminoma should be considered as intermediate grade germ cell cancer (GCC). Eur J Cancer 1995;31A: 1392–1394.
51. Petersen PM, Skakkebaek NE, Rorth M, Giwercman A. Semen quality and reproductive hormones before and after orchiectomy in men with testicular cancer. J Urol 1999;161:822–826.
52. Heidenreich A, Holtl W, Albrecht W, et al. Testis-preserving surgery in bilateral testicular germ cell tumours. BJU Int 1997;79:253–257.
53. Heidenreich A, Weißbach L, Höltl W, et al. Organ sparing surgery for malignant germ cell tumor of the testis. J Urol 2001;166:2161–2165.
54. International Germ Cell Cancer Collaborative Group. International Germ Cell Consensus Classification: a prognostic factor-based staging system for metastatic germ cell cancers. J Clin Oncol 1997;15:594–603.
55. Greene FL, Page DL, Fleming ID, et al. AJCC Cancer Staging Manual, Sixth Edition. New York: Springer, 2002.
56. Baniel J, Sella A. Complications of retroperitoneal lymph node dissection in testicular cancer: primary and post-chemotherapy. Semin Surg Oncol 1999;17: 263–267.
57. Nasser A, Janetschek G. laparoscopic retroperitoneal lymph node dissection in the management of clinical stage I and II testicular cancer. J Endourol 2005;19:683–692.
58. Holtl L Peschel R, Knapp R, et al. Primary lymphatic metastatic spread in testicular cancers occurs ventral to the lumbar vessels. Urology 2002;59:114–118.
59. Satoh M, Ito A, Kaiho Y, et al. Intraoperative radio-guided sentinel lymph node mapping in laparoscopic lymph node dissection for stage I testicular carcinoma. Cancer 2005;103:2067–2072.
60. Petersen PM, Giwercman A, Daugaard G, et al. Effect of graded testicular doses of radiotherapy in patients treated for carcinoma-in-situ in the testis. J Clin Oncol 2002;20:1537–1543.
61. Christensen TB, Daugaard G, Geersten PF, von der Maase H. Effect of chemotherapy on carcinoma in situ of the testis. Ann Oncol 1998;9:657–660.
62. Warde P, Specht L, Horwich A, et al. Prognostic factors for relapse in stage I seminoma managed by surveillance: a pooled analysis. J Clin Oncol 2002;20(22):4448–4452.
63. Oliver RTD, Mason MD, Mead GM, et al. Radiotherapy versus singe-dose carboplatin in adjuvant treatment of stage 1 seminoma: a randomised trial. Lancet 2005; 366(9482):293–300.

64. Foster RS and Roth BJ. Clinical stage I nonseminoma: surgery versus surveillance. Sem Oncol 1998;25:145–153.

65. Freedman L, Oliver R, Peckham M. Prognostic factors in advanced non-seminomatous germ cell testicular tumours: results of a multicentre study. Lancet 1985;1: 8–11.

66. Freedman L, Parkinson MC, Jones WG, et al. Histopathology in the prediction of relapse of patients with stage I testicular teratoma treated by orchidectomy alone. Lancet 1987;2:294–298.

67. Cullen MH, Stenning SP, Parkinson MC, et al. Short-course adjuvant chemotherapy in high-risk stage I nonseminomatous germ cell tumors of the testis: a Medical Research Council report. J Clin Oncol 1996;14:1106–1113.

68. Williams SD, Stablein DM, Einhorn LH, et al. Immediate adjuvant chemotherapy versus observation with treatment at relapse in pathological stage II testicular cancer. N Engl J Med 1987;317(23):1433–1438.

69. Spermon JR, Roeleveld TA, van der Poel HG, et al. Comparison of surveillance and retroperitoneal lymph node dissection in stage I nonseminomatous germ cell tumors. Urology 2002;59(6):923–929.

70. Gels ME, Hoekstra HJ, Sleijfer DT, et al. Detection of recurrence in patients with clinical stage I nonseminomatous testicular germ cell tumors and consequences for further follow-up: a single-center 10-year experience. J Clin Oncol 1995;13:1188–1194.

71. Chung PW, Gospodarowicz MK, Panzarella T, et al. Stage II testicular seminoma: patterns of recurrence and outcome of treatment. Eur Urol 2004;45(6):754–759; discussion 759–760.

72. Bokemeyer C, Kollmannsberger C, Stenning SP, et al. Metastatic seminoma treated with either single agent carboplatin or cisplatin-based combination chemotherapy: a pooled analysis of two randomised trials. Br J Cancer 2004;91(4):683–687.

73. Patterson H, Norman AR, Mitra SS, et al. Combination carboplatin and radiotherapy in the management of stage II testicular seminoma: comparison with radiotherapy treatment alone. Radiother Oncol 2001;59(1):5–11.

74. Warde P, Gospodarowicz M, Panzarella T, et al. Management of stage II seminoma. J Clin Oncol 1998;16:290–294.

75. Fossa SD, Oliver RT, Stenning SP, et al. Prognostic factors for patients with advanced seminoma treated with platinum-based chemotherapy. Eur J Cancer 1997;33: 1380–1387.

76. Duchesne GM, Stenning SP, Aass N, et al. Radiotherapy after chemotherapy for metastatic seminoma—a diminishing role. MRC Testicular Tumour Working Party. Eur J Cancer 1997;33(6):829–835.

77. Stephenson AJ, Sheinfeld J. Management of patients with low-stage nonseminomatous germ cell testicular cancer. Review. Curr Treat Options Oncol 2005;6(5):367–377.

78. Xiao H, Mazumdar M, Bajorin DF, et al. Long-term follow up of patients with good-risk germ cell tumors treated with etoposide and cisplatin. J Clin Oncol 1997; 15(7):2553–2558.

79. De Wit RJ, Roberts T, Wilkinson PM, et al. Equivalence of three or four cycles of bleomycin, etoposide, and cisplatin chemotherapy and of a 3- or 5- day schedule in good prognosis germ cell cancer: a randomized study of the European Organization for Research and Treatment of Cancer Genitourinary Tract Cancer Cooperative Group and the Medical Research Council. J Clin Oncol 2001;19(6):1629–1640.

80. Fossa SD, de Wit RJ, Roberts JT, et al. Quality of life in good prognosis patients with metastatic germ cell cancer: a prospective study of the European Organization for

Research and Treatment of Cancer Genitourinary Group/Medical Research Council Testicular Cancer Study Group (30941/TE20). J Clin Oncol 2003;21:1107–1118.

81. Schmoll HJ, Souchon R, Krege S, et al. European consensus on diagnosis and treatment of germ cell cancer: a report of the European Germ Cell Cancer Consensus Group (EGCCCG). Ann Oncol 2004;15(9):1377–1399.

82. Bower M, Newlands ES, Holden L, et al. Treatment of men with metastatic non-seminomatous germ cell tumours with cyclical POMB/ACE chemotherapy. Ann Oncol 1997;8(5):477–483.

83. Christian JA, Huddart RA, Norman A, et al. Intensive induction chemotherapy with CBOP/BEP in patients with poor prognosis germ cell tumors. J Clin Oncol 2003; 21(5):871–877.

84. Lange PH, Chang WY, Fraley EE. Fertility issues in the therapy of nonseminomatous germ cell tumours. Urol Clin North Am 1987;14(4):731–747.

85. Whitelaw GP, Smithwick RH. Some secondary effects of sympathectomy—with particular reference to disturbance of sexual function. N Engl J Med 1951;245: 121–130.

86. Steele GS, Richie JP. Current role of retroperitoneal lymph node dissection in testicular cancer. Oncology 1997;11:717–729.

87. Baniel J, Foster RS, Rowland RG, et al. Complications of post-chemotherapy retroperitoneal lymph node dissection. J Urol 1995;153(3 pt 2):976–980.

88. Fizazi K, Tjulandin S, Salvioni R, et al. Viable malignant cells after primary chemotherapy for disseminated nonseminomatous germ cell tumors: prognostic factors and role of postsurgery chemotherapy-results from an international study. J Clin Oncol 2001;19:2647–2657.

89. Fossa SD, Stenning SP, Gerl A, et al. Prognostic factors in patients progressing after cisplatin-based chemotherapy for malignant non-seminomatous germ cell tumours. Br J Cancer 1999;80(9):1392–1399.

90. Fléchon A, Culine S, Théodore C, Droz J-P. Pattern of relapse after first line treatment of advanced stage germ-cell tumors. Eur Urol 2005;48:957–964.

91. Motzer RJ, Sheinfeld J, Mazumdar M, et al. Paclitaxel, Ifosfamide and cisplatin second line therapy for patients with relapsed testicular germ cell cancer. J Clin Oncol 2000;18:2413–2418.

92. Einhorn LH. Ifosfamide in germ cell tumors. Oncology 2003;65(suppl 2):73–75.

93. Loehrer PJ Sr, Gonin R, Nichols CR, et al. Vinblastine plus ifosfamide plus cisplatin as initial salvage therapy in recurrent germ cell tumor. J Clin Oncol 1998;16:2500–2504.

94. Farmakis D, Pectasides M, Pectasides D. Recent advances in conventional-dose salvage chemotherapy in patients with cisplatin-resistant or refractory testicular germ cell tumors. Eur Urol 2005;48:400–407.

95. Kondagunta GV, Bacik J, Donadio A, et al. Combination of paclitaxel, ifosfamide and cisplatin is an effective second-line therapy for patients with relapsed testicular germ cell tumors. J Clin Oncol 2005;27:8549–8555.

96. Beyer J, Bokemeyer C, Rick O, et al. Salvage treatment in germ cell tumors using Taxol, ifosfamide, cisplatin (TIP) followed by high dose carboplatin, etoposide and thiotepa (HDCET): first results. Proc Am Soc Clin Oncol 1998:17:322a.

97. El-Helw LM, Naik JD, Chester JD, et al. High-dose chemotherapy with haemopoietic stem-cell support in patients with poor prognosis, relapsed or refractory germ cell tumours. Br J Urol Int 2006;98:519–525.

98. de Giorgi U, Rosti G, Papiani G, Marangolo M. The status of high-dose chemotherapy with hemopoietic stem cell transplantation in patients with germ cell tumor. Haematologica 2002:87:95–104.

99. Bokemeyer C, Kuczyk MA, Kohne H, et al. Haematopoietic growth factors and treatment of testicular cancer: biological interactions, routine use and dose-intensive chemotherapy. Ann Haematol 1996;72:1–9.

100. Miller KD, Loehrer PJ, Gonon R, et al. Salvage chemotherapy with vinblastine, cisplatin in recurrent seminoma. J Clin Oncol 1997;15:1427–1431.

101. Viale PH. Integrating aprepitant and palonosteron into clinical practice: a role for the new antiemetics. Clin J Oncol Nurs 2005;9:77–84.

102. Gregg RW, Molepo JM, Monpetit VJ, et al. Cisplatin neurotoxicity: the relationship between dosage, time and platinum concentration in neurologic tissues, and morphologic evidence of toxicity. J Clin Oncol 1992;10:795–803.

103. Jules-Elysee K, White D. Bleomycin-induced pulmonary toxicity. Clin Chest Med 1990;11:1–20.

104. Saxman SB, Nichols CR, Einhorn LH. Pulmonary toxicity in patients with advanced germ cell tumors receiving bleomycin with or without granulocyte colony stimulating factor. Chest 1997;111:657–660.

105. Dirix LY, Libura M, Libura J, et al. In vitro toxicity studies with mitomycin and bleomycin on endothelial cells. Anticancer Drugs 1997;8:859–868.

106. Weijl NI, Rutten MF, Zwinderman AH, et al. Thromboembolic events during chemotherapy for germ cell cancer: a cohort study and review of the literature. J Clin Oncol 2000;18:2169–2178.

107. Oliver RTD, Ong J, Berney D, Nargund V, et al. Testis conserving chemotherapy in germ cell cancer: its potential to increase understanding of the biology and treatment of carcinoma-in-situ. APMIS 2003;111:86–92.

108. Berger CC, Bokemeyer C, Schneider M, et al. Secondary Raynaud's phenomenon and other late vascular complications following chemotherapy for testicular cancer. Eur J Cancer 1995;31A (13–14):2229–2238.

109. Sagstuen H, Aass N, Fossa SD, et al. Blood pressure and body mass index in long-term survivors of testicular cancer. J Clin Oncol 2005;23(22):4980–4990.

110. Fossa SD, Aass N, Harvei S, Tretli S. Increased mortality rates in young and middle-aged patients with malignant germ cell tumours. Br J Cancer 2004;90:607–612.

111. Travis LB, Fosså SD, Schonfeld SJ, et al. Second cancers among 40,576 testicular cancer patients: focus on long-term survivors. J Natl Cancer Inst 2005;97(18): 1354–1365.

112. Kaasa S, Aass N, Mastekaasa A, Lund E, Fossa SD. Psychosocial well-being in testicular cancer patients. Eur J Cancer 1991;27(9):1091–1095.

113. Mykletun A, Dahl AA, Haaland CF, et al. Side effects and cancer-related stress determine quality of life in long-term survivors of testicular cancer. J Clin Oncol 2005; 23:3061–3068.

114. Bosl GJ, Motzer RJ. Testicular germ cell cancer. N Engl J Med 1997;337:242–253.

115. Bokemeyer C, Nichols CR, DrozJ-P, et al. Extragonadal germ cell tumours of the mediastinum and retroperitoneum: results from an international analysis. J Clin Oncol 2002;20(7):1864–1873.

116. Chaganti RSK, Houldsworth J. Genetics and biology of adult human male germ cell tumours. Cancer Res 2000;60:1475–1482.

117. Freeman DA. Steroid-hormone producing tumors in man. Endocr Rev 1986;7: 204–220.

118. Gabrilove JI, Freiberg EK, Leiter E, et al. Feminizing and nonfeminizing Sertoli cell tumours. J Urol 1980;124:757–767.

17.2
Radiotherapy in the Management of Testicular Germ Cell Tumors

Dag Josefsen and Sophie D. Fosså

Radiotherapy as a routine treatment in patients with germinal cell cancers is offered to patients with early stages of seminomatous testicular cancers including clinical stage I and stage IIA and limited stage IIB disease. The rationale for radiotherapy in the management of seminoma with limited lymph node metastasis is its extreme sensitivity to radiotherapy, and the stepwise dissemination of tumor cells through lymphatics in the retroperitoneum (1). Radiotherapy, therefore, induces high cure rates in patients with low-volume seminomatous disease. Principles of management of various stages of testicular germ cell tumors (TGCTs), including relapse, is discussed in Chapter 17.1.

Carcinoma In Situ

It is generally agreed that carcinoma in situ (CIS) is the precursor of all germ cell tumors (GCTs) except spermatocytic seminoma. Patients with CIS, therefore, are at high risk of getting invasive GCTs, with nearly 50% of them becoming invasive lesions within 5 years of diagnosis (2). The standard treatment for CIS is local radiotherapy (20 Gy in single fractions of 2 Gy) after counseling about infertility and endocrine changes that occur after the treatment. Other management modalities include orchiectomy and surveillance (see Chapter 17.1).

Management of Seminoma Stage I Disease

Radiotherapy to the paraaortic and iliac lymph nodes has been the standard treatment of patients with seminoma for many years. The actuarial risk of relapse in these patients at 3 years is around 15% (3) and at 15 years 20% (4), with most relapses being infradiaphragmatic.

The use of infradiaphragmatic radiotherapy is a safe adjuvant treatment modality, but it increases the risk of late side effects, including secondary malignancies and cardiovascular disease (5–7). Recently published data demonstrate a similar relapse-free survival and overall survival rates using one cycle of carboplatin instead of radiotherapy (8). Thus, today we have several options in management of seminoma stage I disease, including surveillance, radiotherapy, and chemotherapy (9).

Using radiotherapy as the treatment in patients with seminoma stage I disease, target doses of 25 to 30 Gy have been applied. Prior to inguinal surgery, paraaortic lymph nodes represent the first site of lymphatic spread. If these lymph nodes are tumor free, it is extremely unlikely that iliac lymph node metastases are found. This has led to a study by the Medical Research Council (in the United Kingdom) comparing the relapse rates in patients with seminoma stage I disease treated with the conventional "dog-leg" radiotherapy with that in patients treated with the paraaortic strip technique (10). Relapse rates in both treatment arms were similar, though there were more pelvic recurrences in the paraaortic strip arm.

A subsequent trial assessed the target dose comparing 30 versus 20 Gy in stage I seminoma (11). After a median time of 61 months, no difference in survival was found between the two treatment alternatives. Thus, the standard adjuvant radiotherapy in patients with stage I seminoma without prior inguinal surgery is paraaortic strip radiotherapy with a target dose of 20 Gy. The upper border is set between thoracic vertebra 10 and 11, whereas lower field margin is set below lumbar vertebra 5. Lateral field margins include the transverse processes of the included vertebrae. Gonadal shielding is unnecessary in patients receiving paraaortic strip radiotherapy.

If inguinal surgery or scrotal violation has previously been performed, the ipsilateral iliac lymph nodes should also be included, and the remaining testis is to be shielded from scattered irradiation. The relapse rates after radiotherapy for stage I seminoma are less than 5%. The relapses are generally supradiaphragmatic or rarely in inguinal regions. As indicated earlier, supradiaphragmatic relapse is managed by a standard cisplatin-containing chemotherapy combination.

Treatment of Patients with Low-Volume Metastatic Seminomatous Disease (Clinical Stages IIA and IIB)

Radiotherapy is a standard treatment in patients with seminoma stage IIA/IIB disease. Chung et al. (12) demonstrated that radiation of infradiaphragmatic lymph nodes, including paraaortic and ipsilateral (with or without contralateral) pelvic lymph nodes (dose of 25 to 35 Gy), yielded a 5-year relapse-free rate of 91%. Classen et al. (1) found that radiotherapy targeting paraaortic and high ipsilateral iliac lymph nodes (doses of 30 Gy for stage IIA and 36 Gy for stage IIB) demonstrated a 6-year relapse-free survival of 95.3% and 88.9% for stage IIA and stage IIB (2 to 5 cm), respectively. The target volume should include the paraaortic strip, as mentioned above, as well as the ipsilateral iliacal lymph nodes with a lower field margin at the upper border of acetabulum. In addition, when deciding the lateral margins in the paraaortic region, the metastatic lymph node needs to be encompassed with an adequate margin. Patterson and coworkers (13) found that combination of carboplatin (one cycle) with radiotherapy in patients with stage IIA-B testicular seminoma yielded a 5-year relapse-free survival of 96.9%. In addition, minimal additional toxicity was seen compared to that in patients who received radiotherapy alone. However, these results should be confirmed by multicenter phase III randomized trials. Alternatively, patients with stage IIA-B seminomatous disease could be treated with three cycles of bleomycin, etoposide, and Platinol (cisplatin) (BEP), or four courses of etoposide and cisplatin (EP) (9).

Among 10-year survivors of testicular cancer initially given radiotherapy, the relative risks of solid tumors at sites included in typical infradiaphragmatic fields were considerably higher than those at sites not in the field (7).

Effects of Radiation

Acute effects of radiation are rare due to the low dosage of radiotherapy involved. Upper gastrointestinal (GI) symptoms like nausea and vomiting are not uncommon. Lethargy may last for a few days after completion of the treatment. Lower GI symptoms may include diarrhea.

Chronic GI problems include peptic ulceration and diarrhea. Increased incidence of cardiac disease and second malignancy was observed in a study by Gunar et al. (14). The effects of direct radiation to the testis cause infertility and loss of Leydig cell function.

Postchemotherapy Radiotherapy

Radiotherapy after chemotherapy is no longer routinely used as a treatment modality in patients with testicular cancer. However, in patients with advanced, widespread disease, including brain metastases, radiotherapy might be included as a treatment modality in addition to other treatment modalities.

References

1. Classen J, Schmidberger H, Meisner C, et al. Radiotherapy for stages IIA/B testicular seminoma: final report of a prospective multi-center clinical trial. J Clin Oncol 2003;21:1101–1106.
2. von der Maase H, Rorth M, Walbom-Jorgensen S, et al. Carcinoma in situ of contralateral testis in patients with testicular germ cell cancer: study of 27 cases in 500 patients. Br Med J 1986;293(6559):1398–1401.
3. Duchesne GM, Horwich A, Dearnley DP, et al. Orchidectomy alone for stage I seminoma of the testis. Cancer 1990;65(5):1115–1118.

4. Choo R, Thomas G, Woo T, et al. Long-term outcome of postorchidectomy surveillance for stage I testicular seminoma. Int J Radiat Oncol Biol Phys 2005;61(3): 736–740.

5. Fossa SD. Long-term sequelae after cancer therapy—survivorship after treatment for testicular cancer. Acta Oncol 2004;43(2):134–141.

6. Huddart RA, Norman A, Shahidi M, et al. Cardiovascular disease as a long-term complication of treatment for testicular cancer. J Clin Oncol 2003;21(8):1513–1523.

7. Travis LB, Fossa SD, Schonfeld SJ, et al. Second cancers among 40,576 testicular cancer patients: focus on long-term survivors. J Natl Cancer Inst 2005;97:1354–1365.

8. Oliver RT, Mason MD, Mead GM, et al. Radiotherapy versus single-dose carboplatin in adjuvant treatment of stage I seminoma: a randomised trial. Lancet 2005; 366(9482):293–300.

9. Schmoll HJ, Souchon R, Krege S, et al. European consensus on diagnosis and treatment of germ cell cancer: a report of the European Germ Cell Cancer Consensus Group (EGCCCG). Ann Oncol 2004;15(9):1377–1399.

10. Fossa SD, Horwich A, Russell JM, et al. Optimal planning target volume for stage I testicular seminoma: A Medical Research Council randomized trial. Medical Research Council Testicular Tumor Working Group. J Clin Oncol 1999;17(4):1146.

11. Jones WG, Fossa SD, Mead GM, et al. Randomized trial of 30 versus 20 Gy in the adjuvant treatment of stage I testicular seminoma: a report on Medical Research Council Trial TE18, European Organization for the Research and Treatment of Cancer Trial 30942 (ISRCTN 18525328). J Clin Oncol 2005;23(6):1200–1208.

12. Chung PW, Warde PR, Panzarella T, et al. Appropriate radiation volume for stage IIA/B testicular seminoma. Int J Radiat Oncol Biol Phys 2003;56(3):746–748.

13. Patterson H, Norman AR, Mitra SS, et al. Combination carboplatin and radiotherapy in the management of stage II testicular seminoma: comparison with radiotherapy treatment alone. Radiother Oncol 2001;59(1):5–11.

14. Gunar K. Zagars, Matthew T, et al. Mortality after cure of testicular seminoma. J Clin Oncol 2004;22(4):640–647.

18
Prostate

18.1
Epidemiology, Pathology, and Pathogenesis

Sheilagh V. Reid and Freddie C. Hamdy

Structure of the Prostate Gland

Anatomically the prostate is described as having anterior, posterior, and lateral surfaces with a narrow apex inferiorly and a broad base superiorly in continuity with the bladder. It is composed of approximately 70% glandular and 30% fibromuscular stroma containing collagen and smooth muscle.

The glandular elements of the prostate are described in three distinct zones: transition, central, and peripheral (1,2) (Fig. 18.1.1). These zones correlate with location of their ducts in the urethra, with the pathology, and to some extent with the embryological origin. The transition zone (TZ) normally accounts for 5% to 10% of prostatic glandular tissue. Its ducts arise at the angle dividing the prostatic and preprostatic urethra (i.e., where the urethra angles anteriorly) and pass beneath the preprostatic sphincter to travel on its lateral and posterior sides. This zone is the location for benign prostatic hyperplasia (BPH) and 20% of prostatic cancers. The ducts of the central zone (CZ) arise circumferentially around the openings of the ejaculatory ducts. The glands of CZ are thought to be wolffian in origin, and in keeping with this they are structurally and immunohistochemically different from the rest of the prostate. Only 1% to 5% of cancers arise from this zone.

The peripheral zone (PZ) (Fig. 18.1.1) accounts for 70% of glandular tissue covering the posterior and lateral parts of the gland, also accounting for 70% of cancers. Its ducts drain into the prostatic sinus along the entire length of the prostatic urethra. The anterior fibromuscular stroma is the nonglandular part of the prostate and accounts for up to one third of the prostate mass. It is rarely invaded by carcinoma.

Incidence and Epidemiology

Worldwide more than half a million men are diagnosed with prostate cancer annually, accounting for a tenth of all new male cancers. It is the third most common cancer in men after lung and stomach (3). The highest incidence is in

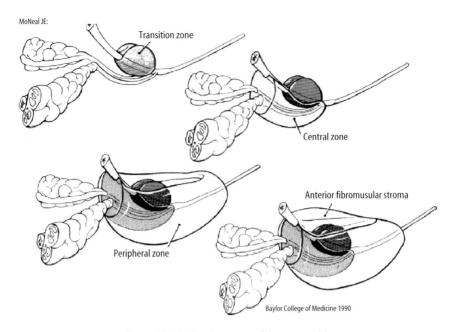

FIGURE 18.1.1. Zonal anatomy of the prostate (2).

the developed world, with the lowest in Africa and Asia. The incidence is particularly high in the United States (104 per 100,000), possibly increased by high rates of prostate-specific antigen (PSA) testing, with blacks having a higher incidence than white Americans (Fig. 18.1.2).

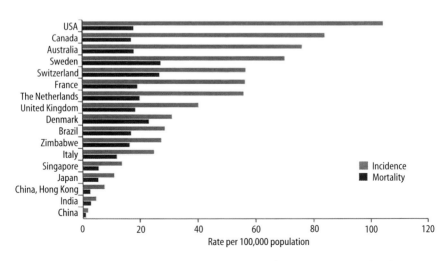

FIGURE 18.1.2. World age standardized incidence and mortality for prostate cancer in selected countries, 2000. [From Toms, 2004 (4), with permission.]

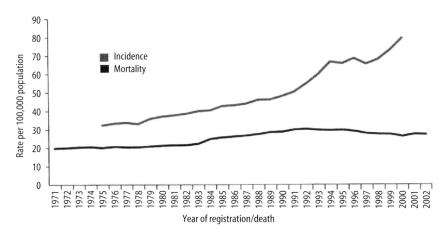

FIGURE 18.1.3. European age standardized prostate cancer mortality and incidence rates in Great Britain from 1971 to 2002. [From Toms, 2004 (4), with permission.]

In 2000 there were 27,149 new cases of prostate cancer in the United Kingdom (4). The incidence is 40 per 100,000 men, rising steeply with age, and most deaths (93%) occur in men older than 64 years of age (5). The lifetime risk of a man of 50 years of age having microscopic evidence of prostate cancer is 42%, while his risk of dying from the disease is only 3% (6). It is worth noting that men with total PSA (tPSA) levels less than or equal to 4 ng/mL (which has been considered the upper limit of normal) have been found to have a rate of prostate cancer on biopsy of 15.2% (7).

The rising incidence in prostate cancer reported in recent years is at least in part due to two factors, the increasing use of transurethral resection of the prostate (TURP) during the 1980s and PSA testing in the 1990s. Prostate cancer is an incidental finding in the tissue removed by TURP in around 10% of patients (8).

The number of prostate cancer cases can also be expected to rise as the population at risk (older men) grows with increasing life expectancy in the Western world. It is interesting to note that mortality rates have increased significantly less than incidence (Fig. 18.1.3).

Screening

The purpose of screening for prostate cancer is to identify a group of asymptomatic men with early-stage organ-confined disease who would benefit from early radical intervention. The benefit from radical intervention can be expressed only in terms of prolonged survival or improved quality of life. To date there is no evidence that these benefits can be obtained by the establishment of mass screening programs.

The key principles that a disease should satisfy before introducing screening as a public health policy were established in 1968 by Wilson and Jungner (9). The most important of these in relation to prostate cancer are the following:

1. The disease should be an important health problem. The high incidence and mortality was discussed in the preceding section.

2. There should be a preclinical state more amenable to successful treatment than clinical disease. This is unclear in prostate cancer with the majority of screen-detected cases with low PSA levels being stage T1c. An important reservation about prostate cancer screening is that it leads to overdetection of many cancers that might never have become clinically relevant. Not only would this not increase survival, but it would significantly increase morbidity. There is at present no way of differentiating these cancers from those that would become clinically relevant. The issue of high-grade prostatic intraepithelial neoplasia (HGPIN), associated in approximately 50% of cases with invasive cancer and thought to be a precursor of cancer (10), is discussed below (see Pathology).

3. There should be an acceptable screening instrument for the disease. The combination of digital rectal examination (DRE), serum PSA, transrectal ultrasound (TRUS), and prostate biopsy remains conventional for diagnosing and staging the disease. However, it is now accepted that neither DRE nor TRUS should be included in screening. The PSA has a sensitivity of 70% to 80% when a threshold level of 4 ng/mL is used (11). This compares favorably with mammography for breast cancer with a sensitivity of 63.2% to 83.8% (12). Specificity, however, is not as good, with up to two thirds of men with elevated PSA levels not having prostate cancer (13).

4. There should be an accepted and effective treatment. The evidence that aggressive treatment of screen-detected prostate cancer is effective in improving survival and quality of life is still awaited from clinical trials. The most substantive evidence of effectiveness of radical prostatectomy comes from a Scandinavian trial (14,15). The trial randomized 695 men with clinically localized prostate cancer to watchful waiting (WW) or radical prostatectomy (RP). The first paper reported a median 6.2-year follow-up, with the most important finding being a 50% reduction in disease-specific mortality in favor of RP, but no difference in overall mortality and significant surgical morbidity. However, the second paper had a median 8.2-year follow-up and showed a modest reduction in overall mortality alongside reduction in disease-specific mortality, risks of metastasis, and local progression. This study has a number of limitations and did not recruit men with screen-detected cancers specifically. The effectiveness of treatment in screen-detected cancer therefore remains unproven, and results from ongoing trials are awaited.

5. The natural history of the disease should be known. The natural history of prostate cancer is really only known in relation to the pre-PSA era. It was recognized in the 1960s that unless a man had a minimum 10-year life expectancy, competing comorbidity was more likely to be the cause of death than prostate cancer (16). Two recent studies have examined the long-term natural history of early prostate cancer. A Swedish study (17) followed 223 patients from diagnosis

with an average follow-up of 21 years. Overall 91% of patients died, with 16% of the whole cohort dying of prostate cancer, and 40% experienced progression of the disease. Progression and mortality rates were similar over the first 15 years but increased approximately threefold higher in the 49 men still alive beyond 15 years. A U.S. study (18) looked at 20-year follow-up of 767 men treated with androgen withdrawal or observation alone. It showed that men with low-grade prostate cancers (Gleason grades 2 to 4) have a minimal risk of dying from prostate cancer over 20 years and those with high grade (Gleason grades 8 to 10) had a high risk within 10 years. This study did not show increased progression or mortality rates after 15 years. The data from both these studies were collected from patients diagnosed with prostate cancer before the PSA era. Patients diagnosed with PSA have the added element of lead-time bias, which is the time between screen detection and clinical detection of a disease so that patients have a diagnosis earlier, which can falsely imply longer survival. It is estimated that lead-time bias using PSA screening is 12.3 years (age 55) to 6 years (age 75) (19).

There are two ongoing major randomized trials using the PSA as a detection tool to investigate the benefits of screening for prostate cancer—the Prostate, Lung, Colon, Ovary Screening Trial (PLCO) in the U.S. (20), and the European Randomized Study of Screening for Prostate Cancer (ERSCP) (21,22) in Europe. Two others trials are investigating the effectiveness of treatment in screen-detected cancers.

In the U.S., the Prostate Cancer Versus Observation Trial (PIVOT) has been recruiting and randomizing men under the age of 75 years to a trial of treatment, comparing radical prostatectomy with expectant management, using all-cause mortality as a primary end point. The trial has closed, having recruited 731 men (23).

In the U.K. the Prostate Testing for Cancer and Treatment (ProtecT) study is recruiting 130,000 men aged 50 to 69 years and randomizing approximately 2000 patients with clinically localized prostate cancer to a trial comparing active monitoring, radical prostatectomy, and three-dimensional conformal external beam radiotherapy. The main aim is to investigate the effectiveness of treatment in terms of survival at 10 years and quality of life. It is likely that screening issues will also be informed by the trial (24).

A recent review prepared for the Prostate Cancer Risk Management Program concluded, "There is insufficient evidence to launch a national program of national cancer screening" (4). The main concerns are the lack of evidence that screening would reduce mortality. It is necessary to await the results from the ongoing trials.

Etiology and Risk Factors

The etiology of prostate cancer is not clear. Common, although not absolute, factors in this disease are increased prevalence with age, requirement for the presence of androgens (i.e., the disease does not occur in men castrated before puberty), and response to androgen deprivation.

Risk factors include family history, race, hormones, aging, diet, and environmental agents. Unlike many other malignancies, there is inadequate evidence to link smoking and prostate cancer. Reports of association between vasectomy and prostate cancer have been misleading, with inconsistent results between studies. A major flaw of those studies reporting a positive association is that of detection bias (i.e., men who have vasectomies are more likely to see urologist) (25).

Family History

Family history has an association with prostate cancer, with increased risk associated with greater genetic linkage and with greater number of relatives with the disease (26,27). Risk has been quoted as two to three times more likely in a man with an affected first-degree relative (28) and up to an 11-fold greater risk with more than three first- or second-degree relatives (26) (see Hereditary Prostate Cancer, below).

Race

There are some differences in prostate cancer risk in different races. The highest rates are in African-American men, cited as 180 per 100,000 compared to white Americans, 134 per 100,000 from the same study, with higher stage specific mortality in black men (29,30).

Hormones

Dihydrotestosterone (converted from testosterone by 5α-reductase) is necessary for growth and maintenance of the prostate, and androgen suppression causes cancer regression. Despite this, evidence is conflicting regarding the association of low or high levels of androgens with prostate cancer. It is worth remembering that the peak age for prostate cancer in the older male is when androgen levels are declining. The role of chemoprevention is discussed in Chapter 18.6.

Aging

The incidence of prostate cancer rises with age. These age-related malignant changes are thought to be due to accumulation of DNA damage, with cellular oxidants such as free radicals being the main suspects.

Diet

There is a strong correlation between prostate cancer incidence and dietary fat consumption (31,32). The relationship is complex, and proposed mechanisms include oxidation of DNA and proteins, and alteration in hormone profiles. Results of one study (33) showed that the *AMACR* (α-methyl-coenzyme A remarcase) gene is upregulated and overexpressed in prostates with malignancy but not in those without. *AMACR* plays a key part in peroxisomal oxidation of dietary branched fatty acids, which generate hydrogen peroxide, a potential source of carcinogenic oxidative damage. Dairy products are a major source of dietary branched fatty acids, and upregulation of *AMACR* may explain some of the association between high-fat diet and prostate cancer.

Some dietary factors may have a protective effect against prostate cancer including vitamin E, lycopene, and selenium. A Finnish prevention trial reported a significantly decreased risk of developing and dying from prostate cancer for male smokers receiving α-tocopherol (vitamin E) supplements compared to those receiving placebo (34,35). The Nutritional Prevention Cancer Trial in the U.S. found a 65% reduction in prostate cancer incidence in those receiving selenium supplementation compared to those receiving placebo (36,37). However, a more recent study using nail clippings to measure selenium concentration found no association between selenium concentration and prostate cancer risk (38). A large prospective randomized controlled trial—the Selenium and Vitamin E Cancer and Prevention Trial (SELECT)—is currently underway in the U.S. to investigate the effects of selenium and vitamin E on the risk of developing prostate cancer in the general population. The antioxidant lycopene (which is a carotenoid) is found in tomatoes and tomato-based products. Frequent consumption of these products was found to reduce prostate cancer risk in a cohort of healthy men (39).

Vitamin D deficiency may be a risk factor for prostate cancer. The hormonal form of vitamin D, 1,25- dihdyroxyvitamin D (1,25-D), has been shown to inhibit invasiveness of prostate cancer cells in vitro (40), and low levels were associated clinically with an increased risk of clinically detected prostate cancer among older men (41). However, other studies have refuted an association between vitamin D and prostate cancer (42,43) (see Chapter 13).

The prostate has a higher concentration of zinc than any other organ in the human body. Its concentration is lower in older than in younger men (44). Prostates containing cancers have lower levels of zinc than those without (45). Currently the relationship between dietary zinc and prostate cancer is uncertain.

Environmental

Endocrine-disrupting chemicals (EDCs) are environmental agents that alter hormone activity. Estrogen agonists, particularly when exposure occurs during fetal life, may be involved in imprinting (turning genes on or off) and have an effect on future prostate cancer risk (46).

Pathogenesis

The pathogenesis of prostate cancer has multiple mechanisms. There are five unique characteristics of prostate cancer that contribute to its clinical behavior (46):

1. The disease tends to be slow growing, with a typical doubling time of 3 to 4 years.

2. It is age-related, rarely appearing in men younger than 40 years. This suggests an accumulation of oxidative damage, perhaps resulting from a number of endogenous and exogenous factors.

3. It is usually multifocal.

4. There does not appear to be a unique genetic pathway for prostate cancer to occur, and virtually the whole genome participates in the carcinogenesis, suggesting multiple pathways and mechanisms.

5. It has the highest prevalence of any non-skin human cancer. Similar rates of neoplastic foci are found in the prostates of men all around the world regardless of diet, occupation, or lifestyle (29). Essentially most men with circulating androgens will develop microscopic prostate cancer if they live long enough.

Pathology

Prostatic intraepithelial neoplasia (PIN) (Fig. 18.1.4) consists of architecturally benign prostatic acini or ducts lined by cytologically atypical cells. The reporting of so-called low-grade PIN is no longer appropriate, as it does not correlate with malignancy, and PIN should only refer to high grade. There is a significant association between PIN and malignancy, and its presence on biopsy should prompt a repeat biopsy. The risk of cancer for a patient with PIN on subsequent biopsy is approximately 50% (10).

Adenocarcinoma accounts for the vast majority of prostate cancers. The location they arise from corresponds to McNeal's (2) zones: peripheral (70%), transitional (20%), and central (1–5%). It is multifocal in more than 85% of cases.

The Gleason system is based on the glandular pattern of the tumor as identified at relatively low magnification (Fig. 18.1.4). Cytologic features including nuclear atypia play no role in the grade of the tumor. Both the primary (predominant) and the secondary (second most prevalent) architectural patterns are identified and assigned a grade from 1 to 5, with 1 being the most differentiated and 5 being the least differentiated.

The other pattern that has been recognized is tertiary grade in needle biopsies. For example, in a patient with Gleason grades of 3 (primary), 4 (secondary), and 5 (tertiary), the overall grading comes to 8.

More aggressive but rare forms of adenocarcinoma include mucinous adenocarcinoma and prostatic duct adenocarcinoma. They tend to present late due to difficulty in diagnosis because of normal PSA levels and DRE (47). Other forms of prostate malignancy include transitional cell carcinoma of the prostate without bladder involvement, small cell carcinoma, lymphoma, and sarcoma.

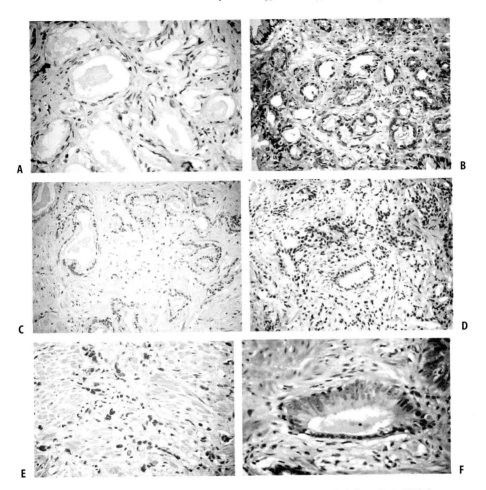

FIGURE 18.1.4. Gleason grading system for high-grade prostatic intraepithelial neoplasia (PIN) {hematoxylin and eosin). (A) Grade 1. (B) Grade 2. (C) Grade 3. (D) Grade 4. (E) Grade 5. (F) High-grade PIN. (Courtesy of Dr. Sohail Baithun, Royal London Hospital, Whitechapel, London.)

Staging

Staging is done in the following ways:

1. Tumor, node, metastasis (TNM) staging system 2002 (Table 18.1.1): The most accurate staging can only be done after radical prostatectomy, and the most important criteria predictive of prognosis are tumor grade, surgical margin status, and the presence of extracapsular disease, seminal vesicle invasion, or involvement of pelvic lymph nodes.

2. Digital rectal examination (DRE): The DRE has poor sensitivity as a staging tool. Data from the European randomized study of screening for

TABLE 18.1.1. Tumor, node, metastasis (TNM) staging 2002

Malignancy	Stage	Characteristics
Primary tumor (T)	Tx	Primary tumor cannot be assessed
	T0	No evidence of primary tumor
	T1	Clinically inapparent tumor not palpable or visible by imaging
	T1a	Tumor incidental histological finding in <5% of tissue resected
	T1b	Tumor incidental histological finding in >5% of tissue resected
	T1c	Tumor identified by needle biopsy (e.g., because of elevated PSA)
	T2	Palpable tumor confined within prostate
	T2a	Tumor involves one lobe
	T2b	Tumor involves both lobe
	T3	Tumor extends through prostatic capsule
	T3a	Extracapsular extension (unilateral on bilateral)
	T3b	Tumor invades seminal vesicle(s) (SV)
	T4	Tumor is fixed or invades adjacent structures other than the SV bladder neck, external sphincter, rectum, levator muscle, or pelvic wall
Pathologic primary tumor (pT2)	pT2	Organ confined
	pT2a	Unilateral
	pT2b	Bilateral
	pT3	Extraprostatic extension
	pT3a	Extraprostatic extension
	pT3b	Seminal vesicle invasion
	pT4	Invasion of bladder or rectum
Regional lymph node metastases	NX	Regional lymph nodes cannot be assessed
	N0	No regional lymph node metastasis
	N1	Metastasis in regional lymph node or nodes
Distant metastases	MX	Distant metastasis cannot be assessed
	M0	No distant metastasis
	M1	Distant metastasis
	M1a	Nonregional lymph nodes
	M1b	Bone(s)
	M1c	Other site(s)

prostate cancer (ERSPC) have shown poor performance of DRE at PSA levels less than 4 ng/mL (48); however, it is more useful for detecting more advanced disease and worth noting that in some high-grade tumors with normal PSA, DRE may be the only means to detect them (49).

3. Radiological imaging is generally unhelpful in staging. Transrectal ultrasound is used by some as an adjunct to DRE staging. A bone scan should be performed in patients with PSA levels greater than 10 ng/mL, and in the presence of high-grade disease to exclude bone metastasis. There is a limited role for magnetic resonance imaging (MRI), magnetic resonance spectroscopy (MRS), and computed tomography (CT) scanning, but they are not part of routine staging. They are specifically performed to exclude lymph node metastasis and prior to radiotherapy. The current indication for prostate MRI and MRS is in the evaluation of men with moderate or high risk of extracapsular extension.

4. The PSA is presently the only tumor marker in widespread clinical use for staging. Studies have shown that 80% of men with prostate cancer with tPSA values <4 ng/mL have pathologically organ-confined disease (50,51), two of three men with PSA levels between 4 and 10 ng/mL have organ-confined cancer, and more than 50% of men with PSA levels above 10 ng/mL have disease beyond the prostate.

5. Risk stratification and nomograms: The inherent biological heterogeneity of prostate cancer makes prostate cancer management decisions difficult. Currently, clinical parameters, including PSA, Gleason score, clinical staging, and percentage core biopsies, do not help to distinguish lethal and nonlethal prostate cancers or to predict response to various therapies (52). Nomograms are based on clinical and pathological data at presentation, which can help in predicting patient outcomes, thereby aiding clinicians and patients in making therapeutic decisions (52) (see Chapter 18.3).

6. Surgical staging: Frozen section biopsies of pelvic lymph nodes is performed prior to radical prostatectomy if the Gleason score of the tumor on biopsy is greater than 7 or if the PSA is higher than 10 ng/mL. Radical prostatectomy is conventionally abandoned if frozen section confirms the presence of lymph node metastasis.

Prostate-Specific Antigen

The PSA is an androgen-regulated serine protease secreted as a proenzyme (ProPSA) by the prostatic ductal and acinar epithelium. ProPSA is activated to mature PSA by human kallikrein-2 (HK-2). Its physiological function is to digest the seminal seminogelins and fibronectin, thus liquefying the seminal clot shortly after ejaculation (53).

Measurement of serum PSA has become the most common event leading to the diagnosis of prostate cancer and one of the most commonly used biochemical test for cancer detection.

For the past decade a PSA value of 4.0 ng/mL has been considered to be the upper limit of normal. This was based on two studies in the early 1990s that found detection rates of cancer in 22% and 26% in men with PSA levels of 4 to 10 ng/mL and 67% and 50% in those with PSA >10 ng/mL (54,55). However, Thompson et al. (7) recently demonstrated that men with a PSA less than or equal to 4 ng/mL have an overall prostate cancer prevalence of 15.2%, with those having a PSA consistently <0.5 ng/mL showing a prevalence of 6.6% and those with PSA levels between 3.1 and 4 ng/mL having a prevalence of 26.9%. More than 25% of this latter group had prostate cancers with Gleason scores of 7 or more.

Whatever the upper limit of normal, there remains problems with PSA used as a screening tool. In an effort to improve the sensitivity and specificity, various PSA-related indices have been studied: PSA density, PSA velocity, age-adjusted PSA values, total PSA, PSA isoforms, and PSA kinetics.

Density

The PSA density is defined as the tPSA level (ng/mL) divided by the TRUS-determined prostate volume (cc). Higher levels of tPSA are found in men with large prostates, and the rationale for using density measurements would be to differentiate between cancer and benign hyperplasia in men with intermediate tPSA levels. However, there are limitations with the use of PSA density, first due to observer variability in the accurate estimation of volume, and second, because epithelium-to-stromal ratios vary with individuals and only glandular epithelium produces PSA. Attempts have been made to correct PSA for prostate size to improve specificity in men with large prostates and sensitivity in those with smaller prostates (56). Despite these efforts, conflicting results were obtained, and therefore the usefulness of PSA density has not been corroborated in further studies (57–59).

Velocity

The PSA velocity monitors the change in tPSA with time. Patients with BPH have a linear increase in PSA levels with age, whereas those with cancer will eventually have an exponential increase. Carter et al. (60) reported on PSA velocity in 1992, finding a greater PSA velocity in men with than without prostate cancer 5 years before diagnosis. At least two PSA measurements should be obtained during a 2-year period or at least 12 to 18 months apart to obtain maximal benefit from PSA velocity. There are limitations to using PSA velocity, as it is difficult to calculate and there is variability in PSA levels including confounding factors, irrespective of the presence of BPH or cancer. Despite all this an annual increase of 0.75 ng/mL per year or greater was found in 72% of patients with cancer and only 5% of those with benign disease alone. High annual PSA velocity also has implications for survival when subsequent radical prostatectomy is performed. A recent study from the U.S. demonstrated that a rise in PSA of greater than 2 ng/mL in the 12 months preceding radical prostatectomy was associated with lymph node metastasis, high-grade disease, advanced pathological stage, and high risk of death from prostate cancer (61).

Age Adjusted

The PSA increases with age (62,63). This means that the upper limits of normal will change with age. The standard age-adjusted PSA levels that general practitioners use in the U.K., to prompt urgent referral to urology on a suspected cancer 2-week wait scheme, for further investigation are listed in Table 18.1.2. These cutoff levels give a high specificity for the Caucasian population described in the study by Oesterling et al. (62), but not for black Afro-Caribbeans. The issue of race on PSA levels may be significant, with reports that PSA levels are higher in black than white men even when controlling for age, clinical stage, and Gleason grade (64,65).

TABLE 18.1.2. Age-related PSA levels

Age (years)	PSA ng/mL
40–49	>2.5
50–59	>3.5
60 69	>4.5
70–79	>6.5

Regardless of race there will be some prostate cancers missed at these levels of PSA. Once again, referring to the data produced by Thompson et al. (7), in men aged 62 to 91 years even with PSA levels less than 0.5 ng/mL the PSA prevalence was 6.6%.

Isoforms

The PSA is secreted into prostatic ducts, and 30% to 40% of it is cleaved in seminal fluid by proteolytic enzymes. This process is called nicking, and the cleaved PSA therefore is called nicked PSA, which can be detected by assays. Very little PSA escapes into the circulation under normal circumstances. However, in cancer the tissue architecture is deranged with the loss of direct contact with prostatic ducts, so PSA is secreted directly into the extracellular fluid and the circulation.

In the serum about 5% to 35% of the PSA remains unbound or free (fPSA). The majority binds to α_1-antichymotrypsin (ACT), a protease inhibitor, forming the PSA-ACT complex (66,67). The proportion of PSA-ACT is higher and that of free PSA lower in patients with prostate cancer than those with normal prostates or BPH. About 1% to 2% of PSA occurs in complex with α_1-protease inhibitor (API; also called α_1-antitrypsin) and 5% to 10% in complex with α_2-macroglobulin (A2M). The proportion of these complexes is higher in the serum of patients with BPH compared to those with prostate cancer. The isoforms of PSA in the serum have been found to be different in BPH and prostate cancer. In BPH the PSA in the serum originates mostly from reabsorption from the semen or from extracellular fluid. It therefore contains a larger proportion of nicked PSA and a higher proportion of free PSA than in serum from prostate cancer patients. In prostate cancer patients a high proportion of the PSA has gone directly into the vascular system, and therefore a higher proportion of PSA becomes complexed (68,69).

Assays

There are three commercially available assays: tPSA (measures total PSA), fPSA (free PSA), and cPSA (complexed PSA). Assays for PSA-A2M are not generally available, but PSA-ACT and PSA-API are detected by assays for both tPSA and cPSA. Assays for cPSA, therefore, detect PSA-ACT and PSA-API without free PSA. It is increased in prostate cancer despite the fact that the PSA-API portion is actually decreased, but this portion is small. The tPSA assay is sensitive for prostate cancer detection but suffers from low specificity, meaning that it generates a large number of negative biopsies.

Using the ratio of free to total PSA appears to have greater specificity than using tPSA alone. This ratio has been found to be associated inversely with the risk of prostate cancer with cutoff levels varying between 0.14 and 0.28. A prospective study reported that a ratio cutoff of 0.3 would detect 90% of cancers, eliminating 50% of repeat biopsies (68). The cPSA assay appears more specific than tPSA, as specific as free-to-total ratio and less costly than the latter. Kellog and Partin (70) have even gone so far as to recommend that cPSA should replace tPSA. Further research is underway to evaluate the role of PSA and its isoforms in the diagnosis and staging of prostate cancer.

Doubling Time

Doubling time (DT) is the time required for the PSA to double in value. In initial phases of prostate cancer, the PSA rise seems to be in a linear fashion followed by an exponential phase (71). A short DT is a surrogate for rapid tumor growth, and a longer period of DT would indicate a slow-growing prostate cancer. With PSA velocity, PSA-DT is useful in monitoring disease recurrence and progression following failure of primary treatment (72).

Hereditary Prostate Cancer

Hereditary susceptibility is considered the strongest risk factor for prostate cancer and accounts for 5% to 10% of prostate cancer cases (73). Although hereditary prostate cancer (HPC) has an earlier onset than sporadic cases, there are no differences in clinical characteristics or survival between them (74). The generally accepted definition includes nuclear families with three cases of prostate cancer in each of three generations in the paternal or maternal lineage, and families with two men diagnosed with the disease before the age of 55 years (75).

The genetic mechanisms of prostate cancer have been more difficult to unravel than any other hereditary cancer syndromes (76).

Proposed Candidate Hereditary Prostate Cancer Genes

Although many susceptibility loci have been reported and retested only the *HPC1* linkage seems to have strong evidence confirming its linkage to prostate cancer (Table 18.1.3).

TABLE 18.1.3. Summary of candidate hereditary prostate cancer (HPC) genes

Gene	Location	Comments
HPC1	1q24–25	The prostate cancer susceptibility locus on chromosome has been extensively studied (74); linked to one third of families studied
PCAP	1q42.2–q43	Chromosome accounts for small proportion of cases (77)
HPCX	Xq27–28	Identified by a large international linkage study of 360 families; higher risk for brothers than for sons of men with CaP (78)
CAPB	1p36	Rare (79)
HPC2/ELAC2	17p12	Uncharacterized gene family; has been cloned rare cause for CaP (80)
HPC20	20q13	Linkage more common in late-onset disease (81)
MSR1 (macrophage scavenger receptor 1)	8p22–23	A macrophage specific receptor that binds to HDL, apoptotic cells, and bacteria (82,83)
BRCA2		Breast cancer families: male carriers of BRCA2 mutations are at a higher risk of prostate cancer (84)
CHEK2		Upstream regulator of p53 in the DNA damage signaling pathway (85)

CaP, cancer of the prostate; HDL, high-density lipoprotein.

References

1. McNeal JE. The prostate and prostatic urethra: a morphologic synthesis. J Urol 1972; 107:1008–1016.
2. McNeal JE. Normal histology of the prostate. Am J Surg Pathol 1988;12:619–633.
3. Ferlay J, Bray F, Pisani P, et al. Globocan 2000: Cancer, Incidence, Mortality and Prevalence Worldwide, Version 1.0: IARC Cancer Base No. 5. Lyon, France: IARC Press, 2001.
4. Toms JR, ed. Cancer Research UK. Cancer Stats Monograph 2004. London: Cancer Research UK, 2004.
5. Melia J. The burden of prostate cancer, its natural history, information on the outcome of screening and estimates of ad hoc screening with particular reference to England and Wales. BJU Int 2005;95(suppl 3):4–15.
6. Whitmore N. Localised prostate cancer: management and detection issues. Lancet 1994;343:1263–1267.
7. Thompson IM, Pauler KP, et al. Prevalence of prostate cancer among men with a PSA level <4 ng/mL. N Engl J Med 2004;350:2239–2246.
8. Horwich A, Waxman J, Schroder FH. Tumours of the prostate. In: Peckham M, Pinedo HM, Veronesi U, eds. Oxford Textbook of Oncology, vol 2. Oxford: Oxford University Press, 1995:1498–1530.
9. Wilson JMG, Jungner G. Principles and Practice of Screening for Disease. Public health papers No. 34. Geneva: World Health Organization, 1968.
10. Haggman MJ, Macoska JA, Wojno KJ, Oesterling JE. The relationship between PIN and prostate cancer: critical issues. J Urol 1997;158:12–22.
11. Helzlsouer KJ, Newby J, Comstock GW, et al. PSA levels and subsequent prostate cancer: potential for screening. Cancer Epidemiol Biomarkers Prev 1992;1; 537–540.

12. Kerlikowski K, Carney PA, Geller B, et al. Performance of screening mammography among women with and without a first-degree relative with breast cancer. Ann Intern Med 2000;133:855–863.

13. Klotz L. PSA dynia and other PSA-related syndromes; a new epidemic—a case history and taxonomy. Urology 1997;50:831–832.

14. Holmberg L, Bill-Axelson A, Helgessen F, et al. A randomised trial comparing radical prostatectomy with watchful waiting in early prostate cancer. N Engl J Med 2002; 347:781–789.

15. Bill-Axelson A, Holmberg L, Ruute M, et al. Radical prostatectomy versus watchful waiting in early prostate cancer. N Engl J Med 2005;352:1977–1984.

16. Barnes RW. Survival with conservative therapy. JAMA 1969;210:331.

17. Johanssen JE, Andren O, et al. Natural history of early localized prostate cancer. JAMA 2004;291:2713–2758.

18. Albertson PC, Hanley JA, Fine J. 20–year outcomes following conservative management of clinically localized prostate cancer. JAMA 2005;293;17;2095–2101.

19. Draisma G, Boer R, Otto SJ, et al. Lead times and over detection due to PSA screening: estimates from the European Randomized Study of Screening for Prostate Cancer. J Natl Cancer Inst 2003;95:868–878.

20. Gohagan JK, Prorok PC, Hayes RB. The Prostate, Lung, Colorectal, and Ovarian (PLCO) Cancer Screening Trial of the National Cancer Institute: history, organization and status. Control Clin Trials 2000;21(suppl 6):251S–72S.

21. Auvinen A, Rietbergen JB, Denis LJ, et al. Prospective evaluation plan for randomised trials of prostate cancer screening. The International Prostate Cancer Screening Trial Evaluation Group. J Med Screen 1996;3;97–104.

22. Schroder FH, Denis LJ, Roobol M, et al. The story of the ERSPC. BJU Int 2003;92(suppl 2):1–13.

23. Wilt TJ, Brawer MK, PIVOT. Oncology 1997;11:1133–1139.

24. Donovan J, Hamdy F, Neal D, et al. ProtecT Study Group, ProtecT feasibility study. Health Technol Assess 2003;7:188.

25. Howards SS, Peterson HB, Vasectomy and prostate cancer. Chance, bias or a causal relationship? JAMA 1993;269:913–914.

26. Steinberg GD, Carter BS, Beaty TH, Child B, Walsh PC. Family history and the risk of prostate cancer. Prostate 1990;17:337–347.

27. Cussenot O, Valeri A, Berthon P, Fournier G, Mangin P. Hereditary prostate cancer and other genetic predispositions to prostate cancer. Urol Int 1998;60(suppl 2): 30–34.

28. Glover FE, Coffey DS, Douglas LL, et al. Familial study of prostate cancer in Jamaica. Urology 1998;52:441–443.

29. Pienta KJ, Demers R, Hoff M, et al. Effect of age and race on the survival of men with prostate cancer in the Metropolitan Detroit tricounty area, 1973–1987. Urology 1995; 45:93–101.

30. Hoffman RM, Gilliland FD, Eley JW, et al. Racial and ethnic differences in advanced-stage prostate cancer: the Prostate Cancer Outcomes Study. J Natl Cancer Inst 2001;93:388–395.

31. Howell MA. Factor analysis of international cancer mortality data and per capita food consumption. Br J Cancer 1974;29:328–336.

32. Armstrong B, Doll R. Environmental factors and cancer incidence and mortality in different countries, with special reference to dietary practices. Int J Cancer 1975:15; 617–631.

33. Luo J, Zha S, Gage WR, et al. Alpha-methylacyl-CoA racemase: a new molecular marker for prostate cancer. Cancer Res 2002;62:2220–2226.
34. Hartman TJ, Albanes D, Raultalhati M, et al. Physical activity and prostate cancer in the Alpha-Tocopherol, Beta-Carotene (ATBC) Cancer Prevention Study (Finland). Cancer Causes Control 1998;9:11–18.
35. HeinonenOP, Albanes D, Virtamo J, et al. Prostate cancer and supplementation with alpha-tocopherol and beta-carotene: incidence and mortality in a controlled trial. J Natl Cancer Inst 1998;90:440–446.
36. Li H, Stampfer MJ, Giovannucci EL, et al. A prospective study of plasma selenium levels and prostate cancer risk. J Natl Cancer Inst 2004;90:630–639.
37. Clark LC, Combs GF Jr, Turnbull BW, et al. Effects of selenium supplementation for cancer prevention in patients with carcinoma of the skin. A randomized controlled trial. Nutritional Prevention of Cancer Study Group. JAMA 1996;276:1957–1963.
38. Allen NE, Morris JS, Ngwenyama RA, et al. A case control study of selenium in nails and prostate cancer risk in British men. Br J Cancer 2004;90:1392–1396.
39. Giovannucci E, Ascherio A, Rimm EB, et al. Intake of carotenoids and retinol in relation to the risk of cancer. J Natl Cancer Inst 1995;87:1767–1776.
40. Schwartz GG, Whitlatch LW, Chen TC, et al. Human prostate cells synthesise 1,25–dihydroxyvitamin D3 from 25–hydroxyvitamin D3. Cancer Epidemiol Biomarkers Prev 1998;7:391–395.
41. Giovannucci E. Dietary influences of 1,25(OH)2 vitamin D in relation to prostate cancer: a hypothesis. Cancer Causes Control 1998;9:567–582.
42. Gann PH, Ma J, Hennekens CH, et al. Circulating vitamin D metabolites in relation to subsequent development of prostate cancer. Cancer Epidemiol Biomarkers Prev 1996;5:121–126.
43. Braun MM, Helzlsouer KJ, Hollis BW, Comstock GW, Prostate cancer and pre-diagnostic levels of serum vitamin D metabolites. Cancer Causes Control 1995;6:235–239.
44. Tvedt KE, Halgunset J, Kopstad G, Haugen OA. Intracellular distribution of calcium and zinc in normal, hyperplastic and neoplastic human prostate: x-ray microanalysis of freeze dried cryosections. Prostate 1989;15:41–51.
45. Feustel A, Wennrich R. Zinc and cadmium plasma and erythrocyte levels in prostatic carcinoma, BPH, urological malignancies and inflammations. Prostate 1986;8:75–79.
46. Bostwick DG, Burke HB, Djakiew D, et al. Human prostate cancer risk factors. Cancer 2004;101;2371–2490.
47. Epstein JI, Lieberman P. Mucinous adenocarcinomas of the prostate gland. Am J Surg Pathol 1985;9:299–307.
48. Schroder FH, Maas P, Beemsterboer P, et al. Evaluation of digital rectal examination as a screening test for prostate cancer. J Natl Cancer Inst 1998;90:1817–1823.
49. Catalona WJ, Richie JP, Ahmann FR, et al. Comparison of DRE and PSA in the early detection of prostate cancer: results of a multicenter clinical trial of 6630 men. J Urol 1994;151:1283–1290.
50. Catalona WJ, Smith DS, Ornstein DK. Prostate cancer detection in men with PSA concentrations of 2.6–4ng/ml and benign prostate examinations: enhancement of specificity with free PSA measurement. JAMA 1997;277:1452–1455.
51. Rietbergen JB, Hoedemaeker RF, Kruger AE, et al. The changing pattern of prostate cancer at the time of diagnosis: characteristics of screen detected prostate cancer in a population based screening study. J Urol 1999;161:1192–1198.

52. Taplin M-E, Kantoff PW. The ingredients for prostate cancer nomograms: the addition of biomarkers sets the table for future recipes. J Clin Oncol 2003;19: 3552–3553.
53. Lilja H. A kallikrein-like serine protease in prostatic fluid cleaves the predominant seminal vesicle protein. J Clin Invest 1985;76;1899–1903.
54. Catalona WJ, Smith DS, Ratliff TL. Measurement of PSA in serum as a screening test for prostate cancer. N Eng J Med 1991;324:1156–1161.
55. Brawer MK, Chetner MP, Beatie J, et al. Screening for prostate cancer with PSA. J Urol 1992;147;841–845.
56. Benson MC, Whang IS, Olsson CA, et al. The use of PSA density to enhance the predictive value of intermediary levels of serum PSA. J Urol 1992:147;817–821.
57. Brawer MK, Aramburu EA, Chen GL, et al. The inability of PSA index to enhance the predictive value of PSA in the diagnosis of prostatic carcinoma. J Urol 1993;150 (2 pt 1):369–373.
58. Catalona WJ, Richie JP, deKernion JB, et al. Comparison of PSA concentration versus PSA density in the early detection of prostate cancer: receiver operating characteristic curves. J Urol 1994;152:2031–2036.
59. Polascik TJ, Oesterling JE, Partin AW. PSA: a decade of discovery—what we have learned and where we are going [review article]. J Urol 1999;162:293–306.
60. Carter HB, Pearson JD, Metter EJ, et al. Longitudinal evaluation of PSA levels in men with and without prostate disease. JAMA 1992;267:2215–2220.
61. D'Amico AV, Chen MH, Roehl KA, Catalona WJ, Preoperative PSA velocity and the risk of death from prostate cancer after radical prostatectomy. N Engl J Med 2004; 351:125–135.
62. Oesterling JE, Jacobsen SJ, Chute CG, et al. Serum PSA in a community-based population of healthy men: establishment of age-specific reference ranges. JAMA 1993;270: 860–864.
63. Gustafsson O, Mansour E, Norming U, et al. PSA, PSA density and age-adjusted PSA reference values in screening for prostate cancer—a study of a randomly selected population of 2400 men. Scand J Urol Nephrol 1998;32:373–377.
64. Morgan TO, Jacobsen SJ, McCarthy WF, et al. Age-specific reference ranges for PSA in black men. N Engl J Med 1996;335:304–310.
65. Moul JW, Sesterhenn IA, Connelly RR, et al. PSA values at the time of diagnosis in African-American men, JAMA 1995;274;1277–1281.
66. Lilja H, Christensson A, Dahlen U, Matikeinen MT, et al. PSA in serum occurs predominately in complex with alpha 1 antichymotrypsin. Clin Chem 1991;37: 1618–1625.
67. Stenman UH. PSA, clinical use and staging: an overview. Br J Urol 1997;1:52–60.
68. Stenman UH, Leinonen J, Zhang WM, Finne P. PSA prostate-specific antigen. Semin Cancer Biol 1999;9:83–93.
69. Djavan B, Zlotta A, Remzi M, et al. Optimal predictors of prostate cancer on repeat prostate biopsy: a prospective study of 1051 men. J Urol 2000;163:1148–1149.
70. Kellog JP, Partin AW. Applying complexed PSA to clinical practice. Urology 2004; 63:815–818.
71. Pearson JD, Carter HB. Natural history of changes in prostate specific antigen in early stage prostate cancer. J Urol 1994;152:1743–1748.
72. Klotz L, Teahan S. Current role of PSA kinetics in the management of patients with prostate cancer. Eur Urol 2006;suppl 5:472–478.
73. Bratt O. Hereditary prostate cancer: clinical aspects. J Urol 2002;168:906–913.

74. Bratt O, Damber JE, Emmanuelsson M, Gronberg H. Hereditary prostate cancer: clinical characteristics and survival. J Urol 2002;167:2423–2426.
75. Carter BS, Bova GS, Beaty TH, et al. Hereditary prostate cancer: epidemiologic and clinical features. J Urol 1993;150:797–802.
76. Smith JR, Freije D, Crepten JD, et al. Major susceptibility locus for prostate cancer on chromosome 1 suggested by genome-wide search. Science 1996;274:1371–1374.
77. Gibbs M, Chakrabarti L, Stanford JL, et al. Analysis of chromosome 1q42.2–43 in 152 families with high risk of prostate cancer. Am J Hum Genet 1999;64(4):1087–1095.
78. Xu J, Meyers D, Freije D, et al. Evidence for a prostate cancer susceptibility locus on the X chromosomes. Nat Genet 1998;20:175–179.
79. Gibbs M, Stanford JL, McIndoe RA, et al. Evidence for a rare prostate cancer susceptibility locus at chromosome 1p36. Am J Hum Genet 1999;64:776–787.
80. Tavtigian SV, Simard J, Teng DH, et al. A candidate prostate cancer susceptibility gene at chromosome 17p. Nat Genet 2001;27(2):172–180.
81. Berry R, Schroeder JJ, French AJ, et al. Evidence for a prostate cancer susceptibility locus on chromosome 20. Am J Hum Genet 2000;67:82–91.
82. Xu J, Zheng SL, Komiya A, et al. Germline mutations and sequence variants of the macrophage scavenger receptor 1 gene are associated with prostate cancer risk. Nat Genet 2002;32:321–325.
83. Seppala EH, Ikonen T, Autio V, et al. Germ-line alterations in MSR1 gene and prostate cancer risk. Clin Cancer Res 2003;9(14):5252–5256.
84. Edwards SM, Kote-Jerai Z, Meitz J, et al. Two percent of men with early-onset prostate cancer harbor germline mutations in the BRCA2 gene. Am J Hum Genet 2003; 72:1–12.
85. Dong X, Wang L, Taniguchi K, et al. Mutations in CHEK2 associated with prostate cancer risk. Am J Hum Genet 2003;72(2):270–280.

18.2
Clinical Presentation, Diagnosis, and Staging

Vinod H. Nargund

Clinical Features

Prostate cancer runs a protracted course, and most patients with early disease are likely to be asymptomatic. As most cancers arise in the posterior part of the peripheral zone well away from the urethra, obstructive symptoms are not common in the early stages. Bladder outflow symptoms suggest locally advanced disease into the urethra or bladder neck.

Incidental Finding of Prostate Cancer

Unsuspected and nonpalpable prostate cancer may be detected in cystoprostatectomy and transurethral resection of the prostate (TURP) specimens. Prostate cancer found in cystoprostatectomy may not be clinically significant unless the apical area of the prostate has foci of carcinoma, which has implications on prognosis and the future management of the patient (1). It is important to note that TURP specimens mostly represent tissue from the transition zone (TZ), bladder neck, and fibromuscular stroma in the anterior region, and not from the peripheral zone. The TZ tumors generally have lower Gleason scores and small tumor volume. T1a tumors may be followed with watchful waiting (2). Rectal examination for nonurological reasons may also reveal a suspicious nodule/area leading to the diagnosis.

Lower Urinary Tract Symptoms

Men in their 50s or 60s are likely to have outflow symptoms due to benign prostatic enlargement. The symptoms may include frequency, weak urinary flow, painful micturition (dysuria), sensation of incomplete voiding, hesitancy, urinary incontinence, urinary retention, and renal failure. Bladder irritative symptoms like urgency, frequency, and urge incontinence may be present. Assessment in these cases may unravel prostate cancer.

Hematuria

Microscopic or frank hematuria may occur as a result increased vascularity due to carcinoma or associated benign hypertrophy of prostate. Hematospermia is another recognized manifestation of carcinoma of the prostate. Men presenting with hematospermia, therefore, should be screened for prostate cancer (3) (see Chapter 4).

Erectile and Ejaculatory Symptoms

Decreased ejaculation is likely to be due to obstructed ejaculatory ducts. Erectile dysfunction may indicate a locally advanced disease involving neurovascular bundles.

Metastatic Prostate Cancer

Nearly 70% of patients with advanced disease develop bony metastasis (4). As prostate cancer mostly involves the axial skeleton, patients may present with severe back pain and spinal cord compression (see Chapter 11). Skeletal metastasis in weight-bearing bones may cause pathological fractures, which can adversely affect prognosis (5).

Paraneoplastic Syndromes

Metastatic prostate cancer may rarely present as a paraneoplastic syndrome. A number of conditions and neurological syndromes including peripheral neuropathy, cerebellar ataxia, and brainstem and limbic encephalopathy have been described in relation to prostate cancer (6).

Signs

A palpable prostate cancer is felt as an induration on digital rectal examination (DRE). Suspicious findings warrant further assessment with prostate-specific antigen (PSA) measurement and transrectal ultrasound (TRUS) biopsy. It must be noted, however, that DRE in a low PSA setting (<4 ng/mL) has no diagnostic value as a screening tool for prostate cancer (7), but DRE should be done in all men as part of clinical examination (8). In patients with PSA ≥4 ng/mL with associated abnormal DRE and TRUS findings, the incidence of cancer could be as high as 75% (9). Weight loss and anemia may be evident on physical examination in men who have widespread metastasis.

Diagnosis of Prostate Cancer

Prostate-Specific Antigen

The basics of the PSA and its indices are discussed in Chapter 18.1. The PSA estimation is routinely done for men presenting with prostate-related lower urinary tract symptoms (LUTSs), erectile dysfunction, hematuria, or hematospermia. The risks, benefits, and the course of management in relation to various PSA levels should be explained to patients for ethical, medical, and legal reasons (10). Interpretation of PSA levels (normal or abnormal) and a need for biopsy depends on the urologist treating the patient and clinical findings relevant to that patient.

Transrectal Ultrasound Biopsy of Prostate

The main role of transrectal ultrasound is to provide visual guidance for the needle biopsy. It is not helpful as a tool for local staging of prostate cancer. Transrectal ultrasound has a limited capacity to identify prostate cancer due to variability in the ultrasonic appearance of cancers and lack of specificity (11). In addition to biopsying, TRUS guidance is also used in brachytherapy, cryotherapy, high-intensity focused ultrasound (HIFU), and radiofrequency tumor ablation (RTA).

Indications for TRUS-Guided Prostate Biopsy

Rising PSA

Serum total PSA (tPSA) levels ≥4.0 ng/mL have been traditionally considered as an indication for biopsy since 1990 (12). There is growing evidence to suggest that there is no definite cutoff point for PSA as a significant number of men with PSA values below the level of 4 ng/mL have prostate cancer. In the Prostate Cancer Prevention Trial (PCPT), Thompson et al. (13) found an incidence of 15% in men with PSA levels below 4.0 ng/mL and 15% of these men had Gleason scores of 7 or higher. Similar findings were noted in the European Randomized Study of Screening for Prostate Cancer (ERSPC), which originally adopted 4.0 ng/mL as a threshold PSA level for biopsy. It is now reduced to 3.0 ng/mL (14). In other studies on men with a tPSA range of 2.6 to 4 ng/mL, the incidence of cancer was 25% (15,16). Total PSA with either a fixed (3.0 ng/mL) or age-specific range for the time being remains the best method for evaluating men for prostate cancer (8).

Abnormal Digital Rectal Examination

As already mentioned, an abnormal nodule/area on the prostate should be considered as an important indication for biopsy even if the PSA is within normal limits (17).

Repeat Biopsies for Prostatic Intraepithelial Neoplasia or Atypia

Between 4% and 25% of men who undergo TRUS biopsy for high PSA or abnormal DRE have prostatic intraepithelial neoplasia (PIN) (18). As the natural history of PIN is not clear, there is no strategy for repeat biopsy in such patients. High-grade PIN (HGPIN) has a higher predictive value for carcinoma on a subsequent biopsy, as nearly 27% to 100% of patients with PIN have prostate cancer on repeat biopsy (19). Men with lower PSA levels and negative biopsy should be advised to have repeat biopsy if there is evidence of HGPIN, abnormal DRE, and family history of cancer of the prostate (CaP) (20).

Age-Adjusted PSA Levels (see Table 18.1.2) and Other PSA Parameters

Age-adjusted PSA levels were introduced to improve cancer detection sensitivity in younger men and specificity in older men (21). It is important to note that PSA thresholds based solely on age-specific ranges may lead to underdiagnosis of prostate cancer in patients who have prostate cancer (22,23).

Percent free PSA (fPSA) may help in determining the need for biopsy, as it is decreased in patients with prostate cancer (24).

Using 25% fPSA as the cutoff for recommending biopsy, 95% of cancers are likely to be detected while avoiding 20% of unnecessary biopsies in men with a tPSA of 4 to 10 ng/mL (25). The percent fPSA measurement, however, is less robust in discriminating between benign prostatic disease and CaP at tPSA ranges of 2.6 to 4 ng/mL (26).

Repeat TRUS Biopsy

The TRUS biopsy has significant false-negative rates. The importance of a missed cancer diagnosis is not known. Biopsy also has a low sensitivity rates in younger patients with low PSA and in early disease probably due to small volume disease (27).

In one study, men with smaller prostates (≤20 cc) and persistently elevated tPSA had a higher incidence of CaP (28). The same study also showed that men with larger prostates (>70 cc) with one set of negative sextant biopsies were less likely to have cancer. Repeat biopsies particularly in the far lateral PZ are likely to increase the diagnostic yield by 30% to 35% (29,30).

Post–Radical Prostatectomy Prostatic Fossa Biopsy

The role of biopsy is not clear in detecting the local recurrence after radical prostatectomy. The prostatic fossa biopsy is avoided in patients with normal DRE or ultrasound results and PSA levels below 0.5 ng/mL (31). However, TRUS-guided needle biopsy of prostatic fossa biopsy is considered more sensitive than a DRE for detecting local recurrence, especially with low PSA levels (32). Biopsy in the region of the vesicourethral anastomotic area is likely to yield more information. Negative biopsy of the fossa does not rule out recurrence, and a positive biopsy does not exclude systemic metastasis (32).

Prostate Biopsy After Radiotherapy

Postradiotherapy (RT) prostate biopsies are likely to pose problems in histological interpretation. False negatives due to sampling error, false positives due to delayed tumor regression, and indeterminate biopsies showing radiation effect in residual tumor of uncertain viability are common occurrences (33).

Predictors of a Positive Biopsy

The main aims of the TRUS biopsy are not only to diagnose prostate cancer but also to determine its aggressiveness. The relative specificity of sextant biopsy can be assessed by PSA indices discussed above (PSA density, velocity, free/total ratio, age-adjusted PSA). Nam et al. (34) categorized six risk groups including patient age, ethnicity, family history of prostate cancer, previous negative biopsy, voiding symptoms, and prostate volume, and concluded that PSA is highly accurate in predicting prostate cancer. Age-specific PSA levels, percent fPSA ratio, and HGPIN also provide useful information and have been already discussed.

Prostate Biopsy Technique

Transrectal ultrasound–guided biopsy is the preferred method except in patients who had the rectum and anus excised, in which case the biopsy is performed by the transperineal route. Transrectal ultrasound is carried out by using a 5- to 8-MHz handheld high-resolution probe with capabilities of sagittal and transverse (coronal) imaging. A disposable adaptor is fitted on the probe that will direct the biopsy needle into various regions of the prostate as guided by ultrasound imaging.

Principles of the TRUS Examination

Informed Consent

Alternatives, consequences, and complications of biopsy are discussed prior to the procedure. Patients should have clear directions in dealing with the complications of a TRUS biopsy.

Antibiotic Prophylaxis

Oral aminoquinolones in the form of Ciproxin or norfloxacin are sufficient in uncomplicated cases. Patients with cardiac valve problems should receive intravenous antibiotics.

Anticoagulation

These medications are discontinued for several days prior to the biopsy. In high-risk patients, hospitalization and parenteral heparin cover may be necessary.

Digital Rectal Examination

Digital rectal examination should be performed prior to the biopsy to make sure that rectum is empty and to rule out rectal pathology. In some centers, an enema is routine prior to TRUS biopsy. In addition, DRE will help to note any abnormal areas in the prostate and the presence of a nodule. These areas are included in the biopsies.

Pain Relief

Patients feel pain and discomfort because of the ultrasound probe and needle passage through the prostate gland, particularly below the dentate line in the anorectum (35). Patients also experience considerable psychological stress because of the fear of impending cancer diagnosis. The pain induced during the procedure can lead to contraction of pelvic floor muscles causing exacerbation of pain. Periprostatic infiltration with 1% to 2% lignocaine significantly decreases the pain during the procedure (35).

Biopsy

The anatomy of the prostate, bladder, seminal vesicles, and ampulla of vas is examined for asymmetry and distortion. This is followed by examination of the prostate for abnormal shadows, hypoechoic areas, erosion of capsule, and volume measurement. The gland is scanned in both the sagittal and coronal planes. The width of the prostate is measured in the axial (coronal) plane and the length of the prostate is measured in the sagittal plane. Most of the TRUS machines have the capability for calculation of volume. At this stage if the operator is interested in Doppler evaluation (color and power) this could be done to identify hypervascular areas for biopsy.

The zonal anatomy of the prostate was described in Chapter 18.1. The details of various zones as seen in sagittal section on ultrasound are diagrammatically shown in Figure 18.2.1. As 70% of cancers occur in the peripheral zone and nearly 25% occur in the central zone, biopsies of the posterior part of the prostate seem logical, and for biopsy purposes the prostate gland can be divided into base, midregion, and apex (Fig. 18.2.1). The transition zone is included in repeat biopsies. Sextant biopsy of the prostate has been a gold standard and

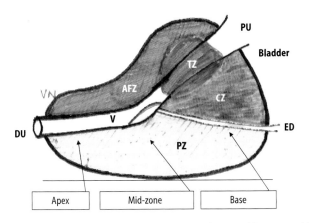

FIGURE 18.2.1. Zonal anatomy of prostate in sagittal section and sextant biopsy areas (diagrammatic). AFZ, anterior fibromuscular zone; CZ, central zone; DU, distal urethra; ED, ejaculatory ducts; PU, proximal urethra; PZ, peripheral zone; TZ, transition zone; V, verumontanum.

involves taking three paired biopsies of the prostate from the base, midzone, and apex in the midlobar parasagittal planes (36). The needle tip is placed near the region of the intended biopsy and the gun is fired to get the sample. The length of the biopsy core also determines the detection rate in sextant biopsy, particularly at the apex (37), with a longer core giving higher detection rates. Each core is sent to the laboratory in a separate container properly labeled for histological diagnosis.

Extended TRUS Biopsy

After sextant biopsy, more biopsies are taken from far lateral areas of the prostate at the base, midlobe, and apex. The five-region biopsy involves sextant biopsies (six cores), four far lateral biopsies, and three midline biopsies (29). By including these extra biopsies this technique reduces the false-negative rate by 35%.

Limitations of Sextant Biopsy

The sextant biopsy was described in relation to palpable or suspicious areas in prostate. In the present PSA era, with nonpalpable lesions the sextant biopsy does not adequately sample the prostate gland, particularly the peripheral zone (PZ). In a study of 137 men undergoing two consecutive sets of sextant biopsies in a single setting, Levine et al. (38) demonstrated that 22% of patients had prostate cancer and another 13% had cancer diagnosed on the second set of biopsies. Stamey (39), based on cancer mapping on radical prostatectomy specimens, suggested that biopsies near the midzone and base should be directed into the anterolateral region of the prostate (PZ). By including the PZ, the biopsy should increase the sensitivity of TRUS-guided biopsy. Many studies have shown a significant increase (14–35%) in detection rates with extended biopsy (40,41). For larger glands at least 12 cores should be obtained with more biopsies from the lateral horns.

Role of Transition Zone Biopsies

Most of the TZ tumors are diagnosed following transurethral resection biopsy. In men with previously negative biopsies, TRUS-guided TZ biopsy should be done to exclude the cancer.

Complications

Transrectal guided prostate biopsy is not without risks and complications. Taking more biopsy cores does not necessarily increase the complication rates (42). Most of the following complications are minor and self-limiting but can cause considerable anxiety to the patients:

Bleeding: urethral bleeding/hematuria (35%), hematochezia (9%), and hematospermia (5%) are usually self-limiting and do not need any active treatment (43).

Infections: prostatitis, epididymitis, and septicemia; sepsis is the most dangerous complication as it can be life-threatening in elderly patients.

Outflow symptoms: painful micturition. Urine should be tested for infection
and appropriate antibiotics usually improve symptoms. Urinary retention
could be precipitated by the biopsy due to hemorrhage and edema. Catheterization is done to relieve the obstruction and a trial removal can be done
10 days later.

Staging Investigations

Prostate cancer spreads locally within its zones and into the ejaculatory ducts,
seminal vesicles, and neurovascular bundles. Distal spread includes lymphatic
(to internal iliac lymph nodes) and hematogenous routes to bones, lungs, and
other organs. The bony metastasis involves bones of the axial skeleton. Visceral
metastasis is rarely seen in newly diagnosed patients and rarely seen even in
patients dying of prostate cancer (44).

For clinical staging the extent of the prostate cancer is assessed by DRE, PSA,
TRUS, and Gleason histological grading. For example, in patients with stage T1c
or less disease with a total Gleason score of 4 to 6 and a PSA of less than 10 ng/
mL, no further staging investigations would be required unless there is a specific
indication. Currently no single imaging study can demonstrate the evidence of
capsular breach. Nodal involvement requires further imaging or histological
identification by lymph node dissection.

Selective cross-sectional imaging modalities like computed tomography (CT)
and magnetic resonance imaging (MRI) and bone scan help to assess the extent
of spread and are mainly performed for the following reasons:

1. To determine lymph node status in high risk patients
2. Apical disease
3. Suspected locally advanced disease
4. Prior to radiotherapy

The risk of metastasis can be quantified by PSA levels and clinical and TRUS
biopsy findings (see Chapter 18.3).

Magnetic resonance imaging has a number of advantages over CT in prostate
cross-sectional imaging. It helps in the detailed evaluation of prostatic, periprostatic, and pelvic anatomy (45), and therefore mostly is used as a staging
study in men with biopsy-proven prostate cancer.

Magnetic resonance imaging findings in extracapsular extension include a
focal irregular capsular bulge, asymmetry or invasion of neurovascular bundles,
and obliteration of rectoprostatic angle (46). Magnetic resonance spectroscopy
(MRS) is an advanced form of MRI in that it uses the property of hydrogen
ions known as chemical shift. The MRI uses strong magnetic fields to induce
spinning of hydrogen protons, generating a map of proton signal intensity.
The hydrogen protons in different molecules have different frequencies—the

TABLE 18.2.1. Investigations and their limitations in the diagnosis of prostate cancer

Imaging modality	Current indications	Limitations and future scope
TRUS	Biopsy of prostate and seminal vesicles; blood flow studies may increase chances of cancer diagnosis	Not possible to localize tumor in all cases; not used for staging, although in late stages distortion of SV and asymmetry may be seen; role of 3D and 4D still under investigation
CT	Not indicated in early disease; may be useful in T3 tumors with PSA >20 ng/mL and Gleason 4 to 5; mainly to study extraprostatic spread	Not recommended for local staging due to its low diagnostic accuracy; it is more useful in detecting local extraprostatic spread (e.g., levator ani infiltration or lateral wall involvement, LN involvement)
MRI and MRS	Currently the most useful technique in staging after TRUS biopsy; detailed evaluation of prostatic, preprostatic, and pelvic anatomy	Useful in detecting extraprostatic disease; high diagnostic specificity can be achieved by variation in techniques (38); its role in posttreatment (surgery and radiotherapy) follow-up is not established
Isotope bone scan	In high-risk patients with high PSA or raised alkaline phosphatase; PSA >10 ng/mL in newly diagnosed and >20 ng/mL in follow-up patients	
PET scan	Not used as it does not differentiate between BPH and prostate cancer (8)	Low sensitivity because of decreased glucose utilization (44); may have a role in lymph node metastasis detection after primary local therapy
PSMA scan	No clear diagnostic indication (48)	May have therapeutic value

CT, computed tomography; MRI, magnetic resonance imaging; MRS, magnetic resonance spectroscopy; PET, positron emission tomography; PSMA, prostate-specific membrane antigen; TRUS, transrectal ultrasound.

chemical shift (47). The main advantage of MRS is supposed to be its increased staging accuracy for less experienced readers and reduction of interobserver variability (47). Current investigations and their limitations are summarized in Table 18.2.1.

Bone Scan

Serum PSA levels can predict the results of radionuclide bone scan in newly diagnosed patients. In patients with a PSA of <20 ng/mL and no bony pain, the likely chance of bony metastasis is less than 0.3% (49). The technical details are given in Chapter 5.

References

1. Revelo MP, Cookson MS, Chang SS, et al. Incidence and location of prostate and urothelial carcinoma in prostates from cystoprostatectomies: implications for possible apical sparing surgery. J Urol 2004;171(2 pt 1):646–651.

2. Rogers E, Eastham JA, Ohori M, et al. Impalpable prostate cancer: clinicopathological features. Br J Urol 1996;77(3):429–432.

3. Han M, Brannigan RE, Antenor JA, Roehl KA, Catalona WJ. Association of hemospermia with prostate cancer. J Urol 2004;172(6 pt 1):2189–2192.

4. Coleman RE. Biphosphonates: clinical experience. Oncologist 2004;9:14–27.

5. Oefelein MG, Ricchiuti V, Conrad W, Resnick MI. Skeletal fractures negatively correlate with overall survival in men with prostate cancer. J Urol 2002;168:1005–1007.

6. Benjamin R. Neurological complications of prostate cancer. Am Family Phys 2002; 65:834–840.

7. Schroder FH. Re: Lest we abandon digital rectal examination as a screening test for prostate cancer. J Natl Cancer Inst 1999;91:1331–1332.

8. Teillac P. The global state of prostate cancer: new diagnostic tools, minimal requirements for diagnosis and staging, and guidelines in the second millennium. BJU Int 2004:94(suppl 3):3–4.

9. Rietbergen JB, Hoedemaeker RF, Kruger AE, et al. The changing pattern of prostate cancer at the time of diagnosis: characteristics of screen detected prostate cancer in a population based screening study. J Urol 1999;161:1192–1198.

10. Machia RJ. Editorial: biopsy of prostate-an ongoing evolution. J Urol 2004;171: 1487–1488.

11. Klein EA, Zippe CD. Editorial: transrectal ultrasound guided prostate biopsy – defining a new standard. J Urol 2000;163:179–180.

12. Cooner WH, Mosley BR, Rutherford CL Jr, et al. Prostate cancer detection in a clinical urological practice by ultrasonography, digital rectal examination and prostate specific antigen. J Urol 1990;167:966–973.

13. Thompson IM, Pauler DK, Goodman PJ, et al. Prevalence of prostate cancer among men with a prostate specific antigen level ≤4 ng per milliliter. N Engl J Med 2004; 350:2239–2246.

14. Schroder FH, Gosselaar C, Roemling S, et al. PSA and the detection of prostate cancer after 2005. Part I. Eur Urol 2005;suppl 4(1):2–12.

15. Roehl KA, Antenor JAV, Catalona WJ. Robustness of free prostate specific antigen measurements to reduce unnecessary biopsies in 2.6 to 4 ng/mL range. J Urol 2002; 168:922–925.

16. Babian RJ, Johnston DA, Naccarto W, et al. The incidence of prostate cancer in a screening population with a serum prostate specific antigen between 2.5 and 4.0 ng/ mL: relation to biopsy strategy. J Urol 2001;165:757–760.

17. Carvalhal GF, Smith DS, Mager DE, et al. Digital rectal examination for detecting prostate cancer at prostate specific antigen levels of 4 ng/mL or less. J Urol 1999;16: 835–839.

18. Bostwick DG. Prostatic intraepithelial neoplasia is a risk factor for cancer. Sem Urol Oncol 1999;17:187–198.

19. Lefkowitz GK, Taneja SS, Brown J, et al. Follow up interval prostate biopsy 3 years after diagnosis of high grade intraepithelial neoplasia is associated with high likelihood of prostate cancer, independent of change in prostate specific antigen levels. J Urol 2002;168:1415–1418.

20. Eggner SE, Roehl KA, Catalona WJ. Predictors of subsequent prostate cancer in men with a prostate specific antigen of 2.6 to 4.0 ng/mL and an initially negative biopsy. J Urol 2005;174:500–504.

21. Matlaga BR, Eskew LA, McCullough DL. Prostate biopsy: indications and technique. J Urol 2003;169:12–19.

22. Catalona WJ, Hudson MA, Scardino PT, et al. Selection of optimal prostate specific antigen cutoffs for early detection of prostate cancer: receiver operating characteristic curves. J Urol 1994;152:2037–2042.

23. Morgan TO, Jacobsen SJ, McCarthy WF, et al. Age-specific reference ranges for serum prostate-specific antigen in black men. N Engl J Med 1996;335:304–310.

24. Catalona WJ, Smith DS, Wolfert RL, et al. Evaluation of percentage of free serum prostate-specific antigen to improve specificity of prostate cancer screening. JAMA 1995;274:1214–1220.

25. Catalona WJ, Partin AW, Slawin KM, et al. Use of the percentage of free prostate-specific antigen to enhance differentiation of prostate cancer from benign prostatic disease:a prospective multicenter clinical trial. JAMA 1998;279:1542–1547.

26. Roehl KA, Antenor JA, Catalona WJ. Robustness of free prostate specific antigen measurements to reduce unnecessary biopsies in the 2.6 to 4.0 ng/mL range. J Urol 2002;168:922–925.

27. Aus G, Bergdahl S, Hugosson J, et al. Outcome of laterally directed sextant biopsies of the prostate in screened males aged 50–66 years. Eur Urol 2001;39:655–661.

28. Zackrisson B, Aus G, Lilja H, et al. Follow up of men with elevated prostate-specific antigen and one set of benign biopsies at prostate cancer screening. Eur Urol 2003; 43:327–332.

29. Eskew LA, Bare RL, McCullough DL. Systemic 5 region prostate biopsy is superior to the sextant method of diagnosing prostate carcinoma of prostate. J Urol 1997;157: 199–203.

30. Levine MA, Ittman M, Melamed J, Lepor H. Two consecutive sets of transrectal ultrasound guided sextant biopsies of the prostate for the detection of prostate cancer. J Urol 1998;159:471–476.

31. Scattoni V, Montorsi F, Picchio M, et al. Diagnosis of local recurrence after radical prostatectomy. BJU Int 2004;93(5):680–688.

32. Naya Y, Okihara K, Evans RB, Babaian RJ. Efficacy of prostatic fossa biopsy in detecting local recurrence after radical prostatectomy. Urology 2005;66:350–355.

33. Crook J, Malone S, Perry G, et al. Postradiotherapy prostate biopsies: what do they really mean? Results for 498 patients. Int J Radiat Oncol Biol Phys 2000;48(2): 355–367.

34. Nam RK, Toi A, Trachtenberg J, et al. Making sense of prostate specific antigen: improving its predictive value in patients undergoing prostate biopsy. J Urol 2006; 175:489–494.

35. Autorino R, De Sio M, Di Lorenzo G, et al. How to decrease pain during transrectal ultrasound guided prostate biopsy: a look at the literature. J Urol 2005;174: 1091–1097.

36. Hodge KK, McNeal JE, Terris MK, Stamey TA. Random systemic versus directed ultrasound guided transrectal core biopsies of prostate. J Urol 1989;142:71–74.

37. Iczkowski KA, Casella G, Seppala RJ, et al. Needle core length in sextant biopsy influences prostate cancer detection rate. Urology 2002;59:698–703.

38. Levine MA, Ittman M, Melamed J, et al. Two consecutive sets of transrectal ultrasound guided sextant biopsies of the prostate for the detection of prostate cancer. J Urol 1998;159:471–476.

39. Stamey TA. Making the most out of six systematic sextant biopsies. Urology 1995; 45:2–12.

40. Chang JJ, Shinohara K, Hovey RM, et al. Prospective evaluation of lateral biopsies of the peripheral zone for prostate cancer detection. Urology 1998;52:89–93.

41. Eskew LA, Bare RL, McCullough DL. Systematic 5-region prostate biopsy is superior to sextant method for diagnosing carcinoma of the prostate. J Urol 1997;157: 199–202.

42. Berger AP, Gozzi C, Steiner H, Frauscher F, et al. Complication rate of transrectal ultrasound guided prostate biopsy: a comparison among 3 protocols with 6, 10 and 15 cores. J Urol 2004;171:1478–1481.

43. Rifkin MD. Biopsy techniques. In: Rifkin MD, ed. Ultrasound of the Prostate, 2nd ed. Philadelphia: Lippincott-Raven, 1997:236–262.

44. Yu KK, Hawkins RA. The prostate: diagnostic evaluation of metastatic disease. Radiat Clin North Am 2000;38(1):139–157.

45. Coakley FV, Qayyum A, Kurhanwicz J. Magnetic resonance imaging and spectro-scopic imaging of prostate cancer. J Urol 2003;170:S69–S76.

46. Yu KK, Scheidler J, Hricak H, et al. Prostate cancer: prediction of extracapsular exten-sion with endorectal MR imaging and three-dimensional proton MR spectroscopic imaging. Radiology 1999;213:481–488.

47. Yu KK, Hricak H. Imaging prostate cancer. Rad Clin North Am 2000;38(1):59–85.

48. Nargund V, Al Hashmi D, Kumar P, et al. Imaging with radiolabelled monoclonal antibody (MUJ591) to prostate-specific membrane antigen in staging of clinically localized prostate carcinoma: comparison with clinical, surgical and histological staging. BJU Int 2005;95:1232–1236.

49. Oesterling JE, Martin SK, Bergstrahl EJ, et al. The use of prostate specific antigen in staging with newly diagnosed prostate cancer. JAMA 1993;269:57–60.

18.3
Surgical Management of Carcinoma of the Prostate

Vinod H. Nargund

This chapter discusses patient selection and treatment by radical prostatectomy, and the principles of various other operative procedures used in the management of prostate cancer.

Radical Surgery

Surgical Anatomy of the Prostate Gland

Knowledge of the fascial layers and neurovascular bundle is crucial in understanding the principles of radical surgery of the prostate gland. The prostate is situated deep in the lesser pelvis below the urinary bladder and in front of the rectum, and measures on average 4.0 to 4.5 cm in transverse diameter. The gland develops its adult morphology during puberty, and its structure gets distorted by disease (e.g., benign prostatic hypertrophy, BPH) by the fifth decade (1), and the variety of shape and size can be anticipated due to the associated BPH. The gland has its own capsule and fascia. The Denonvilliers fascia, which is situated between the prostate and the rectum, continues laterally with pararectal fascia posteriorly and lateral pelvic fascia anteriorly. The lateral pelvic fascia anteriorly becomes less prominent and gets attached to the capsule of the prostate (2). The neurovascular bundle (NVB) is posterolateral to the prostate in front of the rectum and is related to the lateral pelvic, prostatic, and Denonvilliers fascia (Fig. 18.3.1) (3). The nerves are particularly vulnerable near the apex, where they lie very close to the prostatic capsule at the 5 and 7 o' clock positions (4). The NVBs contain cavernosal nerves branching from the pelvic plexus, which is formed by parasympathetic (pelvic splanchnic) and sympathetic (hypogastric) nerves (5). The nerves become more condensed at the midprostate level. The nerve bundles should be released from the apical region prior to urethral transection. Careful apical dissection is important because of its closeness to the external sphincter and variations in the shape of prostate apex (6). The arterial supply comes from the inferior vesical artery, and venous drainage is from Santorini's plexus. The blood vessels and nerves run between the lateral

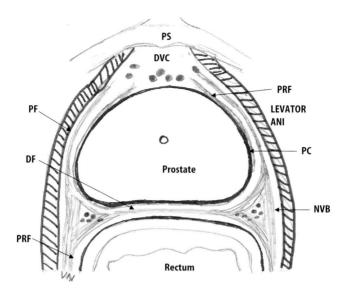

FIGURE 18.3.1. Anatomical arrangement of fascial layers and neurovascular bundles (diagrammatic). DF, Denonvilliers fascia; DVC, dorsal venous complex; NVB, neurovascular bundle; PC, prostatic capsule; PF, pelvic fascia; PS, pubic symphysis; PRF, pararectal fascia.

pelvic and the prostatic fascia. Due to the close relationship between vessels and nerves, diathermy ideally should be avoided while dissecting in this area in nerve-sparing prostatectomy.

The radical prostatectomy (RP) consists of removal of the prostate gland with its capsule, seminal vesicles and ampulla of vas with or without the pelvic lymph nodes followed by anastomosis of the bladder neck with the urethra. The procedure may be accomplished by nerve preservation (cavernous nerve sparing) in selected cases. The RP is accomplished by the retropubic (open or laparoscopic/robotic) or perineal route.

Preoperative Considerations

The PSA, Gleason grading, and clinical assessment by the digital rectal examination (DRE) are the information available prior to surgery, and additional investigations are considered on an individual basis. Radical surgery is curative only if the tumor is confined to the prostate with intact capsule (stages T1a,b,c and T2). The operative mortality for RP is less than 1% in organ-confined cancer of the prostate (CaP), and it offers the best disease-free survival rates (80% to 90% in 10 to 15 years in several series).

Preoperative exclusion of locally advanced or distal metastatic disease is therefore of utmost importance. High-risk patients need further imaging studies, mainly magnetic resonance imaging (MRI). Current clinical parameters and investigations, however, do not answer important questions in relation to RP, such as how to distinguish between significant and insignificant prostate cancers, and how to predict the outcome of surgery (7). Although the tables and nomograms may be useful adjuncts, they are still in the evolutionary stage (see below).

A multidisciplinary conference consisting of a group of clinicians, pathologists, and statisticians was organized by the College of American Pathologists in 1999 to assess the existing predictive factors on the strength of published evidence. The predictive factors were ranked into three categories:

Category I: factors that are of prognostic importance and useful in clinical management, like preoperative total prostate-specific antigen (tPSA) tumor, node, metastasis (TNM) stage grouping, histological grade, and surgical margin status.

Category II: factors that have been extensively studied clinically and biologically, but their importance remains to be validated in statistically robust studies, such as tumor volume, histological type, and DNA ploidy.

Category III: other factors whose prognostic value is not evident enough to show their prognostic value, such as perineural invasion, neuroendocrine differentiation, microvessel density (angiogenesis), nuclear roundness, chromatin texture, other karyometric factors, proliferation markers, PSA derivatives, and other factors (oncogenes, tumor suppressor genes, apoptosis genes, etc.) (8). For all intents and purposes only category I factors are used for the decision-making process.

Predictive Factors for Radical Prostatectomy

Category I factors should be carefully considered before discussing the cancer management with patient.

Gleason Grade

The likelihood of extracapsular disease increases with higher Gleason grades (Table 18.3.1). The Gleason grade is a critical prognostic factor to predict the biochemical failure, capsular involvement, local recurrences, lymph node involvement. and distant metastasis.

The Gleason grades between transrectal ultrasound (TRUS) and RP specimens may be different due to multifocality of the tumor and limited tissue material being available to the pathologist after TRUS biopsy. The agreement in Gleason grading between TRUS biopsy and RP specimen varies widely (31% to 81%) (10,11). In addition, there can be interobserver and intraobserver variation.

TABLE 18.3.1. Risk of positive margins in relation to Gleason grades (9)

Gleason grade	Capsular penetration (%)	Positive surgical margins (%)
8–10	85	59
7	62	48

Tumor Characteristics at PSA Values Above ≥10 ng/mL

There is evidence to suggest that cancers presented with tPSA levels of more than 10 ng/mL often have signs of advanced disease, such as capsular invasion, involvement of adjacent organs, high tumor volume, high Gleason grade, and lymph node involvement. This is demonstrated in a large multicenter study by Partin et al. (12), who reported the following findings in men with PSA of ≥10 ng/mL: 29% had organ-confined disease (<T2c), 46% had extraprostatic disease (T3a), 13% had seminal vesicle involvement (pT3b), and 11% had lymph node involvement (N1).

The percent of positive cores in the TRUS biopsy has been shown to be indicative of adverse pathology and biochemical failure after RP. In a study of more than 1000 patients, Freedland et al. (13) found the percent of positive biopsy cores to be a significant prognostic factor for adverse pathology and biochemical recurrence. They categorized the percent of positive biopsy cores into three levels for risk stratification: <34% low risk, 34% to 50% intermediate risk, and >50% high risk.

Tumor Volume

There is evidence to suggest that tumor volume is an independent prognostic factor in patients undergoing RP (14).

Lymph Node Metastasis

Lymph node metastasis in clinically localized CaP is a poor prognostic indicator for biochemical recurrence and survival (15,16).

Miscellaneous

Like other oncological surgical procedures, the outcome of RP also depends on meticulous surgical technique, in particular control of bleeding during surgery, which can damage the capsule and other adjacent structures.

Decision-Making Process

Once the diagnosis of localized prostate cancer is made, patients should have the benefit of counseling in conjunction with their spouse, close relative, or friend if possible. The factors that are taken into account to consider radical surgery are summarized in Table 18.3.2.

Imaging is needed in selected cases, as described in Chapter 18.2. Most patients with early disease and low-risk category would be suitable for nerve-sparing RP.

Selected patients with T3 disease can be treated by radical surgery, for example, in patients with small T3, PSA of <20 ng/mL, Gleason score of <8, and a life expectancy of more than 10 years (17).

TABLE 18.3.2. Factors taken into account prior to considering a patient for radical prostatectomy (RP)

Patient factors
Age: Surgery is generally reserved for patients younger than 70 years
Life expectancy: >10 years
Marked obstructive outflow symptoms
Comorbidity: There should be few or no comorbid conditions
Patient's preference/physician's preference
Other treatment options available in the center

Tumor factors
PSA levels
Gleason grading
Clinical staging: T1a, N0, M0/ T1b, N0, M0 / T1c, N0, M0 / T2, N0, M0, any Gleason grade
In carefully selected patients with T3NX M0: RP + pelvic lymphadenectomy

Information about all the treatment modalities that are available in a specific center with the available data on survival, success rates, complications, and cancer control for each treatment should be discussed (Table 18.3.3). When evaluating treatment options, it is important to discuss (1) the advantages and disadvantages, (2) the indications and contraindications, and (3) the availability of each treatment and expertise.

TABLE 18.3.3. Advantages and disadvantages with different forms of management for localized carcinoma of the prostate (CaP)

Advantages	Disadvantages
Radical surgery	
a. Radical excision of the growth with long-term cancer control	a. Hospitalization and anesthesia required
b. Accurate histopathological grading and staging	b. Major surgical procedure: blood loss, injury to pelvic organs; incomplete excision
c. In case of local recurrence further treatment with other modalities [e.g., external beam radiation therapy (EBRT) is available]	c. Urinary incontinence, bladder neck stenosis, and erectile dysfunction
	d. Lymphocele and wound complications
	e. Local recurrence
Radiotherapy	
a. Outpatient treatment	a. Delayed occurrence of urinary incontinence and erectile dysfunction
b. No anesthesia and other immediate postoperative complications	b. Bowel and bladder problems
c. Further local treatment possible with cryotherapy/high-intensity focused ultrasound (HIFU)	c. Salvage surgery is risky
	d. No ways of assessing disease control
	e. Uncertain long-term cancer control
Watchful waiting	
a. No surgery or radiotherapy side effects or complications; quality of life maintained	a. Patient compliance required
b. Normal urinary and erectile functions may be maintained	b. Local advancement and distant metastasis may be missed
c. Various treatment options can be considered with progression of the disease	c. Ongoing psychological stress to the patient that the disease is present

Nomograms

Nomograms are multivariate models based on the clinical and pathological data at presentation calibrated and validated to evaluate their accuracy. They are useful in predicting patient outcomes, and thereby can be used as discrimination tools in predicting outcome of the treatment (18). Nomograms or other models, however, are not a substitute or surrogate for doctor–patient interaction. There are a number of nomograms to predict prostate cancer recurrence after definitive local therapy (19). The proponents cite many reasons for adding nomograms to the traditional decision-making process. Doctors generally decide the treatment modality depending on risk assessment based on their past clinical experience, which is likely to be the preferred outcome rather than actual probability. Clinicians do not recall all cases they have treated and also have difficulty in learning from their past mistakes (19).

Partin's tables are based on information obtained from large cohorts of men who have undergone radical prostatectomy, with precise determination of pathologic stage. In their updated version, Partin et al. (20) from John Hopkins Hospital used multinomial log-linear regression analysis to estimate the likelihood of organ-confined disease, extraprostatic extension, seminal vesicle, or lymph nodal status from the preoperative PSA stratified as 0 to 2.5, 2.6 to 4.0, 4.1 to 6.0, 6.1 to 10.0, and >10 ng/mL, clinical stage (T1c, T2a, T2b, or T2c) [American Joint Committee on Cancer (AJCC) tumor, node, metastasis (TNM) classification, 1992], and biopsy Gleason score stratified as 2 to 4, 5 to 6, 3 + 4 = 7, 4 + 3 = 7, or 8 to 10 among 5079 men (mean age 58 years) treated only with radical prostatectomy (without neoadjuvant therapy) between 1994 and 2000. The tables give a probability of organ-confined disease, capsular penetration, seminal vesicle involvement, and lymph node involvement for individual patients (see Appendix D at end of book). The specificity and sensitivity of the Partin tables have been validated in subsequent studies (21,22).

Kattan Nomograms

Kattan et al. (23,24) have described preoperative and postoperative nomograms by modeling clinical and pathological data and disease follow-up by Cox proportional hazards regression analysis. More recently, their group has published a postoperative nomogram predicting the 10-year probability of recurrence after RP (25) (see Appendix D).

The artificial neural networks (ANNs) are becoming popular in studying diagnosis, staging, and progression of prostate cancer. They are artificial intelligence tools inspired by biological neuronal systems that identify arbitrary nonlinear multiparametric discriminant functions directly from the clinical data (26). They have the potential to combine many factors including various biochemical markers and details of imaging studies, and are still being evaluated.

Preoperative Preparation

Preoperative preparation entails the following:

1. Selection of patients: age, comorbid conditions, life expectancy, Gleason grading, and clinical staging are taken into account in selecting the patients, and have been discussed already.
2. Explain to the patient the anatomical extent of the excision and the possible complications, and ave him sign an informed consent form.
3. Clear knowledge of the pathological anatomy for the operator: the shape, size, and apical involvement of the prostate, and the histology.
4. Bowel preparation for the patient.
5. Autologous blood storage where possible or grouping and crossmatching.

Pelvic Lymph Node Dissection

The pelvic lymph node dissection (PLND) is usually carried out at the time of the retropubic prostatectomy. In patients undergoing perineal prostatectomy, the PLND is carried out as a separate procedure if indicated. The procedure can be carried out laparoscopically or by open procedure.

In men with a tPSA of <10 ng/mL with a low Gleason sum, the incidence of lymph node metastasis is likely to be low (27,28). Due to increased detection rates of early prostate cancer, the contemporaneous prevalence of lymph node metastasis in a clinically localized prostate varies from 3% (well differentiated) to 9% (poorly differentiated) (29,30). These data contrast with a series of 452 patients in 1983 in the pre-PSA era by Smith et al. (31) who reported metastases rates of 24% to 53% (stages T1 to T3). The same study showed correlation between and histological differentiation and lymph node metastases: well differentiated prostate cancer, 10%; moderately differentiated, 24%; and poorly differentiated, 54%.

The indications, extent, and benefits of PLND, however, are a subject of intense debate, particularly in regard to low-risk prostate cancer. It is also worth noting that PLND is not without risks. Injury to the obturator nerve, iliac, and obturator vessels during pelvic dissection are potential complications. In addition there are also delayed complications associated with lymph node dissection elsewhere, including lymphocele formation, fistulas, and lymphedema, which are independent of cancer treatment. Other possible complications include deep vein thrombosis and wound infection. The aim of PLND should be threefold: (3) to stage the disease accurately, (2) to assess the risk of progression, and (3) to remove micrometastases to improve survival (32,33). There is evidence to suggest that pelvic nodal disease increases the risk of progression of prostate cancer (34). In summary, advanced Gleason sum and clinical stage and high tPSA are reliable predictors of lymph node metastasis (35).

The PLND is indicated in men with Gleason score of >7, PSA level of >20, and advanced T stage independently or in combination (36).

The next vexing question is the extent of the lymph node dissection. Traditionally the PLND includes removal of lymphatic tissue medial to the external iliac vein, obturator, and hypogastric region. In extended PLND all lymph nodes below the common iliac bifurcation are cleared (obturator, internal iliac, and its branches). Long-term follow-up of these patients has not yet been reported. The role of extended PLND or the number of lymph nodes removed is currently unsettled and is debated (37,38).

Radical Prostatectomy

Retropubic (Open; Radical Retropubic Prostatectomy): Nerve Sparing and Non–Nerve Sparing

Nearly 90% of RPs are performed by the retropubic route. Obturator lymph node sampling is done if indicated by making an incision through the posterior peritoneum between the obliterated umbilical artery and the internal ring. The dissection continues proximally to the bifurcation of the common iliac artery on the medial side of the external iliac artery vein. The posterior dissection continues to include the obturator pocket. The pelvic fascia is incised lateral to the prostate, and the puboprostatic ligaments are defined. After division of the puboprostatic ligaments, the dorsal venous complex is divided. The apical dissection, mobilization of the prostate, with or without preservation of the NVB, and dissection of the seminal vesicles completes the excision. This is followed by division of the urethra and a urethrovesical anastomosis. The bladder neck is everted and anastomosed to the urethra. The wound is closed with a retropubic drain. This is done either by open or laparoscopic approach (see Chapter 7).

Perineal (Radical Perineal Prostatectomy)

This approach is suitable for prostates weighing less than 100 g. The cancer control is equally effective by this route. The advantages of radical perineal prostatectomy (RPP) are a relatively avascular field, clear apical exposure, and good exposure for the urethravesical anastomosis. Similar to RRP there are nerve-sparing and non–nerve-sparing approaches. Blood loss is relatively less as the dorsal venous complex is generally not divided. It is a preferred route in patients who have undergone previous abdominal surgery. The main disadvantage is the inability to carry out simultaneous lymph node dissection; however, this should not be a problem, as most patients do not need PLND (see above).

Contraindications for RPP

Patients with a previous history of retropubic or transvesical prostatectomy are not candidates for RPP. Massive obesity and restricted mobility in the hip joint are relative contraindications.

Open vs. Laparoscopic/Robotic Prostatectomy

Early results from laparoscopic RP and robot-assisted RP are comparable to those of open RRP. Blood loss and transfusion rates are much lower than in the open procedure. The recovery time is much shorter than in the open procedure. Financial costs, however, are higher than in the open procedure. The long-term oncological outcomes are awaited (39).

Complications of Radical Prostatectomy

Early

Hemorrhage

Intraoperative bleeding is one of the major problems during prostatic surgery. Bleeding can occur from the dorsal venous complex or vascular pedicles, and during lymph node dissection. Excessive bleeding can further lead to injuries to other structures such as the rectum, ureters, and obturator nerve.

Deep vein thrombosis (DVT) and pulmonary embolism occur in less than 0.4% of patients (40). The incidence of DVT increases with PLND (41).

Rectal Injury and Rectourethral Fistula

Although not common, rectal injury can occur, and recognition at the time of surgery is extremely important. Primary repair is carried out in two layers followed by an omental flap (42). Rectourethral fistula is a rare complication. Patients with iatrogenic rectourethral fistula following RP are managed by urinary and fecal diversion after radical retropubic prostatectomy or radiation. This is followed by closure of the fistula with muscle transposition. The urinary and fecal continuity are reestablished after successful closure of the fistula (43).

Lymphocele

Pelvic lymph node dissection is associated with a slightly higher incidence of lymphoceles, although it is a rare problem after RRP without PLND (41). The diagnosis is usually by ultrasound. Small lymphoceles may not need any treatment, while large ones are drained under ultrasound control or by laparoscopic marsupialization.

Urinary Leak

This is an extremely rare complication and is usually managed by prolonged catheterization, catheter traction, passive drainage, and active catheter suction (44).

Anastomotic Stricture

This is a well-recognized complication with an incidence up to 32% (45). Various risk factors including previous transurethral resection, urinary extravasation, and symptomatic bacteriuria predispose to stricture formation at anastomotic site (46). The anastomotic stricture is managed by cold knife incision or by dilatation (46).

Erectile Dysfunction

Between 16% and 82% of patients undergoing RP and 2% to 34% receiving external beam radiation develop erectile dysfunction (ED) (47). Patients undergoing nerve-sparing RP often experience ED, which may be due to neuropraxia of the cavernosal nerves. Absent erections may lead to poor oxygenation and corporeal fibrosis, leading to veno-occlusive ED (48).

It has also been suggested from animal experiments that apoptosis in penile smooth muscle cells is enhanced by nerve injury (49). The cavernous nerve reconstruction using the sural nerve has been suggested for prevention of post-RT impotence; RP may also affect orgasmic sensation. It is important to start anti-ED drugs early to prevent corporeal damage, even in patients who had nerve-sparing RP (50).

Stress Urinary Incontinence

Up to 30% of patients have urinary leakage after RP and nearly 5% have persistent leakage (51). Various causes cited for incontinence include sphincter damage, detrusor dysfunction, and poor bladder compliance. Urodynamic studies show mixed findings regarding the degree of contribution between detrusor and urethral factors.

Detrusor instability is an important cause in the early postoperative period (4 weeks to 6 months) and is treated with anticholinergic medication and physiotherapy (52). Pelvic floor reeducation is undertaken with positive feedback protocol (53). Persistent incontinence (after 1 year) is usually severe, does not respond to physiotherapy, and may have a devastating effect on the patient's quality of life. In these patients retrograde injection of substances like collagen, Teflon, or autologous fat into the external sphincter region may help in the short-term. Cummings et al. (54) reported an overall satisfaction rate of 58% with these options (mean follow-up 10.4 months). The last option is insertion of an artificial urinary sphincter (AUS). It has satisfaction rates ranging between 80% and 90% (55,56).

Summary of Operative Factors

The following operative factors improve surgical outcome and prevent complications:

1. Early effective control of dorsal venous complex
2. Protection of neurovascular bundles
3. Nerve bundle release before urethral transaction; as mentioned above, in surgical anatomy a urethral transaction is carried out only after making sure that the nerve bundles have been released
4. Sphincter preservation

5. Preservation of pelvic floor
6. Excellent lighting, including the judicious usage of a headlight, and surgical loupe magnification and "sponge sticks" in the retraction of the gland during dissection (open procedure)

Other Surgical Procedures for CaP

Salvage Prostatectomy

The rate of recurrence after radiotherapy is not clear, and younger patients with a life expectancy of more than 10 years and localized recurrence need further treatment (57). Some of the treatments suggested include cryotherapy, radical cystoprostatectomy, and radical prostatectomy (57). Salvage radical prostatectomy, however, is not widely accepted because of its associated morbidity and high recurrence rate (58). For example, the incontinence rates could be as high as 58% and other major complications up to 33% (59).

Transurethral Resection of the Prostate for Outflow Obstruction

This procedure is generally indicated in patients who have retention with advanced prostate cancer. The resection is usually limited, and a narrow channel is created for relieving the obstruction. Transurethral resection of the prostate (TURP) has also been advocated in men with multiple negative prostate biopsies, but the diagnostic yield is low (60). In patients who develop severe outflow symptoms after brachytherapy, TURP is usually delayed for 6 months (61).

Bilateral Subcapsular Orchiectomy

Removal of testicular tissue had been widely practiced before the introduction of antiandrogen therapy. The procedure can be done under local or general anesthesia. There is a decline in the number of bilateral subcapsular orchiectomies (BSOs) done due to a shift to earlier stages and younger ages at diagnosis, and the development of antiandrogens. It may be of value in a patient with metastatic prostate cancer with poor patient compliance and economic reasons.

Cystoscopy and JJ Stenting

Patients with prostate cancer can present with renal failure due to bilateral ureteric obstruction. Immediate relief is achieved by percutaneous nephrostomy or antegrade or retrograde stenting. Cystoscopy is indicated when there is hematuria both as a diagnostic and therapeutic aid when bleeding is from the prostate.

References

1. McNeal JE. The prostate gland: morphology and pathobiology. Mono Urol 1983; 4:3–35.

2. Walsh PC, Lepor H, Eggleston JC. Radical prostatectomy with preservation of sexual function: anatomical and pathological considerations. Prostate 1983;4:473–485.
3. Schlegel PN, Walsh PC. Neuroanatomical approach to radical cystoprostatectomy with preservation of sexual function. J Urol 1987;138:1402–1406.
4. Brooks JD. Anatomy of the lower urinary tract and male genitalia. In: Walsh PC, Retik AB, Vaughan, Jr ED, Wein AJ, eds. Campbell's Urology. Philadelphia: WB Saunders, 2002:41–80.
5. Walsh PC, Donker PJ. Impotence following radical prostatectomy: insight into aetiology and prevention. J Urol 1982;128:492–497.
6. Myers RP, Goellner JR, Cahill DR. Prostate shape, external striated urethral sphincter and radical prostatectomy: the apical dissection. J Urol 1987;138:543–550.
7. Remzi M, Waldert M, Djavan B. Preoperative nomograms and artificial neural networks (ANNs) for identification of surgical candidates. Eur Urol EAU Update Series 2005;3:63–71.
8. Bostwick DG, Grignon D, Hammond EH, et al. Predictive factors in prostate cancer. College of Pathologists consensus statements 1999. Arch Pathol Lab Med 2000;124: 996–1000.
9. Oestrling JE, Brendler CB, Epstein JI, et al. Correlation of clinical stage, serum prostatic acid phosphatase and preoperative Gleason grade with final pathological stage in 275 patients with clinically localized Adenocarcinoma of the prostate. J Urol 1987; 138:92–98.
10. Babaian RJ, Grunow WA. Reliability of Gleason grading system in comparing prostate biopsies with total prostatectomy specimens. Urology 1985;25:564–567.
11. Steinberg D, Sauvageot J, Epstein JI. Correlation of prostate needle biopsy and radical prostatectomy: Gleason grade in academic and community settings. Mol Pathol 1996; 9:83A.
12. Partin AW, Kattan MW, Subong EN, et al. Combination of prostate-specific antigen, clinical stage, and Gleason score to predict pathological stage of localized prostate cancer. A multi-institutional update. JAMA 1997;277:1445–1451.
13. Freedland SJ, Aronson WJ, Terris MK, et al. Percent of prostate needle biopsy cores with cancer is significant independent predictor of prostate specific antigen recurrence following radical prostatectomy: results from SEARCH database. J Urol 2003; 169:2136–2141.
14. Nelson BA, Shappell SB, Chang SS, et al. Tumour volume is an independent predictor of prostate specific antigen recurrence in patients undergoing radical prostatectomy for clinically localized prostate cancer. BJU Int 2006;97:1169–1172.
15. Cheng L, Zincke H, Blute ML, Bergstrahl EJ, et al. Risk of prostate carcinoma death in patients with lymph node metastasis. Cancer 2001;91:66–73.
16. Daneshmand S, Quek ML, Stein JP, Lieskovsky G, et al. Prognosis of patients with lymph node positive prostate cancer following radical prostatectomy: long-term results. J Urol 2004;172:2252–2255.
17. Aus G, Abbou CC, Pacik D, et al. EAU working group on Oncological urology. EAU guidelines on prostate cancer. Eur Urol 2001;40:97–101.
18. Stephenson AJ, Kattan MW. Nomograms for prostate cancer. BJU Int 2006;98:39–46.
19. Ross PL, Scardino PT, Kattan MW, et al. A catalogue of prostate cancer nomograms. J Urol 2001;165:1562–1568.
20. Partin AW, Mangold LA, Lamm DM, et al. Contemporary update of prostate cancer staging nomograms (Partin tables) for the new millennium. Urology 2001;58(6): 843–848.

21. Blute ML, Bergstralh EJ, Partin AW, et al. Validation of Partin tables for predicting pathological stage of clinically localized prostate cancer. J Urol 2000;164(5): 1591–1595.

22. Graefen M, Augustin H, Karakiewicz PI, et al. Can predictive models for prostate cancer patients derived in the United States of America be utilized in European patients? A validation study of the Partin tables. Eur Urol 2003;43(1):6–10; discussion 11.

23. Kattan MW, Eastham JA, Stapleton AMF, Wheeler TM, Scardino PT. A preoperative nomogram for disease recurrence following radical prostatectomy for prostate cancer. J Natl Cancer Inst 1998;90(10):766–771.

24. Kattan MW, Wheeler TM, Scardino PT. Postoperative nomogram for disease recurrence after radical prostatectomy for prostate cancer. J Clin Oncol 1999;17: 499–507.

25. Stephenson AJ, Scardino PT, Eastham JA, et al. Preoperative nomogram predicting the 10-year probability of prostate cancer recurrence after radical prostatectomy. J Natl Cancer Inst 2006 7;98(10):715–717.

26. Remzi M, Djavan B. Artificial neural networks in Urology 2004. Eur Urol 2004;suppl 3:33–38.

27. Narayan P, Fournier G, Gajendran V, et al. Utility of preoperative prostate-specific antigen concentration and biopsy Gleason score in predicting risk of pelvic lymph node metastases in prostate cancer. Urology 1994;44:519–524.

28. Alagiri M, Colton MD, Seidmon EJ, et al. The staging lymphadenectomy: implications as an adjunctive procedure for clinically localized prostate cancer. Br J Urol 1997; 80:243–246.

29. Petros JA, Catalona WJ. Incidence of unsuspected lymph node metastasis in 521 consecutive patients with clinically localized prostate cancer. J Urol 1992;147: 1574–1575.

30. Danella JF, DeKernion JB, Smith RB, Steckel J. The contemporary incidence of lymph node metastases in prostate cancer. Implications for laparoscopic lymph node dissection. J Urol 1993;149:1488–1491.

31. Smith JA Jr, Seaman JP, Gleidman JB, Middleton RG. Pelvic lymph node metastases from prostatic cancer. Influence of tumor grade and stage in 452 consecutive patients. J Urol 1983;130(2):290–292.

32. Barth PJ, Gerharz EW, Ramaswamy A, Riedmiller H. The influence of lymph node counts on the detection of pelvic lymph node metastasis in prostate cancer. Pathol Res Pract 1999;195:633–636.

33. Weckermann D, Goppelt M, Dorn R, et al. Incidence of positive pelvic lymph nodes in patients with prostate cancer, a prostate-specific antigen (PSA) level of ≥10 ng/mL and biopsy Gleason score ≤6, and their influence on PSA progression-free survival after radical prostatectomy. BJU Int 2006;97:1173–1178.

34. Masterson TA, Bianco FJ Jr, Vickers AJ, et al. The association between total and positive lymph node counts, and disease progression in clinically localized prostate cancer. J Urol 2006;175(4):1320–1324; discussion 1324–1325.

35. Cagiannos I, Karakiewicz P, Eastham JA, et al. A preoperative nomogram identifying decreased risk of positive pelvic lymph nodes in patients with prostate cancer. J Urol 2003;170:1798–1803.

36. Hoenig DM, Chi S, Porter C, et al. Risk of nodal metastasis at laparoscopic pelvic lymphadenectomy using PSA, Gleason score and clinical stage in men with localized prostate cancer. J Endourol 1997;11:263–265.

37. DiMarco DS, Zincke H, Sebo TJ, et al. The extent of lymphadenectomy for pTxNo prostate cancer does not affect prostate cancer outcome in the prostate specific antigen era. J Urol 2005;173:1121–1125.
38. Schumacher MC, Burkhard FC, Thalmann GN, et al. Is pelvic lymph node dissection necessary in patients with serum PSA <10 ng/ml undergoing radical prostatectomy for prostate cancer? Eur Urol 2006;50:272–279.
39. Bollens R, Roumeguere T, Vanden Bossche M, et al. Comparison of laparoscopic radical prostatectomy techniques. Curr Urol Rep 2002;3(2):148–151.
40. Lepor H, Nieder AM, Ferrandino MN. Intraoperative and postoperative complications of radical retropubic prostatectomy in a consecutive series of 1,000 cases. J Urol 2001;166:1729–1733.
41. Augustin H, Hammerer P, Graefen M, et al. Intraoperative and perioperative morbidity of contemporary radical retropubic prostatectomy in a consecutive series of 1243 patients: results of a single center between 1999 and 2002. Eur Urol 2003;43: 113–118.
42. Katz R, Borkowski T, Hoznek A, et al. Operative management of rectal injuries during laparoscopic radical prostatectomy. Urology 2003;62(2):310–313.
43. Nyam DC, Pemberton JH. Management of iatrogenic rectourethral fistula. Dis Colon Rectum 1999;42(8):994–997; discussion 997–999.
44. Moinzadeh A, Abouassaly R, Gill IS, Libertino JA. Continuous needle vented Foley catheter suction for urinary leak after radical prostatectomy. J Urol 2004;171(6 pt 1):2366–2367.
45. Davidson PJ, van den Ouden D, Schroeder FH. Radical prostatectomy. Prospective assessment of mortality and morbidity. Eur Urol 1996;29:168–173.
46. Surya BV, Provet J, Johanson K-E, Brown J. Anastomotic strictures following radical prostatectomy: risk factors and management. J Urol 1990;143:755–758.
47. Siegel T, Moul J, Speval M, et al. The development of erectile dysfunction in men treated for prostate cancer. J Urol 2001;165:430–435.
48. Moreland RB. Is there hypoxia in penile fibrosis? A viewpoint presented to the society for the study of impotence. Int J Impot Res 1998;10:113–120.
49. User HM, Hairston JH, Zelner DJ, et al. Penile weight and cell subtype changes in a postradical prostatectomy model of erectile dysfunction. J Urol 2003;169: 1175–1179.
50. Montorosi F, Guazzoni G, Strambi LF, et al. Recovery of spontaneous erectile function after nerve-sparing radical retropubic prostatectomy with or without early intracavernosus injections of alprostadil results of a prospective randomized trial. J Urol 1997;158:1408–1410.
51. Peyromaure M, Ravery V, Boccon-Gibod L. The management of stress urinary incontinence after radical prostatectomy. BJU Int 2002;90:155–161.
52. Chao R, Mayo M E. Incontinence after radical prostatectomy: detrusor or sphincter causes. J Urol 1995;154:16–18.
53. Franke JJ, Barrit Gilbert W, Grier J, et al. early post-prostatectomy pelvic floor biofeedback. J Urol 2000;163:191–193.
54. Cummings JM, Boullier JA, Parra RO. Transurethral collagen injections in the therapy of post-radical prostatectomy stress incontinence. J Urol 1996;155:1011–1013.
55. Fleshner N, Herschorn S. The artificial urinary sphincter for post-radical prostatectomy incontinence. Impact on urinary symptoms and quality of life. J Urol 1996;155: 1260–1264.

56. Klijn AJ, Hop WCJ, Mickisch G, et al. The artificial urinary sphincter in men incontinent after radical prostatectomy: 5-year actuarial adequate function rates. Br J Urol 1998;82:530–533.

57. Vaidya A, Soloway MS. Salvage radical prostatectomy for radiorecurrent prostate cancer revisited. J Urol 2000;164:1998–2001.

58. Seitz C, Remzi M, Djavan B. Immediate treatment after PSA progression. Eur Urol Suppl 2005;4:28–42.

59. Rogers E, Ohori M, Kassabian VS, et al. Salvage radical prostatectomy: outcome measured by serum prostate specific antigen levels. J Urol 1995;153:104–110.

60. Zigeuner R, Schips L, Lipsky K, et al. Detection of prostate cancer by TURP or open surgery in patients with previously transrectal prostate biopsies. Urology 2003;62: 883–887.

61. Flam TA, Peyromaure M, Chauveinc L, et al. Post-brachytherapy transurethral resection of the prostate in patients with localized prostate cancer. J Urol 2004;172: 108–111.

18.4
Expectant Management of Early Prostate Cancer

Nicholas J. Van As and Christopher C. Parker

Expectant management of most cancers would lead to certain disease progression, disfigurement, and death. Prostate cancer is different. While prostate cancer *can* follow an aggressive and ultimately fatal course, similar to that of other cancers, in most cases it behaves in an indolent fashion, with no effect either on health or longevity. For such patients, definitive treatment, with its attendant risks, would be worse than the so-called disease. The challenge of managing early prostate cancer is to distinguish patients with clinically relevant cancers who require treatment from the remainder who do not, or, in other words, to tell the "tigers" from the "pussy cats."

It is important at the outset to distinguish between the two contrasting methods of expectant management. The term *watchful waiting* has been used for decades to describe a policy of observation with the use of palliative treatment for symptomatic progression. In more recent years, a quite distinct policy has evolved in which the choice between radical treatment and continued observation is based on evidence of disease progression, with progression defined by the rate of rise of the prostate-specific antigen (PSA) or "upgrading" at repeat biopsy. This latter method of expectant management has been termed "active surveillance" or "expectant management with curative intent." The aim of active surveillance is to identify cases for treatment long before any symptoms or overt clinical signs of tumor progression are evident. Whereas watchful waiting involves relatively lax observation with late, palliative treatment for those who develop symptoms of progressive disease, active surveillance involves close monitoring with early, radical treatment in those with biochemical or histologic signs of progression.

Traditional Watchful Waiting

Whereas patients with any other curable cancer would automatically be offered radical treatment, watchful waiting has long been a recognized approach to managing prostate cancer, with excellent long-term results in selected patients (1).

In fact, the first good evidence that radical treatment of localized prostate cancer improves on the outcome of watchful waiting has only recently become available. From 1989 to 1999, the Scandinavian Prostatic Cancer Group Study randomized 695 men with localized disease between radical prostatectomy and watchful waiting (2). Patients had a mean age of 65 years, a mean PSA of 13 ng/ml, and the grade mix was 68% Gleason score (GS) <7, 26% GS 7, and 6% GS 8 to 10.

At a median follow-up of 8.2 years, randomization to radical prostatectomy was associated with a benefit both in terms of disease-specific mortality [hazard ratio (HR) 0.56; 95% confidence interval (CI) 0.36–0.88; p = .01], and overall mortality (HR 0.74; 95% CI 0.56–0.99; p = .04). This translated into 10-year overall survival of 73% versus 68% (p = .04) for radical prostatectomy versus watchful waiting, respectively (2–4). This is a very important result, and demonstrates beyond doubt that some patients with localized prostate cancer benefit from surgery, as opposed to traditional watchful waiting. However, there are at least three reasons why expectant management remains a valid option, and why immediate radical treatment should not be uncritically accepted as the standard of care for all men with localized prostate cancer:

1. Patients need to weigh the survival benefit of immediate radical treatment against the risk of adverse consequences. The 5% absolute improvement in 10-year survival was achieved at the expense of a 35% absolute increase in the risk of erectile dysfunction and a 28% absolute increase in the risk of urinary leakage (4). Faced with these figures, some patients would choose surgery, but many would choose watchful waiting (5). An individual's treatment decision depends not only on trial results, but also on his personal values, and in particular the relative importance he places on prolonging life versus preserving lifestyle.

2. The outcome data from this trial were based largely on clinically detected prostate cancer, and should not be applied to men with screen-detected disease. Only 12% of patients in the Scandinavian trial had stage T1c disease, and as many as 19% of patients had a PSA greater than 20 ng/mL. Prostate-specific antigen screening results in overdetection (of cases that would not otherwise have been detected within the patient's lifetime) and introduces a lead time (the time difference between screen detection and clinical detection in the absence of screening), which may be of the order of 10 years or more (6). It follows that, in the absence of treatment, the natural history of screen-detected prostate cancer will be more favorable than that of clinically detected prostate cancer.

This is an important consideration for men faced with the choice between conservative management and curative treatment. In comparison with clinically detected disease, men with screen-detected cancers will have longer to endure any adverse effects of curative treatment, and longer to wait for any beneficial effect on survival to emerge. One attempt to model the magnitude of this effect is illustrated in Figure 18.4.1.

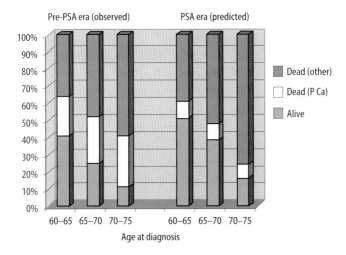

FIGURE 18.4.1. Influence of prostate-specific antigen (PSA) screening on the 15-year outcome of watchful waiting for localized prostate cancer, with a Gleason score of 6. The pre-PSA era data are those reported by Albertsen et al. (1), and the data from the PSA era are those modeled by Nicholson and Harland (12).

3. Watchful waiting is not the same as active surveillance. The Scandinavian trial compared surgery versus watchful waiting (with delayed hormone treatment for symptomatic progression). There remain no completed clinical trials to date comparing surgery versus active surveillance (with radical treatment targeted to those with biochemical or histologic progression). The Scandinavian trial results have proven that radical treatment for all is more effective than radical treatment for none. It remains possible that targeting radical treatment to those who are most likely to benefit would be just as effective as treating all comers, while reducing the burden of side effects from unnecessary intervention.

In light of the above, traditional watchful waiting remains a valid treatment option for men with asymptomatic localized prostate cancer who consider the benefit of treatment to be outweighed by the risk of harm.

It is an attractive option for men with low-grade (Gleason score ≤3 + 4) prostate cancer who have a life expectancy of less than 10 years (by virtue of age or comorbidities). It is also a valid choice for younger, fitter men with an extreme aversion to the risks of incontinence and impotence associated with radical treatment, and who place little value on their longevity.

Active Surveillance

The concept of active surveillance was first described by Choo et al. (7) from Toronto. From 1995 onward, they recruited 299 patients with stage T1/2a disease, Gleason score <3 + 4, and PSA <15 to a prospective study of active surveillance.

Patients were monitored with PSA assay and digital rectal examination (DRE) every 3 months for 2 years and then every 6 months if PSA was stable. Ten to twelve core biopsies were repeated at 1 year and then every 3 years until the age of 80. Patients were free to choose radical treatment at any point. Radical treatment was advised if the PSA doubling time was less than 3 years, or if the repeat biopsies showed an upgrading to Gleason 7 (4 + 3) or higher. With a median follow-up of 5 years, 198 patients are still on surveillance and 101 patients have had interventions. Forty-four patients (15%) had a PSA doubling time less than 3 years, nine patients (3%) had clinical progression, 12 patients (4%) had histological upgrading on repeat biopsy, and 36 patients (12%) elected to have radical treatment without having fulfilled any of the criteria for disease progression. Two of the 299 patients have died of prostate cancer and disease-specific survival at 8 years is 99.2% (8). It is interesting to compare the 8-year disease-specific mortality of just 1% with the 10-year disease-specific mortality of 15% for traditional watchful waiting in the Scandinavian trial.

A similar prospective cohort study of active surveillance is being conducted at the Royal Marsden Hospital (United Kingdom). The study opened in 2002, and has recruited 300 patients with untreated, clinically localized, low to intermediate-risk prostate cancer. They have been followed using frequent serum PSA monitoring and with repeat prostate biopsy performed after 18 to 24 months. The repeat biopsy results on the first 119 patients were presented at the American Society of Clinical Oncology (ASCO) Prostate Cancer Symposium in 2006. For the purposes of the analysis, histological disease progression on repeat biopsy was arbitrarily defined as either primary Gleason grade ≥ 4, or positive cores >50%, or an increase in GS from ≤ 6 to ≥ 7. Histological disease progression on repeat biopsy was seen in 33 of the 119 cases (28%). Of these, 21 cases were upgraded, and 12 had >50% of the repeat biopsy cores involved. On multivariate analysis, significant predictors of disease progression were PSA density and PSA velocity.

It is noteworthy that PSA density, derived from the initial PSA level at the time of diagnosis, was the single most important predictor of adverse findings at repeat biopsy performed 18 to 24 months later. This suggests that sampling error on the original diagnostic biopsy may be a significant cause of so-called histological disease progression.

In light of these observations, there is a good case for immediate, rather than delayed, repeat biopsy in patients who wish to pursue active surveillance for apparently low-risk disease based on T stage, Gleason score, and PSA level, but who have a PSA density greater than 0.2 ng/mL/mL. Conversely, it is possible that patients with a favorable PSA density (e.g., less than 0.15 ng/mL/mL) and PSA velocity (e.g., less than 0.5 ng/mL/yr) could be managed by active surveillance without the need for repeat biopsies.

Several other smaller active surveillance series have been reported, which confirm the feasibility of this approach to the management of favorable-risk localized prostate cancer. These studies differ from one another in relation to patient eligibility, methods of monitoring, and indications for intervention,

TABLE 18.4.1. Authors' current approach to active surveillance

Eligibility
    Clinical stage T1/T2a
    Gleason score ≤7 (3 + 4)
    PSA ≤15
    Less than 50% of the biopsies positive (minimum of 10 cores)
    PSA density ≤0.25 ng/mL/mL
Monitoring
    Serum PSA and DRE every 3 months for the first 2 years
    Repeat biopsy at 1 year, and then every 2 years
    Serum PSA and DRE every 6 months after 2 years
Indications for radical treatment
    PSA velocity >1 ng/mL/year (based on minimum of four PSA values)
    Gleason score ≥4 + 3, or >50% cores involved on repeat biopsy

which serves to emphasize that there is no consensus on the optimum method of active surveillance. In the absence of a good evidence base, Table 18.4.1 summarizes our own current approach to active surveillance, which is necessarily modified in individual cases according to life expectancy and patient wishes. Ultimately, the choice between observation on the one hand, or radical treatment on the other, cannot be reduced to a formula based on cancer characteristics, and needs to be considered in the context of the individual patient's values.

Ongoing Randomized Trials of Expectant Management

Three ongoing randomized trials aim to compare definitive treatment with expectant management in PSA screen-detected disease. The Prostate Cancer Intervention Versus Observation Trial (PIVOT) compares radical prostatectomy versus watchful waiting and has completed enrollment with 731 patients (9). The Prostate Testing for Cancer and Treatment (ProtecT) study compares radical prostatectomy, external beam radiotherapy and active monitoring, and aims to recruit over 2000 patients (10). The National Cancer Institute of Canada (NCIC) PR11 trial compares immediate radical treatment versus active surveillance and opened in 2006. The results of these trials will be critically important in helping to determine the relative merits of definitive treatment and expectant management of early prostate cancer.

    The PIVOT trial is in many ways similar to the Scandinavian trial of radical prostatectomy versus watchful waiting, but in a different patient population. On the one hand, PIVOT will likely include a greater proportion of men with PSA screen-detected cancers with a more favorable natural history and less potential to benefit from definitive treatment. On the other hand, patients with high-grade disease for whom the opposite is true were eligible for PIVOT, but not for the Scandinavian trial. One important limitation of PIVOT is that the approach to expectant management, with palliative treatment for symptomatic progression, is very different from expectant management as it is now widely practiced, with radical treatment for those patients with biochemical or histological progression. If radical treatment for all turns out to improve survival compared with radical treatment for none, it will beg the question as to whether radical treatment for some, selected for example according to PSA kinetics, would have been as effective but less morbid.

The ProtecT study opened in 1999, supported by the U.K. Department of Health, and was expected to recruit over 2000 patients by 2006—an outstanding achievement. It promises to be the single most important trial comparing expectant management and definitive treatment of PSA screen-detected prostate cancer. The active monitoring arm of the trial might be considered intermediate between traditional watchful waiting and active surveillance. Patients randomized to active monitoring are followed with PSA tests every 3 months in the first year and then every 3 to 6 months. Repeat prostate biopsies are not routinely performed. Prostate-specific antigen progression is suspected if there is a 50% increase in PSA within any 12-month period.

Suspected progression will prompt restaging investigations, and the decision whether to proceed to curative treatment will be "based on full participant information and joint decision-making." It will be interesting to see what proportion of patients in the active monitoring arm do proceed to curative treatment. A 50% increase in PSA within 12 months is the equivalent of a PSA doubling time of shorter than 20 months. Only a very small proportion of patients with localized prostate cancer have such a rapid rate of rise of PSA (7), suggesting that this active monitoring policy may be similar in effect to traditional watchful waiting.

The NCIC PR11 trial aims to recruit up to 2000 men with low-risk localized prostate cancer to be randomized between immediate radical treatment and active surveillance. The surveillance policy is based on the Toronto experience described earlier. Patients randomized to immediate radical treatment, and those with disease progression on the surveillance arm of the trial, will have a choice between radical prostatectomy or radical radiotherapy.

Future Directions

At present, there is no consensus on the optimum approach to expectant management. Uncertainties include the frequency of PSA testing, the need for repeat biopsies, the role of imaging investigations, and the criteria used to define disease progression requiring radical treatment. As the approach to active surveillance is optimized, so our ability to target treatment to those who stand to benefit should improve. In the future, one can envisage that active surveillance could be combined with low-toxicity interventions designed not to eradicate the disease but to alter its natural history. This is an attractive possibility, not least because incidental prostate cancer is an extremely common postmortem finding even in those countries with the lowest rates of clinically significant disease (11), suggesting that environmental factors, such as diet, may influence prostate cancer progression, rather than initiation. Nutritional interventions require further study, but could become a middle way between definitive treatment and traditional approaches to expectant management.

The long-standing debate concerning the relative merits of expectant management and definitive intervention rests to a large extent on the extraordinary degree of interpatient variation in prostate cancer behavior, together with our inability to predict that behavior in individual cases. While we know beyond reasonable doubt that half the men diagnosed with early prostate cancer do not need treatment, at present we do not know which half. As our understanding of the molecular pathology of prostate cancer advances, it is likely that we will identify new and better predictors of prostate cancer behavior.

In the long-term, the use of such biological predictors could revolutionize our ability to select patients for definitive treatment, on the one hand, or expectant management, on the other.

Acknowledgments. This work was undertaken at the Royal Marsden National Health Service (NHS) Trust, which received a proportion of its funding from the NHS Executive. The views expressed in this publication are those of the authors and not necessarily those of the NHS Executive. This work was supported by the Institute of Cancer Research, the Cancer Research UK Section of Radiotherapy (CUK) grant C46/A2131, and National Cancer Research Institute (NCRI) South of England Prostate Cancer Collaborative.

References

1. Albertsen P, Gleason D, Barry M. Competing risk analysis of men aged 55 to 74 years at diagnosis managed conservatively for clinically localized prostate cancer. JAMA 1998;280(11):975–980.
2. Bill-Axelson A, Holmberg L, Ruutu M, et al. Radical prostatectomy versus watchful waiting in early prostate cancer. N Engl J Med 2005;352(19):1977–1984.
3. Holmberg L, Bill-Axelson A, Helgesen F, et al. A randomized trial comparing radical prostatectomy with watchful waiting in early prostate cancer. N Engl J Med 2002; 347(11):781–789.
4. Steineck G, Helgesen F, Adolfsson J, et al. Quality of life after radical prostatectomy or watchful waiting. N Engl J Med 2002;347(11):790–796.
5. Singer PA, Tasch ES, Stocking C, et al. Sex or survival: trade-offs between quality and quantity of life. J Clin Oncol 1991;9(2):328–334.
6. Draisma G, Boer R, Otto S, et al. Lead times and overdetection due to prostate-specific antigen screening: estimates from the European Randomized Study of Screening for Prostate Cancer. J Natl Cancer Inst 2003;95(12):868–878.
7. Choo R, DeBoer G, Klotz L, et al. PSA Doubling time of prostate carcinoma managed with watchful observation alone. Int J Radiat Oncol Biol Phys 2001;50(3):615–620.
8. Klotz L. Active surveillance with selective delayed intervention using PSA doubling time for good risk prostate cancer. Eur Urol 2005;47(1):16–21.

9. Wilt TJ, Brawer MK. The Prostate Cancer Intervention Versus Observation Trial (PIVOT). A randomized trial comparing radical prostatectomy versus expectant management for the treatment of clinically localised prostate cancer. Cancer 1995; 75(suppl 7):1963–1968.

10. Donovan J, Hamdy F, Neal D, et al. Prostate Testing for Cancer and Treatment (ProtecT) feasibility study. Health Technol Assess 2003;7(14):1–88.

11. Yatani R, Shiraishi T, Nakakuki K, et al. Trends in frequency of latent prostate carcinoma in Japan from 1965–1979 to 1982–1986. J Natl Cancer Inst 1988;80(9): 683–687.

12. Nicholson PW, Harland SJ. Survival prospects after screen-detection of prostate cancer. BJU Int 2002;90(7):686–693.

18.5
Radiation Therapy for Clinically Localized Prostate Cancer

Michael A. Papagikos and W. Robert Lee

Radiation therapy (RT) is one of the two main local treatments for clinically localized prostate cancer; radical prostatectomy (RP) is the other. The treatment options that are available for a particular patient are extensive and can include expectant management, RP, external beam radiation therapy (EBRT), interstitial brachytherapy (IB), androgen deprivation therapy (ADT), or any combination of these.

This chapter discusses the role of radiation therapy in the management of clinically localized prostate cancer as definitive therapy and as an adjuvant therapy following RP. Expectant management, surgery, and management of metastatic disease are discussed in Chapters 18.3 and 18.4.

Statement of Data

Randomized clinical trials (RCTs) are the gold standard of evidence-based medicine, and special emphasis is given to data from RCTs, when available. When it is not available, retrospective data will be provided along with appropriate cautions regarding interpretation. The RCTs have been reported addressing the role of radiation dose escalation, the addition and timing of androgen deprivation therapy to radiation, and postoperative radiation. No RCT of RT versus surgery or external radiation versus brachytherapy has been reported.

Risk Group Definitions

A number of variables have been consistently reported as independent predictors of biochemical relapse-free survival (BRFS) following radiation therapy (EBRT or IB) for clinically localized prostate cancer. These variables include Gleason score, pretreatment prostate-specific antigen (PSA) level, and clinical T stage. These variables have been combined by various authors to form risk groupings that predict BRFS. The most commonly used risk stratification

TABLE 18.5.1. D'Amico risk group definitions

Risk group	Combination of pretreatment variables
Low	≤T2a and PSA <10 ng/mL and GS ≤6
Intermediate	T2b or PSA 10–20 ng/mL or GS =7
High	≥T2c or PSA >20 ng/mL or GS ≥8

schema was first described by D'Amico et al. (1). Patients are classified as low, intermediate, or high risk (Table 18.5.1). This classification has been shown to provide accurate assessments of BRFS for patients regardless of treatment (RP, EBRT, or IB) and to correlate with prostate cancer specific survival. When possible, the results of radiation therapy will be discussed in the context of these risk groupings.

Biochemical Relapse-Free Survival as an End Point and American Society of Therapeutic Radiology and Oncology Criterion

Due to the long natural history of prostate cancer, it is difficult to demonstrate a beneficial effect of any therapeutic intervention. D'Amico et al. (2) quantified prostate cancer–specific mortality (PCSM) in men with clinically localized T1–2 prostate cancer treated with RP or EBRT in the PSA era. This analysis included more than 7000 men from 44 different institutions. The rate of PCSM was dependent on risk groupings and primary treatment. In men treated with EBRT and with low-risk disease, the 8-year rate of PCSM was <5% and approximately 10% for intermediate risk patients. If aggressive local therapy is to impact survival, especially for low-risk patients, large patient numbers with long follow-up will be required. Additionally, many men are diagnosed with prostate cancer beyond the age of 65 and thus have competing medical comorbidities, likely making detection of treatment-related improvements difficult. More than 50% of men treated in Radiation Therapy Oncology Group (RTOG) prostate trials between 1975 and 1992 died of nonprostate causes. For these reasons, researchers have sought a surrogate for survival when conducting clinical research. Using the posttreatment PSA level as a surrogate has gained acceptance, and the BRFS is the most commonly reported end point used. The American Society of Therapeutic Radiology and Oncology (ASTRO) convened a consensus panel to discuss the role of PSA measurements after radiotherapy. The result of this conference was the publication of the ASTRO Consensus Definition (ACD) of biochemical failure. The ACD defines biochemical failure as three consecutive rises from the nadir value, and the time to failure is defined as the midpoint between the nadir value and the first rise. This definition has its strengths and weaknesses and has not been universally adopted; however, most researchers report their findings using this definition, and this chapter relies on the ACD unless stated otherwise.

External Beam Radiation Therapy Monotherapy

Patient Selection

External beam radiation therapy as monotherapy is appropriate for most men with low-risk disease and some men with intermediate-risk disease. It is not appropriate for men with high-risk or locally advanced cancer.

International Commission of Radiation Units and Measurements Target Definition

The gross tumor volume (GTV) is defined as the tumor that is palpable or visible on imaging. The clinical target volume (CTV) includes the GTV plus any additional areas that are thought to be at risk for microscopic involvement (i.e., seminal vesicles, pelvic lymph nodes). The planning target volume (PTV) includes the CTV plus an expansion to account for organ motion and daily setup uncertainties (Table 18.5.2).

Many clinicians use nonuniform margins with the smallest CTV to PTV margins posteriorly in the vicinity of the rectum. A variety of beam arrangements have been described ranging from a coplanar, four-field technique to a non-coplanar seven-field approach. Immobilization devices are commonly used to decrease setup error, reducing the CTV to PTV margin. In an attempt to reduce the CTV to PTV margin further, a number of investigators have localized the prostate daily prior to delivering treatment. Common techniques include transabdominal ultrasound localization of the prostate and the use of implanted fiducial markers.

Three-Dimensional Conformal Radiation Therapy

Three-dimensional conformal radiation therapy (3D-CRT) requires a computed tomography (CT) scan of the treatment area and specialized treatment planning software. The basic process involves obtaining a CT scan with the patients immobilized in the treatment position. The prostate and surrounding tissues are then segmented, and the data are reconstructed into high-resolution 3D images. This method gives the radiation oncologist the ability to use beam's eye view (BEV) planning, and optimizes the radiation field size shape and gantry/table angles. Numerous reports have been published that document the outcome

TABLE 18.5.2. Volume recommendations of the International Commission of Radiation Units and Measurements (ICRU Report 50)

Parameter	Definition
Gross tumor volume (GTV)	Palpable or visible extent of tumor
Clinical target volume (CTV)	GTV + margin for subclinical disease
Planning target volume (PTV)	CTV + margin for organ motion and daily setup error

TABLE 18.5.3. Therapy for T1-2 prostate cancer according to prognostic group

Author	No. of patients	Treatment dates	Median follow-up (years)	Median dose (Gy)	Prognostic group	5-year BRFS
Shipley	1765	1988–1995	4.1	69.4	I	81
					II	69
					III	47
					IV	29
Zelefsky	743	1988–1995	3	75.6	Favorable	85
					Intermediate	65
					Unfavorable	35
Kupelian	628	1990–1998	4.3	70.2	Favorable	90 (8-yr)
					Unfavorable	59 (8-yr)
D'Amico	381	1988–2000	3.8	70.4	Low	78
					Intermediate <34%	65
					Intermediate ≥34%	35
					High	40

of patients with localized prostate cancer managed with this technique (Table 18.5.3). Summarizing this information, it is clear that pretreatment variables can be combined to create prognostic groups. In men with favorable risk disease, EBRT is associated with 5-year BRFS of 78% to 90%. Men with intermediate- and high-risk features experience 5-year BRFS of approximately 65% and 35%, respectively. The use of EBRT alone to conventional doses (70 Gy) appears insufficient in men with T1–2 disease and intermediate- or high-risk features.

External Beam Dose Escalation

With the evolution from two-dimensional treatment planning to 3D-CRT, data have emerged that support the concept that higher radiation doses yield better clinical outcomes with acceptable toxicity profiles. Three RCTs have addressed the role of external beam dose escalation.

The study by Shipley et al. (3) included only men with locally advanced disease. This study spanned the development of PSA, and as such PSA was not part of the stratification process. All patients were clinically staged T3-4 and all received 50.4 Gy of pelvic radiation followed by a proton boost. Proton radiation oncology group (PROG) 95-09 included T1b-T2b stage disease with PSA values <15 ng/mL (4). All patients received 50.4 Gy via photons to the prostate and seminal vesicles followed by a prostate-only boost. Androgen deprivation therapy was not allowed prior to biochemical recurrence.

It is important to note that this study did not include any stage T3 patients, and only 8% would be classified high-risk using the D'Amico classification. Subset analysis by risk group was performed for low- and intermediate-risk groups, and the absolute magnitude of benefit was identical.

A more mature RCT investigating dose escalation was reported by Pollack et al. (5) from the M.D. Anderson Cancer Center. Patients with T1-3 disease were included. Again it should be noted that this study was primarily of intermediate-risk patients, with only 20% of patients entered having clinically staged T3 disease. The utilization of intensity modulated radiation therapy (IMRT) is increasing dramatically. This technique enables significant dose escalation to doses ranging from 76 to 86 Gy. None of the above studies incorporated IMRT as a means of escalating the dose to the prostate, and randomized trials with adequate follow-up and attention to toxicity will be needed before such high doses can routinely be recommended.

Intensity Modulated Radiation Therapy

Intensity modulated radiation therapy is a type of 3D-CRT that relies on volumetric imaging to deliver thousands of tiny radiation beamlets that enter the body from many angles and all intersect at the tumor. The intensity of each beamlet (as opposed to each beam in standard 3D-CRT) can be controlled, and thus the radiation dose can conform around normal tissue, create concave shapes, and have rapid falloff turning corners. The aim is to deliver a higher radiation dose to a tumor with less damage to nearby healthy tissue. The improved conformality of IMRT compared to 3D-CRT offers the possibility of further dose escalation without an increase in normal tissue injury.

One of the largest experiences with this new approach has been described by Zelefsky et al. (6). In this report, the early toxicity and biochemical results from 772 men treated at one hospital between 1996 and 2001 are outlined. Ninety percent of these men were treated to a dose of 81 Gy and 10% were treated to 86.4 Gy.

The late rectal and urinary toxicity was much lower than expected. The actuarial probability of grade 2 or greater rectal toxicity was 4%, while the analogous rate of grade 2 or greater urinary toxicity was 15%, with most of the urinary toxicity manifest as urethra symptoms requiring medication.

Although the follow-up is relatively short (24 months), the BRFS is encouraging. The 3-year rate of BRFS is 92%, 86%, and 81% for the low-, intermediate-, and high-risk groups, respectively. Preliminary results from other institutions are available, but longer follow-up is required to assess 5- to 10-year BRFS and long-term morbidity.

Complications

The complications of EBRT for prostate cancer depend on the dose and volume of tissue irradiated. The four main categories of complications are gastrointestinal, urinary, sexual, and other, and these each are divided into acute and late phases.

Acute intestinal toxicity can manifest during RT as enteritis and is dependent on the volume of bowel irradiated with symptoms resolving typically by 6 weeks.

Symptoms (diarrhea, tenesmus, rectal/anal strictures, and/or hematochezia) will persist in approximately 3% and be labeled chronic radiation proctitis.

Acute urinary toxicity (urinary frequency, dysuria, and urgency) manifests in most patients during RT and usually resolves by 3 weeks after completion. Late genitourinary (GU) toxicity is rare with modern techniques, with approximately 5% of men developing urethral stricture, cystitis, hematuria, or bladder spasm. About half of late GU toxicities are strictures that can be managed with outpatient dilatation. The rate of urinary incontinence has been reported at 0.3% following RT.

Sexual function following treatment of prostate cancer depends on the treatment, baseline potency, and age of the patient. Modern series have reported that approximately one third of men who are potent pre-RT develop impotency after RT, with the frequency increasing over time.

Radiation-induced secondary malignancies are potentially the most important complication following EBRT to the prostate. The incidence of rectal cancer is increased in men treated with EBRT compared to men treated with radical prostatectomy. This increased risk is equivalent to having a first-degree relative diagnosed with rectal cancer. Radiation-induced bladder cancers and sarcomas are also possible.

Combined Modality Therapy (External Beam Radiation Therapy and Androgen Deprivation Therapy)

There is a large and growing body of evidence to suggest that biochemical outcomes as well as overall survival are improved when radiation therapy is combined with ADT. The details and results of the following RCTs are detailed in Table 18.5.4:

TABLE 18.5.4. Randomized controlled trials of external beam radiation therapy (EBRT) and androgen deprivation therapy (ADT)

Study	n	Length of ADT (months)	RT (Gy)	Median follow-up (years)	Results
EORTC	415	36 vs 0	50 WP 70 P	5.5	5-yr OS increased from 62% to 78% with ADT
85–31	977	24 vs 0	44–46 WP 65–70 P	7.6	10-yr OS increased from 39% to 49% with ADT
86–10	471	4 vs 0	44–46 WP 65–70 P	6.7	Improved PCSM; OS benefit only for GS ≤6 with ADT
D'Amico	206	6 vs 0	70 P	4.5	5-yr OS increased from 78% to 88% with ADT
92–02	1554	28 vs 4	44–46 WP 65–70 P	5.8	Improved BRFS; OS benefit only seen for GS ≥8 with LTAD

BRFS, biochemical relapse-free survival; LTAD, long term androgen deprivation; OS, overall survival; P, prostate; PCSM, prostate cancer specific mortality; WP, whole pelvis.

1. RTOG 86-10: Eligibility included patients with T2-4 disease with or without positive pelvic lymph nodes.
2. RTOG 85-31: Inclusion criteria included clinical T3 disease or regional lymphatic involvement or pathologic T3a or T3b disease postprostatectomy.
3. European Organization for Research and Treatment of Cancer (EORTC): The EORTC study included high-grade T1-2 or T3/T4 disease. Approximately 90% of the patients had ≥T3 disease and 10% had high-grade T1-2 disease.
4. RTOG 92-02: Patients with T2c-4 disease and PSA <150 ng/mL were eligible. Fifty-five percent of patients had ≥T3 disease with a median PSA of 20 ng/mL.
5. D'Amico: This single-institution RCT included men with PSA >10 ng/mL, or GS ≥7, or had radiographic evidence of extraprostatic disease.

Interstitial Brachytherapy

Brachytherapy is a general term used to describe the placement of a radioactive source(s) into or near a tumor. The source can be placed permanently or reside temporarily. The present widespread utilization of permanent prostate brachytherapy is the result of prostate screening and improved technology that currently allows for an outpatient procedure that generally can be accomplished in 1 to 2 hours.

Low Dose Rate Monotherapy

Treatment Planning

Brachytherapy treatment planning determines the optimal radiation dose distribution for an individual patient, depending on the size and shape of the prostate gland. Most practitioners use a peripheral loading scheme to reduce the dose to the urethra and maximize the dose to the peripheral zone. Transrectal ultrasound images are generally used for treatment planning. The two radioisotopes most commonly used are iodine 125 and palladium 103. Each of these isotopes possesses a low dose rate and low energy relative to the isotope used for temporary brachytherapy (iridium 192). The radiation dose prescribed differs according to the isotope and whether brachytherapy is used alone (monotherapy) or combined with external beam radiation therapy (combined modality therapy, CMT) (Table 18.5.5).

TABLE 18.5.5. Prescription doses (Gy) for permanent prostate brachytherapy (PPB) according to isotope

Radioisotope	Dose (Gy) PPB alone	Dose (Gy) PPB plus EBRT*
Iodine 125	144	100–110
Palladium 103	115–125	80–90

EBRT, external beam radiation therapy.
*Combined with EBRT (40–50 Gy).

The low energy of the sources simplifies radiation protection precautions, and patients can be discharged from the hospital immediately.

Source Placement

The radioactive sources are usually placed transperineally using some form of perineal template and ultrasound guidance, although magnetic resonance (MR)-guided and computed tomography (CT)-guided approaches have been described. Close monitoring of the source deposition process enables the operator to recognize and adjust for changes that may occur intraoperatively (prostate gland movement, prostate gland swelling, and source movement).

Postimplant Evaluation

Some form of postprocedure dosimetric evaluation is mandatory. Most investigators use CT for this assessment. Commercially available software is available to import CT images and outline the prostate gland and nearby structures (urethra, rectum, penile bulb, etc.). Based on the delineation of the prostate and the location of the sources, isodose distributions can be calculated and dose-volume histograms created. A standard definition of a good implant has yet to be universally accepted by the brachytherapy community. There is early evidence that delivering at least 90% of the prescription dose to 90% of the prostate gland results in improved biochemical relapse-free survival. Although preliminary work is emerging, acceptable doses to normal tissues (urethra, rectum, penile bulb) are much less clear.

Complications

Toxicity from prostate brachytherapy is mainly gastrointestinal (GI) and GU in nature. Acute GU complications include urinary frequency, urgency, and dysuria, and these symptoms tend to occur several days following the implant, with prior transurethral resection of the prostate (TURP) and large gland size increasing this risk.

Approximately 5% to 10% of men develop acute urinary retention requiring catheterization. Late toxicity can include any of the following: impotence, urinary incontinence or retention, persistent irritative symptoms, rectal urgency, bowel frequency, rectal bleeding, rectal ulceration, and prostatorectal fistula. The incidence of persistent urinary retention requiring self-catheterization is 1% to 5%. Physician-reported potency retention is approximately 85% following prostate brachytherapy (PB), with patient-reported results in the 50% range.

Combined External Beam Radiation Therapy and Brachytherapy

Brachytherapy has been combined with EBRT in the treatment of pelvic cancers for many decades. The combination has been used in the treatment of prostate cancer, but the vast majority of published results include only patients with low- and intermediate-risk features. Retrospective data have suggested that

TABLE 18.5.6. Biochemical relapse-free survival following PPB combined with EBRT for T1–2 prostate cancer

Author	No. of patients	Isotope(s)	Implant dose (Gy)	EBRT dose	EBRT fields	Follow-up (years)	BRFS (year)
Ragde	82	^{125}I	110	45 Gy	4-field: P-SV	10	79% (10)
Blasko	231	^{125}I	110	45 Gy	4-field: P-SV	5	79% (9)
Lederman	348	^{125}I	110	45 Gy	4-field	4	77% (6)
		^{103}Pd	90				
Critz	689	^{125}I	120	45 Gy	P-SV-PPT	4	88% (6)
Dattoli	124	^{103}Pd	90	41 Gy	Limited pelvic	3.8	76% (4)

monotherapy with low dose rate (LDR) brachytherapy is inferior to EBRT or radical prostatectomy (RP) for high-risk patients and has not been advocated for this patients population.

The results from five centers with a significant experience with combined modality therapy [permanent prostate brachytherapy (PPB) plus EBRT] are outlined in Table 18.5.6. All patients in these reports were treated after 1986 and have had continuous PSA follow-up available. The closed transperineal method of PPB was used in all cases. Three reports originate from centers where combined modality therapy (CMT) is used in all prostate cancer cases and two are from institutions that select CMT for higher risk patients, reserving PPB alone for patients with low risk disease.

Ragde et al. (7)

All men were treated between January 1987 and December 1989 so that the follow-up is quite long (median 122 months). These patients were selected for CMT based on high-risk features. The vast majority of men (84%) had palpable disease, although only four men were felt to have clinical extracapsular disease (T3). The mean PSA in this group was 14.7 ng/Ml, and 18 men (24%) had a Gleason score above 6. Androgen deprivation therapy was not used.

Blasko et al. (8)

The median follow-up was 58 months. During this period some men were treated with monotherapy, and the use of supplemental EBRT was at the discretion of the physician. The mean PSA was 15.6 ng/mL and 35% or patients presented with a Gleason score above 7. No patients received ADT. The results of BRFS were provided according to the prognostic groupings of Zelefsky. In this report the authors compared the results with CMT to monotherapy according to risk group and found no group that benefited from the addition of EBRT.

Lederman et al. (9)

In this report PPB was performed prior to EBRT. No patient received ADT. The median follow-up was 44 months. One hundred sixty-four (47%) men had a pretreatment PSA above 10 ng/mL and 119 (34%) were assigned a Gleason score between 7 and 10. Only 17 (4.9%) men had T3 disease. The ACD was not used to define BRFS. Instead, biochemical failure was defined as the use of ADT anytime following treatment, or a serum PSA >5.0 ng/mL at last follow-up, or two consecutive rises in serum PSA greater than 0.5 ng/mL. The authors divided patients into risk groups according to pretreatment PSA, T stage, and Gleason score.

Radiotherapy Clinics of Georgia: Critz et al. (10)

The median follow-up was 4 years. Twenty-eight men (4%) had a Gleason score above 7 and 44 (6%) had a pretreatment PSA above 20. No patient received ADT. As is the custom with these investigators, the ACD was not used to calculate BRFS. Instead, an absolute value of ≤0.2 was used to define cure. Patients are censored if the PSA is declining (but not ≤0.2) at the time of analysis.

Dattoli et al. (11)

This reports includes only patients with high-risk features. The PPB was performed 4 weeks following EBRT. The median follow-up for non-failing patients was 7 years. Approximately 25% of patients had a pretreatment PSA above 20. Approximately 20% of the patients were assigned a Gleason score above 7. The ACD was not used to calculate BRFS. Instead, a PSA level of ≤0.2 ng/mL defined the absence of disease (11).

Summary of Studies

Although the amount of information is small it appears that patients with favorable and intermediate-risk disease do well with CMT but patients with high-risk features do not fare nearly as well suggesting that they may benefit from effective systemic therapy combined with local therapy.

Postprostatectomy External Beam Radiation Therapy

Approximately 80,000 to 100,000 RPs are performed in the United States each year, and 30,000 of these patients have a PSA failure. Sixty-five percent will develop bone metastases by 10 years without any salvage therapy (12).

Approximately one third of the clinically staged T1 or T2 tumors will be upstaged (i.e., to pT3) after RP. The PSA should be undetectable by 1 to 2 months post-RP and there is a positive biopsy rate as high as 40% if PSA is detectable. A PSA elevation predates clinical recurrence by several years, with the median time from PSA rise to palpable disease of 7 to 9 years. A PSA reduction occurs in 80% of patients treated with EBRT after RP and remains undetectable in 30% to 50%. There are two approaches to postprostatectomy radiotherapy: salvage and adjuvant.

The risk factors for distant failure after prostatectomy include the following:

High grade
PSA nadir that does not reach zero
Rapid PSA doubling time (PSADT)
Short disease-free interval
Negative surgical margins

The risk factors for local failure after prostatectomy include the following:

Low grade
PSA nadir of zero
Slow PSADT
Long disease-free interval
Positive surgical margins

Adjuvant External Beam Radiation Therapy

Adjuvant EBRT is delivered soon after radical prostatectomy based on adverse pathologic factors such as positive margins, extracapsular extension, and seminal vesicle involvement. The EORTC performed an RCT of observation versus immediate RT for high-risk postprostatectomy prostate cancer patients (13). Eligibility included clinical T1–3N0M0, age <75 years old and a good performance status. Pathologic risk factors were capsule invasion, positive margins, or seminal vesicle invasion (SVI). External beam radiation therapy (60 Gy) had to start within 4 months of surgery. A total of 1005 patients accrued between 1992 and 2001 with a median age of 65, median pretreatment PSA of 12.3, and median postoperative PSA of 0.2. The 5-year BRFS rate was 74% versus 53% in favor of RT ($p < .0001$). Clinical progression free survival (PFS) and local control were also improved with RT. Further follow-up is needed to determine an effect on overall survival.

Salvage

Salvage radiation therapy is given in response to a rising PSA after radical prostatectomy. Stephenson et al. (14) performed a retrospective review of 501 patients who received salvage RT for rising PSA after RP from 1987 to 2002. All patients were thought to have local failure (21% had biopsy proven local disease). One third of patients never reached an undetectable PSA following surgery. The median RT dose was 64.8 Gy, with 17% receiving neoadjuvant ADT. The median follow-up time was 45 months. Biochemical failure (BF) was defined as PSA >0.1 over the nadir confirmed by a second and increasing PSA. Fifty percent of patients developed disease progression, 10% developed distant metastases, 4% died from prostate cancer, and 4% dead from other causes. The 4-year PFS rate was 45%. Multivariate analysis showed GS 8 to 10, pre-RT PSA level >2 ng/mL, negative surgical margins, SVI, and PSADT <10 months to all be independently associated with an increased risk of PSA progression following salvage RT. A patient with no adverse features based on the above factors has a 77% 4-year PFS rate. This drops to 12% for those with the highest risk factors.

Conclusion

External beam radiation therapy alone (utilizing 3D-CRT or IMRT techniques) or permanent prostate brachytherapy are acceptable treatments for men with low-risk prostate cancer. Randomized clinical trials support the use of higher than conventional doses (>70 Gy) in men treated with EBRT. Randomized trials support the use of ADT plus EBRT in men with high-risk disease. Randomized clinical trials support the use of postprostatectomy RT in men with adverse pathologic risk factors.

References

1. D'Amico AV, Schultz D, Loffredo M, et al. Biochemical outcome following external beam radiation therapy with or without androgen suppression therapy for clinically localized prostate cancer. JAMA 2000;284(10):1280–1283.
2. D'Amico AV, Moul J, Carroll PR, et al. Cancer-specific mortality after surgery or radiation for patients with clinically localized prostate cancer managed during the prostate-specific antigen era. J Clin Oncol 2003;21(11):2163–2172.
3. Shipley WU, Thames HD, Sandler HM, et al. Radiation therapy for clinically localized prostate cancer: a multi-institutional pooled analysis. JAMA 1999;281(17): 1598–1604.
4. Zietman AL, DeSilvio ML, Slater JD, et al. Comparison of conventional-dose vs high-dose conformal radiation therapy in clinically localized adenocarcinoma of the prostate: a randomized controlled trial. JAMA 2005;294(10):1233–1239.
5. Pollack A, Zagars GK, Starkschall G, et al. Prostate cancer radiation dose response: results of the M. D. Anderson phase III randomized trial. Int J Radiat Oncol Biol Phys 2002;53:1097–1105.
6. Zelefsky MJ, Fuks Z, Hunt M, et al. High-dose intensity modulated radiation therapy for prostate cancer: early toxicity and biochemical outcome in 772 patients. Int J Radiat Oncol Biol Phys 2002;53(5):1111–1116.
7. Ragde H, Korb LJ, Elgamal AA, Grado GL, Nadir BS. Modern prostate brachytherapy. Prostate specific antigen results in 219 patients with up to 12 years of observed follow-up. Cancer 2000;89(1):135–141.
8. Blasko JC, Grimm PD, Sylsvester JE, Cavanagh W. The role of external beam radiotherapy with I-125/Pd-103 brachytherapy for prostate carcinoma. Radiother Oncol 2000;57(3):273–278.
9. Lederman GS, Cavanagh W, Albert PS, et al. Retrospective stratification of a consecutive cohort of prostate cancer patients treated with a combined regimen of external-beam radiotherapy and brachytherapy. Int J Radiat Oncol Biol Phys 2001;49(5): 1297–1303.
10. Critz FA, Williams WH, Levinson AK, et al. Simultaneous irradiation for prostate cancer: intermediate results with modern techniques. J Urol 2000;164(3 pt 1): 738–741.
11. Dattoli M, Wallner K, True L, Cash J, Sorace R. Long-term outcomes after treatment with external beam radiation therapy and palladium 103 for patients with higher risk prostate carcinoma: influence of prostatic acid phosphatase. Cancer 2003;97(4): 979–983.

12. Pound CR, Partin AW, Eisenberger MA, et al. Natural history of progression after PSA elevation following radical prostatectomy. JAMA 1999;281(17):1591–1597.
13. Bolla M, van Poppel H, Collette L, et al. Postoperative radiotherapy after radical prostatectomy: a randomised controlled trial (EORTC trial 22911). Lancet 2005; 366(9485):572–578.
14. Stephenson AJ, Shariat SF, Zelefsky MJ, et al. Salvage radiotherapy for recurrent prostate cancer after radical prostatectomy. JAMA 2004;291(11):1325–1332.

18.6
Endocrine Manipulation

Shandra S. Wilson and E. David Crawford

Androgen Deprivation Therapy

Charles B. Huggins won the Nobel Prize in medicine in 1966 for establishing the relationship between testosterone and prostate cancer. Since then, androgen deprivation therapy (ADT) and its apoptotic effect on the prostate epithelium have continued to be an important component in the adjuvant as well as palliative treatment of prostate cancer.

Endocrinology

Luteinizing hormone–releasing hormone (LHRH, also known as gonadotropin-releasing hormone, GnRH) is a hypothalamic neurohumoral decapeptide produced in a pulsatile manner from its precursor prohormone. It stimulates the secretion of follicle-stimulating hormone (FSH) and luteinizing hormone (LH), which in turn help to release inhibin and testosterone from Sertoli cells and Leydig cells respectively. The testicular hormones directly regulate LHRH, FSH, and LH secretion. Continuous administration of LHRH analogues initially stimulates the secretion of LH and FSH and subsequently blocks the downregulation of LHRH receptors. The suppression effect on LH synthesis leads to inhibition of testosterone synthesis.

Testosterone is converted into 5α-dihydrotestosterone (DHT) by 5α-reductase isoenzymes in the prostate. Testosterone deprivation leads to apoptosis of prostate epithelial cells. Androgens (both testosterone and dihydrotestosterone) mediate their action through the androgen receptor (AR), which is a phosphoprotein, although dihydrotestosterone has a higher affinity than testosterone; AR is found in abundance in male genital tissue including prostate. The cancer cells rely on androgens for growth and to avoid apoptosis. The therapies based on this principle include the following:

(1) orchiectomy (removal of source of testosterone surgically); (2) LHRH analogues (androgen ablation); (3) blockade of androgen receptor (flutamide and bicalutamide); and (4) maximum androgen blockade (combination of 2 and 3, above). Although most tumors respond to these treatments initially, they

subsequently become refractory (androgen-independent). There are many mechanisms by which tumor cells become androgen-refractory. This could be due to AR mutation, amplification of the AR gene, mutated AR responding to small amounts of androgens or even to antiandrogens, activation of AR by adrenal androgens, and bypassing of AR mechanism (1).

Hormone Manipulation with Major Modalities of Treatment

Radiotherapy

Although the optimal time for neoadjuvant treatment is still being debated and no study has ever been completed comparing ADT plus external beam radiation therapy (EBRT) to ADT alone, androgen deprivation should be used for most patients undergoing EBRT. Several studies have shown improved overall and cancer-specific survival with this combination (2–6).

Brachytherapy

Androgen deprivation therapy does not appear to be as important for cancer control with brachytherapy. A recent retrospective study found that neoadjuvant androgen deprivation (NAAD) does not appear to be an independent predictor of relapse in men undergoing transperineal brachytherapy for prostate cancer (7). This retrospective study found the 5-year biochemical relapse-free survival (BRFS) to be 87.1% in men who had been treated with NAAD and 86.9% in those who had not (7). Androgen deprivation therapy is occasionally used with brachytherapy to downsize large glands or decrease the risks of lower urinary tract obstruction after the treatment. Based on previous prospective evaluation, the prostate volume reduction seen with ADT is 33% at 3.7 months and 46% at 12 months (8,9).

Postradical Prostatectomy

Androgen deprivation prior to radiation may also be helpful in the postprostatectomy salvage setting, but again the data are limited. Katz et al. (10) have shown that the salvage disease-free survival was improved for men being treated with combination therapy when radical prostatectomy specimens showed negative surgical margins, no extracapsular extension, and absent seminal vesicle invasion.

Cryotherapy

Androgen deprivation therapy prior to cryotherapy has also been used. This has resulted in a reported 1-year salvage BRFS of 66%, but no randomized controlled trials have defined the use of ADT with primary or salvage cryotherapy to date (11).

Androgen deprivation prior to radical prostatectomy has been clearly evaluated in several large trials. In general, men treated with neoadjuvant androgen deprivation prior to prostatectomy have fewer positive margins, smaller prostate volumes, and less extracapsular extension. Despite these findings, no prospective study (with the exception of a subgroup of one Canadian study of men with PSA values greater than 20 ng/mL) has shown an increased survival rate in men treated with NAAD (12–15).

Management of Rising Prostate-Specific Antigen After Primary Therapy

In spite of improvements in surgical technique and radiation dosimetry over the last decade, the risk of requiring secondary treatment after localized therapy is estimated to be between 10% and 41%, for a total United States incidence of 50,000 men with recurrent disease per year (16,17). The definition of biochemical recurrence with definitive treatment is controversial. A study from the Mayo Clinic of 2700 men found 0.4 ng/mL to be the most reliable prostate-specific antigen (PSA) value in defining true prostate cancer recurrence after surgery (18).

The American Society for Therapeutic Radiology and Oncology (ASTRO) now defines postradiation recurrence as a rise of 2 ng/mL or more above the nadir PSA (19).

Gleason score, PSA, pathological stage (20), nadir after treatment (21), a PSA doubling time of <10 months (22), and recurrence within 2 years of definitive treatment (23,24) each have a significant independent impact on the outcome. With EBRT, a PSA nadir ≤1 ng/mL has been shown to be an independent predictor of a significantly improved disease-free survival.

When a biochemical recurrence is detected, staging is difficult to accomplish but is important for determining therapy. Studies on the sensitivity and specificity of bone scan and computed tomography (CT) have found that these imaging modalities are not cost-effective in patients with a PSA of less than 20 to 40 ng/mL, although both are generally recommended (25,26). Similarly, biopsy of the prostatic fossa has a false-negative rate of 45.6% following radiation and a false-positive result reported to be highly likely in men who have undergone radiation within the previous 3 years (27). The ProstaScint scan uses a radiolabeled monoclonal antibody against prostate-specific membrane antigen (PSMA) to detect the potential extent and location of recurrent disease. Unfortunately, the sensitivity of this test is around 62%, the specificity 72%, and the overall accuracy 68% (28).

Adjuvant radiation therapy is the most effective modality used to treat rising PSA after radical prostatectomy. If radiation is given in a salvage setting, outcomes are improved when treatment is given prior to serum PSA values rising above 1 ng/mL (29). A report on a small cohort of 73 men who received postoperative radiation after prostatectomy (T3 or margin positive), radiotherapy was associated with a lower risk of relapse and undetectable PSA levels, with two patients developing grade 3 urinary complications (30).

Adjuvant treatment following radiation includes salvage prostatectomy, cryotherapy, and brachytherapy, provided that the initial prostate cancer was localized prior to radiation therapy. Series from Michigan and from Memorial Sloan-Kettering Cancer Center found the 3-year disease-free survival after salvage prostatectomy to be 68% for PSA <10, and 83% for PSA <4, with 75% of patients free of surgical complications (such as incontinence or need for colostomy) in men undergoing salvage prostatectomy in the modern era (31,32).

Salvage cryotherapy is a minimally invasive option emerging for recurrent prostate carcinoma after radiation therapy. In a study from MD Anderson, with a median follow-up of 5.7 years, 46.9% of patients appeared to have a durable response to salvage cryotherapy. More importantly, many of these patients had advanced stage disease (43%) and none were treated with concominent androgen deprivation. In general, cryotherapy is tolerated well, is minimally invasive, and rarely results in severe complications (such as rectourethral fistulas).

Salvage brachytherapy is an additional treatment modality for treating patients with recurrent prostate cancer after radiation. This treatment also can be effective, but should be used with caution. Data from one retrospective study of 49 patients found a 5-year biochemical disease-free survival of 34%. The risk of incontinence at 3 years in this study was 6% (in which a prior transurethral resection of the prostate was a risk factor in each case). Additionally, two patients had rectal ulcers, and one required a colostomy (34).

Maximum Androgen Blockade, Early Androgen Deprivation, Intermittent Hormone Therapy, and Antiandrogen Monotherapy

Many randomized controlled trials have evaluated the benefit of combining an antiandrogen with an LHRH agonist to block adrenal androgens in addition to suppressing testicular function. Most studies have shown a small survival advantage using the combined regimen. In 2000, an article was published in *The Lancet* that typifies urologists' and urologic oncologists' attitudes about combined androgen blockade. This study evaluated the results from 8275 patients involved in 27 randomized trials and found a 2% to 3% improvement in the 5-year overall survival in men with advanced prostate cancer treated with combined androgen blockage over LHRH agonist alone (35). Although this benefit may be even greater when considering that many men were on steroidal antiandrogens, which may not have as potent an effect, the financial (estimated to be around $100,000 per quality-adjusted life year) and possible adverse-event cost associated with antiandrogen therapy for extended periods of time may not justify such a small survival advantage. Some do continue to point out the flaws of metaanalysis and point out that in the National Cancer Institute trial addressing this question, men with minimal disease on combined androgen deprivation experienced a two-year improvement in overall survival, and point out that combined androgen deprivation can be recommended for men with a very aggressive disease.

As for early versus delayed therapy, two studies warrant mention. The Medical Research Council (MRC) study of 987 patients with advanced prostate cancer randomized to early lifelong ADT versus treatment upon progression found a survival advantage in men started upon the diagnosis of prostate cancer (46% vs. 30% at 10 years), with the greatest advantage seen in those with less advanced disease.

Although this study is criticized for men dying in the observation arm prior to the initiation of therapy, a clear benefit was also seen in decreased cord compression, skeletal fractures, ureteral/urethral obstruction, and extraskeletal metastases, and is generally used to justify early treatment with LHRH agonists (36). The other randomized trial evaluating early versus late initiation of androgen deprivation also showed a survival advantage when androgen deprivation therapy was initiated early when lymph node metastases were confirmed during radical prostatectomy. In this study of 98 men, those who received immediate, lifelong androgen deprivation had a much higher cancer-specific survival (30.8% vs. 4.3%) and progression-free rate (75% vs. 18.8%) than those who were treated only upon disease progression (37).

Intermittent androgen deprivation (IAD) is supposed to work on the assumption that apoptotic potential by successive rounds of androgen suppression and withdrawal would delay tumor growth. Preliminary studies have demonstrated improvement in the quality of life while off treatment (although the time to normalization can take up to a year following cessation of androgen deprivation) (38), as well as decreased risk of developing elevated chromogranin A, which may be associated with the development of bony metastases 38% vs. 6% (39,40). However, other preliminary data demonstrate that although the overall survival is the same, the time to progression is decreased in men on intermittent androgen deprivation (41). A large prospective, randomized, controlled trial coordinated by the Southwest Oncology Group addressing this issue is currently underway.

Antiandrogens used as monotherapy offer advantages of retained sexual function, cognition, and bone mineral density due to maintained serum testosterone levels. However, as testosterone can undergo aromatization to estrogen, the development of gynecomastia is not unusual with this regimen. Short courses of breast radiation prior to initiation of antiandrogen monotherapy or coadministration of tamoxifen (an antiestrogen) or Arimidex (an aromatase inhibitor) have been seen to minimize this effect (42,43). Although antiandrogens alone may not offer an improved or equivalent cancer-specific survival rate (44) when compared to combined androgen deprivation therapy, the Early Prostate Cancer Prevention Trial found that this regimen, when used adjuvantly in 8113 men with T1-4 Nx/N0 M0 prostate cancer undergoing standard therapy for prostate cancer resulted in an improvement in disease progression by 42%.

The greatest benefits were seen in those men being observed with localized prostate cancer (47% improvement vs. 37% in men undergoing prostatectomy or radiation). Additionally, bicalutamide monotherapy decreased the incidence of bony metastases or death by 33% (45). At this time both intermittent androgen deprivation and antiandrogen monotherapy are considered investigational and should be considered only under the umbrella of a clinical trial.

Complications of Androgen Deprivation Therapy

The complications of androgen deprivation therapy are numerous, including hot flushes, osteoporosis, anemia, erectile dysfunction, muscle wasting, fatigue, depression, decline in physical activity, increase in fat apposition, and decline in cognitive function.

Hot Flushes

Hot flushes are experienced by 80% of patients on LHRH and are thought to be related to an increased catecholamine secretion due to decreased end-organ response to LHRH, resulting in stimulation of the thermoregulatory center of the hypothalamus. Symptoms are fairly well controlled with progestins (Megace), estrogen (adverse events should be carefully monitored), antidepressants (venlafaxine), and possibly with soya or vitamin E (46,47).

Fractures

It is estimated that 50% of men with hip fractures have evidence of hypogonadism and that the risk of fracture in a hypogonadal men is five times that of their eugonadal counterparts (48). Important work has evaluated the use of intravenous bisphosphonates in men being treated with hormone withdrawal for prostate cancer. In a multicenter, double-blinded, placebo-controlled trial of men beginning androgen deprivation regimens for prostate cancer, the mean bone mineral density increased an average of 5.6% at 1 year with intravenous bisphosphonates given every 3 months, versus a decrease of 2.2% for those on ADT alone (49). Another double-blinded study with metastatic androgen-insensitive prostate cancer found that patients treated with zoledronic acid (an intravenous bisphosphonate given at a dosage of 4 mg every 3 weeks for 15 months) had a decrease in skeletal-related events (44.2% vs. 33.2%), time to first skeletal-related even (not reached vs. 321 days), and decrease in pain and bone resorption markers with treatment (50). Skeletal-related events are significantly and independently linked to increased mortality in patients on androgen deprivation for prostate cancer. It is important to screen for and consider bisphosphonate treatment (in conjunction with calcium and vitamin D) in men with decreasing bone mineral density on ADT. Encouragingly, a recent randomized study found bone marrow density to be significantly better in men on zoledronic acid treated just once and measured one year after treatment than controls on androgen deprivation alone (51).

Anemia

Anemia is also encountered as a result of decreased stimulation of erythroid precursors by DHT in men on ADT. In a study by Strum et al. (52), 90% of patients experienced a 10% drop in hemoglobin levels. This change occurred as early as 1 month and at a nadir at 6 months after initiating treatment. This phenomenon may contribute to the fatigue experienced by men on ADT therapy and can be corrected by recombinant human erythropoietin when severe. Anemia resolution by bone marrow production following the cessation of ADT may take at least 1 year.

Decreased Muscle Mass

Serum testosterone has been seen to correlate with increased muscle mass, and men on ADT frequently complain of decreased muscle mass or strength as well as increased body fat deposition. A striking jump in triglycerides can also be seen in patients treated with androgen deprivation (26.5% in 1 year by one study) (53). Studies are ongoing to evaluate the effect of various exercise regimes in men maintained on ADT.

Cognitive Function

The effect of ADT on cognitive function is difficult to quantify and has been verified in some studies but discounted in others. Androgen deprivation therapy may have an effect on a man's spatial ability, verbal memory, and fluency. It is well known that testosterone levels less than $50\,ng/mL$ are known to cause a decrease in sexual desire and function.

Second-Line Hormonal Manipulations in the Management of Androgen-Independent Cancer of the Prostate: Definitions and Classifications

The definition of androgen-independent cancer of the prostate (AICP) (or hormone refractory prostate cancer, HRPC) is the demonstration of two or three serial rises in serum PSA obtained at least 2 weeks apart during castrate serum testosterone levels. Imaging, including a CT and bone scan, is generally recommended at the onset of AICP.

The mechanism of the development of AICP is controversial. Although it was previously assumed that androgen receptors became downregulated with the development of AICP, in fact the pathophysiology is much more complex, with data supporting alterations of androgen receptor cofactors, receptor promoter hypermethylation, and androgen receptor mutation with hyperactivation (54,55). Obviously research is critical in assessing and preventing these changes in order to improve the survival of men with advanced prostate cancer and is ongoing.

Androgen-independent prostate cancer can be present in a variety of situations. Some men develop AICP when minimal disease is present following definitive treatment and salvage androgen deprivation therapy has been initiated (biochemical AICP). Others have high volume, widely metastatic disease. Previous studies found the median time to symptomatic progression in biochemical AICP once a PSA reaches $4\,ng/mL$ is 6 to 8 months, and the median time to death thereafter is 18 months (56).

Further stratification based on 160 patients followed retrospectively can be predicted based on three independent risk factors: nadir of PSA on ADT, time to PSA recurrence, and PSA doubling time. The observed median cancer-specific survival times were 14, 38, and 89 months for patients in low-, intermediate-, and high-risk groups using these three variables, respectively. In general, a PSA doubling time of 6 months, or time to recurrence >7 months following androgen deprivation, and PSA nadir ≤ 0.1 are all positive predictors of improved survival in men with AICP, with PSA doubling time being the most important (57). Prostate-specific antigen, alkaline phosphatase, lactate dehydrogenase, hemoglobin, Gleason score, Eastern Cooperative Oncology Group (ECOG) performance status, and presence or absence of visceral metastases can also help predict an individual's risk of mortality in those with more advanced AICP (58).

Various treatments may be tried when patients begin to progress on ADT. When the antiandrogen is withdrawn in patients maintained on combined androgen deprivation, a 15% to 30% response is seen, for a mean duration of 3 to 5 months (59). Additional data support the use of flutamide after failure using bicalutamide, as this may bind to the receptor differently (60). Ketoconazole also may have activity on PSA in AICP, even in men with castrate levels of testosterone on traditional therapy, but does not appear to change overall survival rates (61).

An ECOG intergroup trial is currently ongoing, randomizing men with nonmetastatic prostate cancer with castrate levels of testosterone and rising PSA to ketoconazole and hydrocortisone or docetaxel and estramustine. PC-SPES, an over-the-counter herbal combination, found to contain estrogenic components, was also demonstrated to be effective in AICP. Unfortunately, this treatment is no longer available due to toxicity and inconsistency of product content (62). Oral estrogen therapy combined with anticoagulation prophylaxis has also been effective in small trials of men with androgen insensitive prostate cancer and is inexpensive, well-tolerated, and easy to administer (63).

Clearly the evaluation that is underway of the modification of signaling proteins and cytokines that lead to the development and progression of AICP is important and will be a focus for several years to come.

Chemotherapy

Approximately 30,000 men die of prostate cancer annually in the United States, most whom have developed AICP. In general, AICP is chemoresistant, with early studies demonstrating only an 8% to 15% response to treatment, with no change in overall survival, and a median survival of 1 year (64).

Data showing that mitoxantrone combined with steroids improved the quality of life in men with metastatic AICP (although no change in survival was seen) led to the Food and Drug Administration (FDA) approval in the 1990s for mitoxantrone as the agent of choice in this setting (65). Mitoxantrone is an anthraquinone, developed in an effort to create a compound with similar activity to, but less cardiotoxicity than, doxorubicin. Currently a multiinstitutional, randomized trial coordinated by the Southwest Oncology Group (SWOG) is evaluating the efficacy of mitoxantrone when used immediately following prostatectomy in men with high-risk prostate cancer treated with prostatectomy and adjuvant androgen deprivation.

Estramustine has an estrogenic as well as microtubule cytotoxic effect and was developed in the hopes of fighting breast cancer. Although it was not as effective as was hoped for with breast cancer, estramustine does appear to have activity in AICP. Low-dose warfarin or aspirin is recommended in combination with estramustine to counteract the thromboembolic-inducing potential of this drug. Docetaxel similarly effects microtubules and also has been seen to have activity in AICP (45% of patients experiencing a 50% decrease in PSA). Toxicity appears less when patients are dosed on an every third week schedule as opposed to a weekly schedule (66). Steroids are used to decrease fluid retention with treatment.

For the first time ever, a study (coordinated by SWOG) recently found a survival advantage in AICP patients treated with chemotherapy. This trial randomized 666 patients to docetaxel plus estramustine or mitoxantrone and prednisone. Patients on the docetaxel/estramustine regimen realized a mean 18-month overall survival compared to 15 months in the mitoxantrone/prednisone arm, confirming docetaxel and estramustine as the standard-of-care treatment for men with AICP (67). Another phase 3 clinical trial compared docetaxel in two dosage regimens (weekly vs. every 3 weeks) against mitoxantrone and prednisone, and again found a survival advantage as well as improved pain palliation in men treated with docetaxel and prednisone on the 21-day schedule (68).

Carboplatin may also be a synergistic agent to the docetaxel/estramustine combination (68% of patients with a 50% or greater decline in PSA) (69). Calcitriol may be an additional synergistic chemotherapeutic agent with docetaxel and estramustine (81% of patients experiencing a 50% or greater decline in PSA values) and has recently been evaluated in a phase 2/3 trial evaluating the triplet to the doublet combination (70). Using an entirely different strategy, bevacizumab (a vascular endothelial growth factor inhibitor) has been evaluated in a phase II trial as a single agent in men with AICP, and no patient achieved a 50% decline in PSA (71). Although a dramatic improvement has not been realized, the fact that any agent is affecting the overall survival of men with prostate cancer, and that newer agents are showing activity in the disease, offers hope for men with AICP. Excitingly, a phase III randomized controlled study has lead to FDA approval for "Provenge," a recombinant of autologous dendritic cells "loaded" with prostatic acid phosphatase and fused with granulocyte-macrophage colony stimulating factor (GM-CSF). In this study of 127 men with metastatic disease, 4.4% of those randomized to immunotherapy had a decline of 50% or greater in their PSA, while none had this decline in the control group. More importantly, the mean survival for men treated with Provenge was 25.9 months versus 21.4 months for controls (72). Also exciting as a new modality of treatment, Satroplatin, a novel, orally bioavailable chemotherapy has shown activity in prostate cancer as well (73).

Endocrine Therapy for Localized Prostate Cancer with or Without Radical Prostatectomy

Many quality studies have evaluated the effect of NAAD on surgical outcome. It is clear that patients treated with NAAD have fewer positive surgical margins and have smaller prostate volumes, and the percentage with extracapsular extension may be decreased (74–78). No study has shown an increased survival rate despite these positive findings, with the exception of a small subgroup analysis of men with a PSA greater than 20 in a study performed by the Canadian Urologic Oncology Group (79).

It is possible that further dedicated evaluation of high risk men with PSA values greater than 20 ng/mL, or men with metastatic disease treated nonconventionally with adjuvant androgen deprivation as well as focal therapy, have improved survival rates or an improved quality of life (80).

As mentioned already, cryotherapy is an emerging area of treatment in prostate cancer. Although formal randomized studies have not been performed to prove the efficacy of NAAD for primary or salvage treatment of prostate cancer, one of the largest experiences comes from Columbia University. As reported above, the 2-year survival reported for salvage cryotherapy using this protocol is 74% (33). It is not clear if NAAD therapy is necessary when performing primary cryotherapy for prostate cancer, but most urologists do not use androgen deprivation for primary definitive cryotherapy.

Neoadjuvant androgen deprivation, however, acts synergistically with radiation and improves disease-free and overall survival in various groups of men who undergo radiation therapy for prostate cancer. A prospective, Radiation Therapy Oncology Group (RTOG) trial (number 85-31) showed disease-free survival rates clearly favored men with early and continuous androgen deprivation treated definitively with EBRT over radiation alone (60% vs. 44% at 5 years, $p <.001$). This study included 977 men with T3 disease or nodal metastases. Overall survival rates were significantly higher in men treated with adjuvant androgen deprivation who had Gleason 8 to 10 prostate cancers as well (66% vs. 55% $p = .03$) (81). Another trial coordinated by the RTOG (number 86-10) showed that disease-free survival was also improved in patients who underwent brief NAAD followed by EBRT compared to radiation alone (46% vs. 21% at 5 years, $p <.001$). This study included 233 men with bulky T2 and T3 prostate cancer who were treated with 2 months of neoadjuvant and 2 months of adjuvant combined androgen blockade during radiation (82). Seven-year follow-up data showed this improved disease-free survival in patients treated with NAAD prior to radiation was durable ($p = .004$) (5). A prospective multiinstitutional study from Europe confirmed these findings in 415 men with Gleason 8-10 or T3-4 or node-positive prostate cancer. These men were randomized to treatment with combined androgen blockade beginning 1 week prior to radiation therapy and continuing for 3 years after treatment versus radiation therapy alone. The disease-free survival at 5 years was 74% in the androgen deprivation group versus 40% in the radiation alone group ($p = .0001$). In addition to demonstrating an improvement in disease-free survival, a significant overall survival improvement in the patients treated with NAAD was seen as well (78% vs. 62% at 5 years, $p = .0002$) (83).

Patients undergoing brachytherapy as the sole treatment for prostate cancer may not require NAAD. This may be secondary to the low-risk nature of prostate cancer treated by this modality or secondary to the higher doses able to be delivered to the prostate. Neoadjuvant androgen deprivation, however, prior to brachytherapy, can be useful in decreasing the size of prostates greater than 50 to 60 cc in volume to decrease pubic arch interference and improve dosimetry. A prostate volume reduction of 33% is generally seen at a mean of 3½ months (83).

Chemoprevention of Prostate Cancer and Its Mechanism

Relatively recently, the data from the Prostate Cancer Prevention Trial were released. This study randomized 18,882 men with normal serum PSA to daily finasteride or placebo. At an interim analysis that resulted in early termination the study found that cancer was detected in 803/4368 (18.3%) men in the finasteride arm and 1147/4692 (24.4%) men in the placebo group (a 24.8% cancer reduction, p <.001). Unfortunately, high-grade tumors (Gleason sum ≥7) were more common in patients who had been on finasteride (6.4% of tumors vs. 5.1% of tumors), but some authors suggest that this finding may be attributed to increased difficulty with grading tumors after relative hormonal manipulation and improved sampling due to decreased total prostate size (84). Importantly, the cancer detection rate of 24.4% in men over age 55 who underwent biopsy is significantly higher than the traditionally reported incidence of prostate cancer found in men who undergo biopsy with screening. Although there is a significant risk of finding indolent cancers in men with normal PSAs and digital rectal examination (DREs), 15% of cancers found in the Prostate Cancer Prevention Trial were identified in men with a PSA <2.5 ng/mL and were Gleason's sum 7 to 10 (85).

Soybean isoflavones are "natural" 5α-reductase inhibitors. Epidemiological data also suggest a link between increased soy consumption and decreased incidence of prostate cancer, which has been supported by animal studies (86–89). A phase II randomized, placebo controlled trial has recently been developed by the National Cancer Institute (NCI) to investigate the effect of supplementation with dietary soy in patients with PSA greater than 4 ng/mL. Additionally, soy is being evaluated in combination with vitamin E and selenium in patients with high-grade prostatic intraepithelial neoplasia in a prospective study in Canada (90). Not surprisingly the effect of dual 5α-reductase inhibitor (Dutasteride) in prostate cancer prevention is being investigated.

Other prostate cancer prevention efforts focus on selenium, vitamin E, vitamin D, and lycopene. A secondary analysis of the Nutritional Prevention of Cancer Trial revealed that selenium supplementation does appear to reduce the risk of prostate cancer in men, particularly in those with a prostate-specific antigen (PSA) ≤4 ng/mL who are in the lowest two tertiles of base serum selenium concentrations (91). Investigation has demonstrated that selenium does not change testosterone (T) levels, DHT levels, or DHT/T ratios, and that one of the mechanisms of selenium may be to reduce oxidative damage to cells.

Properly powered, prospective randomized studies are underway to evaluate the possible benefit of selenium in patients with prostatic intraepithelial neoplasia (PIN) (SWOG trial 9917). Other trials to evaluate the benefit of selenium with or without vitamin E, against vitamin E alone, and against placebo for men with a PSA ≤4 ng/mL are also underway (SELECT trial 00-1092). Investigation continues to evaluate the efficacy of deltanoids (or vitamin D analogues) in the prevention of prostate cancer (92). Finally, further investigation is planned to follow-up on early epidemiological studies showing an inverse association between prostate cancer risk and dietary intake of lycopene (the degradation products of which enhance gap junction cell signaling). Preliminary investigations at Wayne State University found that a small group of men randomly assigned to receive a tomato extract (30 mg lycopene) daily for 3 weeks prior to surgery were more likely to have smaller tumors (80% vs. 45% volume <4 ml), negative surgical margins were seen, and less extracapsular extension (73% vs. 18%) (93). Laboratory studies corroborate the phytochemical retardation of prostate tumor growth in rats (94).

Serum testosterone levels, body mass index, and prostate cancer risk are still areas of considerable controversy. The Health Professionals Follow-Up Study subset analysis showed that a low body mass index (BMI) may be a risk factor for developing prostate cancer in men with a familial disease. The authors speculated that a decreased BMI results in decreased circulating sex hormone–binding globulin (SHBG) and, therefore, more bioavailable plasma testosterone, which actually may increase certain men's risk for prostate cancer (95). Raivio et al. (96), however, compared the sera of 101 men with benign prostatic hypertrophy (BPH) to those with prostate cancer and found the androgen bioactivity levels to be significantly *lower* in men with prostate cancer than in those with BPH (3.0 nM vs. 3.2 nM, $p < .005$). It is also well established that total testosterone levels decline approximately 1.6% per year (97) while BMI (and therefore SHBG) increase, implying a decline in free testosterone levels with age, which correlates with patterns of prostate cancer prevalence.

Other investigators, though, continue to support the traditional indirect evidence of the tumor-stimulating effect of testosterone, but suspect the stimulation may be due to the relationship between testosterone and insulin-like growth factor-I (IGF-I), insulin, or leptin rather than testosterone itself (98).

Similarly, tradition teaches that estrogens treat prostate cancer; however, a small body of data suggests that estrogen may induce mitogens that stimulate prostate cancer. A phase II clinical trail using the antiestrogen toremifene citrate for prostate cancer chemoprevention is currently underway (99). Clearly the effect of steroid hormones on prostate cancer has yet to be fully elucidated.

Selective cyclooxygenase-inhibiting nonsteroidal antiinflammatory drugs (NSAIDs), in general, appear to have a detrimental effect on cancer growth, perhaps through inhibition of Akt and ERK-2. Research will likely continue in this arena, particularly using nonselective NSAIDs despite previous controversies (100).

Molecular Epidemiology

Further work continues on genetics and prostate cancer. The *RNASEL* gene (on HPC1) mediates the apoptotic activity of interferons by cutting double-stranded RNA. Polymorphic changes within this gene may be associated with increased risk of familial but not sporadic prostate cancer (101). At this time it is estimated that 9% of newly diagnosed prostate cancer can be traced to heredity, and it has been estimated that 44% may be due to genetic factors (102). Models that combine genetic susceptibility as well as environmental pressures are being evaluated (103). Research continues on DNA hypo- and hypermethylation as well as altered histone acetylation, which have all been observed in prostate cancer (104). An interesting study from New Mexico found that decreased telomere content in tissue obtained from radical prostatectomy predicted prostate cancer recurrence when controlling for Gleason sum and grade, suggesting possible genomic instability with decreased telomere DNA content (105). More importantly, RNA analysis for PCA3 has been found to be helpful in diagnosing prostate cancer, with a ROC (receiver operating characteristic) curve equal to 0.68 for urine PCA3 compared to 0.52 for serum PSA (106). Clearly the future for prostate cancer diagnosis and treatment appears to be advancing.

References

1. Grossman ME, Huang H, Tindall DJ. Review: androgen receptor signaling in androgen-refractory cancer. J Natl Cancer Inst 2001;93:1687–1697.
2. Kupelian PA, Mohan DS, Lyons J, et al. Higher than standard radiation doses (>72 Gy) with or without androgen deprivation in the treatment of localized prostate cancer. Int J Radiat Oncol Biol Phys 2000;46:567–574.
3. D'Amico AV, Schultz D, Loffredo M, et al. Biochemical outcome following external beam radiation therapy with or without androgen suppression therapy for clinically localized prostate cancer. JAMA 2000;284:1280–1283.
4. Pilepich MV, Winter K, et al. Phase III Radiation Therapy Oncology Group (RTOG) Trial 86–10 of androgen deprivation adjuvant to definitive radiotherapy in locally advanced carcinoma of the prostate. Int J Radiat Oncol Biol Phys 2001;50:1243–1252.
5. Bolla M, Gonzales D, Warde P, et al. Improved survival in patients with locally advanced prostate cancer treated with radiotherapy and goserelin. Lancet 2002; 360(9327):103–106.
6. Zelefsky MJ, Leibel SA, Kutcher GJ, et al. Three-dimensional conformal radiotherapy and dose escalation: where do we stand? Semin Radiat Oncol 1998;8: 107–114.
7. Potters L, Torre T, Ashley R, et al. Examining the role of neoadjuvant androgen deprivation in patients undergoing prostate brachytherapy. J Clin Oncol 2000; 18:1187–1192.
8. Kucway R, Vicini F, Huang R, et al. Prostate volume reduction with androgen deprivation therapy before interstitial brachytherapy. J Urol 2002;167(6):2443–2447.
9. Lilleby W, Fossa SD, Knutsen BH, et al. Computed tomography/magnetic resonance based volume changes of the primary tumor in patients with prostate cancer with or without androgen deprivation. Radiat Oncol 2000;57:195–200.
10. Katz MS, Zelefsky MJ, Venkatraman ES, et al. Predictors of biochemical outcome with salvage conformal radiotherapy after radical prostatectomy for prostate cancer. J Clin Oncol 2003;21(3):483–489.
11. de la Taille A, Hayek O, Benson MC, et al. Salvage cryotherapy for recurrent prostate cancer after radiation therapy: the Columbia experience. Urology 2000;55:79–84.
12. Soloway MS, Pareek K, Sharifi R, et al. Neoadjuvant androgen ablation before radical prostatectomy in cT2bNxM0 prostate cancer: 5-year results. J Urol 2002;167:112.
13. Aus G, Abrahammsson PA, Ahlgren G, et al. Hormonal treatment before radical prostatectomy: a 3-year follow-up. J Urol 1998;159:2013.

14. Meyer F, Bairate I, Bedard C, et al. Duration of neoadjuvant androgen deprivation therapy before radical prostatectomy and disease-free survival in men with prostate cancer. Urology 2001;58:71.

15. Schulman CC, Debruyne FMJ, Forster G, et al. 4-year follow-up results of a European Prospective Randomized Study on neoadjuvant hormonal therapy prior to radical prostatectomy in T2–3N0M0 prostate cancer. European Study Group on Neoadjuvant Treatment of Prostate Cancer. Eur Urol 2000;38(6):706–713.

16. Klotz LH, Godenberg SL, Jewett MAS, et al. Long-term follow-up of a randomized trial of 0 versus 3 months of neoadjuvant androgen ablation before radical prostatectomy. J Urol 2003;170:791–794.

17. Nasr R, Goldenberg S. Rising prostate specific antigen after radical prostatectomy: a case based review. Can J Urol 2001;8:1306–1313.

18. Amling C, Blute M, Bergstralh E, et al. Long-term hazard of progression after radical prostatectomy for clinically localized prostate cancer: continued risk of biochemical failure after 5 years. J Urol 2000;164:101–105.

19. Roach M 3rd, Hanks G, Thames H Jr, et al. Defining biochemical failure following radiotherapy with or without hormonal therapy in men with clinically localized prostate cancer: recommendations of the RTOG-ASTRO Phoenix Consensus Conference. Int J Radiat Oncol Biol Phys 2006;65:965–974.

20. Pound CR. Partin AW. Epstein JI. Walsh PC. Prostate-specific antigen after anatomic radical retropubic prostatectomy. Patterns of recurrence and cancer control. Urol Clin North Am 1997;24(2):395–406.

21. Akduman B, Crawford E. The management of high risk prostate cancer. J Urol 2003;169(6):1993–1998.

22. Shipley WU, Thames HD, Sandler HM, et al. Radiation therapy for clinically localized prostate cancer: a multi-institutional pooled analysis. JAMA 1999;281(17):1598.

23. Pound CR, Partin AW, Eisenberger MA, et al. Natural history of progression after PSA elevation following radical prostatectomy. JAMA 1999;281(17):1591–1597.

24. Coetzee LJ, Hars V, Paulson DF. Postoperative prostate-specific antigen as a prognostic indicator in patients with margin-positive prostate cancer, undergoing adjuvant radiotherapy after radical prostatectomy. Urology 1996;47(2):232–235.

25. Johnstone P, Tarman G, Riffenburgh R, et al. Yield of imaging and scintigraphy assessing biochemical failure in prostate cancer patients. Urol Oncol 1997;3:108.

26. Dotan ZA, Bianco FJ Jr, Rabbani F, et al. Pattern of prostate-specific antigen (PSA) failure dictates the probability of a positive bone scan in patients with an increasing PSA after radical prostatectomy. J Clin Oncol 2005;23(9):1962–1968.

27. Svetec D, McCabe K, Peretsman S, et al. Prostate rebiopsy is a poor surrogate of treatment efficacy in localized prostate cancer. J Urol 1998;159:1606.

28. Ponsky L, Cherullo E, Starkey R, et al. Evaluation of preoperative ProstaScint scans in the prediction of nodal disease. Prostate Cancer Prostatic Dis 2002;5(2):132–135.

29. Cotton C, Gospodarowicz M, Warde P, et al. Adjuvant and salvage radiation following radical retropubic prostatectomy for adenocarcinoma of the prostate. Radiother Oncol 2001;59:51–60.

30. Choo R, Hruby G, Hong J, et al. Positive resection margin and/or pathologic T3 adenocarcinoma of the prostate with undetectable postoperative PSA after prostatectomy: to irradiate or not? Int J Radiat Oncol Biol Phys 2002;52:674–680.

31. Chen BT, Wood DP Jr. Salvage prostatectomy in patients who have failed radiation therapy or cryotherapy as primary treatment for prostate cancer. Urology 2003; 62(suppl 1):69–78.

32. Garzotto M, Wajsman Z. Androgen deprivation with salvage surgery for radiorecurrent prostate cancer: results at 5-year follow-up. J Urol 1998;159(3):950–954.

33. Spiess PE, Lee AK, Leibovici D, Wang X, Do KA, Pisters LL. Presalvage prostate-specific antigen (PSA) and PSA doubling time as predictors of biochemical failure of salvage cryotherapy in patients with locally recurrent prostate cancer after radiotherapy. Cancer 2006;107:275–280.

34. Grado GL, Collins JM, Kriegshauser JS, et al. Salvage brachytherapy for localized prostate cancer after radiotherapy failure. Urology 1999;53(1):2–10.

35. Prostate Cancer Trialists' Collaborative Group. Maximum androgen blockade in advanced prostate cancer: an overview of the randomized trials. Lancet 2000; 355:1491–1498.

36. Medical Research Council. Br J Urol 1997;79:235–246.

37. Messing E, Crawford E, Sarosdy M, et al. Immediate hormonal therapy compared with observation after radical prostatectomy and pelvic lymphadenectomy in men with node-positive prostate cancer. N Engl J Med 1999;341:1781–1788.

38. Bruchovsky N, Klotz LH, et al. Intermittent androgen suppression for prostate cancer: Canadian prospective trial and related observations. Mol Urol 2000;4:191–199.

39. Sciarra A, Monti S, Genitle V, et al. Variation in chromogranin A serum levels during intermittent versus continuous androgen deprivation therapy for prostate adenocarcinoma. Prostate 2003;55:168–179.

40. Tarle M, Ahel MZ, Kovicic K. Acquired neuroendocrine-positivity during maximal androgen blockade in prostate cancer patients. Anticancer Res 2002;22:2525–2529.

41. Olsson CA, Dennis JJ, Miller GL, et al. 2003 Annual Meeting Convention Highlights. Med Assoc Comm 2003;15.

42. Olsson CA, Dennis JJ, Miller GL, et al. 2003 Annual Meeting Convention Highlights. Med Assoc Comm 2003;4.

43. Widmark A, Fossa SD, Lundmo P, et al. Does prophylactic breast irradiation prevent anti-androgen-induced gynecomastia? Evaluation of 253 patients in the randomized Scandinavian trial SPCG-7/SFUO-3. Urology 2003;61(1):145–151.

44. Iversen P, Tammela TL, Vaage S, et al. Scandinavian Prostatic Cancer Group (SPCG). A randomised comparison of bicalutamide ("Casodex") 150 mg versus placebo as immediate therapy either alone or as adjuvant to standard care for early non-metastatic prostate cancer. First report from the Scandinavian Prostatic Cancer Group Study No. 6. Eur Urol 2002;42(3):204–211.

45. Boccardo F, Barichello M, Battaglia M, et al. Bicalutamide monotherapy versus flutamide plus goserlin in prostate cancer: updated results of a multicentric trial. Eur Urol 2002;42(5):481–490.

46. Loprinzi CL, Michalak JL, Quella SK, et al. Megestrol acetate for the prevention of hot flashes. N Engl J Med 1994;331:347–352.

47. Loprinzi CL, Kugler CL, Sloan J, et al. Venlaflaxine in management of hot flashes in survivors of breast cancer: a randomized controlled trial. Cancer 2000;356:2059–2061.

48. Morote J, Martinez E, Trilla E, et al. Osteoporosis during continuous androgen deprivation: influence of the modality and length of treatment. Eur Urol 2003; 44:661–665.

49. Smith MR, Estham J, Gleason DM, et al. Randomized controlled trial of zolendronic acid to prevent bone loss in men receiving androgen deprivation therapy for non-metastatic prostate cancer. J Urol 2003;169:2008–2012.

50. Saad F, Gleason DM, Murray R, et al. A randomized, placebo-controlled trial of zolendronic acid in patients with hormone-refractory metastatic prostate carcinoma. J Natl Cancer Inst 2002;94:1458–1468.

51. Michaelson MD, Kaufman DS, Lee H, et al. Randomized controlled trial of annual zoledronic acid to prevent gonadotropin-releasing hormone agonist-induced bone loss in men with prostate cancer. J Clin Oncol 2007;25:1038–1042.

52. Strum SB, McDermed JE, Scholz MC, et al. Anaemia associated with androgen deprivation in patients with prostate cancer receiving combined hormone blockade. Br J Urol 1997;79:933–941.

53. Smith MR, Finklestein JS, McGovern FJ, et al. Changes in body composition during androgen deprivation therapy for prostate cancer. J Clin Endocrinol Metab 2002; 87:599–602.

54. Suzuki H, Ueda T, Ichikawa T, Ito H. Androgen receptor involvement in the progression of prostate cancer. Endocr Rel Cancer 2003;10:209–216.

55. Heinlein CA, Chang C. Androgen receptor (AR) coregulators: an overview. Endocr Rev 2002;23:175–200.

56. Robson M, Dawson N. How is androgen dependent metastatic prostate cancer best treated? Hematol/Oncol Clin North Am 1996;10:727–747.

57. Shulman MJ, Benaim EA. The natural history of androgen independent prostate cancer. J Urol 2004;172(1):141–145.

58. Wyatt RB, Sanchez-Ortiz RF, Wood CG, et al. Prognostic factors for survival among Caucasian, African-American and Hispanic men with androgen-independent prostate cancer. J Natl Med Assoc 2004;96(12):1587–1593.

59. Small EJ, Srinivas S. The antiandrogen withdrawal syndrome. Experience in a large cohort of unselected patients with advanced prostate cancer. Cancer 1995;76: 1428–1434.

60. Joyce R, Fenton MA, Rode P, et al. High dose bicalutamide for androgen independent prostate cancer: effect of prior hormonal therapy. J Urol 1998;159:149–153.

61. Small EJ, Halabi S, Picus J, et al. Antiandrogen withdrawal alone or in combination with ketoconazole in androgen-independent prostate cancer patients: a phase III trial (CALGB 9583). J Clin Oncol 2004;22(6):1025–1033.

62. Walsh PC. Prospective, multicenter, randomized phase II trial of the herbal supplement, PC-SPES, and diethylstilbestrol in patients with androgen-independent prostate cancer. J Urol 2005;173:1966–1967.

63. Siddiqui K, Abbas F, Biyabani SR, et al. Role of estrogens in the secondary hormonal manipulation of hormone refractory prostate cancer. JPMA 2004;54(9):445–447.

64. Eisenberger MA, Simon R, et al. A reevaluation of nonhormonal cytotoxic chemotherapy in the treatment of prostatic carcinoma. J Clin Oncol 1985;3:827–841.

65. Tannock IF, Osoba D, Stockler MR, et al. Chemotherapy with mitoxantrone plus prednisone or prednisone alone for symptomatic hormone-resistant prostate cancer: a Canadian randomized trial with palliative end points. J Clin Oncol 1996; 14:1756–1764.

66. Picus J, Schultz M. Docetaxel (Taxotere) as monotherapy in the treatment of hormone-refractory prostate cancer: preliminary results. Semin Oncol 1999;26: 14–18.

67. Petrylak D, Tangen C, Hussain M, et al. Immediate verses deferred treatment for advanced prostate cancer: initial results of the Medical Research Council Trial. Proc Am Soc Clin Oncol 2004;23:2.

68. Eisenberger M, De Wit R, Berry W, et al. A multicenter phase III comparison of docetaxel + prednisone and mitoxantrone + prednisone in patient with hormone refractory prostate cancer. Cancer 2003;98:2592–2598.

69. Oh WK, Halabi S, Kelly WK, et al. A phase II study of estramustine, docetaxel, and carboplatin with granulocyte-colony-stimulating factor support in patients

with hormone-refractory prostate carcinoma-cancer and leukemia group B 99813. Cancer 2003;98:2592–2598.

70. Picus J, Halabi S, Rini BI, et al. The use of bevacizumab (B) with docetaxel (D) and estramustine (E) in hormone refractory prostate cancer (HRPC): initial results of CALGB 90006. Proc Am Soc Clin Oncol 2003;22:1578A.

71. Reese DM, Fratesi P, Cory M, et al. A phase II trial of humanized antivascular endothelial growth factor antibody for the treatment of androgen-independent prostate cancer. Prostate J 2001;3:65–70.

72. Lim AM, Hershberg RM, Small EJ. Immunotherapy for prostate cancer using prostatic acid phosphatase loaded antigen presenting cells. Urol Oncol 2006;24:434–441.

73. Choy H. Satraplatin: an orally available platinum analog for the treatment of cancer. Expert Rev Anticancer Ther 2006;6:973–982.

74. Aus G, Abrahammsson PA, Ahlgren G, et al. Hormonal treatment before radical prostatectomy: a 3-year follow-up. J Urol 1998;159:2013.

75. Meyer F, Bairate I, Bedard C, et al. Duration of neoadjuvant androgen deprivation therapy before radical prostatectomy and disease-free survival in men with prostate cancer. Urology 2001;58:71.

76. Schulman CC, Debruyne FMJ, Forster G, et al. 4-year follow-up results of a European Prospective Randomized Study on neoadjuvant hormonal therapy prior to radical prostatectomy in T2–3N0M0 prostate cancer. European Study Group on Neoadjuvant Treatment of Prostate Cancer. Eur Urol 2000;38(6):706–713.

77. Klotz LH, Godenberg SL, Jewett MAS, et al. Long-term follow-up of a randomized trial of 0 versus 3 months of neoadjuvant androgen ablation before radical prostatectomy. J Urol 2003;170:791–794.

78. Crawford ED. Retrospective review of SWOG patients treated with and without prostatectomy in the face of metastatic disease. Personal communication, 2006.

79. Gleave ME, Goldenberg SL, Chin JL, et al. Randomized comparative study of 3 versus 8 month neoadjuvant hormonal therapy before radical prostatectomy: biochemical and pathological effects. J Urol 2001;166:500–505.

80. Pilepich MV, Caplan RW, Byhardt CA, et al. Phase III trial of androgen suppression using goserelin in unfavorable-prognosis carcinoma of the prostate treated with definitive radiotherapy: report of the Radiation Therapy Oncology Group Protocol 85–31. J Clin Oncol 1997;15(3):1013–1021.

81. Pilepich MV, Winter K, Roach M, et al. RTOG Trial 86–10 of androgen deprivation before and during radiotherapy in locally advanced carcinoma of the prostate. Am Int J Rad Onc Bio Phy 2001;50:1243–1252.

82. Bolla M, Collette L, Blank L, et al. Long-term results with immediate androgen suppression and external irradiation in patients with locally advanced prostate cancer (an EORTC study): a phase III randomised trial. Lancet 2002;360(9327): 103–106.

83. Gelblum DY, Potters L, Ashley R, et al. Urinary morbidity following ultrasound-guided transperineal prostate seen implantation. Int J Radiat Oncol Biol Phys 1999;45:59–67.

84. Thompson IM, Phyllis JG, Tangen CM, et al. The influence of finasteride on the development of prostate cancer. N Engl J Med 349(3):213–222.

85. Thompson IM, Pauler DK, Goodman PJ, et al. Prevalence of prostate cancer among men with PSA ≤4.0 ng/ml. N Engl J Med 2004;350(22):2239–2249.

86. Moyad MA. Soy, disease prevention, and prostate cancer. Semin Urol Oncol 1999; 17:97.

87. Lamartiniere CA, Cotroneo MS, Fritz WA, et al. Genistein chemoprevention: timing and mechanisms of action in murine mammary and prostate. J Nutr (suppl) 2002; 132:552S.

88. Pollard M, Wolter W. Prevention of spontaneous prostate-related cancer in Lobund-Wistar rats by a soy protane isolate/isoflavone diet. Prostate 2000;45:101.

89. Barqawi A, Thompson I and Crawford ED. Prostate cancer chemoprevention: an overview of the United States Trials. J Urol 2004;171(2 of 2):S5–8.

90. Duffield-Lillico AJ, Dalkin BL, et al. Selenium supplementation, baseline plasma selenium status and incidence of prostate cancer: an analysis of the complete treatment period of the Nutritional Prevention of cancer Trial. BJU Int 2003;91(7): 608–612.

91. El-Bayoumy K, Richie JP Jr, Boyiri T, et al. Influence of selenium-enriched yeast supplementation of biomarkers of oxidative damage and hormone status in healthy adult males: a clinical pilot study. Cancer Epidemiol Biomarkers Prev 2002;11: 1459–1465.

92. Guyton KZ, Kensler TW, Posner GH. Vitamin D and vitamin D analogs as cancer chemopreventive agents. Nutr Rev 2003;61(7):227–238.

93. Kucuk O, Sarkar FH, Djuric Z, et al. Effects of lycopene supplementation in patients with localized prostate cancer. Exp Biol Med (Maywood) 2002;227(10):881–885.

94. Campbell JK, Canene-Adams K, Linshield BL, et al. Tomato phytochemicals and prostate cancer risk. J Nutr 2004;134:3486S–3489S.

95. Giovannucci E, Rimm EB, Liu Y, et al. Body mass index and risk of prostate cancer in U.S. health professionals. J Natl Cancer Inst 2003;95(16):1240–1244.

96. Raivio T, Santti H, Schatzl G, et al. Reduced circulating androgen bioactivity in patients with prostate cancer. Prostate 2003;55(3):194–198.

97. Juul A, Skakkebaek NE. Androgens and the ageing male. Hum Reprod Update 2002; 8(5):423–433.

98. Kaaks R, Lukanova A, Rinaldi S, et al. Interrelationships between plasma testosterone, SHBG, IGF-I, insulin and leptin in prostate cancer cases and controls. Eur J Cancer Prev 2003;12(4):309–315.

99. Raghow S, Hooshdaran MZ, Katiyar S, et al. Toremifene prevents prostate cancer in the transgenic adenocarcinoma of mouse prostate model. Cancer Res 2002;62:1370.

100. Sabichi AL, Lippman SM. COX-2 inhibitors and other nonsteroidal anti-inflammatory drugs in genitourinary cancer. Semin Oncol 2004;31(2 suppl 7):36–44.

101. Van Gils CH, Bostick RM, Stern MC, et al. Differences in base excision repair capacity may modulate the effect of dietary antioxidant intake on prostate cancer risk: an example of polymorphisms in the XRCC1 gene. Cancer Epidemiol Biomarkers Prev 2002;11(11):1279–1284.

102. Gronberg H, Isaacs SD, Smith JR, et al. Characteristics of prostate cancer in families potentially liked to the hereditary prostate cancer 1 (HPC1) locus. JAMA 1997; 278:1251.

103. Casey G, Neville PJ, Plummer Y, et al. RNASEL Arg462Gln variant is implicated in up to 13% of prostate cancer cases. Nat Genet 2002;32:581–583.

104. Li LC, Carroll P, Dahiya R. Epigenetic changes in prostate cancer: implication for diagnosis and treatment. J Natl Cancer Inst 2005;97(2):103–115.

105. Fordyce CA, Heaphy CM, Joste NE, et al. Association between cancer-free survival and telomere DNA content in prostate tumors. J Urol 2005;173(2):61.

106. Marks LS, Fradet Y, Deras IL, et al. PCA3 molecular urine assay for prostate cancer in men undergoing repeat biopsy. Urology 2007;69:532–535.

18.7
Hormone-Refractory Prostate Cancer: A Rational Approach to Chemotherapy

Derek Raghavan

One of the important issues in the use of cytotoxic chemotherapy is the timing of treatment. When considering chemotherapy for "hormone-refractory" prostate cancer, one must ensure that the cancer is really resistant to the impact of castration. Adrenal androgens contribute to the hormonal environment, so that some tumors that appear to be resistant or refractory to the castrate, testosterone-depleted setting, may actually be receiving stimulation from adrenal hormones, and will thus respond to second-line adrenal blockers, such as aminoglutethimide or ketoconazole. These remissions sometimes may be sustained for months to years.

Thus, important factors to consider before implementing chemotherapy include the following:

- Adherence: is the patient taking the prescribed medications, or are other medications interfering with absorption or function of the treatment, thus interfering with the process of medical castration?
- Is there a late, agonist effect from peripheral androgen blockers, such as flutamide or bicalutamide?
- Is there a significant component of adrenal or other androgenic function?
- Is this truly adenocarcinoma, or is there a neuroendocrine outgrowth?
- Is this a second malignancy?

These issues can be assessed by taking a careful history and doing a physical examination and appropriate tests, such as measurement of gonadotrophins, testosterone, and adrenal androgens. In some cases, where there is no evidence of rapid, symptomatic tumor progression, a therapeutic trial of second-line hormone therapy with an adrenal blocker may yield another remission, and this should be considered before the initiation of chemotherapy.

Changing Precision of Assessment of Outcomes

The utility of chemotherapy for patients with advanced, hormone-refractory prostate cancer has been the subject of controversy (1,2). However, it has become clear that there is a defined role for cytotoxics in advanced, symptomatic, hormone-refractory disease, leading to improved quality of life and a survival benefit (3,4). Analogous to the management of breast cancer, it seems likely that chemotherapy will be introduced earlier into clinical practice, in the context of neoadjuvant or adjuvant therapy, and will then realize its fullest impact.

In the early days of chemotherapy, investigators attempted to define criteria for the assessment of response, culminating in attempts to identify patient benefit within the broad category of disease stabilization (5). The National Prostatic Cancer Project (NPCP) documented the variability in response patterns, and found that stable disease often correlates with prolongation of survival, leading to the project's unique allocation of criteria of response. As the category of stable disease included both patients with very indolent disease and those with a genuine slowing of tumor growth rate, the NPCP system was heavily criticized (1) and fell into some disrepute. This was unfortunate, as the basic system was predicated on sound reasoning, but characterized by a seminal flaw in execution (the bracketing of induced stable disease with inherently slowly progressive tumor).

Surrogate Markers of Response

In recent times, the availability of surrogate markers of response has facilitated the assessment of chemotherapy for prostate cancer, addressing the heterogeneity of outcome within the category of stable disease. With the introduction of serial measurement of prostate-specific antigen (PSA), a response category that requires reduction in circulating levels of PSA by 50% or more has been used to identify patients within the stable clinical disease category who have actually shown an improvement after chemotherapy (6,7). The National Cancer Institute convened an expert panel to attempt to achieve consensus on the use of PSA measurements as a surrogate for tumor response in phase II trials (8). This panel identified four groups of patients who would be suitable for entry into phase II clinical trials, including a category with rising PSA only and no other evidence of disease. They also required proof of effective castration (via measurement of serum testosterone) at the time of progression to constitute "hormone-refractory" disease.

However, the inclusion of patients with a minimum PSA level of only 5 ng/mL has made the interpretation of data more difficult. This lower limit allows the presence in these trials of patients with lower volume disease and also of those with predominant neuroendocrine or small cell anaplastic differentiation (which is characterized by lower PSA levels and the presence of other markers). More recently, there have been a series of meetings convened by the Food and Drug Administration and the National Cancer Institute to rationalize and update the use of surrogate markers. It is clear that the approach to the use of surrogate markers is changing, and we are still learning to use measurement of quality of life and assessment of a range of surrogate markers in the evaluation of novel therapies.

For example, reporting a study from the Southwest Oncology Group, we have recently demonstrated that maintenance at 3 months of PSA remission is the most powerful surrogate marker for patients with advanced hormone-refractory disease, treated by mitoxantrone or docetaxel-based regimens (9). Furthermore, in this study we have questioned the utility of 50% PSA reduction as a useful surrogate marker.

Quality-of-Life Assessments: A Confounding Variable?

The assessment of chemotherapy outcomes is also confounded by the introduction of other new end points. The tools for the measurement of the quality of life (QOL) of patients with prostate cancer have improved somewhat, but are still imperfect. This parameter is being incorporated more often into the assessment of new treatments, despite the current flaws in methodology. In inexperienced hands, this may constitute a much less robust surrogate end point, leading to artificially high response rates. It is important that validated purpose-designed instruments be employed for prostate chemotherapy trials (10).

It should not be forgotten that many patients who receive chemotherapy for prostate cancer have already been castrated, have intercurrent diseases, and are elderly. Thus it may be difficult to define the side effects of chemotherapy accurately, given that these situations may be associated with major symptoms of their own.

Nonetheless, with the broader acceptance of structured QOL assessment, the Food and Drug Administration approved the use of mitoxantrone for the indication of advanced prostate cancer, based largely on QOL comparisons in a large Canadian randomized trial (11). In this study, mitoxantrone was compared to mitoxantrone plus prednisone (11). The primary index of clinical benefit was improved QOL, based on a well-validated model (10).

Although this trial was an important paradigm shifting study, there are still substantial problems in the methodology of QOL assessment (12), and it is my belief that the primary index for the assessment of novel compounds in the management of advanced hormone-refractory prostate cancer should still be objective tumor regression or survival.

Stage Migration

Stage migration is a phenomenon in clinical trials in which the amount of tumor in patients presenting for these trials changes over time because of improved staging technology or changes in treatment patterns.

This usually contributes to increasing proportions of patients with lesser tumor volume and thus a better prognosis within the mix of patients entered into more recent trials. This has confounded interpretation of these studies (Table 18.7.1).

TABLE 18.7.1. Comparable series of treatment of hormone-refractory prostate cancer

Parameter	Raghavan et al., 1996 (24)	Tannock et al., 1996 (11)	Kantoff et al., 1999 (25)	Ernst et al., 2003 (26)	Berry et al., 2002 (27)	Raghavan et al., 2005 (14)
Age						
Median	64	69	72	71	70	73
Interquartile range	50–77*	63–75	67–75	64–75	49–87	
ECOG PS						
0	48%	6%	85%	13%	75%**	4%
1	52%	57%	15%	62%	23%**	79%
≥2		37%		25%	2%**	18%
Metastases						
Bone	90%	98%	91%	Not stated	86%	93%
Lung	10%	4%	21%		2%	10%
Liver	6%		9%		4%	17%
Nodes	16%	22%	9%		18%	28%
PSA (ng/mL)						
Median	Not stated	209	150	150	57	210
Interquartile range		66–678	52–362	45–361	4–2375*	77–430
Alkaline phase Median	Not stated	2.0 (S.I. units)	167 105–317	229 150–495	Not stated	355 44–3018
Range		1.0–5.3				
% with pain	Not defined	99%	Not defined	100%	0%	100%
% with narcotic analgesics	Not defined		Not defined	22%	0%	100%
2-year actuarial survival		~15%	~20%***	~15–17%	~15%***	21%**

ECOG PS, Eastern Cooperative Oncology Group prostate cancer stage.
*Total (not interquartile) range.
**Actual, not actuarial survival.
***Stage migration influences survival (25), with less extent of tumor.

For example, the availability of PSA monitoring after primary therapy or hormonal manipulation has now led to the identification of relapsing patients earlier. In the 1980s, prior to the routine use of PSA monitoring, the first evidence of clinical relapse or metastasis was often pain, a pathological fracture, or some other indication of more advanced cancer. This change has resulted in the inclusion of patients with lower tumor mass than in the chemotherapy studies conducted two to three decades ago. This leads to the potential artifact of interpretation where new drugs appear to yield better outcomes than old drugs. For example, the median survival of patients treated with mitoxantrone and prednisone for hormone-refractory prostate cancer has increased 50% in the past 20 years, presumably due to stage migration and better supportive care (9). In this context, it has required randomized trials to show definitively that a survival benefit can be achieved by the use of chemotherapy (3,4).

Importance of Randomized Clinical Trials in Assessment of Chemotherapy

In view of all these variables in the assessment of new treatments, one must bring rigor and structure to the assessment of progress in this field, which is best done through the use of randomized trials. There is no doubt that noncomparative phase I to II trials have been critically important in identifying the potential role of the conventional and novel cytotoxic agents for advanced prostate cancer (1,2,13,14). The following drugs have been shown to have some anticancer effect against bone-dominant, hormone-refractory prostate cancer when used as single agents: doxorubicin, cyclophosphamide, cisplatin, carboplatin, mitoxantrone, paclitaxel, docetaxel, and mitomycin C. Each produces objective response rates of about 10% to 20%, sometimes with improved quality of life.

The problem is that new end points of assessment (e.g., PSA response) or changes in the population of patients treated (e.g., with lower tumor mass) could easily lead to misinterpretation of the extent of benefit from these new agents, as compared to the utility of some of the older drugs studied in the trials of the 1980s and 1990s. Ultimately the only reliable way to prove that novel agents are achieving more than older compounds is through randomized clinical trials.

Through this vehicle, direct comparison has shown that mitoxantrone improves QOL compared to noncytotoxic treatment (10,11), and that docetaxel is more active against prostate cancer than is mitoxantrone (at the expense of more toxicity) (3,4). This paradigm will be essential to the accurate evaluation of novel agents for prostate cancer.

Emerging Role of Cytotoxic Chemotherapy

Although single-agent chemotherapy has been shown to improve QOL and yield a modest survival benefit, randomized trials have not yet proven the superiority of combination chemotherapy over single agents. Some promising combination regimens have recently been reported, suggesting that combination chemotherapy may increase patient benefit, despite the problems of stage migration and altered end points. The combination of paclitaxel or docetaxel plus estramustine gives subjective response in approximately 50% to 60%, PSA response in 40% to 75%, and objective tumor response in up to 30%, depending on whether patients with soft tissue disease dominate the population of patients (15–17). Others have reported that the addition of carboplatin to the paclitaxel-estramustine doublet adds to clinical activity, claiming higher objective and PSA response rates (18,19). However, these data have not been validated by randomized trials.

Biochemical modulation of chemotherapeutic agents and the structural modification of established drugs are currently being evaluated in clinical trials. For example, we have recently suggested that tesmilifene, a tamoxifen analogue that modulates function of cytochrome P-450 and the multidrug resistance pump, may cause mitoxantrone to be a more effective agent against prostate cancer (14). In a small phase II trial, we tested this combination in 29 patients with narcotic-dependent pain, hormone refractory metastases and grossly elevated PSA levels, and recorded a PSA reduction of 75% in 48% of patients, and a 2-year survival of 21% (14). These data appeared to be highly unusual, meriting a formal randomized trial. Such a trial has been designed by the Southwest Oncology Group and is awaiting formal review by staff of the Clinical Trials Evaluation Program of the U.S. National Cancer Institute.

Another modulation of function has been achieved by the use of the protease function of PSA to activate doxorubicin. This has been tested in prostate cancer at a preliminary level, suggesting a possible enhanced anticancer effect (20).

A novel class of compounds that have some functional similarity to the taxanes, the epothilone B analogues, are being tested against prostate cancer. Ixabepilone, one of these agents, has recently been shown to induce objective response in up to 30% of cases, and a 50% PSA reduction in 48% of patients (21). This finding will require further testing to compare this agent's activity with that of docetaxel and to evaluate its utility in combination regimens.

Recently, nano-engineering methods have been used to alter the structure of paclitaxel, facilitating its entry into cancer cells without the need for cremophore dissolution. This new agent, Abraxane, is entering clinical trials in the treatment of prostate cancer at the Cleveland Clinic Taussig Cancer Center.

In view of the clear evidence of anticancer efficacy of cytotoxics in hormone refractory disease, chemotherapy is now being assessed earlier, analogous to the progression of studies in breast cancer 30 years ago. For example, Waxman's group has suggested that adjuvant mitoxantrone chemotherapy adds to the impact of castration, when started at the same time (22). While the published data are provocative, case selection bias may have influenced the results, and this has led to formal testing of the concept in a randomized trial by the Southwest Oncology Group (SWOG); SWOG trial 9921 compares castration versus castration plus mitoxantrone and prednisone in patients who have undergone radical prostatectomy for locally extensive disease. It seems likely that, predicated on the results of SWOG trial 9916, comparing docetaxel and mitoxantrone, studies assessing the utility of adjuvant docetaxel will also be started, although these may be harder to implement, given the greater toxicity of docetaxel and the relatively modest difference in outcome.

Another variant of this approach, neoadjuvant chemotherapy, has been to test novel cytotoxics in patients with untreated, locally extensive disease who are about to undergo radical prostatectomy (23). In preliminary studies of neoadjuvant docetaxel, reductions of PSA have been documented, although major tumor lysis has not been identified (23), and more extensive phase II to III trials will be required to validate this approach. It should be noted that cases of acute leukemia have been identified in SWOG 9921, among patients receiving adjuvant hormones plus mitoxantrone, and accordingly the trial has been closed prematurely. It is not yet known whether the small number of cases represents a true increase in incidence, but prudence has dictated early closure, with observation of all patients. This serves to illustrate the importance of randomized clinical trials in the implementation of novel strategies, especially for patients with potentially good prognosis.

Future Directions

Promising new data require validation in carefully structured comparative clinical trials to ensure that real progress is being made in the use of chemotherapy for prostate cancer, and that improved results are not just a reflection of improved supportive care, earlier diagnosis, and stage migration. Rigor in clinical testing is essential, especially as several new concepts are being tested in early-phase trials, including biochemical modulation, application of nano-technology, and the use of targeted therapies that are directed to the determinants of cellular turnover. We seem to be on the verge of a major step forward, the result of 50 years of meticulous, structured investigation.

References

1. Tannock IF. Is there evidence that chemotherapy is of benefit to patients with carcinoma of the prostate? J Clin Oncol 1985;3:1013–1021.
2. Raghavan D. Non-hormone chemotherapy for prostate cancer: principles of treatment and application to the testing of new drugs. Semin Oncol 1988;15:371–389.
3. Petrylak D, Tangen CM, Hussain MH, et al. Docetaxel and estramustine compared with mitoxantrone and prednisone for advanced refractory prostate cancer. N Engl J Med 2004;351:1513–1520.
4. Tannock IF, deWit R, Berry WR, et al. Docetaxel plus prednisone or mitoxantrone plus prednisone for advanced prostate cancer. N Engl J Med 2004;351:1502–1512.
5. Slack NH. Results of chemotherapy protocols of the US National Prostatic Cancer Project (NPCP). Clin Oncol 1983;2:441–459.
6. Kelly WK, Scher HI, Mazumdar M. Prostate specific antigen as a measure of disease outcome in metastatic hormone-refractory prostate cancer. J Clin Oncol 1993;11: 607–615.
7. Sridhara R, Eisenberger MA, Sinibaldi V, Reyno LM, Egorin MJ. Evaluation of prostate-specific antigen as a surrogate marker for response of hormone-refractory prostate cancer to suramin therapy. J Clin Oncol 1995;13:2944–2953.
8. Bubley GJ, Carducci M, Dahut W, et al. Eligibility and response guidelines for phase II clinical trials in androgen-independent prostate cancer: recommendations from the Prostate-Specific Antigen Working Group. J Clin Oncol 1999;17:3461–3467.
9. Petrylak D, Ankerst D, Jiang C, et al. Evaluation of post treatment PSA declines for surrogacy using Prentice's criteria in patients treated on SWOG 99–16. J Natl Cancer Inst 2006;98:516–521.
10. Osoba D, Tannock IF, Ernst DS, Neville AJ. Health-related quality of life in men with metastatic prostate cancer treated with prednisone alone or mitoxantrone and prednisone. J. Clin. Oncol 1999;17:1654–1663.
11. Tannock IF, Osoba D, Stockler MR, et al. Chemotherapy with mitoxantrone plus prednisone or prednisone alone for symptomatic hormone-resistant prostate cancer:

a Canadian randomized trial with palliative end points. J Clin Oncol 1996;14: 1756–1764.

12. Browman GP. Science, language, intuition, and the many meanings of quality of life. J Clin Oncol 1999;17:1651–1653.

13. Beer T, Raghavan D. Chemotherapy for hormone-refractory prostate cancer: beauty is in the eye of the beholder. Prostate 2000;45:184–193.

14. Raghavan D, Brandes LJ, Klapp K, et al. Phase II trial of tesmilifene plus mitoxantrone and prednisone for hormone refractory prostate cancer: high subjective and objective response in patients with symptomatic metastases. J Urol 2005;174:1808–1813.

15. Hudes GR, Nathan F, Khater C, et al. Phase II trial of 96-hour paclitaxel plus oral estramustine phosphate in metastatic hormone-refractory prostate cancer. J Clin Oncol 1997;15:3156–3163.

16. Savarese D, Taplin ME, Halabi S, et al. A phase II study of docetaxel (Taxotere), estramustine, and low-dose hydrocortisone in men with hormone-refractory prostate cancer: Preliminary results of Cancer and Leukemia Group B trial 9780. Semin Oncol 1999;26(suppl 17):39–44.

17. Petrylak DP, Shelton GB, England-Owe C, et al. Response and preliminary survival results of a phase II study of docetaxel (D) + estramustine (E) in patients (Pts) with androgen-independent prostate cancer (AIPCA). Proc ASCO 2000;19:334a(abstract 1312).

18. Kelly WK, Curley T, Slovin S, et al. Paclitaxel, estramustine phosphate, and carboplatin in patients with advanced prostate cancer. J Clin Oncol 2001;19:44–53.

19. Urakami S, Igawa M, Kikuno K, et al. Combination chemotherapy with paclitaxel, estramustine and carboplatin for hormone refractory prostate cancer. J Urol 2002; 168:2444–2450.

20. DiPaola RS, Rinehart J, Nemunaitis J, et al. Characterization of a novel prostate-specific antigen-activated peptide-doxorubicin conjugate in patients with prostate cancer. J Clin Oncol 2002;20:1874–1879.

21. Galsky MD, Small EJ, Oh WK, et al. Multi-institutional randomized phase II trial of the epothilone B analog ixabepilone (BMS-247550) with or without estramustine phosphate in patients with progressive castrate metastatic prostate cancer. J Clin Oncol 2005;23:1439–1446.

22. Wang J, Halford S, Rigg A, et al. Adjuvant mitozantrone chemotherapy in advanced prostate cancer. BJU Int 2000;86:675–680.

23. Dreicer R, Magi-Galluzzi C, Zhou M, et al. Phase II trial of neoadjuvant docetaxel before radical prostatectomy for locally advanced prostate cancer. Urology 2004; 63:1138–1142.

24. Raghavan D, Coorey G, Rosen M, Page J, Farebrother T. Management of hormone-resistant prostate cancer: an Australian trial. Semin Oncol 1996;23(suppl 14):20–23.

25. Kantoff PW, Halabi S, Conaway M, et al. Hydrocortisone with or without mitoxantrone in men with hormone-refractory prostate cancer: results of the Cancer and Leukemia Group B 9182 study. J Clin Oncol 1999;17:2506–2513.

26. Ernst DS, Tannock IF, Winquist EW, et al. Randomized, double-blind, controlled trial of mitoxantrone/prednisone and clodronate versus mitoxantrone/prednisone and placebo in patients with hormone-refractory prostate cancer and pain. J Clin Oncol 2003;21:3335–3342.

27. Berry W, Dakhil S, Modiano M, Gregurich M, Asmar L. Phase III study of mitoxantrone plus low dose prednisone versus low dose alone in patients with asymptomatic, hormone refractory prostate cancer. J Urol 2002;168:2451–2453.

18.8
Investigational Therapies for Prostate Cancer

Suresh Radhakrishnan and Frank Chinegwundoh

Universal agreement has not been reached as to the best treatment for cancer of the prostate (CaP) at any stage. Radical prostatectomy, external-beam radiation therapy, and brachytherapy are potentially curative in patients with clinically localized disease. Despite the widespread use of prostate-specific antigen (PSA) in early detection and screening, significant numbers of cases are not diagnosed until the disease has advanced or metastasized beyond the reach of these local treatment modalities. Hormonal therapy and chemotherapy are the only other systemic treatments available at the present time. Because of the limitations of current local and systemic therapies for prostate cancer, there is a continued interest in the development of new treatment modalities. This chapter discusses some of the therapies and their principles that are being investigated in CaP.

Gene Therapy for Prostate Cancer

In recent years, gene therapy has emerged as a new frontier in the management of cancer. As prostate cancer represents the accumulation of genetic mutations that causes the prostate cell to lose its ability to control growth, reversal or correction of the genetic defects through gene therapy seems to be a promising method in treating prostate cancer. The term *gene therapy* broadly refers to the transfer of genetic material into human cells and the expression of that material in these cells for a therapeutic purpose (1). With respect to cancer, the goal of gene therapy is to prevent or treat disease by using the therapeutic information encoded in the DNA sequences.

Evidence suggests that tumor formation is caused by the overexpression of oncogenes or by mutations in suppressor genes in the presence or absence of cancer-causing environmental agents. The first human experiment of gene therapy can be attributed to Anderson and coworkers (2), who successfully transferred the gene for adenosine deaminase in a 4-year-old girl with severe combined immunodeficiency due to adenosine deaminase deficiency. Subsequently, gene therapy has been studied in the field of cancer prevention and treatment. When considering gene therapy as a treatment approach for prostate cancer, the questions that arise are what genes to insert and how to deliver the genes. Two major categories of gene therapy are cytoreductive gene therapy and corrective gene therapy. Cytoreductive gene therapy includes treatment strategies designed to selectively destroy malignant cells either directly (e.g., toxic genes) or indirectly (e.g., genes that stimulate immune responses). Corrective gene therapy involves replacing or inactivating defective genes in preneoplastic or neoplastic cells with genes that can slow or reverse the loss of growth-control mechanisms (e.g., tumor suppressor genes). These therapeutic genetic modifications can be performed either ex-vivo or in vivo, depending on the strategy. The concepts and strategies are shown in Figure 18.8.1.

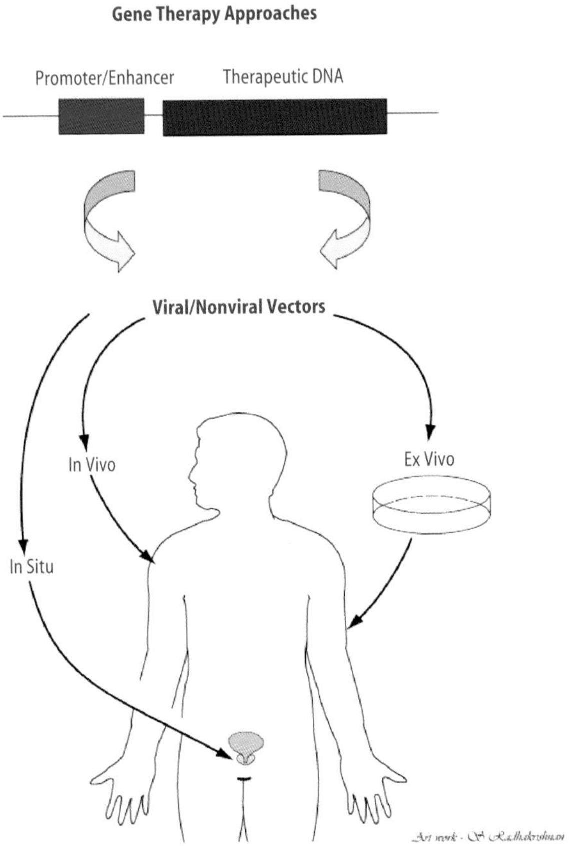

FIGURE 18.8.1. Gene therapy strategies.

What Genes to Insert?

Cytoreductive Gene Therapy

The most thoroughly evaluated form so far involves stimulation of antitumor immune response against a cancer by vaccinating affected patients with genetically modified tumor cells (3). This approach is discussed later.

Yet another approach for cytoreductive gene therapy was to direct the action of chemotherapeutic agents to target cancerous cells alone by using a prodrug that gets activated only in the cancerous cells, and thus the active drug is formed in active concentration only in the target cancerous cells sparing the normal cells [gene-directed enzyme prodrug delivery (GDEPT)]. The selectivity is achieved by identifying the genetic changes in the cancerous cells during carcinogenesis, and the prodrug is delivered to these cells by an adenovirus vector carrying the prodrug, thus sparing the normal cells. Freytag et al. (4) conducted a phase I trial by intraprostatic injection of viral particles combining 5-fluorocytosine and valganciclovir prodrug and adenovirus carrying the cytosine deaminase/herpes simplex virus thymidine kinase fusion gene at 1, 2, or 3 weeks along with conventional three-dimensional conformal radiotherapy (3D-CRT). This study showed that the patients who received more than 1 week of prodrug therapy had a shorter mean PSA half-life than the patients receiving prodrug therapy for 1 week (0.6 vs. 2.0 months). The results demonstrate that replication-competent adenovirus-mediated double-suicide gene therapy can be combined safely with conventional-dose 3D-CRT in patients with intermediate- to high-risk prostate cancer.

Corrective Gene Therapy

The mutated genes in prostate cancer can be restored to the normal genome so that the cancer formation or progression is prevented. The *p53* gene is commonly mutated in human cancers at a frequency varying between 5% to 65% (5). The *p53* gene replacement is a particularly attractive therapeutic strategy because in vitro restoration of wild-type *p53* in many tumor cell lines causes growth arrest or apoptosis. However, there are limitations in the use of this approach for treating prostate cancer. In metabolic diseases in which a single gene defect has been identified as the cause of the disease state, such as in cystic fibrosis, replacing the defective gene product is a promising treatment approach. However, the main problem in cancer is that there is no single oncogene or tumor suppressor gene defect. Table 18.8.1 lists many different genes mutated in prostate cancer that can act as potential gene therapy targets.

How to Deliver the Genes

The key factor in gene therapy is the development of a safe, reliable vector that can insert the desired gene into the target. Vectors are engineered DNA or RNA

TABLE 18.8.1. Some common gene therapy targets for treating prostate cancer

Genes	Clinical/lab studies
Tumor suppressor genes	
p53	Pisters et al. (6), Mikata et al. (7)
Rb	
pTEN	Tanaka et al. (8)
	Rosser (9)
KAI 1	
p16	
Oncogenes	
Myc	Iversen (10)
Bcl2	Shi (11)
Growth factors	
Transforming growth factor-β	Cao (12)
PSA	Cheng (13)
Antiangiogenic genes	
Endostatin	Li et al. (14)
Angiostatin	
Proapoptotic gene	
BAX	

sequences into which a therapeutic gene can be inserted. Some common vectors are given in Table 18.8.2

The Future of Gene Therapy

The first gene therapy trial occurred in 1990 at the National Institutes of Health in the United States. As of January 2006, there were 1145 approved gene therapy/transfer protocols for both cancer and noncancerous conditions, and 67% of these were for cancer treatment (15). To date, at least 15 phase I or phase I/II clinical trials on gene therapy for prostate cancer have been started. The future of gene therapy in prostate cancer or other cancers depends on the development of new vectors that would increase transgene size capacity, better immunogenic properties, better transduction efficiency, and a better understanding of the genes involved in tumor induction and proliferation. Research into the molecular mechanisms has improved our knowledge of genes involved in the development and progression of CaP.

However, a broad range of molecular alterations including progression of prostate cancer into androgen independence is a major problem in the development of the treatment strategies. New viruses with better oncolytic potential are being studied along with development of safe delivery system.

TABLE 18.8.2. Vectors for gene therapy

Viral vector	Advantages	Disadvantages
Retrovirus	Easy to produce	Targets only dividing cells
	Efficient transfer	Risk of replication
	Small genome	Carries small DNA sequences only
	Biology well understood	Low transduction efficiency
	Nontoxic to host cells	Integration with potential oncogenesis
	High-efficiency genomic integration	
Adenovirus	Highly efficient transfer	Possible host immune reaction
	Targets nondividing cells	Risk of replication
	Nontoxic to host cell	Carries small DNA sequences only
	High transduction efficiency	Low potential oncogenesis
	Immunogenicity	No integration
		Transient expression
Adeno-associated virus	Less likely to produce immune reactions	Small capacity
	Targets nondividing cells	Immunogenic
	Nonpathogenic in humans	Risk of replication
	Efficient transfer	
	Good in vivo delivery	
	Integrates into genome	
Vaccinia virus	High titer	Immunogenicity
	Large insert size	Toxicity
Herpes simplex virus	Large insert size	Toxicity

Nonviral vectors	Advantages	Disadvantages
Plasmid DNA	No size limitation	Low efficiency
Liposome	Easy to produce	Low efficiency
	Safety features	
	Less likely to produce immune response	
	No limitation on size and type of nucleic acid	

Vaccine Therapy in Prostate Cancer

Tumor contains many antigens that are not expressed in normal cells but are recognized as foreign proteins by the immune system, which thereby surmounts a defense mechanism killing the cancer cells. But unlike immunotherapy by vaccination against infectious diseases, clinical immunotherapy of cancer has achieved limited success to date. The immune response to tumor cells is generally inadequate, and cancer eventually proliferates in individuals with normal immune function. It is possible that cancer cells have multiple mechanisms to evade immune system. Attempts have been made to modulate the immune system to overcome tumor defense and escape mechanisms, fighting cancer with high efficacy and specificity. The earliest evidence of the anticancer potential of the immune system came from William Coley, who noted that several sarcomas regressed after an inflammatory response to local bacterial infections (16).

Antitumoral immunotherapy may be either passive or active. Passive immunotherapy typically involves the transfer of immunological agents into a tumor-bearing host. In contrast, active immunotherapy involves the administration of agents that elicit an antitumoral response directly from host immune system.

The prevailing techniques of tumor immunotherapy can be broadly divided into two groups: nonspecific and antigen-specific therapies. The latter technique can be achieved by either adoptive transfer or vaccination. In adoptive transfer the actual components of the immune system that are already capable of producing a specific immune response are transferred to the patient. Vaccination, on the other hand, involves the administration of a particular antigen to induce a specific immune response in the host.

Whole Cell Vaccine

In simple terms, whole cell vaccines use whole tumor cells for vaccination. In the ex vivo vaccine approach, tumor cells are removed from the patient at surgery, grown in cell culture, and transfected with cytokine genes that stimulate an immune response to antigens present on the tumor cell vaccine. The gene-modified tumor vaccine is then irradiated to prevent subsequent tumor growth and reinjected into the patient in an attempt to generate either a local or systemic immune response against the remaining tumor burden in the patient. The immune response activated by vaccination can then act systemically eradicating or slowing down the growth of distant micrometastatic cells that share antigens with the genetically engineered vaccine cell. Early clinical studies with this whole cell vaccine approach were met with limited success. Probably one of the early works on vaccines in carcinoma of the prostate was done by Sanda et al. They found that therapy using gene-modified, irradiated vaccine cells genetically transduced to secrete granulocyte-macrophage colony-stimulating factor (GM-CSF) prolonged survival in animals with prostate cancer. There were numerous technical difficulties in the preparation of autologous cells that represented a significant limitation to this method, and individualized preparation of the vaccine was labor-intensive. These persistent problems have shifted the focus of research to allogeneic vaccines, which are readily available from established prostate cancer cell lines.

Granulocyte-macrophage colony-stimulating factor gene transduced irradiated prostate cancer vaccine cells (GVAX) is a vaccine composed of allogeneic prostate cancer cell lines (PC-3 and LNCaP) genetically modified to secrete GM-CSF (3,17). A single-institution phase I/II trial in hormone therapy–naive patients with PSA relapse following radical prostatectomy and absence of radiologic metastases has show that at 20 weeks after the first treatment, 16 of 21 (76%) patients showed a statisti-cally significant decrease in PSA velocity (slope) compared with prevaccination (17).

Onyvax-P consists of the irradiated allogeneic prostate cancer cell lines ONYCAP23, P4E6 and LNCaP, which are representative of different stages of the cancer and express prostate-associated antigens administered at a dose of $8 \times$

10^6 cells. Patients were administered the vaccine in three cycles biweekly then monthly up to 12 months from the initiation of vaccination (18). Eleven of 26 patients had decreased PSA velocities and a median time to disease progression of 58 weeks, as compared with an historic value of 28 weeks (19,20). No significant toxicities were observed.

Dendritic Cell–Based Vaccines

Dendritic cells (DCs) are rare leukocytes that have a unique ability to present antigen to T cells. Growing evidence indicates that DCs mediate a crucial role in priming antigen-specific immune responses (21). The DCs are well suited to this purpose, as they express diverse receptors that mediate the acquisition of antigens in peripheral tissues, process this material efficiently into the major histocompatibility complex (MHC) class I and II presentation pathway, upregulate co-stimulatory molecules on maturation, and migrate to secondary lymphoid tissues. The delineation of specific properties of DCs that elicit high levels of antitumor activity provides important guidelines for optimizing the therapeutic use of these cells for cancer immunotherapy.

Sipuleucel-T (APC 8015, Provenge) is an autologous, dendritic cell-based vaccine. It contains autologous antigen-presenting cells (APCs) loaded with PA2024, a recombinant prostatic acid phosphatase/GM-CSF fusion protein, as the immunogen. It stimulate T-cell immunity against prostatic acid phosphatase. Patients are typically administered three intravenous (IV) infusions of the vaccine over a 1-month period as a complete course of therapy.

A phase II trial was conducted to assess the PSA-modulating effects of APC8015 in patients with androgen-dependent prostate cancer with biochemical progression (22). Patients with nonmetastatic recurrent disease as manifested by increasing PSA levels (0.4 to 6.0 ng/mL) and who had undergone previous definitive surgical or radiation therapy were enrolled. Therapy consisted of APC8015 infusion on weeks 0, 2, and 4. Prostate-specific antigen was measured at baseline and monthly until disease progression, defined as a doubling of the baseline or nadir PSA value (whichever was lower) to ≥ 4 ng/mL or development of distant metastases. Thirteen of 18 patients demonstrated an increase in PSA doubling time (PSADT) with a median increase of 62% (4.9 months before treatment vs. 7.9 months after treatment).

A recent phase III placebo-controlled study enrolled a total of 127 patients with asymptomatic metastatic hormone-refractory prostate cancer to receive three infusions of sipuleucel-T ($n = 82$) or placebo ($n = 45$) every 2 weeks in a 2:1 ratio (23). Of the 127 patients, 115 patients had progressive disease. The median time to disease progression for sipuleucel-T was 11.7 weeks compared with 10.0 weeks for placebo, and median survival was 25.9 months for sipuleucel-T and 21.4 months for placebo.

APC8015 combined with bevacizumab (recombinant antibody against vascular endothelial growth factor, a proangiogenic protein with inhibitory effects on APC) has been evaluated, and the study treated 22 patients. It showed that one patient achieved a $\geq 50\%$ decrease in PSA. Nine patients exhibited some decrease in PSA from baseline, ranging from 6% to 72%, with the PSA of three patients decreasing at least 25%. The median pretreatment PSADT for the 20 evaluable patients was 6.9 months, and the median posttreatment PSADT was 12.7 months. All patients demonstrated induction of an immune response against PA2024.

Antigen Vaccines

Antigen vaccines stimulate the immune system by using individual antigens, rather than whole tumor cells. There are many known targets in prostate cancer that have been utilized including PSA, prostatic acid phosphatase (PAP), prostate-specific membrane antigen (PSMA), and MUC1 protein. The PSA, owing to its restricted expression in prostate cancer and normal prostatic epithelial cells, is one of the potential targets for a vaccine. A number of PSA-specific epitopes have been identified that can activate cytotoxic T lymphocytes and, in turn, result in the killing of tumor targets by the peptide-specific cytotoxic T lymphocytes.

DNA Vaccines

MVA-MUC1-IL-2 (TG4010), a viral suspension of a recombinant vaccinia vector containing the coding for MUC1 (an epithelial antigen that is overexpressed in prostate cancer), and interleukin-2 (IL-2) were evaluated in a randomized phase II trial of 40 patients that compared two schedules of the vaccine (24). MUC-1–specific immune responses and significant lengthening of PSA doubling times were observed.

The Eastern Cooperative Oncology Group (ECOG) have reported a phase II trial of 65 patients designed to evaluate the tolerability and feasibility of a prime/boost vaccine strategy using vaccinia virus and fowlpox virus expressing human PSA in patients with PSA progression after definitive local therapy (25); PSA progression-free survival at 19.1 month occurred in 45.3%, and 78.1% demonstrated clinical progression-free survival.

High-Intensity Focused Ultrasound

High-intensity focused ultrasound (HIFU) is a technology that has moved from being used for benign prostatic disease (26) to the treatment of prostate cancer. Gelet et al. (27) first applied HIFU for treatment of prostate cancer.

Mechanism of Action

Focused ultrasound holds promise in a large number of therapeutic applications. It has long been known that HIFU can kill tissue through coagulative necrosis. Tissue destruction in the target zone is attributable to three phenomena: coagulation, cavitation, and heat. Absorption of the ultrasound energy creates an increase in temperature (to between 70°C and 100°C), which destroys the tissue within the focal area. However, it is only in recent years that practical clinical applications are becoming possible, with the development of high-power ultrasound arrays and noninvasive monitoring methods. In the last decade, HIFU has been adapted and used to treat localized prostate cancer.

Indications and Advantages

High-intensity focused ultrasound is intended to destroy prostate tissue without damaging intervening and surrounding tissue, thus eliminating the need for incisions, transfusions, general anesthesia, and their resulting complications. Rebillard et al. (28) analyzed studies published up to July 2004, totaling 5084 sessions of HIFU. They suggested that indications for HIFU treatment include well to moderately differentiated localized prostate cancer (T1–2 N0M0) with a baseline PSA value ≤15 ng/mL in men with an estimated life expectancy between 5 and 15 years and those who are not candidates for radical prostatectomy, obese, or with comorbidities.

For patients with a localized tumor associated with an intermediate or low risk of recurrence, the preliminary results of HIFU are comparable to those of other treatment options such as radical surgery and radiotherapy. The use of HIFU as the second-line treatment of a localized tumor after failure of radio-therapy appears to be promising (29).

Certain characteristics of HIFU make it particularly promising in the therapy of malignant tumors. It is noninvasive and treats the inner tumor without damaging the body. It can pass through tissues and accurately damage target tissues. The boundary between therapy zone and the nontherapy zone is clear, and tissue beyond the target zone is hardly destroyed (30,31). High-intensity focused ultrasound can be used in real time, enabling accurate targeting and monitoring, and thus facilitating estimating the therapeutic effect and adjusting the dosage (32).

High-intensity focused ultrasound treatment has many advantages. It causes less pain, entails minimal damage, has fewer influences on splanchnic function, and results in faster recovery for the body (32). The treatment can also be repeated if necessary.

It is not advisable to use HIFU in glands of more than 40 cc because of the limited focal length of HIFU (33). However, this problem can be overcome by downsizing the gland with transurethral resection of the prostate (TURP) or by luteinizing hormone–releasing hormone (LHRH) agonist therapy (33). Anticoagulation medication is a relative contraindication, and it needs to be stopped 10 days prior to the treatment. Patients who have rectal problems or had abdomino perineal (AP) resection of rectum are not suitable for HIFU.

Technique

High-intensity focused ultrasound for prostate cancer is usually carried out under spinal or general anesthesia. With the patient lying on his right side, an

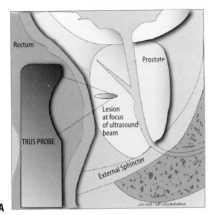
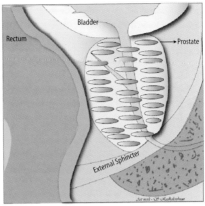

FIGURE **18.8.2.** High-intensity focused ultrasound (HIFU) treatment. (A) Creation of lesion. (B) Lesions at end of procedure. TRUS, transrectal ultrasound.

endorectal probe incorporating an ultrasound scanner and a HIFU treatment applicator is inserted, allowing visualization and definition of the target area. The probe emits a beam of ultrasound, which is focused to reach a high intensity in the target area; the sudden and intense absorption of the ultrasound beam creates a sudden elevation of the temperature and coagulative necrosis. By repeating the shots, and moving the focal point between each shot, it is possible to destroy a volume that includes the whole tumor (400 to 600 shots). The treatment duration varies according to prostate volume (1 to 2 hours). Figure 18.8.2 shows a HIFU applicator and the lesions created. By moving the probes to different areas of the prostate, the entire gland can be treated. A cooling balloon surrounding the probe protects the rectal mucosa from the high temperature. A urethral/suprapubic catheter is left in situ after the procedure.

Results

A systematic review (34), including eight case series, reported a negative biopsy rate of 60% (35), and 80% in a study with 3 year follow-up (36). In three further studies in the review, the proportion of patients without clinical or biochemical evidence of disease ranged from 56% at 24 months to 66% at 19 months (27).

In 1995, Madersbacher et al. (37) reported the ability of HIFU (using the older Sonablate 200 system) to destroy entire tumors in an experimental study of 10 patients with localized disease.

Gelet et al. (27,38) reported their preliminary experience of HIFU using the Ablatherm prototype 1.0 (EDAP-Technomed, Lyon, France) for treating localized prostate cancer, and their results showed a complete response in two thirds of the patients, with no residual cancer, and no patient had three consecutive increases in PSA level. Chaussy and Thuroff (39) have reported that the combination of TURP before HIFU reduced the treatment-related morbidity, including catheter duration, incontinence, and urinary infection. In addition, they summarized the clinical outcome using the American Society for Therapeutic Radiology and Oncology (ASTRO) definition, an 84% stability rate in the HIFU group, and an 80% rate in the TURP and HIFU group. In their study Beerlage et al. (35) found that there is extensive coagulation necrosis in treated areas, and they stressed the importance of targeting the lesion. A more recent study with 63 patients (40) found 3-year biochemical disease-free survival rates for patients with a PSA level before HIFU of <10, 10.01 to 20, and >20 ng/mL of 82%, 62%, and 20%, respectively, using the ASTRO consensus criteria. It found an overall biochemical disease-free rate of 75%. The major published studies are listed in Table 18.8.3.

Side Effects and Complications

Chaussy and Thuroff (36) reported the following complications in 315 patients who underwent HIFU treatment with Ablatherm: six patients had stress incontinence of grade 1, five patients had a rectourethral fistula, eight patients had stress incontinence after a repeat treatment, and three patients had stress incontinence of grade 2 and above. Urinary retention occurs due to a swollen gland and coagulation necrosis of an adenoma, and is treated by suprapubic catheterization. Other complications included urge incontinence, urgency, bladder neck stenosis, urethral stenosis, urethritis, prostate abscess, epididymitis, asymptomatic rectal burns, and chronic pelvic pain.

However, there are no randomized studies on the efficacy of HIFU and only case series has been published. The latest published results suggest that HIFU treatment is a valuable option for well-differentiated and moderately differentiated tumors, as well as for local recurrence after external-beam radiation therapy. Long-term results are still awaited regarding survival benefit.

Cryotherapy

Cryotherapy is another treatment modality that has been added to the armamentarium of the management of localized prostate cancer. It selectively freezes the tissue causing tissue destruction in a controlled fashion. It is also used in cases of recurrent prostate cancer following radiotherapy.

Mechanism of Action

Cryotherapy is based on the ablation of tissue by local induction of extreme cold temperatures. Tissue destruction is achieved by disruption of cell membranes by ice crystal formation during freezing and vascular damage leading to thrombosis and ischemia. The tissue effects vary with the temperature and freezing time. Once below 0°C, extracellular fluid begins to crystallize, which

TABLE 18.8.3. Major published studies on high-intensity focused ultrasound

Author	Center	Year	No of patients	Mean follow-up	Device	Disease control	Post-HIFU-negative biopsy rates
Beerlage et al. (35)	Netherlands and Germany	1999	111	12 months	Ablatherm	PSA nadir <0.5 ng/mL in 55% in globally treated group vs. 19%, in selectively treated patients	Residual cancer spots in 72% of cases in the selectively treated group and in 32% in the globally treated group
Chaussy and Thuroff (36)	Germany	2000	184		Ablatherm	The nadir PSA < 4 ng/mL in 97%, including 61% who had values <0.5 ng/mL	80% Cancer free
Gelet et al. (38)	France	2001	102	19 months	Ablatherm	Overall disease-free survival = 66%	Negative biopsy: 75% (76/102)
Thuroff et al. (41)	European Multicentric Study Prospective	2003	402	407 days		Overall mean nadir PSA (ng/mL) for patients with 6-month follow-up =1.8	Overall negative biopsy of 87.2%
Chaussy and Thuroff (39)	Germany	2003	271	Follow-up: HIFU = 18.7 months TURP and HIFU = 10.9 months	Ablatherm	Stable PSA at last follow-up: HIFU = 84.2% TURP and HIFU = 80.0%	Negative biopsy at last follow-up: HIFU = 87.7% TURP and HIFU = 81.6%
Blana et al. (42)	Germany	2004	146	22.5 months	Ablatherm	PSA nadir <1.0 ng/mL: 92%	Negative biopsies: 93.4%
Kiel et al. (43)	Germany	2000	62	Median 15 months		Complete response—no tumor on biopsy and PSA < 4: 68.7%	
Uchida et al. (40)	Hachioji, Japan	2006	63	Median 22 months	Sonablate	Overall biochemical disease-free rate was 75% according to ASTRO consensus criteria	87% patients cancer free at 3 years

ASTRO, American Society for Therapeutic Radiology and Oncology.

increases the osmotic pressure from the remaining unfrozen fluid in the extra cellular space. This drags fluid from the cells and leads to changes in the intra-cellular pH and protein denaturation. Below −15°C, all the extracellular fluid is frozen, trapping cells. Subsequent expansion of the ice crystals results in mechanical disruption of protein and cell membranes. Further temperature reduction causes intracellular freezing with further damage. Stasis in blood vessels adds hypoxia as a further cell damage mechanism. Not all damage relates to freezing, and further cellular insults occur during thawing. Fluids shift back into the intracellular space, causing the cell to burst. As a general rule maximum tissue death occurs with rapid freezing to the lowest possible temperature followed by slow thawing.

As cryotherapy damages surrounding tissues, the procedure is monitored with ultrasound, which can localize the position of the ice ball. The ice ball is created using pressurized argon or nitrogen gas with single or multiple hollow needles. Multiple needles result in a conformal ice ball similar to the treatment area provided by brachytherapy.

James Arnott (Brighton, UK) was the first physician to use hypothermia to treat cancer. He used a mixture of ice and saline to reduce morbidity, especially pain, of women with advanced uterine and breast cancer. Solid carbon dioxide became widely used to treat various dermatological diseases in the early 20th century.

The first prostate cryosurgery was performed by Gonder et al. (44) in 1966 using a single 26-French transurethral liquid N_2 probe to treat bladder outlet obstruction from an enlarged prostate. Complications were common, particularly urethral sloughing and rectal fistula due to lack of proper monitoring. Currently, argon is used for cryotherapy, with lower complication rates. Perineal approaches in the past were associated with significant complications, mainly in the form of urethral fistula (1% to 3%) and incontinence (8%) (45,46). Other complications reported in the literature include impotence (72%) and perineal and rectal pain (18%).

The most significant development, which led to the resurgence of interest in cryosurgery, was the introduction of real-time transrectal ultrasound-guided placement of the probes and continuous monitoring of the iceball progression by Onik et al. (47) in 1993 (second-generation cryosurgery). The sound waves reflect off the frozen-unfrozen interface and appear as an advancing hyperechoic rim with an anechoic shadow behind it (47). One of the limitations of ultrasound is the inability to provide information about the temperature distribution within the iceball. The introduction of thermosensors (48) in 1994 enabled the operator to precisely monitor the iceball temperature. This has resulted in a more efficient freeze with a significant rise in the success rates (49). Another key advance of modern cryosurgery has been urethral mucosal protection with a warming catheter. This has led to a major reduction in sloughing and incontinence rates (50). The recent third-generation cryosurgical technique uses compressed gases—argon to freeze and helium to thaw the tissue in a freeze-thaw cycle.

Technique

The procedure is usually carried out under spinal anesthesia. A warming catheter is inserted into the bladder and kept distended and warmed to 38°C. The catheter remains in place for 2 hours following the procedure.

Multiple small-diameter cryoprobes are placed through the perineum into the prostate tissue at selected spatial intervals. Transrectal ultrasound is used to position the cylindrical probes before activation of the argon cooling element, which lowers the tissue temperature below –40°C. Tissue effect is monitored by transrectal ultrasound changes as well as thermocouples placed in the tissue. Thermocouples or temperature monitor probes are placed adjacent to the neurovascular bundles, the apex, the Denonvilliers space, and the external sphincter. A double freeze-thaw process is initiated with the anterior cryoprobes being activated first, followed by the posterior probes. The aim is to freeze the entire gland. A suprapubic catheter is left in place and open for at least 4 days postoperatively.

Selection of Patients

Patients with low PSA (≤ 10 ng/mL), low Gleason score, and T1-2 disease may respond well to cryotherapy. It can also be used in a salvage setting for local recurrence after radiotherapy and radical prostatectomy.

Results

The initial enthusiasm for cryoablation of previously untreated prostate cancer waned when many centers failed to achieve sustained satisfactory biochemical outcome. The lack of evidence to date from randomized controlled clinical trials confirming its long-term efficacy, however, has led some groups to limit the use of cryoablation primarily to the salvage situation of tumor relapse after radiation therapy given with curative intent. However, with recent developments in the techniques, many centers have renewed their interest in using cryosurgery as a primary therapy.

Pisters et al. (51) studied the efficacy and complication rates of salvage cryotherapy as a treatment modality for 150 patients with locally recurrent prostate cancer following full-dose radiation therapy or systemic therapy. They also compared efficacy of single versus double freeze-thaw cycles using post-treatment PSA levels and prostate biopsies as end points; 31% of patients had persistently undetectable PSA. The main complications of salvage cryotherapy were urinary incontinence (73% of the patients), obstructive symptoms (67%), impotence (72%), and severe perineal pain (8%). They found that a double freeze-thaw cycle appears more effective than a single cycle. Like salvage prostatectomy, salvage cryotherapy causes significant morbidity (52). Table 18.8.4 lists some of the published studies in cryosurgery used either as primary or salvage therapy.

TABLE 18.8.4. Some published results in cryosurgery of the prostate

Author	Center	Year of study	Year of publication	No of patients	Follow-up period	Primary or salvage	PSA control	Postprocedure negative biopsy rates	Complications
Shinohara et al. (53)	California	1993–1995	1996	102	6 months	Primary	48% had undetectable PSA at 6 months	77%	57% (excluding impotence rate of 84%)
Wong et al. (50)	Alhambra, California	1993–1995	2000	83	30 months	Primary	Median PSA 0.3 at 30 months	90% (n = 71) at 30 months in patients where urethral warmer was used	46% with urethral warmer
Cohen et al. (54)	Pittsburgh	1990–1994	1996	239	Minimum 21 months	Primary		69% after one treatment and 82% following one or more treatments	Urethral tissue sloughing in 10% of patients
Koppie et al. (55)	San Francisco	1993–1998	1999	176	Mean 30.8 months	Primary	Nadir PSA undetectable in 49% patients	63% in patients with at least 24 months follow-up	
Long et al. (56)	Boston	1993–1998	2001	975	Median 24 months	Primary	5-year BDFS 36–61%	Overall 18% positive biopsy rate	Impotence 93% Incontinence 7.5%
Pisters et al. (51)	Houston	1992–1995	1997	150	Mean 17.3 months for single freeze-thaw cycle and 10 months for double freeze-thaw cycle	Salvage	Over all 31% had persistently undetectable PSA	93% for double and 71% for single freeze-thaw cycle	Incontinence 73% Obstructive symptoms 67%
Bahn et al. (57)	California	1993–2001	2003	59	7 years	Salvage	BDFS rate using a PSA cutoff of 0.5ng/mL was 59%		

BDFS, biochemical disease-free survival.

Radiofrequency Treatment in Prostate Cancer

Thermal therapy is used to kill tumors by heating them to temperatures greater than 50°C for an extended period of time. Cell death results from thermal coagulation. Radiofrequency ablation involves percutaneous or intraoperative insertion of an electrode into a lesion under ultrasonic guidance. The energy sources available for this approach include radiofrequency electrodes, microwave antennas, laser fiber optics, and ultrasound transducers. Each of these modalities has the potential to be delivered in a minimally invasive manner, and many theoretical and experimental investigations of these devices have been performed.

Most mammalian cells do not survive temperature exceeding 42°C. If tissues are exposed to temperatures between 42° and 46°C, coagulative necrosis occurs. Death begins to occur with in 4 to 6 minutes at 50°C and occurs more rapidly with increasing temperature. It becomes nearly instantaneous above 60°C. At 100°C, the cell membrane melts, intracellular water vaporizes, and tissue gets desiccated and charred.

Radiofrequency treatment is usually divided into a lower frequency band (3 kHz to 30 MHz) and a higher frequency microwave band (300 MHz to 300 GHz). The radiofrequency band is a low-energy alternating current, requiring direct contact with tissues for its effect to occur.

Radiofrequency interstitial tumor ablation (RITA) uses high-frequency current alternating rapidly at approximately 480 KHz (within range of radio transmission). It is delivered to the tumor tissue via a needle electrode. As the current alternates, the ions in the vicinity of the needle tip rapidly change direction (ionic agitation), which causes frictional heating of the tissue (resistive heating) and cell death by coagulative necrosis. Thus, the tissue itself is the source of heat rather than the electrode tip. The amount of heat deposited in the tissue is proportional to the strength of the current and the resistance of the tissue, and falls off approximately at the inverse fourth power of the distance. With the present system, usually a sphere of 4.5 to 5 cm of hyperthermia is created at the tip. Since the temperature falls off drastically at the periphery, the goal of the procedure is to include a margin of 1 cm of normal tissue within the sphere. Small vessels less than 3 mm in diameter are cauterized during the procedure. This reduces the risk of hemorrhage during the procedure. Also the ensuing tissue hypoxia contributes to the complete ablation of tumor. The cells become scar tissue and eventually shrink.

Radiofrequency Interstitial Tumor Ablation

A high-frequency radiator has been developed for the treatment of prostate cancer by hyperthermia. The applicator produces a deep-seated hot spot. The radiator has an outer diameter of 20 mm and an insertable length of about 175 mm. A high-frequency cylindrical slot antenna inside the applicator is cooled by water. The frequency used is 433.9 MHz. A control system regulating the power output of the radiator avoids damage to the tissue around the prostate, especially the rectum mucosa and the tissue between the rectum and the prostate (58). Radiofrequency interstitial tumor ablation (RITA) is a promising new technology that proved to be able to induce extensive necrosis, but the follow-up is too short to determine its definite place in the treatment of prostate cancer.

Radiofrequency interstitial tumor ablation has been used alone or combined with other minimally invasive treatments such as external-beam irradiation combined with the use of iridium-192 implants, with the aim of achieving the maximum effect on the prostate tissue (59). Zlotta et al. (60) performed RITA in 15 patients with localized prostate cancer before radical surgery. Radiofrequency energy was delivered to the prostate by active needle electrodes (monopolar or bipolar) placed transperineally under transrectal ultrasonography guidance. Needle electrodes were used with different configurations and in some cases were covered by retractable shields to vary the length and circumference of the thermal lesions created. In eight patients the procedure was performed immediately before radical prostatectomy, in six patients RITA was performed under spinal anesthesia 1 week before surgery, and in one patient no surgery was performed but the patient was followed by serial determinations of PSA. At least two lesions were created in each prostate, including both capsule and peripheral zones. Reduced nicotinamide adenine dinucleotide phosphate (NADPH) and hematoxylin and eosin (H&E) staining were used to assess the extent of the necrotic lesion in the radical prostatectomy specimen. The mean energy delivered was 10.5 kJ, with central temperatures reaching up to 105°C during 12 minutes of ablation; rectal temperature remained at <38°C.

There were no complications. Macroscopic examination showed well-demarcated lesions including the prostatic capsule, up to 2.2 × 1.5 × 4.5 cm. With monopolar energy, the observed lesion size was comparable to the predicted 2 × 2 × 2 cm lesion, while with bipolar energy, lesion size was related to inter-needle distance and uncovered needle length. Microscopic examination showed clearly delineated lesions both with NADPH (in prostates immediately removed after surgery) and H&E (at 1 week after RITA) staining. The lesion size observed on pathological analysis correlated with the predicted lesion size. In one patient, no residual cancer was found in the specimen. In the patient whose entire prostate was targeted and followed by serial PSA measurements, the latter were undetectable at 3 months of follow-up.

Similarly, Shariat et al. (61) reported a pilot study on 11 patients with biopsy-proven, hormone-naive, clinically localized prostate cancer, followed up for 20 months. Serum PSA levels decreased after RITA by >50% in 90% of patients, >70% in 72% of patients, and >80% in 46% of patients. The mean PSA doubling time after RITA was slower than that before RITA (37 ± 22 months vs. 14 ± 13 months, $p = .008$). At 12 months after RITA, 50% of patients with sufficient follow-up had no residual cancer on repeat systematic 12-core biopsy cores and 67% were cancer-free in biopsy cores sampled from the RITA-treated areas. The RITA has been shown to be feasible, but larger, prospective, multicenter clinical studies are needed to confirm these findings.

Magnetic Fluid Hyperthermia

Magnetic fluid hyperthermia (MFH) is a yet another new technique for thermoablation of tumors. After direct intratumoral injection of magnetic fluids into the target region, the particles are selectively heated in an externally applied AC magnetic field. The magnetic fluid contains super paramagnetic iron oxide nanoparticles with a core diameter of 15 nm. Preliminary studies in the Dunning tumor model of prostate cancer have demonstrated the feasibility of MFH in vivo.

Johannsen et al. (62) carried out a systematic analysis of the effects of MFH in the orthotopic Dunning R3327 tumor model of the rat. Treatment animals received two MFH treatments following a single intratumoral injection of a magnetic fluid. At the end the tumor weights in the treatment and control groups were compared. In addition, tumor growth curves were generated and histological examinations and iron measurements in selected organs were carried out. Magnetic fluid hyperthermia led to an inhibition of tumor growth of 44% to 51% over controls. Mean iron content in the prostates of treated and untreated (injection of magnetic fluids but no AC magnetic field exposure) animals was 82.5%, whereas only 5.3% of the injected dose was found in the liver, 1.0% in the lung, and 0.5% in the spleen (62,63). Thus this method is still in the experimental stage, and Johannsen et al. concluded that it is unlikely that hyperthermia alone is sufficient to eliminate prostate tumors, suggesting that combination with radiation should be considered for the clinical treatment of prostate cancer. They also studied the combined effect of MFH and radiotherapy in an orthotopic rat model of prostate cancer (64) and saw an additive effect for the combined treatment at a radiation dose of 20 Gy, which was equally effective in inhibiting tumor growth as radiation alone with 60 Gy.

References

1. Sikora K, Pandha H. Gene therapy for prostate cancer. Br J Urol 1997;79(suppl 2): 64–68.
2. Anderson WF, Blaese RM, Culver K. The ADA human gene therapy clinical protocol: points to consider response with clinical protocol, July 6, 1990. Hum Gene Ther 1990;1(3):331–362.
3. Simons JW, Mikhak B, Chang JF, et al. Induction of immunity to prostate cancer antigens: results of a clinical trial of vaccination with irradiated autologous prostate tumor cells engineered to secrete granulocyte-macrophage colony-stimulating factor using ex vivo gene transfer. Cancer Res 1999;59(20):5160–5168.
4. Freytag SO, Stricker H, Pegg J, et al. Phase I study of replication-competent adenovirus-mediated double-suicide gene therapy in combination with conventional-dose three-dimensional conformal radiation therapy for the treatment of newly diagnosed, intermediate- to high-risk prostate cancer. Cancer Res 2003;63(21): 7497–7506.
5. Downing SR, Russell PJ, Jackson P. Alterations of p53 are common in early stage prostate cancer. Can J Urol 2003;10(4):1924–1933.

6. Pisters LL, Pettaway CA, Troncoso P, et al. Evidence that transfer of functional p53 protein results in increased apoptosis in prostate cancer. Clin Cancer Res 2004; 10(8):2587–2593.

7. Mikata K, Uemura H, Ohuchi H, et al. Inhibition of growth of human prostate cancer xenograft by transfection of p53 gene: gene transfer by electroporation. Mol Cancer Ther 2002;1(4):247–252.

8. Tanaka M, Rosser CJ, Grossman HB. PTEN gene therapy induces growth inhibition and increases efficacy of chemotherapy in prostate cancer. Cancer Det Prev 2005; 29(2):170–174.

9. Rosser CJ, Tanaka M, Pisters LL, et al. Adenoviral-mediated PTEN transgene expression sensitizes Bcl-2–expressing prostate cancer cells to radiation. Cancer Gene Ther 2004;11(4):273–279.

10. Iversen PL, Arora V, Acker AJ, Mason DH, Devi GR. Efficacy of antisense morpholino oligomer targeted to c-myc in prostate cancer xenograft murine model and a Phase I safety study in humans. Clin Cancer Res 2003;9(7):2510–2519.

11. Shi XB, Gumerlock PH, Muenzer JT, deVere White RW. BCL2 antisense transcripts decrease intracellular Bcl2 expression and sensitize LNCaP prostate cancer cells to apoptosis-inducing agents. Cancer Biother Radiopharm 2001;16(5):421–429.

12. Cao G, Su J, Lu W, et al. Adenovirus-mediated interferon-beta gene therapy suppresses growth and metastasis of human prostate cancer in nude mice. Cancer Gene Ther 2001;8(7):497–505.

13. Cheng WS, Kraaij R, Nilsson B, et al. A novel TARP-promoter-based adenovirus against hormone-dependent and hormone-refractory prostate cancer. Mol Ther 2004;10(2):355–364.

14. Li X, Raikwar SP, Liu YH, et al. Combination therapy of androgen-independent prostate cancer using a prostate restricted replicative adenovirus and a replication-defective adenovirus encoding human endostatin-angiostatin fusion gene. Mol Cancer Ther 2006;5(3):676–684.

15. Gene Therapy Clinical Trials Worldwide. New York: Wiley Interscience, 2006. http://www.wiley.co.uk/genetherapy/clinical/.

16. Kaminski JM, Summers JB, Ward MB, Huber MR, Minev B. Immunotherapy and prostate cancer. Cancer Treat Rev 2003;29(3):199–209.

17. Simons JW, Carducci MA, Mikhak B, et al. Phase I/II trial of an allogeneic cellular immunotherapy in hormone-naive prostate cancer. Clin Cancer Res 2006; 12(11pt 1):3394–3401.

18. Michael A, Ball G, Quatan N, et al. Delayed disease progression after allogeneic cell vaccination in hormone-resistant prostate cancer and correlation with immunologic variables. Clin Cancer Res 2005;11(12):4469–4478.

19. Small EJ, Fratesi P, Reese DM, et al. Immunotherapy of hormone-refractory prostate cancer with antigen-loaded dendritic cells. J Clin Oncol 2000;18(23):3894–3903.

20. Carducci MA, Padley RJ, Breul J, et al. Effect of endothelin-A receptor blockade with atrasentan on tumor progression in men with hormone-refractory prostate cancer: a randomized, phase II, placebo-controlled trial. J Clin Oncol 2003;21(4): 679–689.

21. Zeng G, Wang X, Robbins PF, Rosenberg SA, Wang RF. CD4(+) T cell recognition of MHC class II-restricted epitopes from NY-ESO-1 presented by a prevalent HLA DP4 allele: association with NY-ESO-1 antibody production. Proc Nat Acad Sci USA 2001; 98(7):3964–3969.

22. Beinart G, Rini BI, Weinberg V, Small EJ. Antigen-presenting cells 8015 (Provenge) in patients with androgen-dependent, biochemically relapsed prostate cancer. Clin Prostate Cancer 2005;4(1):55–60.

23. Small EJ, Schellhammer PF, Higano CS, et al. Placebo-controlled phase III trial of immunologic therapy with sipuleucel-T (APC8015) in patients with metastatic, asymptomatic hormone refractory prostate cancer. J Clin Oncol 2006;24(19): 3089–3094.

24. Rochlitz C, Figlin R, Squiban P, et al. Phase I immunotherapy with a modified vaccinia virus (MVA) expressing human MUC1 as antigen-specific immunotherapy in patients with MUC1–positive advanced cancer. J Gene Med 2003;5(8):690–699.

25. Kaufman HL, Wang W, Manola J, et al. Phase II randomized study of vaccine treatment of advanced prostate cancer (E7897):a trial of the Eastern Cooperative Oncology Group. J Clin Oncol 2004;22(11):2122–2132.

26. Madersbacher S, Kratzik C, Szabo N, et al. Tissue ablation in benign prostatic hyperplasia with high-intensity focused ultrasound. Eur Urol 1993;23(suppl 1):39–43.

27. Gelet A, Chapelon JY, Bouvier R, et al. Treatment of prostate cancer with transrectal focused ultrasound: early clinical experience. Eur Urol 1996;29(2):174–183.

28. Rebillard X, Gelet A, Davin JL, et al. Transrectal high-intensity focused ultrasound in the treatment of localized prostate cancer. J Endourol 2005;19(6):693–701.

29. Gelet A, Chapelon JY, Poissonnier L, et al. Local recurrence of prostate cancer after external beam radiotherapy: early experience of salvage therapy using high-intensity focused ultrasonography. Urology 2004;63(4):625–629.

30. Wang ZB, Wu F, Wang ZL, et al. Targeted damage effects of high intensity focused ultrasound (HIFU) on liver tissues of Guizhou Province miniswine. Ultrason Sonochem 1997;4(2):181–182.

31. Yang R, Sanghvi NT, Rescorla FJ, et al. Extracorporeal liver ablation using sonography-guided high-intensity focused ultrasound. Invest Radiol 1992;27(10):796–803.

32. Vaezy S, Shi X, Martin RW, et al. Real-time visualization of high-intensity focused ultrasound treatment using ultrasound imaging. Ultrasound Med Biol 2001;27(1): 33–42.

33. Azzouz H, de la Rosette JJMCH. HIFU: local treatment of prostate cancer. Eur Urol 2006;4(EAU series):62–70.

34. Hummel S, Paisley S, Morgan A, Currie E, Brewer N. Clinical and cost-effectiveness of new and emerging technologies for early localised prostate cancer: a systematic review. Health Technol Assess 2003;7(33):iii, ix-x, 1–157.

35. Beerlage HP, Thuroff S, Debruyne FM, Chaussy C, de la Rosette JJ. Transrectal high-intensity focused ultrasound using the Ablatherm device in the treatment of localized prostate carcinoma. Urology 1999;54(2):273–277.

36. Chaussy C, Thuroff S. High-intensity focused ultrasound in prostate cancer: results after 3 years. Mol Urol 2000;4(3):179–182.

37. Madersbacher S, Pedevilla M, Vingers L, Susani M, Marberger M. Effect of high-intensity focused ultrasound on human prostate cancer in vivo. Cancer Res 1995; 55(15):3346–3351.

38. Gelet A, Chapelon JY, Bouvier R, et al. Transrectal high intensity focused ultrasound for the treatment of localized prostate cancer: factors influencing the outcome. Eur Urol 2001;40:124–129.

39. Chaussy C, Thuroff S. The status of high-intensity focused ultrasound in the treatment of localized prostate cancer and the impact of a combined resection. Curr Urol Rep 2003;4:248–252.

40. Uchida T, Ohkusa H, Nagata Y, et al. Treatment of localized prostate cancer using high-intensity focused ultrasound. BJU Int 2006;97(1):56–61.
41. Thuroff S, Chaussy C, Vallancien G, et al. High-intensity focused ultrasound and localized prostate cancer: efficacy results from the European multicentric study. J Endourol 2003;17(8):673–677.
42. Blana A, Walter B, Rogenhofer S, Wieland WF. High-intensity focused ultrasound for the treatment of localized prostate cancer: 5-year experience. Urology 2004;63(2): 297–300.
43. Kiel HJ, Wieland WF, Rossler W. Local control of prostate cancer by transrectal HIFU-therapy. Arch Ital Urol Androl 2000;72(4):313–319.
44. Gonder MJ, Soanes WA, Shulman S. Cryosurgical treatment of the prostate. Invest Urol 1966;3(4):372–378.
45. Flocks RH, Nelson CM, Boatman DL. Perineal cryosurgery for prostatic carcinoma. J Urol 1972;108(6):933–935.
46. Megalli MR, Gursel EO, Veenema RJ. Closed perineal cryosurgery in prostatic cancer. New probe and technique. Urology 1974;4(2):220–222.
47. Onik GM, Cohen JK, Reyes GD, et al. Transrectal ultrasound-guided percutaneous radical cryosurgical ablation of the prostate. Cancer 1993;72(4):1291–1299.
48. Onik G, Cobb C, Cohen J, Zabkar J, Porterfield B. US characteristics of frozen prostate. Radiology 1988;168(3):629–631.
49. Lee F, Bahn DK, McHugh TA, Onik GM, Lee FT Jr. US-guided percutaneous cryoablation of prostate cancer. Radiology 1994;192(3):769–776.
50. Wong WS, Chinn DO, Chinn M, et al. Cryosurgery as a treatment for prostate carcinoma: results and complications. Cancer 1997;79(5):963–974.
51. Pisters LL, von Eschenbach AC, Scott SM, et al. The efficacy and complications of salvage cryotherapy of the prostate. J Urol 1997;157(3):921–925.
52. Ahmed S, Lindsey B, Davies J. Salvage cryosurgery for locally recurrent prostate cancer following radiotherapy. Prostate Cancer Prostatic Dis 2005;8(1):31–35.
53. Shinohara K, Connolly JA, Presti JC Jr, Carroll PR. Cryosurgical treatment of localized prostate cancer (stages T1 to T4): preliminary results. J Urol 1996;156(1):115–220; discussion 20–21.
54. Cohen JK, Miller RJ, Rooker GM, Shuman BA. Cryosurgical ablation of the prostate: two-year prostate-specific antigen and biopsy results. Urology 1996;47(3): 395–401.
55. Koppie TM, Shinohara K, Grossfeld GD, Presti JC Jr, Carroll PR. The efficacy of cryosurgical ablation of prostate cancer: the University of California, San Francisco experience. J Urol 1999;162(2):427–432.
56. Long JP, Bahn D, Lee F, Shinohara K, Chinn DO, Macaluso JN Jr. Five-year retrospective, multi-institutional pooled analysis of cancer-related outcomes after cryosurgical ablation of the prostate. Urology 2001;57(3):518–523.
57. Bahn DK, Lee F, Silverman P, et al. Salvage cryosurgery for recurrent prostate cancer after radiation therapy: a seven-year follow-up. Clin Prostate Cancer 2003;2(2): 111–114.
58. Beerlage HP, Thuroff S, Madersbacher S, et al. Current status of minimally invasive treatment options for localized prostate carcinoma. Eur Urol 2000;37(1): 2–13.
59. Bagshaw MA, Prionas SD, Goffinet DR, et al. External beam irradiation combined with the use of 192–iridium implants and radiofrequency-induced hyperthermia in the treatment of prostatic carcinoma. Prog Clin Biol Res 1991;370:275–279.

60. Zlotta AR, Djavan B, Matos C, et al. Percutaneous transperineal radiofrequency abla-
    tion of prostate tumour: safety, feasibility and pathological effects on human prostate
    cancer. Br J Urol 1998;81(2):265–275.

61. Shariat SF, Raptidis G, Masatoschi M, Bergamaschi F, Slawin KM. Pilot study of
    radiofrequency interstitial tumor ablation (RITA) for the treatment of radio-recur-
    rent prostate cancer. Prostate 2005;65(3):260–267.

62. Johannsen M, Thiesen B, Jordan A, et al. Magnetic fluid hyperthermia (MFH) reduces
    prostate cancer growth in the orthotopic Dunning R3327 rat model. Prostate 2005;
    64(3):283–292.

63. Johannsen M, Jordan A, Scholz R, et al. Evaluation of magnetic fluid hyperthermia
    in a standard rat model of prostate cancer. J Endourol 2004;18(5):495–500.

64. Johannsen M, Thiesen B, Gneveckow U, et al. Thermotherapy using magnetic
    nanoparticles combined with external radiation in an orthotopic rat model of pros-
    tate cancer. Prostate 2006;66(1):97–104.

19
Cancer of the Penis and Scrotum

Simon Horenblas and Bin K. Kroon

Carcinoma of the Penis

Epidemiology

Cancer of the penis is a rare malignancy with incidence rates of 0.3 to 8 per 100,000. High-incidence areas are found in South America, the highest being Brazil (8/100,000). It has a low incidence in countries where circumcision at birth or at a very young age is practiced (e.g. Israel, Middle East) (1,2).

Etiology

Phimosis

A nonretractile foreskin predisposes to penis cancer, probably due to chronic infection of the glans and the prepuce (chronic balanoposthitis) (1,3).

Human Papilloma Virus

Human papilloma virus (HPV) is a sexually transmitted agent that appears to have a role in penile cancer. Persistent infection with high-risk HPV is a major cause of cervical cancer (4). Nearly 30% of cases of penile cancer have HPV-DNA in them (5,6). It accounts for mutations in the retinoblastoma and the *p53* genes through the activity of E6 and E7 viral transcripts (7). The prevalence of high-risk HPV is different in various parts of the world, partially explaining the variation in incidence.

Chronic Inflammatory Conditions

Lichen sclerosis et atrophicus (LSA) is a chronic inflammatory skin disease of unknown etiology. In analogy to vulvar squamous cell carcinoma, 5% to 10% of patients with LSA develop squamous cell carcinoma (3).

Smoking

There seems to be an association of smoking with genital squamous cell carcinoma, although the exact mechanism is not known. Accumulation of nitrosamines in genital secretions has been suggested but not proven (3,8,9).

Premalignant Lesions

Penile Intraepithelial Neoplasia

Like most epithelial malignancies the intraepithelial component is considered a premalignant lesion, especially for cancers associated with HPV. Nearly all penile intraepithelial neoplasia (PIN) lesions have evidence of HPV-DNA in the tumor. However, only 5% to 15% of cases of PIN develop invasive cancer lichen sclerosis et atrophicus (balanitis xerotica). Lichen sclerosis et atrophicus is likely to be the precursor in those cases of cancers that are not associated with HPV infection (3,10).

Natural History

The duration between the development of a PIN lesion and infiltrating tumor is 10 to 15 years. The majority of tumors develop in the sulcus of the glans and prepuce. Local infiltration and regional lymph involvement are the routes of dissemination. Lymphatic spread follows a sequential pathway from inguinal lymph nodes to pelvic lymph nodes. Skip metastasis are hardly found. Hematogenic spread occurs quite late in the course of the disease.

Pathology

Squamous cell carcinoma (SCC) accounts for 95% of the malignant tumors of the penis. The other 5% consists of tumors originating in the skin, including melanoma, basal cell cancer, or soft tissue tumors arising from the elements of cavernous tissue. In rare cases metastases or lymphoreticular malignancies are found (2,11,12).

Staging

The staging is based on the tumor, node, metastasis (TNM) classification (Table 19.1). Grading is mostly based on the work of Broders in 1921, taking into account keratinization, nuclear pleomorphism, and mitosis.

Prognostic Factors

Factors predisposing to local recurrence after treatment are increasing T stage and increased grade of differentiation (13). The most important prognostic factor for survival is the presence or absence of lymph node metastasis (14–16).

TABLE 19.1. Tumor, node, metastasis (TNM) classification: penis cancer

T: Primary tumor
Tx Primary tumor cannot be assessed
T0 No evidence of primary tumor
Tis Carcinoma in situ
Ta Noninvasive verrucous carcinoma
Tl Tumor invades subepithelial connective tissue
T2 Tumor invades corpus spongiosum or cavernosum
T3 Tumor invades urethra or prostate
T4 Tumor invades other adjacent structures

N: Lymph nodes
Nx Regional lymph nodes cannot be assessed
N0 No regional lymph-node metastasis
N1 Metastasis in a single superficial inguinal lymph node
N2 Metastasis in multiple or bilateral superficial inguinal lymph nodes
N3 Metastasis in deep inguinal or pelvic lymph node(s), unilateral or
    bilateral

M: Distant metastasis
Mx Distant metastasis cannot be assessed
M0 No distant metastasis
M1 Distant metastasis

Clinical Features

The main clinical presentation is the presence of the primary lesion. Regional metastasis may present as occult metastases or overt lymph node involvement.

Primary Tumor

The primary lesion mostly originates in the sulcus of the corona glandis. It is clearly visible after retracting the foreskin. The lesion could be papillary, solid, or ulcerating. The lesion may be superficial or infiltrating into various tissue layers of the penis. Foul-smelling penile discharge may be the first sign in patients with a nonretractile prepuce. The tumor can usually be palpated under the foreskin.

Regional Metastases

Unilateral or bilateral enlargement of inguinal lymph nodes may be the main clinical feature. Signs of inflammation (hyperemia, pain, edema) can dominate the clinical picture. Other manifestations include lymphedema due to proximal lymphatic obstruction, flank pain from ureteric obstruction, and bone pain (bone metastases) with or without hypercalcemia.

Diagnosis

Primary Tumor

A biopsy (incisional or excisional) is strongly recommended to establish a correct histological diagnosis. The biopsy is preferably taken from the normal and abnormal tissue encompassing the full thickness of the tumor. This enables the pathologist to assess the depth of infiltration (1,17–19).

Verification of Regional Lymph Node Metastasis

Ultrasound-guided fine-needle aspiration (FNA) is done to determine lymph node metastasis. Removal of a single lymph node is not recommended, unless the proof of lymph node involvement cannot be obtained by repeated FNA (20).

Staging

Primary Tumor

In most cases physical examination may be sufficient. The exact location, size of the lesion, and involvement of tissue planes—skin, subcutaneous tissue, cavernous tissue, urethra, and neighboring tissues—are recorded. The proximal extent is determined by ultrasound and magnetic resonance imaging (MRI) (21–23).

Regional Lymph Nodes

Occult metastases may be detected by imaging. Ultrasound-guided FNA may be of help (24). Recently, lymphotropic nanoparticle-enhanced magnetic resonance imaging (LNMRI) using ferumoxtran-10, an iron oxide, has been used to triage patients for lymphadenectomy (25). The dynamic sentinel node biopsy is quite invasive. In patients with distinct metastases, it is important to record the size, number of lymph nodes, and fixation to the skin or underlying neurovascular structures like the femoral artery/vein or femoral nerve.

Management

The selection of treatment depends on the size, location, invasiveness, and stage of the tumor (Table 19.2).

TABLE 19.2. Stage grouping

Stage 0:	Tis N0 M0; Ta N0 M0
Stage I:	T1 N0 M0
Stage II:	T1 N1 M0; T2 N0, N1 M0
Stage III:	T1 N2 M0; T2 N2 M0; T3 N0, N1, N2 M0
Stage IV:	T4 Any N M0; Any T N3 M0; Any T Any N M1

Primary Tumor

Standard Management

Stage 1 (T1 N0M0). Penis-preserving therapies can be attempted if removal with a minimal margin of 2 to 3 mm of normal tissue can be attained. This is achieved by simple excisional surgery (circumcision) or by microscopically controlled surgery. Laser treatment has been employed successfully in the treatment of carcinoma in situ and in selected cancer cases. The CO_2 laser vaporizes tissue with a minimal depth of infiltration, while the neodymium : yttrium-aluminum-garnet (Nd : YAG) laser has excellent coagulative properties with a depth of infiltration of 3 to 4 mm.

Stage II (T1 N1M0; T2 N0M0; T2 N1M0). These tumors are frequently managed by penile amputation (partial or total); however, tissue-sparing strategies like amputation of the glans only or local excision with split skin graft have been proven to be oncologically safe (26,27). Radiation with surgical treatment is another option. Laser treatment in selected cases may be used.

Stage III (T1 N2M0; T2 N2M0; T3 N0M0; T3 N1M0; T3 N2M0). Surgical treatment is directed by the size and local invasion. The management of lymph nodes is discussed below. Standing voiding is possible after a partial amputation. A perineal urethrostomy behind the scrotum is constructed after total amputation.

In nonsurgical management of the primary tumor, penis preservation can be achieved by external-beam radiation, brachytherapy, or laser coagulation. Brachytherapy is an effective penis-preserving treatment for T1, T2, and selected T3 squamous cell carcinoma (SCC) of the penis (13,28,29).

Regional Lymph Nodes

Management of Clinically Node Negative Patients

This is a controversial issue, with some authors advocating inguinal lymph node dissection in all (with the exception of small primary tumors) and others advocating monitoring (wait-and-see management) in all patients (except those patients with unfavorable prognostic factors). However, there is a uniform consensus for expectant management in patients presenting with carcinoma in situ (stage Tis) and well-differentiated T1 tumors (14,30,31). Similar to melanoma and breast cancer, the so-called dynamic sentinel node biopsy was developed for all other categories (32). A lymph node dissection is done only in patients with positive sentinel node biopsy. Results show acceptable false-negative rates and excellent survival figures compared to a cohort of patients managed conservatively (22,33).

Management of Clinically Node Positive Patients

Treatment in these patients is quite straightforward: inguinal lymph node dissection preceded by confirmation of metastatic involvement by FNA.

Depending on the number of tumor-positive nodes, extracapsular growth and the location of tumor-positive nodes, a complementary iliac lymph node dissection is mandatory. Patients with fixed nodes or presenting with retroperitoneal nodes should undergo preoperative treatment with combination chemotherapy or radiation therapy. After response evaluation, subsequent surgery is scheduled in patients with clinical response. Because of the rarity of this disease, this surgery should be done preferably within the framework of a clinical study (34,35).

Results

Primary Tumor

Penis-preserving treatment is safe, but careful follow-up with self-examination by the patient is of utmost importance. The local recurrence rates vary from 19% to 37% irrespective of the type of local treatment. Local recurrence is treated at the earliest possible moment due to the danger of further spread. Local recurrence after partial or total amputation is rare. The most common complication is stenosis of the neourethra after partial or total amputation (5% to 10%) (13,36).

Standing urination and normal erection are maintained in penis preserving treatments and often after partial amputation, depending on the size of the stump. Standing voiding is not possible after total amputation. Patients do have normal ejaculation after total amputation (37,38).

Patients with a single lymph nodes metastasis have a 5-year disease-specific survival of 70%, in contrast to 50% with bilateral lymph node invasion. This decreases further to 29% in patients with microscopic pelvic lymph node invasion. Patients presenting with fixed inguinal masses or large pelvic lymph nodes do poorly, with hardly any long-term survivors (14,21,34).

Tumors of the Scrotum

Epidemiology

Scrotal tumors are exceedingly rare, with an age-adjusted incidence of 0.2 to 0.3 per 100,000 (39).

Etiology

Historically scrotal cancer was one of the known occupational cancers. The disease was initially described by Percival Pott in the 18th century as a disease common in chimney sweepers. This association led to the discovery of the carcinogenic role of industrial oils, like alkaline ether, and coal tar. Occupation-related and -induced tumors are rare now. Whether human papilloma virus plays a role is unclear (39).

TABLE 19.3. Staging system for scrotal carcinoma

Stage A1	Localized to scrotal wall
Stage A2	Locally extensive tumor invading adjacent structures (testis, spermatic cord, penis, pubis, perineum)
Stage B	Metastatic disease involving inguinal lymph nodes only
Stage C	Metastatic disease involving pelvic lymph nodes without evidence of distant spread
Stage D	Metastatic disease beyond the pelvic nodes involving distant organs

Pathology

The majority of tumors consists of squamous cell carcinoma. Other cancers include basal cell carcinoma and melanoma.

Staging

There is no official TNM classification for scrotal cancer. Another staging system was based on the probability of surgical treatment (Table 19.3).

Prognostic Factors

Just like squamous cell carcinoma of the penis, invasion of regional lymph nodes is the most important prognostic factor for survival.

Clinical Features

Primary Tumor

Clinical presentation is most often a solitary tumor in the scrotal skin. Various benign diseases should be distinguished from cancer, such as sebaceous cyst, dermoid cyst, and cutaneous nevus.

Clinical Features of Regional Metastasis

Patients may present with palpable masses in the inguinal region, especially if the primary tumor remains undetected for a long time.

Management

Primary Tumor

Treatment consists of surgical removal of the affected part of the scrotum. In extensive cases a complete scrotectomy is mandatory. The scrotum can be reconstructed using free skin graft on the tunica vaginalis of the testes (39).

Regional Metastasis

Patients presenting with clinically node-positive disease should undergo a lymph node dissection after confirmation with fine-needle aspiration. Clinically node-negative patients could benefit from a dynamic lymph node biopsy in analogy to squamous cell carcinoma of the penis (33).

Treatment Results

Primary Tumor

Local recurrence rates of 21% to 40% have been reported. However, all reports include very small number of patients (39).

Regional Metastasis

Five-year survival figures can hardly been given based on the scanty published information. However, patients with a minimal amount of metastatic load survive after a lymph node dissection. By contrast, there are hardly any survivors in patients presenting with involved pelvic lymph nodes.

References

1. Misra S, Chaturvedi A, Misra NC. Penile carcinoma: a challenge for the developing world. Lancet Oncol 2004;5(4):240–247.
2. Stancik I, Holtl W. Penile cancer: review of the recent literature. Curr Opin Urol 2003;13(6):467–472.
3. Dillner J, von Krogh G, Horenblas S, Meijer CJ. Etiology of squamous cell carcinoma of the penis. Scand J Urol Nephrol Suppl 2000;205:189–193.
4. Walboomers JM, Jacobs MV, Manos MM, et al. Human papillomavirus is a necessary cause of invasive cervical cancer worldwide. J Pathol 1999;189(1):12–19.
5. Ferreux E, Lont AP, Horenblas S, et al. Evidence for at least three alternative mechanisms targeting the p16INK4A/cyclin D/Rb pathway in penile carcinoma, one of which is mediated by high-risk human papillomavirus. J Pathol 2003;201(1): 109–118.
6. Bezerra AL, Lopes A, Santiago GH, et al. Human papillomavirus as a prognostic factor in carcinoma of the penis: analysis of 82 patients treated with amputation and bilateral lymphadenectomy. Cancer 2001;91(12):2315–2321.
7. Munger K. The role of human papillomaviruses in human cancers. Front Biosci 2002;7:d641–d649.
8. Harish K, Ravi R. The role of tobacco in penile carcinoma. Br J Urol 1995;75: 375–377.
9. Tsen HF, Morgenstern H, Mack T, Peters RK. Risk factors for penile cancer: results of a population-based case-control study in Los Angeles County (United States). Cancer Causes Control 2001;12:267–277.
10. von Krogh G, Horenblas S. Diagnosis and clinical presentation of premalignant lesions of the penis. Scand J Urol Nephrol Suppl 2000;205:201–214.
11. Sanchez-Ortiz RF, Pettaway CA. The role of lymphadenectomy in penile cancer. Urol Oncol 2004;22(3):236–244.

12. Liegl B, Regauer S. Penile clear cell carcinoma: a report of 5 cases of a distinct entity. Am J Surg Pathol 2004;28(11):1513–1517.
13. Horenblas S, van Tinteren H, Delemarre JF, et al. Squamous cell carcinoma of the penis. II. Treatment of the primary tumor. J Urol 1992;147(6):1533–1538.
14. Horenblas S, van Tinteren H, Delemarre JF, et al. Squamous cell carcinoma of the penis. III. Treatment of regional lymph nodes. J Urol 1993;149(3):492–497.
15. Ornellas AA, Seixas AL, Marota A, et al. Surgical treatment of invasive squamous cell carcinoma of the penis: retrospective analysis of 350 cases. J Urol 1994;151: 1244–1249.
16. Lopes A, Hidalgo GS, Kowalski LP, et al. Prognostic factors in carcinoma of the penis: multivariate analysis of 145 patients treated with amputation and lymphadenectomy. J Urol 1996;156(5):1637–1642.
17. Kroon BK, Horenblas S, Deurloo EE, Nieweg OE, Teertstra HJ. Ultrasonography-guided fine-needle aspiration cytology before sentinel node biopsy in patients with penile carcinoma. BJU Int 2005;95:517–521.
18. Singh I, Khaitan A. Current trends in the management of carcinoma penis—a review. Int Urol Nephrol 2003;35(2):215–225.
19. Pizzocaro G, Piva L, Bandieramonte G, Tana S. Up-to-date management of carcinoma of the penis. Eur Urol 1997;32(1):5–15.
20. Horenblas S. Lymphadenectomy for squamous cell carcinoma of the penis. Part 1: diagnosis of lymph node metastasis. BJU Int 2001;88(5):467–472.
21. Horenblas S, van Tinteren H. Squamous cell carcinoma of the penis. IV. Prognostic factors of survival: analysis of tumor, nodes and metastasis classification system. J Urol 1994;151(5):1239–1243.
22. Lont AP, Horenblas S, Tanis PJ, et al. Management of clinically node negative penile carcinoma: improved survival after the introduction of dynamic sentinel node biopsy. J Urol 2003;170(3):783–786.
23. Scardino E, Villa G, Bonomo G, et al. Magnetic resonance imaging combined with artificial erection for local staging of penile cancer. Urology 2004;63(6): 1158–1162.
24. Kroon BK, Horenblas S, Estourgie SH, et al. How to avoid false-negative dynamic sentinel node procedures in penile carcinoma. J Urol 2004;171(6 Pt 1): 2191–2194.
25. Tabatabaei S, Harisinghani M, McDougal WS. Regional lymph node staging using lymphotropic nanoparticle enhanced magnetic resonance imaging with ferumoxtran-10 in patients with penile cancer. J Urol 2005;174(3):923–927.
26. Minhas S, Kayes O, Hegarty P, et al. What surgical resection margins are required to achieve oncological control in men with primary penile cancer? BJU Int 2005;96(7): 1040–1043.
27. Brown CT, Minhas S, Ralph DJ. Conservative surgery for penile cancer: subtotal glans excision without grafting. BJU Int 2005;96(6):911–912.
28. Sagerman RH, Yu WS, Chung CT, Puranik A. External-beam irradiation of carcinoma of the penis. Radiology 1984;152(1):183–185.
29. Crook JM, Jezioranski J, Grimard L, Esche B, Pond G. Penile brachytherapy: results for 49 patients. Int J Radiat Oncol Biol Phys 2005;62(2):460–467.
30. Solsona E, Iborra I, Rubio J, et al. Prospective validation of the association of local tumor stage and grade as a predictive factor for occult lymph node micrometastasis in patients with penile carcinoma and clinically negative inguinal lymph nodes. J Urol 2001;165(5):1506–1509.

31. McDougal WS. Carcinoma of the penis: improved survival by early regional lymphadenectomy based on the histological grade and depth of invasion of the primary lesion. J Urol 1995;154(4):1364–1366.

32. Horenblas S, Jansen L, Meinhardt W, et al. Detection of occult metastasis in squamous cell carcinoma of the penis using a dynamic sentinel node procedure. J Urol 2000; 163(1):100–104.

33. Kroon BK, Horenblas S, Meinhardt W, et al. Dynamic sentinel node biopsy in penile carcinoma: evaluation of 10 years experience. Eur Urol 2005;47(5):601–606.

34. Horenblas S. Lymphadenectomy for squamous cell carcinoma of the penis. Part 2: the role and technique of lymph node dissection. BJU Int 2001;88(5):473–483.

35. Culkin DJ, Beer TM. Advanced penile carcinoma. J Urol 2003;170(2 pt 1):359–365.

36. Windahl T, Andersson SO. Combined laser treatment for penile carcinoma: results after long-term followup. J Urol 2003;169(6):2118–2121.

37. d'Ancona CA, Botega NJ, De Moraes C, Lavoura NS, Jr., Santos JK, Rodrigues Netto N, Jr. Quality of life after partial penectomy for penile carcinoma. Urology 1997;50: 593–596.

38. Opjordsmoen S, Fossa SD. Quality of life in patients treated for penile cancer. A follow-up study. Br J Urol 1994;74(5):652–657.

39. Lowe FC. Squamous-cell carcinoma of the scrotum. Urol Clin North Am 1992; 19(2):397–405.

20
Nonurological Cancers Affecting the Urinary Tract

Julie C. Walther and Melanie E.B. Powell

The bladder and urethra are likely to be affected by cancers of other pelvic viscera by virtue of their close proximity. Secondary tumors may be seen in the kidney but are rare occurrences. This chapter highlights the urological manifestations of pelvic cancers that need urological assessment and intervention, but does not report detailed specialist information. The management of these cancers is multidisciplinary, and it is helpful to know basic anatomical, pathological, and clinical details of pelvic malignancies. For example, the ureter in females is closely related to the cervix, uterine vessels, and vaginal vault, which makes it vulnerable during surgery and in the course of the disease. The ureters also run in close proximity to the rectum and sigmoid colon. The relationship among the prostate, its neurovascular bundles, and the rectum has been described in Chapters 18.1 to 18.8.

Carcinoma of the Endometrium and Cervix

Incidence and Etiology

Cancer of the uterine body predominantly affects postmenopausal women and is the commonest gynecological cancer, with an age-adjusted incidence of 24.7 per 100,000 population (1). Cervical cancer is declining in the West due to screening programs, although in developing countries it remains the main cause of cancer related mortality in women (Table 20.1) (1). Etiological risk factors are listed in Table 20.2.

Spread

The spread of endometrial carcinoma depends on the degree of cellular differentiation, as follows:

1. Local infiltration occurs into the myometrium, cervix, serosa, fallopian tubes, and ovaries. More advanced tumors may invade locally into the bladder or rectum.

TABLE 20.1. Incidence and mortality for endometrial and cervical cancer

	Incidence	Mortality
Endometrium	24/100,000	4.1/100,000
Cervix	9/100,000	2.8/100,000

Source: Surveillance, Epidemiology and End Results Programme (1).

2. Regarding lymphatic spread, certain pathological features such as high tumor grade, depth of myometrial invasion, and lymphovascular space invasion are predictors of nodal involvement. Pelvic node metastases are present in 30% of cases with deep myometrial invasion. Positive paraaortic nodes are unusual in the absence of pelvic nodes and confer a poor prognosis (2,3).

3. Hematogenous spread to the lungs and liver occurs late and is associated with a poor prognosis. Distant bone metastases are rare, but direct invasion may be seen into the lower spine, sacrum, or pelvis. In sarcoma, hematogenous spread to the lung is common even at presentation.

The spread of cervical carcinoma is as follows:

1. Local: The growth can extend laterally into the parametrium and pelvic sidewall, where it may encroach onto the ureter leading to hydronephrosis. More advanced tumors invade the urethra, bladder, or rectum.

2. Lymphatic: Pelvic nodal disease is frequent and related to the size and stage of the tumor as well as tumor differentiation and lymphovascular space invasion. In the presence of positive pelvic nodes, the incidence of paraaortic disease is over 50%. Supraclavicular lymph nodes are a sign of disseminated cancer and confer a poor prognosis.

3. Hematogenous: Once rare, better local control has led to an increase in frequency of metastases to the lung, bone, liver, and brain.

TABLE 20.2. Risk factors for development of endometrial and cervical cancer

Endometrium	Cervix
Early menarche/late menopause	Cervical intraepithelial neoplasia
Diabetes mellitus	Young age at first intercourse
Nulliparity	High parity
Obesity	Human papilloma virus (HPV) infection
Hypertension	(particularly HPV 16/18/33)
Unopposed oestrogen exposure (e.g., polycystic ovaries, advanced liver disease, anovulatory cycles, granulose cell tumour)	Smoking
Tamoxifen	Sexually transmitted disease
	Multiple sexual partners
	Immunosuppression

Pathology

Endometrium

Adenocarcinomas constitute more than 90% of endometrial cancers. Most are endometrioid (papillary, secretory, ciliated cell or adenosquamous). The rest are mucinous, serous, clear cell, or squamous cell, and tend to behave more aggressively.

Other tumors are sarcomas comprising endometrial stromal, leiomyosarcomas, nonspecific mesenchymal and mixed mesodermal tumors.

Cervix

More than 80% of cervical tumors are squamous cell carcinoma. Other tumor types are mainly adenocarcinoma and rarely small cell, neuroendocrine, sarcoma, lymphoma, melanoma, and metastases from other primary cancers.

Clinical Presentation

Gynecological

Patients usually present to a gynecologist with abnormal vaginal bleeding, either postmenopausal or, in younger women, intermenstrual or postcoital. Other symptoms include persistent vaginal discharge and pelvic or back pain.

Urological

Urological symptoms such as urinary frequency, difficulty voiding, dysuria, hematuria, and incontinence may be a presenting feature. These are due to extrinsic pressure on the bladder or urethra or direct infiltration of the bladder. Incontinence may be due to a vesicovaginal fistula and suggests advanced disease.

Ureteric obstruction may occur by direct tumor extension to the pelvic sidewall or pelvic lymphadenopathy. It is often bilateral, and untreated it leads to acute renal failure. Obstructive nephropathy may also be due to tumor infiltrating the bladder or the urethra.

Investigations

Blood

Full blood count, blood biochemistry, and liver function analysis are useful. Testing for human immunodeficiency virus (HIV) should be considered in any patient from a high-risk group.

Imaging

Transvaginal ultrasound to assess the endometrial lining is useful in diagnosing endometrial cancer (biopsy may be done synchronously). Pelvic imaging using either magnetic resonance (MR) or computed tomography (CT) scanning is recommended. The abdomen and chest also should be included in locally advanced or high-risk tumors (e.g., high-grade sarcomas).

Examination Under Anesthesia

Patients with cervical carcinoma require examination under anesthesia (EUA), which includes cystoscopy, sigmoidoscopy, and bimanual examination.

Histopathology

Diagnosis is made by Pipelle biopsy or endometrial curettage for uterine malignancy. Cervical cancer may be diagnosed by biopsy at colposcopy or at EUA.

Staging

The clinically based International Federation of Gynecology and Obstetrics (FIGO) staging system is the most widely used (Table 20.3) (4).

Prognosis

Prognostic factors in endometrial cancer include grade, depth of invasion, lymphovascular space invasion, positive nodes, tumor volume, and cervical involve-

TABLE 20.3. Staging of endometrial and cervical cancers including risk of pelvic nodal metastases [International Union Against Cancer (UICC)/International Federation of Gynecology and Obstetrics (FIGO)]

	Endometrium (% risk nodal metastases)	Cervix (% risk nodal metastases)
I	Confined to corpus	Confined to cervix
	a Endometrium (<10%)	a Microscopic/preclinical
	b Inner half myometrium (10–20%)	1. ≤3 mm deep, ≤7 mm wide (<2%)
	c Extends into outer half myometrium (30%)	2. 3–5 mm deep, ≤7 mm wide (<4%)
		b Clinical
		1. ≤4 cm (15%)
		2. >4 cm (30%)
II	Cervix involved	Beyond cervix (not to pelvic wall or lower one third of vagina)
	a Endocervical glandular involvement only (20%)	a No parametrial spread (20%)
	b Cervical stromal invasion (30%)	b Parametrial spread present (30%)
III	Beyond uterus (within true pelvis)	
	a Serosa and/or adnexae and/or ascites/peritoneal washings	a Lower one third of vagina (30%)
	b Vaginal involvement	b Pelvic side wall/hydronephrosis/nonfunctioning kidney (50%)
	c Pelvic and/or paraaortic nodes	
IV	a Bladder or bowel mucosal spread	a Bladder or bowel mucosa spread or spread beyond pelvis
	b Other distant metastases	b Distant metastases

ment (2,3,5). For cervical cancer they are tumor size and invasion depth, histological type, lymphovascular invasion, lymph node invasion (and number involved), and parametrial invasion (6).

Management of Cervical Cancer

These patients are managed in a specialist cancer center by a multiprofessional team.

Early Disease

Early disease may be treated surgically or with synchronous chemotherapy and radiation. Management should be tailored to avoid the need for both surgery and radiotherapy, as the toxicity of combined treatment is considerable.

Surgical options include cold knife cone biopsy for stage Ia$_1$ tumors and large loop excision of transitional zone (LLETZ) or fertility-sparing trachelectomy (cervical amputation) for stage Ia$_2$ and early stage Ib$_1$ tumors. Wertheim's radical hysterectomy is used for larger Ib$_1$ tumors and IIa disease. Wertheim's hysterectomy involves resection of the uterus, fallopian tubes, ovaries, upper vagina, parametrium, and pelvic lymph nodes.

Chemoradiation

Although radiotherapy and surgery offer equivalent cure rates for early disease (stages Ia, Ib$_1$, and IIa) (7), for more advanced disease (i.e., stage Ib$_2$ and above) chemoradiotherapy is the treatment of choice. Chemoradiation involves the use of a cisplatin-based regimen given concurrently with a course of external-beam treatment. Studies have shown a 12% improvement in 5-year survival compared to radiation alone (8).

Cisplatin is nephrotoxic, and good renal function is a prerequisite for its use as it is mainly excreted through the kidneys. It is essential that renal function be optimized prior to treatment, as delay is detrimental to outcome. Hydronephrosis should be relieved by nephrostomy or JJ-stent placement. Formal assessment of glomerular filtration rate is required.

Radiation fields encompass the uterus, cervix, upper vagina, and pelvic nodes. Paraaortic nodes are not routinely irradiated. Daily treatment over 5 to 6 weeks is given followed by intracavity brachytherapy using a radioactive source, allowing a total dose of at least 75 to 80 Gy to be delivered to the tumor.

Advanced Disease

Chemoradiation is used in locally advanced disease as described, but a planned external-beam boost may be needed rather than brachytherapy. If the patient is frail, shorter radiotherapy schedules may be used without the addition of chemotherapy.

Palliative care input may be useful in addressing symptom control (particularly pelvic pain) and psychological support.

Recurrent or Metastatic Disease

Metastatic disease is incurable, and management is aimed at symptom control. Radiotherapy, chemotherapy, or surgery may all be useful at this time.

Surgery or Radiotherapy Salvage

Following radiotherapy local recurrence may be treated with surgery and vice versa. In surgical salvage, anterior pelvic or total pelvic exenteration may be necessary, which would include urinary diversion.

Chemotherapy

Chemotherapy usually employs platinum-containing regimens. Response rates are about 20%, and duration is usually only months.

Uremia secondary to outflow tract obstruction is not uncommon in advanced pelvic malignancy and nephrostomy or JJ-stenting may be necessary. This may offer a slight increase in life expectancy and provide the opportunity for palliative chemotherapy.

Management of Endometrial Cancer

Early Disease

Surgery

Most women present with stage I disease and are treated with total abdominal hysterectomy and bilateral salpingo-oophorectomy with or without pelvic lymphadenectomy.

Radiotherapy

Stage I patients who are not fit for surgery may be irradiated using a similar technique as described for cervical cancer. Adjuvant vaginal vault brachytherapy with or without external-beam pelvic radiotherapy is often used in stage I disease to reduce the risk of local recurrence (3,9).

Advanced Disease

More advanced disease is usually managed with a combination of surgery and external-beam radiotherapy. Chemotherapy may be used where there is evidence of intraabdominal disease.

Recurrent or Metastatic Disease

Locally recurrent disease may be successfully treated with surgery or, where it has not previously been used, radiotherapy. Systemic treatment may be of palliative value in recurrent or metastatic disease. In tumors with estrogen and progesterone receptors, hormonal manipulation carries a 15% to 30% response rate. Similar findings are seen with chemotherapy (10).

Urological Complications

Surgical Complications

Pelvic surgery may be complicated by damage to the urethra, ureters, or bladder, which can result in hematuria, frequency, urge or stress incontinence, urinary fistula, or obstructive renal failure.

Chemotherapy

Cisplatin is a nephrotoxic drug that can induce both acute and chronic renal failure, due to direct damage of the renal parenchyma, via acute tubular necrosis or tubular interstitial fibrosis (irreversible). These problems can be limited by close monitoring of renal function during treatment and ensuring good hydration and diuresis during chemotherapy administration.

Cisplatin may cause electrolyte imbalances. The most common is hypomagnesemia and extended oral magnesium replacement may be needed hyponatremia and orthostatic hypotension is also seen (see Chapter 12).

Radiotherapy

Early effects include acute radiation toxicity, which is usually mild, lasting about 4 to 6 weeks following completion of treatment. It includes cystitis and urethritis, which are managed symptomatically, and infection must be excluded. Rarely it may be severe enough to interrupt treatment.

Late radiation damage occurs in about 25% of patients; fortunately, less than 5% develop severe problems. The risk of developing radiation toxicity increases with diabetes or vascular and inflammatory bowel disease. Other risk factors include treating large areas of tissue, using large doses per treatment, and concurrent chemotherapy.

Bladder Manifestations

Mild damage to the bladder manifests by pale color of the mucosa. Other changes may be prominent blood vessels (telangiectasia) on the mucosal surface, which can sometimes bleed. More severe toxicity includes mucosal ulceration, hemorrhagic cystitis, fibrosis, and loss of bladder volume and fistula. Clinical manifestations include urgency, frequency, nocturia, hematuria, and incontinence. They may be progressive and, rarely, life threatening. Cystectomy or urinary diversion is occasionally necessary (see Chapters 4 and 11).

Ureteric stenosis may require permanent stenting, and urethral stenosis may need urethral dilatation or intermittent self-catheterization.

Colorectal Cancer

Incidence

Colorectal cancer is the third commonest cancer in both men and women in the United Sates. Between 1998 and 2002, the U.S. incidence was 52 per 100,000 population. Mortality from colorectal cancers have declined by 1.8% during 1998 to 2002 mainly because of increased screening and polyp removal (11). Cancer of the colon and rectum is one of the leading causes of cancer-related morbidity and mortality in most parts of the Western world (12). The incidence of colorectal cancer increases with age, rising sharply after the age of 60. There is a large geographical variation in incidence, with Africa and Asia having a much lower incidence than Western countries. The majority are found in the rectum (almost 40%) and sigmoid colon (20%).

Etiology

The etiology of colorectal cancer includes the following:

1. Polyps: including familial polyposis.
2. Genetic links: About 80% of colorectal cancers are sporadic. Of the rest, 5% are linked to hereditary nonpolyposis colorectal cancer (HNPCC) and 1% to familial adenomatous polyposis (FAP).
3. Inflammatory bowel disease: confers an increased lifetime risk of colorectal cancer, with Crohn's disease having a relative risk of 1.5 to 2 and ulcerative colitis giving a 10% incidence of malignant change at 25 years.
4. Environmental factors: There are thought to be several environmental factors, particularly dietary, with the Western diet, which is high in fat and low in fiber, increasing the risk.

Spread

Most of these cancers develop by malignant transformation of adenomatous polyps. The progression is from mucosal hyperplasia through adenoma and then via growth and dysplasia to malignancy. Advanced disease may present with rectal bleeding and change in bowel habit.

The spread of colorectal cancer is initially by local invasion. Lymph node involvement increases with greater depth of invasion and is seen in 40% to 70% of patients at presentation. Hematogenous spread is to the lungs (more common in rectal tumors), liver (more common in colonic cancers), bone, skin, and brain (rare).

Pathology

Macroscopically tumors may be sessile or pedunculated. They may ulcerate and bleed or produce stenotic lesions and hence obstruction. Microscopically, over 95% are adenocarcinomas. Other histological types are carcinoid, sarcoma, and lymphoma.

Presentation

Colorectal

Up to one fifth present as an emergency, with either obstruction or peritonitis due to perforation. Others present with rectal bleeding, passage of mucus, change in bowel habit, iron deficiency anemia, tenesmus, anorexia, weight loss, or abdominal swelling.

Urological

Urinary symptoms can occur with locally advanced colorectal cancers. Direct extension into the bladder may give rise to cystitis, recurrent infection, or hematuria. Infiltration into the prostate may give rise to prostatic symptoms. Obstructive uropathy is rare and likely to be due to tumor surrounding the ureter.

Investigations

Examination and Endoscopy

Digital examination may reveal rectal tumors, but endoscopic evaluation with biopsy is needed. Assessment of the entire lower gastrointestinal tract is mandatory since about 3% of tumors are associated with synchronous bowel lesions.

Blood Tests

Full blood count, renal function, liver blood tests, and carcinoembryonic antigen (CEA) are routine. Carcinoembryonic antigen is a tumor marker that can aid diagnosis and be useful in serial monitoring following treatment.

Imaging

Colon

For early colon cancers, chest x-ray and liver ultrasound are sufficient to exclude metastases but in more advanced lesions CT imaging of the chest, abdomen, and pelvis is preferable. Laparoscopy and magnetic resonance imaging (MRI) of the liver can be useful in determining resectability of hepatic metastases.

Rectum

Rectal cancers are best assessed for operability with a pelvic MRI and endorectal ultrasound, which determine the depth of mural invasion and the presence of nodal enlargement. Metastases should be excluded with a CT of the chest and abdomen.

Histopathology

Diagnosis is made from an endoscopic biopsy or, in the case of acute presentation, the surgical specimen.

TABLE 20.4. Staging systems for colorectal cancer

	Stage		
TNM	Dukes	UICC	Astler-Coller
T1, N0	A	1	A
T2, N0	A	1	B1
T3, N0	B	2a	B2
T4, N0	B	2b	B3
T1–2, N1	C	3a	C1
T3–4, N1	C	3b	C2
Any T, N2	C	3c	C3
Any T/N, M1	D	4	D

Staging

There are several staging systems in use for colorectal cancer classification, with the tumor, node, metastasis (TNM) classification being the preferred system (13) (Tables 20.4 and 20.5).

Prognosis

Advanced stage, high tumor grade, site of tumor, emergency presentation, and the loss of chromosome 18q are predictors of poor prognosis.

TABLE 20.5. Tumor, node, metastasis (TNM) definitions for colorectal malignancies

TNM	Definition
Tx	Primary tumor cannot be assessed
T0	No evidence of primary tumor
Tis	Carcinoma in situ or invasion into lamina propria
T1	Invades submucosa
T2	Invades muscularis propria
T3	Invades into subserosa, or into nonperitonealized pericolic or perirectal tissues
T4	Invades other organs/structures and/or perforates visceral peritoneum
Nx	Regional lymph nodes cannot be assessed
N0	No regional lymph node involvement
N1	1–3 regional lymph nodes positive
N2	4 or more regional lymph nodes positive
Mx	Distant metastases cannot be assessed
M0	No distant metastases
M1	Distant metastases present

Source: UICC classification of malignant tumors (4)

Management of Colonic Carcinoma

Early Disease

Surgery is the mainstay of treatment. Tumor within a segment of normal bowel and the attached mesentery including the draining lymph nodes are resected. In stage I (Dukes A or Astler-Coller A and B1) cancers, surgery (wide resection and anastomosis) is considered curative.

Adjuvant chemotherapy is known to be beneficial in node-positive tumors. Trials have shown a 40% reduction in risk of recurrence and a 10% absolute survival benefit (14,15). The standard agents are 5-fluorouracil (5-FU) and leucovorin (folinic acid). Drugs such as oxaliplatin and irinotecan and antibody therapies are involved in a number of current trials.

It is considered for those at high risk of recurrence based on pathological findings (15,16).

Radiotherapy is not routine, the site of the tumor maybe difficult to localize, and proximity to the small bowel enhances toxicity. However, it may be used to reduce the risk of local recurrence in T4 tumors with dense adhesions or positive margins (17).

Late Disease

Curative

Some patients who present with liver metastases may still be suitable for curative treatment. Neoadjuvant combination chemotherapy in patients with liver metastases may increase resectability and improve outcome.

Palliative

Palliative treatment employs both surgery and chemotherapy. Surgical interventions include stent placement, palliative resection, bypass operations, or stoma formation. Chemotherapy may improve overall survival by 3 to 6 months without detriment to quality of life if given early. The most active drugs are 5-FU, oxaliplatin, irinotecan, and capecitabine (18). Newer biological agents have also been shown to prolong overall survival when used in combination with irinotecan.

Management of Rectal Carcinoma

A combination of surgery, chemoradiation, and chemotherapy are used.

Surgery

Local excision is possible only in very early tumors. The main surgical procedures used are anterior resection and abdominoperineal resection, both of which should include excision of the entire contents of the mesorectum. In good-prognosis tumors, surgery alone may be sufficient; however, in intermediate or poor prognosis tumors, radiotherapy is also used.

Radiotherapy

Radiotherapy may be used pre- or postoperatively. Preoperative irradiation given as a short 1-week course immediately prior to surgery is used where the mesorectal excision margin appears intact on staging MRI. It can reduce the risk of a positive margin and halve local recurrence (19,20).

Where complete excision is unlikely, long course, 5-week radiotherapy is given with concurrent chemotherapy. Surgery is carried out 6 weeks later.

Postoperative radiotherapy is used to reduce the risk of local recurrence where pathology shows poor prognosis features (21,22).

Adjuvant and Palliative Treatment

Adjuvant and palliative treatment is done as for colon cancers. Palliative radiotherapy may palliate pain, bleeding, and tenesmus.

Urological Complications of Management

As outlined previously with tumors of the cervix and endometrium, pelvic radiotherapy and surgery can result in acute and late toxicity of the urinary tract.

Lymphomas

Incidence

The classification of lymphoproliferative malignancies is complex. In broad terms they can be divided into Hodgkin's lymphoma (HL) and non-Hodgkin's lymphoma (NHL). Between 1998 and 2002, the U.S. incidence was 2.7 and 19.1 per 100,000 population, respectively (1).

Hodgkin's lymphoma has a bimodal age distribution (20–30 and 60–70 years) and is more common in males. The incidence of non-Hodgkin's lymphoma increases with age and is seen equally in male and females.

The majority of urological symptoms are manifested in advanced lymphomas. The rate of involvement of the urinary tract is low (23). Urological intervention is necessary in patients who have renal failure and on occasion to obtain tissue for histological diagnosis.

Etiology

The etiology of HL is unclear, although it has been postulated to have an infective pathology. Epstein-Barr virus (EBV) antigens can be detected in up to 40%

of all HL cases (24). RS cells also express EBV latent membrane antigen protein (LMP-1).

Non-Hodgkin's lymphoma may have an infective etiology and is also seen following radiation exposure. Immunocompromised states such as posttransplant or HIV infection also increase risk of lymphoma, particularly in the later stages of the disease in HIV infection (24).

Spread

Lymphoma may affect any nodal group. Spread is usually contiguous in HL, but in NHL it often skips nodal groups. Extranodal sites are more commonly involved in NHL and may affect any site in the genitourinary tract. Most often affected are the kidney, bladder, testes, and prostate.

Pathology

Non-Hodgkin's Lymphoma

Non-Hodgkin's lymphoma is classified according to the Revised European-American Lymphoma (REAL) 1998 classification that uses the principles of morphology, immunology, genetics, and clinical behavior (25). The main division is between B-and T-cell neoplasms. B-cell neoplasms include entities such as mantle cell, hairy cell, follicular, diffuse large B cell, and Burkitt's lymphoma. T-cell neoplasms are less common and include mycosis fungoides, Sézary syndrome, and natural killer cell lymphoma.

Hodgkin's Lymphoma

The diagnosis of HL is dependent on the presence of Reed-Sternberg cells (giant, atypical, binucleate cells that are CD15 and CD30 positive) in an appropriate pathological background that varies according to subtype. Pathologists currently use the World Health Organization classification, which is as follows (26):

- Nodular lymphocyte predominant HL
- Classical HL
  - Nodular sclerosing HL
  - Lymphocyte rich classical Hodgkin's lymphoma
  - Mixed cellularity HL
  - Lymphocyte depleted HL

Presentation

Nodal Enlargement

Enlarged nodes may be palpable or cause symptoms from compression. Abdominal nodes may cause nonspecific gastrointestinal symptoms, jaundice, or an obstructive uropathy. Pelvic nodes may cause lower limb or genital edema, urinary tract obstruction, or pain.

Systemic B Symptoms

Systemic B symptoms are defined as pyrexia of unknown origin over 38°C, drenching night sweats, and weight loss of more than 10% body weight in the past 6 months.

Urological

Renal impairment may be seen with obstruction of the urinary tract and less commonly with direct involvement of the kidney, ureters, or bladder. It also occurs with urate nephropathy or secondary to hypercalcemia. Hyperuricemia can be seen spontaneously in lymphomas and results in deposition of urate crystals in the distal renal tubules.

Nephrotic syndrome may be seen in lymphomas, particularly HL, where minimal-change glomerulonephritis is the most common pathology. This is best resolved by treating the underlying malignancy. Testicular masses may occur with lymphomatous infiltration (particularly in older men). Lymphoma of the bladder or kidney may present with hematuria.

Investigations

Blood

Full blood count, urea and electrolytes, liver blood tests, erythrocyte sedimentation rate (ESR), lactate dehydrogenase (LDH), β2-microglobulin, and albumin are useful. HIV serology should be considered in at-risk patients.

Imaging

A CT scan of the neck, chest, abdomen, and pelvis is needed for accurate staging. Positron emission tomography (PET)–CT scanning is useful in the diagnosis and follow-up of both NHL and HL.

Histology

Histology requires a biopsy rather than a fine-needle aspirate as architecture is important in arriving at the correct pathological diagnosis. If there is an accessible, enlarged lymph node, it should be excised, otherwise an image-guided Tru-cut biopsy or mediastinoscopy and biopsy may be done. Occasionally laparoscopic biopsy is the only way to obtain tissue.

Testicular masses should be removed at orchidectomy via inguinal incision if malignancy is suspected. In NHL, bone marrow aspirate and trephine (BMAT) is done in all patients except those with stage IA disease. In HL it is only done in advanced disease.

TABLE 20.6. Ann-Arbor staging

I: Single lymph node region involved or localized involvement of a single extralymphatic site (IE)
II: Two or more lymph node regions on the same side of the diaphragm or a single extralymphatic site and its regional lymph nodes with or without lymph nodes on the same side of the diaphragm (IIE)
III: Lymph node regions on both sides of the diaphragm with or without localized involvement of extralymphatic site and/or spleen (IIIE + S)
IV: Multifocal involvement of one or more extralymphatic organs with or without associated lymph nodes or isolated extralymphatic organ involvement with distant lymph nodes
A: No B Symptoms
B: Presence of B Symptoms
E: Extranodal site
Subclassified as follows: S, spleen; O, bone; P, pleura; H, liver; M, bone marrow; L, lung; D, skin
X: Bulk disease (mediastinal mass over one-third chest diameter at the level of T5/6, lymph node mass over 10 cm)

Lumbar Puncture

Central nervous system involvement is more common with testicular, gastrointestinal, or head and neck involvement. These cases and those with HIV, Burkitt's lymphoma, or neurological symptoms should all have the cerebrospinal fluid (CSF) examined.

Staging

Both types of lymphoma are staged according to the Ann Arbor system (Table 20.6).

Prognosis

Prognostic determination depends on histology and stage.

Non-Hodgkin's Lymphoma

The international prognosis index for NHL consists of five factors—age, stage, performance status, number of extranodal sites and LDH (27). Low-risk patients with a score of 0 to 1 have an overall 5-year survival of 73%, whereas high-risk groups with a score of 4 to 5 have an overall 5-year survival of 25%.

Follicular Lymphoma

Follicular lymphoma uses the Follicular Lymphoma International Prognostic Index (FLIPI) classification of five points: hemoglobin, age, stage, number of nodal areas involved, and LDH. A score of 0 to 1 gives a 10-year survival of 70% and 3 or more gives a 10-year survival of 35%.

Hodgkin's Lymphoma

Stage I and II HL can be assessed with the European Organization for the Research and Treatment of Cancer (EORTC) risk factors (28), placing patients into favorable and unfavorable groups. The presence of any of the following places a patient into the unfavorable group: four or more nodal areas, age over 50, or ESR over 50 if asymptomatic or over 30 with B symptoms.

Advanced Hodgkin's Lymphoma

Advanced HL uses the Hasencleaver index with nine factors each giving a score of 1 (29). A score of 4 or more puts patients into a poor prognosis group, and if all are negative, then overall survival is estimated at 84%.

Management of Non-Hodgkin's Lymphoma

High Grade

Early localized (stage IA and nonbulky IIA) disease is treated with three to four cycles of combination chemotherapy, usually a doxorubicin-containing regimen such as cyclophosphamide, hydroxydaunomycin, Oncovin (vincristine) and prednisone (CHOP), followed by radiotherapy treating the prechemotherapy nodal volume (30). If the patient is unfit for chemotherapy, then radiotherapy may be used alone. Prior to chemotherapy, male patients should be offered sperm storage.

Other stages, including primary bladder or testicular lymphoma, are treated with six to eight cycles of combination chemotherapy with the addition of rituximab, a monoclonal anti-CD20 antibody, if the tumor is CD20 positive (31). This addition increases the complete response rate and prolongs event-free and overall survival. Age should not be a contraindication to receiving this treatment. Postchemotherapy radiation may be given if bulky disease was present at diagnosis.

Six to 12 treatments with weekly intrathecal chemotherapy are given if the patient is at high risk of central nervous system (CNS) involvement (see above).

Residual or recurrent disease may be treated with second-line chemotherapy followed by a peripheral blood stem cell autologous transplant if the patient is considered fit enough. Local radiotherapy may also be considered.

Low Grade

Localized Radiotherapy

Localized radiotherapy may be used for stage I disease as curative treatment (32).

Watchful Waiting

Watchful waiting can be used in stage II and above, provided there is a normal full blood count and no B symptoms, compression symptoms, or any nodal mass over 7 cm. Studies have shown this approach to give comparable overall survival as giving chemotherapy at diagnosis (33).

Chemotherapy

If immediate treatment is deemed necessary, many agents have been shown to be effective. The most commonly used drug is oral chlorambucil with response rates of up to 75%. Combination chemotherapy regimes may be preferable if rapid response is necessary for severe symptoms. These tumors are often CD20 positive, and anti-CD20 antibody therapy, alone or in combination, is effective. Radiotherapy may be useful in sites of disease not responding to chemotherapy or where there is localized relapse.

Management of Hodgkin's Lymphoma

Early Disease

This has a high cure rate of over 90%. Usually a combination of chemotherapy and involved field radiotherapy is used; however, in young women upper body radiotherapy is avoided as it may significantly increase the risk of breast cancer.

Radiotherapy Alone

Nonbulky stage Ia lymphocyte-predominant HL can be treated with involved field radiotherapy alone. Otherwise, because of higher relapse rates, combined chemotherapy and radiotherapy is preferred (34).

Combination Chemotherapy and Radiotherapy

Classical HL stages Ia, Ib, and IIa are generally treated with four cycles of combination chemotherapy [Adriamycin (doxorubicin), bleomycin, vinblastine, and dacarbazine (ABVD)] followed by involved field radiotherapy (34).

Advanced Disease

Advanced disease is treated with six to eight cycles of chemotherapy. Radiotherapy should be given to sites of bulk disease (35). High-dose chemotherapy with stem cell rescue may be given if there is progressive disease during initial chemotherapy, if the first relapse is within 1 year, or at second relapse.

Urological Complications of Management

Tumor Lysis Syndrome

Patients often have bulky disease when commencing chemotherapy. Lymphoma is an exceptionally chemosensitive disease, and therefore there is often extensive tumor lysis. This rapid cell breakdown of large volume disease causes metabolic disturbance as intracellular constituents leach into the blood. It is characterized by hyperkalemia, hyperuricemia, hyperphosphatemia, and hypocalcemia. This can result in cardiac arrhythmias, renal failure (from intratubular obstruction causing acute tubular necrosis), and, rarely, sudden death. To prevent this, patients are aggressively hydrated and given allopurinol prior to chemotherapy initiation.

Treatment of uric acid nephropathy (either spontaneous or secondary to tumor lysis) is with hydration (to maintain urine output of >100 mL/h), urinary alkalinization, and allopurinol. In the event of oliguria (where obstruction has been excluded), diuretics are used. Rarely, temporary hemofiltration or hemodialysis is necessary.

Hemorrhagic Cystitis

Chemotherapy with the commonly used drug cyclophosphamide can cause hemorrhagic cystitis. This is unusual with the doses used in treating lymphoma, and can be prevented with aggressive hydration and frequent voiding. This is discussed in Chapter 11.

Chemotherapy-Induced Renal Failure

Where high-dose methotrexate is used, renal failure can occur secondary to precipitation in the tubules and collecting ducts. Adequate prehydration is essential, and alkalinization of urine with intravenous sodium bicarbonate (to maintain urinary pH above 8) may reduce the incidence. Methotrexate renal impairment usually reverses once the drug is stopped, although this may take some weeks.

Hyponatremia

Both cyclophosphamide and vincristine may be associated with a clinical picture similar to the syndrome of inappropriate antidiuretic hormone (SIADH). Treatment is with drug withdrawal, and occasionally fluid restriction is necessary, though this is best avoided as it can precipitate hemorrhagic cystitis.

Radiation Nephritis

If the radiotherapy dose to the kidney is not limited (no more than 50% of each kidney should receive more than 20 Gy), then postradiation nephritis may ensue 6 to 12 months later. This is characterized by hypertension, proteinuria, and microscopic hematuria. Prevention is achieved by careful radiotherapy planning.

References

1. Surveillance, Epidemiology, and End Results (SEER) Program. National Cancer Institute, Surveillance Research Program, Cancer Statistics Branch, released April 2005, based on the November 2004 submission. www.seer.cancer.gov.
2. Hendrickson M, Ross J, Eifel PJ, et al. Adenocarcinoma of the endometrium: analysis of 256 cases with carcinoma limited to the uterine corpus. Pathology review and analysis of prognostic variables. Gynecol Oncol 1982;13(3):373–392.

3. Nori D, Hilaris BS, Tome M, et al. Combined surgery and radiation in endometrial carcinoma: an analysis of prognostic factors. Int J Radiat Oncol Biol Phys 1987;13: 489–497.
4. International Union Against Cancer, Sobin LH, Wittekind Ch, eds. TNM Classification of Malignant Tumours, 6th ed. New York: Wiley-Liss, 2002:154–164.
5. Homesley HD, Zaino R. Endometrial cancer: prognostic factors. Semin Oncol 1994; 21(1):71–78.
6. Zaino RJ, Ward S, Delgado G, et al. Histopathologic predictors of the behavior of surgically treated stage IB squamous cell carcinoma of the cervix. A Gynecologic Oncology Group study. Cancer 1992;69(7):1750–1758.
7. Landoni F, Maneo A, Colombo A, et al. Randomised study of radical surgery versus radiotherapy for stage Ib-IIa cervical cancer. Lancet 1997;350:535–540.
8. Green JA, Kirwan JM, Tierney JF, et al. Survival and recurrence after concomitant chemotherapy and radiotherapy for cancer of the uterine cervix: a systematic review and meta-analysis. Lancet 2001;358:781–786.
9. Creutzberg CL, van Putten WL, et al. for the PORTEC Study Group. Surgery and postoperative radiotherapy versus surgery alone for patients with stage I endometrial carcinoma: multicentre randomised trial. Lancet 2000;355:1404–1411.
10. Thigpen JT, Brady MF, Homesley H, et al. Phase III trial of doxorubicin with or without cisplatin in advanced endometrial carcinoma: a Gynecologic Oncology Group study. J Clin Oncol 2004;22(19):3902–3908.
11. American Cancer Society. Cancer Facts and Figures 2006. Atlanta, Ga: American Cancer Society, 2006. www.cancer.org.
12. Silverberg E, Boring CC, Squires TS. Cancer statistics, 1990. CA Cancer J Clin 1990; 40:9–26.
13. Colon and rectum. In: American Joint Committee on Cancer. AJCC Cancer Staging Manual, 6th ed. New York: Springer, 2002:113–124.
14. Moertel CG, Fleming TR, Macdonald JS et al. Intergroup study of fluorouracil plus levamisole as adjuvant therapy for stage II/Dukes' B2 colon cancer. J Clin Oncol 1995;13(12):2936–2943.
15. Mamounas E, Wieand S, Wolmark N, et al. Comparative efficacy of adjuvant chemotherapy in patients with Dukes' B versus Dukes' C colon cancer: results from four National Surgical Adjuvant Breast and Bowel Project adjuvant studies (C-01, C-02, C-03, and C-04) J Clin Oncol 1999;17:1349–1355.
16. Efficacy of adjuvant fluorouracil and folinic acid in B2 colon cancer. International Multicentre Pooled Analysis of B2 Colon Cancer Trials (IMPACT B2) Investigators. J Clin Oncol 1999;17:1356–1363.
17. Willett CG, Goldberg S, Shellito PC, et al. Does postoperative irradiation play a role in the adjuvant therapy of stage T4 colon cancer? Cancer J Sci Am 1999;5(4): 242–247.
18. Tournigand C, Andre T, Achille E et al. FOLFIRI followed by FOLFOX6 or the reverse sequence in advanced colorectal cancer: a randomized GERCOR study. J Clin Oncol 2004;22:229–237.
19. Kapiteijn E, Marijnen CA, Nagtegaal ID, et al. Preoperative radiotherapy combined with total mesorectal excision for respectable rectal cancer. N Engl J Med 2001; 345(9):638–646.
20. (No authors listed) Improved survival with preoperative radiotherapy in resectable rectal cancer. Swedish Rectal Cancer Trial. N Engl J Med 1997;336(14): 980–987.

21. (No authors listed) Randomised trial of surgery alone versus surgery followed by radiotherapy for mobile cancer of the rectum. Medical Research Council Rectal Cancer Working Party. Lancet 1996;348:1610–1614.

22. (No authors listed) Randomised trial of surgery alone versus radiotherapy followed by surgery for potentially operable locally advanced rectal cancer. Medical Research Council Rectal Cancer Working Party. Lancet 1996;348:1605–1610.

23. Weimer G, Culp DA, Loening S, Narayana A. Urogenital involvement by malignant lymphomas. J Urol 1981;125:230–231.

24. Andersson J. Epstein-Barr virus and Hodgkin's lymphoma. Herpes 2006;13:12–16.

25. Harris NL, Jaffe ES, Armitage JO, et al. Lymphoma classification: from R.E.A.L. to W.H.O. and beyond. Cancer: Principles and Practice of Oncology Updates 1999; 13:1–14.

26. Harris NL. Hodgkin's lymphomas: classification, diagnosis and grading. Semin Hematol 1999;36:220–232.

27. A predictive model for aggressive non-Hodgkin's lymphoma. The International Non-Hodgkin's Lymphoma Prognostic Factors Project. N Engl J Med 1993;329:987–994.

28. EORTC Lymphoma Cooperative Group and GELA. Trial H9 protocol: prospective controlled trial in clinical stages I-II supradiaphragmatic Hodgkin's Disease—evaluation of treatment efficacy, (long term) toxicity and quality of life in two different prognostic subgroups. Brussel: EORTC Lymphoma Cooperative group and GELA, 1999: EORTC protocol 20982.

29. Hasenclever D, Diehl V. A prognostic score for advanced Hodgkin's disease: International Prognostic Factors Project on Advanced Hodgkin's Disease. N Engl J Med 1998;339:1506–1514.

30. Miller TP, Dahlberg S, Cassady JR, et al. Chemotherapy alone compared with chemotherapy plus radiotherapy for localized intermediate- and high-grade non-Hodgkin's lymphoma. N Engl J Med 1998;339:21–26.

31. Coiffier B, Lepage E, Briere J, et al. CHOP chemotherapy plus rituximab compared with CHOP alone in elderly patients with diffuse large-B-cell lymphoma. N Engl J Med 2002;346(4):235–242.

32. Vaughan Hudson B, Vaughan Hudson G, et al. Clinical stage I non-Hodgkin's lymphoma: long-term follow-up of patients treated by the British National Lymphoma Investigation with radiotherapy alone as initial therapy. Br J Cancer 1994;69(6): 1088–1093.

33. Ardeshna KM, Smith P, Norton A, et al. Long-term effect of a watch and wait policy versus immediate systemic treatment for asymptomatic advanced-stage non-Hodgkin lymphoma: a randomised controlled trial. Lancet 2003;362:516–522.

34. Engert A, Schiller P, Josting A, et al. Involved-field radiotherapy is equally effective and less toxic compared with extended-field radiotherapy after four cycles of chemotherapy in patients with early-stage unfavorable Hodgkin's lymphoma: results of the HD8 trial of the German Hodgkin's Lymphoma Study Group. J Clin Oncol 2003; 21:3601–3608.

35. Aleman BM, Raemaekers JM, Tirelli U, et al. Involved-field radiotherapy for advanced Hodgkin's lymphoma. N Engl J Med 2003;348(24):2396–2406.

Appendixes

Appendix A: Abbreviations

ADT: androgen deprivation therapy
AJCC: American Joint Committee on Cancer
ASTRO: American Society for Therapeutic Radiation and Oncology
ATN: acute tubular necrosis
AUA: American Urological Association
AUC: area under the curve
BAUS: British Association of Urological Surgeons
BCG: bacillus Calmette-Guérin vaccine
BMI: body mass index
BPH: benign prostatic hyperplasia/hypertrophy
BRFS: biochemical relapse free survival
CIS: carcinoma *in situ*
CT: computed tomography
EAU: European Association of Urology
EBRT: external-beam radiotherapy
ECOG: Eastern Cooperative Oncology Group; scale for measuring *performance status* from 0 to 4
EGGCT: extragonadal germ cell tumor
EORTC: European Organization for Research and Treatment of Cancer
ER: endoplasmic reticulum
ERSPC: European Randomized Study of Screening for Prostate Cancer
FIGO: International Federation of Gynecology and Obstetrics
FSH: follicle-stimulating hormone
GCT: germ cell tumor
GM-CSF: granulocyte-macrophage colony-stimulating factor
GVHD: graft versus host disease
HGPIN: high-grade prostate intraepithelial neoplasia
IARC: International Agency for Research on Cancer
IB: interstitial brachytherapy
ICRU: *International Commission on Radiation Unit*

IVU: intravenous urography
LDH: lactate dehydrogenase
LH: luteinizing hormone
LOH: loss of heterozygocity
LOI: loss of imprinting
LUTS: lower urinary tract symptoms
MRI: magnetic resonance imaging
MRS: magnetic resonance spectroscopy
NCHCT: noncontrast helical computed tomography
NPCP: National Prostatic Cancer Project
NSAID: nonsteroidal antiinflammatory drugs
NSGCT: nonseminomatous germ cell tumor
PCN: percutaneous nephrostomy
PET: positron emission tomography
PIN: prostatic intraepithelial neoplasia
PLAP: placental alkaline phosphatase
PPS: preprostatic sphincter
PSA: prostate-specific antigen
PTH: parathyroid hormone
RCC: renal cell carcinoma
RCT: randomized controlled trial
RPLND: retroperitoneal lymph node dissection
SLNB: sentinel lymph node biopsy
TCC: transitional cell carcinoma
TGCT: testicular germ cell tumor
TNM: tumor, node, metastasis
TRUS: transrectal ultrasound
TURBT: transurethral resection of bladder tumor
TURP: transurethral resection of the prostate
US: ultrasound
UTI: urinary tract infection
VHL: Von Hippel–Lindau

Appendix B: Tumor, Node, Metastasis Classification

Management of cancer depends on patient and tumor factors. These factors also help in assessing the course of the disease. The patient factors that are likely to influence the course of the disease include age of the patient, duration of symptoms, comorbid conditions, the clinicopathological extent of the disease, and the histological type and grade of the tumor. The tumor, node, metastasis (TNM) system is a worldwide benchmark for staging the cancers and helps in predicting the outcome of patients in patients with cancer (1). The TNM system for classification of malignant tumors was originally developed by Dr. Pierre Denoix at the Institut Gustave-Roussy, France. between 1943 and 1952.

The TNM assessment takes into account three components:

T: The extent of the primary tumor
N: The presence or absence and extent of regional lymph node metastasis
M: The absence or presence of distant metastasis

The objectives of TNM classification are as follows (2):

1. To aid the clinician in the planning of treatment
2. To give some indication of prognosis
3. To assist in evaluation of the results of the treatment
4. To facilitate the exchange of information between treatment centers
5. To contribute to the continuing investigation of human cancer

References

1. Gospodarowicz MK, Miller D, Groome PA, et al., for the UICC report. Improvement of the TNM classification. Cancer 2004;100:1–5.
2. Sobin LH, Wittekind Ch. TNM Classification of Malignant Tumors, 6th ed. New York: Wiley-Liss, 2002.

Appendix C: Performance Status

The well-being of cancer patients is assessed by their performance status, taking into account their ability to perform ordinary tasks. The performance status helps in planning the type of treatment (e.g., chemotherapy). Performance status is also used to assess the quality of life in cancer-related *randomized controlled trials*. The Eastern Cooperative Oncology Group (ECOG) scale score [also known as the World Health Organization (WHO) Zubrod score] ranges from 0 to 5, with 0 denoting perfect health and 5 death (1):

0: Asymptomatic
1: Symptomatic but completely ambulant
2: Symptomatic, <50% in bed during the day
3: Symptomatic, ≥50% in bed, but not bedbound
4: Bedbound
5: Death

Reference

Oken MM, Creech RH, Tormey DC, et al. Toxicity and response criteria of the Eastern Cooperative Oncology Group. Am J Clin Oncol 1982;5:649–655.

Appendix D: Partin Tables and Kattan Nomograms

Tables I to IV are known as the Partin tables, and are reproduced here with permission from Alan Partin (1–3). Figures 1 and 2 demonstrate the Kattan nomograms.

TABLE I. Clinical stage T1c (nonpalpable, PSA elevated)

PSA range (ng/mL)	Pathologic stage	Gleason score				
		2–4	5–6	3 + 4 = 7	4 + 3 = 7	8–10
0–2.5	Organ confined	95 (89–99)	90 (88–93)	79 (74–85)	71 (62–79)	66 (54–76)
	Extraprostatic extension	5 (1–11)	9 (7–12)	17 (13–23)	25 (18–34)	28 (20–38)
	Seminal vesicle (+)	—	0 (0–1)	2 (1–5)	2 (1–5)	4 (1–10)
	Lymph node (+)	—	—	1 (0–2)	1 (0–4)	1 (0–4)
2.6–4.0	Organ confined	92 (82–98)	84 (81–86)	68 (62–74)	58 (48–67)	52 (41–63)
	Extraprostatic extension	8 (2–18)	15 (13–18)	27 (22–33)	37 (29–46)	40 (31–50)
	Seminal vesicle (+)	—	1 (0–1)	4 (2–7)	4 (1–7)	6 (3–12)
	Lymph node (+)	—	—	1 (0–2)	1 (0–3)	1 (0–4)
4.1–6.0	Organ confined	90 (78–98)	80 (78–83)	63 (58–68)	52 (43–60)	46 (36–56)
	Extraprostatic extension	10 (2–22)	19 (16–21)	32 (27–36)	42 (35–50)	45 (36–54)
	Seminal vesicle (+)	—	1 (0–1)	3 (2–5)	3 (1–6)	5 (3–9)
	Lymph node (+)	—	0 (0–1)	2 (1–3)	3 (1–5)	3 (1–6)
6.1–10.0	Organ confined	87 (73–97)	75 (72–77)	54 (49–59)	43 (35–51)	37 (28–46)
	Extraprostatic extension	13 (3–27)	23 (21–25)	36 (32– 40)	47 (40–54)	48 (39–57)
	Seminal vesicle (+)	—	2 (2–3)	8 (6–11)	8 (4–12)	13 (8–19)
	Lymph node (+)	—	0 (0–1)	2 (1–3)	2 (1–4)	3 (1–5)
>10.0	Organ confined	80 (61–95)	62 (58–64)	37 (32–42)	27 (21–34)	22 (16–30)
	Extraprostatic extension	20 (5–39)	33 (30–36)	43 (38–48)	51 (44–59)	50 (42–59)
	Seminal vesicle (+)	—	4 (3–5)	12 (9–17)	11 (6–17)	17 (10–25)
	Lymph node (+)	—	2 (1–3)	8 (5–11)	10 (5–17)	11 (5–18)

PSA, prostate-specific antigen.

TABLE II. Clinical stage T2a (palpable, less than one half of one lobe)

PSA range (ng/mL)	Pathologic stage	Gleason score				
		2–4	5–6	3 + 4 = 7	4 + 3 = 7	8–10
0–2.5	Organ confined	91 (79–98)	81 (77–85)	64 (56–71)	53 (43–63)	47 (35–59)
	Extraprostatic extension	9 (2–21)	17 (13–21)	29 (23–36)	40 (30–49)	42 (32–53)
	Seminal vesicle (+)	—	1 (0–2)	5 (1–9)	4 (1–9)	7 (2–16)
	Lymph node (+)	—	0 (0–1)	2 (0–5)	3 (0–8)	3 (0–9)
2.6–4.0	Organ confined	85 (69–96)	71 (66–75)	50 (43–57)	39 (30–48)	33 (24–44)
	Extraprostatic extension	15 (4–31)	27 (23–31)	41 (35–48)	52 (43–61)	53 (44–63)
	Seminal vesicle (+)	—	2 (1–3)	7 (3–12)	6 (2–12)	10 (4–18)
	Lymph node (+)	—	0 (0–1)	2 (0–4)	2 (0–6)	3 (0–8)
4.1–6.0	Organ confined	81 (63–95)	66 (62–70)	44 (39–50)	33 (25–41)	28 (20–37)
	Extraprostatic extension	19 (5–37)	32 (28–36)	46 (40–52)	56 (48–64)	58 (49–66)
	Seminal vesicle (+)	—	1 (1–2)	5 (3–8)	5 (2–8)	8 (4–13)
	Lymph node (+)	—	1 (0–2)	4 (2–7)	6 (3–11)	6 (2–12)
6.1–10.0	Organ confined	76 (56–94)	58 (54–61)	35 (30–40)	25 (19–32)	21 (15–28)
	Extraprostatic extension	24 (6–44)	37 (34–41)	49 (43–54)	58 (51–66)	57 (48–65)
	Seminal vesicle (+)	—	4 (3–5)	13 (9–18)	11 (6–17)	17 (11–26)
	Lymph node (+)	—	1 (0–2)	3 (2–6)	5 (2–8)	5 (2–10)
>10.0	Organ confined	65 (43–89)	42 (38–46)	20 (17–24)	14 (10–18)	11 (7–15)
	Extraprostatic extension	35 (11–57)	47 (43–52)	49 (43–55)	55 (46–64)	52 (41–62)
	Seminal vesicle (+)	—	6 (4–8)	16 (11–22)	13 (7–20)	19 (12–29)
	Lymph node (+)	—	4 (3–7)	14 (9–21)	18 (10–27)	17 (9–29)

PSA, prostate-specific antigen.

TABLE III. Clinical stage T2b (palpable, one-half or more of one lobe, not on both lobes)

PSA range (ng/mL)	Pathologic stage	Gleason score				
		2–4	5–6	3 + 4 = 7	4 + 3 = 7	8–10
0–2.5	Organ confined	88 (73–97)	75 (69–81)	54 (46–63)	43 (33–54)	37 (26–49)
	Extraprostatic extension	12 (3–27)	22 (17–28)	35 (28–43)	45 (35–56)	46 (35–58)
	Seminal vesicle (+)	—	2 (0–3)	6 (2–12)	5 (1–11)	9 (2–20)
	Lymph node (+)	—	1 (0–2)	4 (0–10)	6 (0–14)	6 (0–16)
2.6–4.0	Organ confined	80 (61–95)	63 (57–69)	41 (33–48)	30 (22–39)	25 (17–34)
	Extraprostatic extension	20 (5–39)	34 (28–40)	47 (40–55)	57 (47–67)	57 (46–68)
	Seminal vesicle (+)	—	2 (1–4)	9 (4–15)	7 (3–14)	12 (5–22)
	Lymph node (+)	—	1 (0–2)	3 (0–8)	4 (0–12)	5 (0–14)
4.1–6.0	Organ confined	75 (55–93)	57 (52–63)	35 (29–40)	25 (18–32)	21 (14–29)
	Extraprostatic extension	25 (7–45)	39 (33–44)	51 (44–57)	60 (50–68)	59 (49–69)
	Seminal vesicle (+)	—	2 (1–3)	7 (4–11)	5 (3–9)	9 (4–16)
	Lymph node (+)	—	2 (1–3)	7 (4–13)	10 (5–18)	10 (4–20)

TABLE III. *Continued*

PSA range (ng/mL)	Pathologic stage	Gleason score				
		2–4	5–6	3 + 4 = 7	4 + 3 = 7	8–10
6.1–10.0	Organ confined	69 (47–91)	49 (43–54)	26 (22–31)	19 (14–25)	15 (10–21)
	Extraprostatic extension	31 (9–53)	44 (39–49)	52 (46–58)	60 (52–68)	57 (48–67)
	Seminal vesicle (+)	—	5 (3–8)	16 (10–22)	13 (7–20)	19 (11–29)
	Lymph node (+)	—	2 (1–3)	6 (4–10)	8 (5–14)	8 (4–16)
>10.0	Organ confined	57 (35–86)	33 (28–38)	14 (11–17)	9 (6–13)	7 (4–10)
	Extraprostatic extension	43 (14–65)	52 (46–56)	47 (40–53)	50 (40–60)	46 (36–59)
	Seminal vesicle (+)	—	8 (5–11)	17 (12–24)	13 (8–21)	19 (12–29)
	Lymph node (+)	—	8 (5–12)	22 (15–30)	27 (16–39)	27 (14–40)

PSA, prostate-specific antigen.

TABLE IV. Clinical stage T2c (palpable on both lobes)

PSA range (ng/mL)	Pathologic stage	Gleason score				
		2–4	5–6	3 + 4 = 7	4 + 3 = 7	8–10
0–2.5	Organ confined	86 (71–97)	73 (63–81)	51 (38–63)	39 (26–54)	34 (21–48)
	Extraprostatic extension	14 (3–29)	24 (17–33)	36 (26–48)	45 (32–59)	47 (33–61)
	Seminal vesicle (+)	—	1 (0–4)	5 (1–13)	5 (1–12)	8 (2–19)
	Lymph node (+)	—	1 (0–4)	6 (0–18)	9 (0–26)	10 (0–27)
2.6–4.0	Organ confined	78 (58–94)	61 (50–70)	38 (27–50)	27 (18–40)	23 (14–34)
	Extraprostatic extension	22 (6–45)	36 (27–59)	48 (37–70)	57 (44–70)	57 (44–70)
	Seminal vesicle (+)	—	2 (1–5)	8 (2–17)	6 (2–16)	10 (3–22)
	Lymph node (+)	—	1 (0–4)	5 (0–15)	7 (0–21)	8 (0–22)
4.1–6.0	Organ confined	73 (52–93)	55 (44–64)	31 (23–41)	21 (14–31)	18 (11–28)
	Extraprostatic extension	27 (7–48)	40 (32–50)	50 (40–60)	57 (43–68)	57 (43–70)
	Seminal vesicle (+)	—	2 (1–4)	6 (2–11)	4 (1–10)	7 (2–15)
	Lymph node (+)	—	3 (1–7)	12 (5–23)	16 (6–32)	16 (6–33)
6.1–10.0	Organ confined	67 (45–91)	46 (36–56)	24 (17–32)	16 (10–24)	13 (8–20)
	Extraprostatic extension	33 (9–55)	46 (37–55)	52 (42–61)	58 (46–69)	56 (43–69)
	Seminal vesicle (+)	—	5 (2–9)	13 (6–23)	11 (4–21)	16 (6–29)
	Lymph node (+)	—	3 (1–6)	10 (5–18)	13 (6–25)	13 (5–26)
>10.0	Organ confined	54 (32–85)	30 (21–38)	11 (7–17)	7 (4–12)	6 (3–10)
	Extraprostatic extension	46 (15–68)	51 (42–60)	42 (30–55)	43 (29–59)	41 (27–57)
	Seminal vesicle (+)	—	6 (2–12)	13 (6–24)	10 (3–20)	15 (5–28)
	Lymph node (+)	—	13 (6–22)	33 (18–49)	38 (20–58)	38 (20–59)

PSA, prostate-specific antigen.

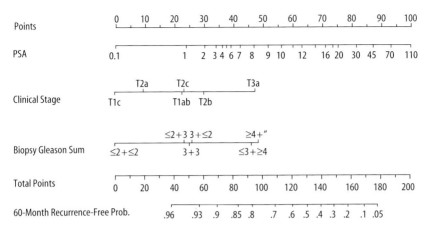

Points 0 10 20 30 40 50 60 70 80 90 100

PSA 0.1 1 2 3 4 6 7 8 9 10 12 16 20 30 45 70 110

Clinical Stage T1c T2a T1ab T2b T2c T3a

Biopsy Gleason Sum ≤2+≤2 ≤2+3 3+≤2 3+3 ≥4+" ≤3+≥4

Total Points 0 20 40 60 80 100 120 140 160 180 200

60-Month Recurrence-Free Prob. .96 .93 .9 .85 .8 .7 .6 .5 .4 .3 .2 .1 .05

<u>Instructions for Physician:</u> Locate the patient's PSA on the **PSA** axis. Draw a line straight upward to the **Points** axis to determine how many points toward recurrence the patient receives for his PSA. Repeat this process for the **Clinical Stage** and **Biopsy Gleason Sum** axes, each time drawing straight upward to the **Points** axis. Sum the points achieved for each predictor and locate this sum on the **Total Points** axis. Draw a line straight down to find the patient's probability of remaining recurrence free for 60 months, assuming he does not die of another cause first.

Note: This nomogram is not applicable to a man who is not otherwise a candidate for radical prostatectomy. You can use this only on a man who has already selected radical prostatectomy as treatment for his prostate cancer.

<u>Instruction to Patient:</u> "Mr. X. if we had 100 men exactly like you, we would expect between <predicted percentage from nomogram −10%> and <predicted percentage +10%> to remain free of their disease at 5 years following radical prostatectomy, and recurrence after 5 years is very rare."

FIGURE 1. Preoperative nomogram based on 983 patients treated at Baylor College of Medicine, Houston, TX, for predicting freedom from recurrence after radical prostatectomy. [Adapted from Kattan et al. (4).]

Postoperative Nomogram for Prostate Cancer Recurrence

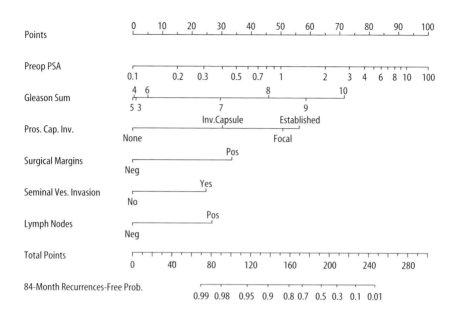

Instructions for Physician: Locate the patient's PSA on the **PSA** axis. Draw a line straight upward to the **Points** axis to determine how many points toward recurrence the patient receives for his PSA. Repeat this process for the other axes, each time drawing straight upward to the **Points** axis. Sum the points achieved for each predictor and locate this sum on the **Total Points** axis. Draw a line straight down to find the patient's probability of remaining recurrence free for 84 months, assuming he does not die of another cause first.

Instructions to Patient: "Mr. X. if we had 100 men exactly like you, we would expect between <predicted percentage from nomogram −10%> and <predicted percentage +10%> to remain free of their disease at 7 years following radical prostatectomy, and recurrence after 7 years is very rare."

FIGURE 2. Postoperative nomogram based on 996 patients treated at Methodist Hospital, Houston, Texas, for predicting prostate-specific antigen (PSA) recurrence after prostatectomy. [Adapted from Kattan et al. (5).

References

1. Partin AW, Kattan MW, Subong EN, et al. Combination of prostate-specific antigen, clinical stage, and Gleason score to predict pathological stage of localized prostate cancer. A multi-institutional update. JAMA 1997;277:1445–1451.
2. Partin AW, Mangold LA, Lamm DM, et al. Contemporary update of prostate cancer staging nomograms (Partin tables) for the new millennium. Urology 2001;58: 843–848
3. Partin AW, Yoo J, Carter HB, et al. The use of prostate specific antigen, clinical stage and Gleason score to predict pathological stage in men with localized prostate cancer. J Urol 1993;150:110–114.

4. Kattan MW, Eastham JA, Stapleton AMF, Wheeler TM, Scardino PT. A preoperative nomogram for disease recurrence following radical prostatectomy for prostate cancer. J Natl Cancer Inst 1998;90(10):766–771.

5. Kattan MW, Wheeler TM, Scardino PT. Postoperative nomogram for disease recurrence after radical prostatectomy for prostate cancer. J Clin Oncol 1999;17: 1499–1507.

Index

•

Printed in Thailand